Behavioral Approaches to Chronic Disease in Adolescence

Behavioral Approaches to Chronic Disease in Adolescence

A Guide to Integrative Care

Editors

William T. O'Donohue

University of Nevada, Reno, NV, USA

Lauren Woodward Tolle

University of Nevada, Reno, NV, USA

Springer

Editors
William T. O'Donohue
Department of Psychology
University of Nevada
Reno NV 89557-0062
USA
wto@unr.edu

Lauren Woodward Tolle
Department of Psychology
University of Nevada
Reno NV 89557-0062
USA
ltolle@unr.nevada.edu

ISBN 978-0-387-87686-3 (hardcover)
e-ISBN 978-0-387-87687-0
ISBN 978-1-4419-8142-4 (softcover)
DOI 10.1007/978-0-387-87687-0
Springer Dordrecht Heidelberg London New York

Library of Congress Control Number: 2009921167

Printed on acid-free paper

Springer is part of Springer Science+Business Media (www.springer.com)

Preface

This book fills a gap in the literature on evidence-based approaches for treating adolescents with chronic illness in an integrated care setting. It is comprehensive in accurately addressing specific considerations inherent in adolescent psychology (therapist burnout, ethical considerations, bringing in the family, cultural considerations, etc.) and in outlining evidence-based practice guidelines for common chronic conditions in adolescence (type I diabetes, asthma, juvenile rheumatoid arthritis, chronic pain, etc.). There are very difficult problems that need to be sorted out and we hope this book, while reflecting the current state of knowledge, will encourage research and intellectual work in this area.

We owe deep gratitude to all our contributing authors who took part in making this a high-quality, integrated resource. We greatly appreciate Ian Marvinney and Janice Stern, our editors at Springer, for their assistance and patience in completing this project. We would also like to thank the wonderful individuals who helped us finish this book, especially Linda Goddard. Finally, we thank our family members Jane Fisher, Katie and Anna, Dennis and Barbara Woodward and Nate Tolle for their unyielding support.

William T. O'Donohue
Lauren Woodward Tolle
Reno, Nevada

Contents

Contributors

Sarah Levin Allen Clinical Psychology Program, Drexel University, Philadelphia, PA, USA

Joan Austin, DNS, RN, FAAN Center for Enhancing Quality of Life in Chronic Illness, Indiana University School of Nursing, Indianapolis, IN, USA

Lamia P. Barakat, Ph.D. Children's Hospital of Philadelphia and University of Pennsylvania School of Medicine, Drexel University, Philadelphia, PA, USA

Julie A. Biller, M.D. Medical College of Wisconsin, Milwaukee, WI, USA

Dedee Caplin, Ph.D. Department of Pediatrics, University of Utah Health Sciences Center, Salt Lake City, UT, USA

Anthony R. Cordaro, Jr., M.D. Department of Psychiatry, The Children's Hospital, University of Colorado at Denver and Health Sciences Center, Aurora, CO, USA

Ivette Cruz, M.S. Department of Psychology, University of Miami, Miami, FL, USA

Carin Cunningham, Ph.D. Case Western Reserve School of Medicine, Cleveland, OH, USA

Lawrence J. D'Angelo, M.D., MPH Division of Adolescent and Young, Adult Medicine, Children's National Medical Center, Washington, DC, USA

W. Hobart Davies, Ph.D. Department of Psychology, University of Wisconsin – Milwaukee, Milwaukee, WI, USA

Alan Delamater, Ph.D. Department of Pediatrics, University of Miami Leonard M. Miller School of Medicine, Miami, FL, USA

Rachel Duchoslav, Ph.D. Department of Psychology, Utah State University, Logan, UT, USA

David W. Dunn, M.D. Department of Psychiatry, Indiana University School of Medicine, Indianapolis, IN, USA

Kathryn Eckert, M.D. Department of Pediatrics, University of Nevada School of Medicine, Reno, NV, USA

Joyce Engel, Ph.D., O.T. Department of Rehabilitation Medicine, University of Washington School of Medicine, Seattle, WA, USA

Clint Field, Ph.D. Department of Psychology, Utah State University, Logan, UT, USA

Judy Garber, Ph.D. Department of Psychology and Human Development, Vanderbilt University, Nashville, TN, USA

M. Elena Garralda, M.D. Division of Neurosciences and Mental Health, Imperial College London, London, UK

Steve Graybar, Ph.D. University of Nevada School of Medicine, Reno, NV, USA

Anthony Hains, Ph.D. Department of Educational Psychology, University of Wisconsin – Milwaukee, Milwaukee, WI, USA

Stuart Hauser, M.D., Ph.D. Harvard Medical School, Judge Baker Children's Center, Boston, MA, USA

Angela Huebner, Ph.D. Department of Human Development, Virginia Tech University, Falls Church, VA, USA

Anne E. Kazak, Ph.D., ABPP Department of Psychology; Department of Pediatrics, University of Pennsylvania School of Medicine, Children's Hospital of Philadelphia, Philadelphia, PA, USA

Annette La Greca, Ph.D. Psychology Department, University of Miami, Coral Gables, FL, USA

Michael Lavin, Ph.D. Psychologist – private practice, Washington, DC, USA

Carol B. Lindsley, M.D. Department of Pediatrics, University of Kansas Medical Center, Kansas City, KS, USA

Vincent A. Loffredo, M.D. Department of Pediatrics, University of Nevada School of Medicine, Reno, NV, USA

Maureen Lyon, Ph.D. Children's National Medical Center, Washington, DC, USA

Eleanor Mackey, Ph.D. Children's National Medical Center, Washington, DC, USA

John D. Mahan, M.D. Nationwide Children's Hospital, The Ohio State University, Columbus, OH, USA

Kristin K. Marciel, Ph.D. Psychology Department, University of Miami, Miami, FL, USA

David A. Maroof, M.A. Ferkauf Graduate School of Psychology, Yeshiva University, Bronx, NY, USA

Michelle A. Meade, Ph.D. Department of Physical Medicine and Rehabilitation, University of Michigan, Ann Arbor, MI, USA

Avani C. Modi, Ph.D. Division of Behavioral Medicine and Clinical Psychology, Cincinnati Children's Hospital, Cincinnati, OH, USA

Ifigenia Mougianis, B.A. Children's Hospital of Philadelphia, Philadelphia, PA, USA

D. Colette Nicolaou, Ph.D. Children's Hospital Los Angeles, Los Angeles, CA, USA

Kathleen O'Connor M.D. Department of Pediatrics, University of Nevada School of Medicine, Reno, NV, USA

William T. O'Donohue, Ph.D. Department of Psychology, University of Nevada, Reno, Reno, NV, USA

Emily A. O'Hara Psychology Department, Drexel University, Philadelphia, PA, USA

Diana Quintero, M.D. Medical College of Wisconsin, Milwaukee, WI, USA

Alexandra L. Quittner, Ph.D. Department of Psychology & Pediatrics, University of Miami, Miami, FL, USA

Michael A. Rapoff, Ph.D. Department of Pediatrics, University of Kansas Medical Center, Kansas City, KS, USA

Helen Rozelman, Ph.D., LMSW Stern College for Women, Yeshiva University, New York, NY, USA; Department of Pediatrics, New York University, School of Medicine, New York, NY, USA

Lisa Schwartz, Ph.D. Children's Hospital of Philadelphia, Philadelphia, PA, USA

Brandyn M. Street Department of Psychology and Human Development, Vanderbilt University, Nashville, TN, USA

Lauren Woodward Tolle, M.A. Department of Psychology, University of Nevada, Reno, NV, USA

Sarah Tornichio MSW, LSW Nationwide Children's Hospital, Columbus, OH, USA

Gary A. Walco, Ph.D. The David Center for Children's Pain and Palliative Care, Hackensack University Medical Center, Hackensack, NJ, USA; Department of Pediatrics, University of Medicine and Dentistry of New Jersey, New Jersey Medical School, Newark, NJ, USA

Marianne Z. Wamboldt, M.D. University of Colorado at Denver and Health Sciences Center, Aurora, CO, USA

Dorothy Warner, Ph.D. Harvard Medical School, Judge Baker Children's Center, Boston, MA, USA

Part I
Basic Issues

Introduction

Adolescents with Chronic Illnesses: Issues and Answers

William O'Donohue and Lauren Woodward Tolle

Adolescence is a difficult period in life, regardless of whether or not there is a chronic illness involved. This period is often marked with distress, strained relationships, and difficulty in navigating new social roles. When individuals enter this developmental stage with a chronic illness, it can be especially trying. Despite how difficult this can be, little research has critically examined optimal, evidence-based ways of treating adolescents with chronic illness within an integrated care setting. Given the long-lasting impact of problems that can arise during this developmental stage (transitioning into adulthood, developing autonomy, creating an identity, creating long-lasting relationships, family functioning, etc.) along with problems that can arise from having a chronic illness (i.e., problems with treatment adherence, social stigma, school functioning, depression, lack of social support, poor coping skills, poor adherence to proper diet/exercise) it seems appropriate and necessary to look at these issues holistically. In addition, adolescence is frequently the time when both positive (i.e., regular exercise, healthful diet, treatment adherence) and negative health behaviors (i.e., poor treatment adherence, smoking, overeating) are initiated and set the tone for future health behaviors (Chesney & Antoni, 2002). This makes this developmental stage an all the more important period to intervene early and implement skills training early to prevent the likelihood of poorer health outcomes later in adulthood.

W. O'Donohue (✉)
Department of Psychology, University of Nevada, Reno, NV, USA

Adolescents display a huge amount of variability. If one says "13-year-old girl," one can gain a rough idea of what that person would be like physically, socially, cognitively, emotionally but still there is wide variability. We want to caution against stereotyping. Each adolescent needs to be viewed ideographically. Nothing in this book implies that easy generalizations can be made about adolescents.

Some of this variability comes from the usual sources: genetics (which also turn on genes at different times, hence different ages for puberty), previous history (an adolescent has already had a decade or so of childhood experiences that produce variability), different current circumstances (family status, economic status, unique cohort effects), and different prospects and goals (family history of attendance of Ivy League schools vs. family history of imprisonment).

A key point is that adolescence is generally the time where the individual needs to take more responsibility for managing their chronic disease. However, this is often not very straightforward. Chronic disease management can require cognitive and behavioral skills (such as self-control, planning, problem solving, empathy) that can be beyond the grasp of adolescence (and all too often key family members). It also can be a time where the individual engages in a lot of risky behaviors, seemingly with little appreciation of the magnitude of these risks. It can also be a time of increased reactivity and counterpliance. Attempts by parents to move in one direction seem to be keys for the adolescent to move in the opposite direction. It is also a time when the child more keenly discerns and responds to the parents' or family's own problems. With the

W.T. O'Donohue, L.W. Tolle (eds.), *Behavioral Approaches to Chronic Disease in Adolescence*,
DOI 10.1007/978-0-387-87687-0_1, © Springer Science+Business Media, LLC 2009

exception of clear abuse and neglect, the infant is relatively oblivious to their parents' deficits, but the adolescent is much more keenly aware (and may even become somewhat of a connoisseur of these). These factors present increased challenges and increased costs of failure for professionals engaged in attempting to help these individuals and their families. Again, we don't wish to stereotype; many adolescents are healthy individuals with good support networks and this often means a more straightforward response to their chronic disease and its management. In general more research is needed in understanding developmental progressions and factors that account for variability in these. The state of the science is itself in its infancy: we have very little nomothetic information to rely on.

But there is a rough developmental progression: infancy to childhood to adolescence, to adulthood, to old age; we believe this "third stage" presents its unique and very challenging problems for the adolescent themselves, for the families of these individuals, and for helpers involved with them. This book attempts to delineate these and to offer some tools for addressing the problems of chronic disease management.

The importance of the book is that it will help equip practitioners with tools necessary to treat psychosocial problems inherently found in adolescents with chronic illness. This book is divided into two parts, the first part outlines the special considerations of adolescent and family psychotherapy within the context of chronic illness. The second part provides detailed descriptions of evidence-based practice guidelines for the major chronic conditions that adolescents face. It is our hope that this book is comprehensive in its ability to accurately address specific considerations inherent in adolescent psychology (therapist burnout, ethical considerations, bringing in the family, cultural considerations, etc.) and to specifically outline evidence-based practice guidelines for common chronic conditions in adolescence (type 1 diabetes, asthma, juvenile rheumatoid arthritis, chronic pain, etc.) such that a clinician can clearly comprehend them and easily use them in an integrated care setting. The strength of this book is the quality and expertise of the contributing authors.

In the second chapter, Huebner sets the scene for this book by providing the reader with an overview of normative adolescent development. He addresses the various aspects of adolescent development by way of an ecological model, focusing on physical development, cognitive development, and psychosocial development. This important chapter highlights how these normative stages might be exacerbated in a case of an adolescent with a chronic illness (i.e., the "it can't happen to me" syndrome or a heightened level of self-consciousness).

The chapter by Warner and Hauser expands off of the second chapter by explicitly discussing how normative adolescent development may be disrupted by the presence of a chronic illness. The chapter follows disease progression from diagnosis and initial adjustment to adherence and living with the illness, the desire for autonomy, and complications in the context of chronic illness, as well as adaptive and maladaptive coping strategies. Warner and Hauser provide empirical evidence for adolescent-focused interventions, family-focused interventions, and finally community and school interventions.

Eckert, Loffredo, and O'Connor, in their chapter, provide detailed information of the important physiological changes occurring in adolescence. Specifically, the chapter first addresses normative physiological changes that occur in adolescence and then addresses specific pediatric conditions (i.e., asthma, type 1 diabetes, cancer, eating disorders, and cystic fibrosis) and how these normative pubertal processes are disrupted and can lead to permanent changes in the adolescent (i.e., short stature or poor bone mineral accretion). This chapter also addresses adolescent brain physiology, the effects of alcohol and antidepressants on the developing brain, and how the developing brain is relevant to issues inherent in chronically ill adolescents (e.g., assisting adolescents in preventing hospitalization by making the connection between cause and effect – the use of preventative inhalers in the case of asthma in preventing hospitalization). Finally, three case examples are provided to illuminate important physiological processes involved in three pediatric illnesses (i.e., lymphocytic leukemia, type 1 diabetes, and asthma).

Field and Duchoslav address the importance of the family and familial influences in adolescents with chronic illness in their chapter. Specifically, they report empirical literature related to family conflict, family cohesion, family relationships, and expressiveness within the family as it relates to adolescent adjustment to chronic illness. The chapter also provides empirical literature concerning family responses to treatment including appraisal of the illness and coping strategies found to be adaptive or maladaptive. Finally, the authors provide findings from literature concerning specific parental factors including maternal maladjustment to the illness and distress as well as overprotection of the adolescent. The chapter concludes with implications for future research and clinical work in providing the best family environment to predict adolescent success in managing their illness.

The next chapter by Lavin provides a thoughtful and interesting perspective on ethical issues that are inherent in treating adolescent patients and provides an example from Shaffer's 1977 play, Equus. Lavin follows this play and includes relevant ethical issues that abound with adolescents and the additional complications when that adolescent has a chronic illness.

Tolle and Graybar, in the seventh chapter, address the inherent problem of burnout in all individuals involved in treating chronic illnesses in adolescents, from the adolescent patient themselves to the family of the adolescent and the medical professionals involved. They provide empirically supported treatment guidelines to treat burnout in the adolescent and family members, as well as structural strategies to prevent burnout and treat compassion fatigue in the mental health care professionals working with this population. A case study is also provided to illuminate the process of working through burnout in a family with an adolescent with type 1 diabetes.

Part II (from the eighth to the twenty-second chapter) of the book provides evidence-based treatment guidelines for specific chronic illnesses commonly found in adolescents. Chapter twenty three is unique in that Quittner, Cruz, Modi, and Marciel provide a review of available assessment tools used in determining quality of life and other health-related constructs in adolescents with chronic health conditions. The contributing authors in Part II are experts in their respective fields and provide cutting-edge information to assist the clinician in an integrated care setting. The chapters follow a consistent outline to provide optimally efficient information. This outline is as follows.

Chapter Outline

1) Description of the chronic condition with adolescents including
   - Epidemiology
     i. Typical age of onset
     ii. Progression
     iii. Percentage of population afflicted with this disease
     iv. Prognosis
   - Symptomatology
     i. Frequency (do they occur all day/every day?)
     ii. Severity (life interference? visible? pain associated?)
     iii. Duration (Does it go away? lifelong?)
     iv. Lethality (Is it or can it be life threatening? If so, how and when?)
     v. Complications
   - Treatment regimen for adolescents (and families where indicated)
     i. Necessary frequency of adherence (what, when, how often)
     ii. Side effects (of medication, etc.)
     iii. Treatment options
     iv. Cost
     v. Insurance coverage
     vi. Frequency of necessary medical attention (checkups, etc.)
2) Common comorbid psychosocial problems:
   - Stigma (how does this affect the given disease, treatment, etc.)
   - Comorbidity (depression, anxiety, substance abuse, body image problems, poor diet, poor physical activity, etc.)
   - Social support
   - Family conflict
   - Treatment adherence issues
   - Cultural considerations
3) How a behavioral health specialist, working within an integrated team, can most effectively target these adolescents:
   - What are the best practices for assessment and treatment?
   - What is the behavioral health clinician's role in most effectively helping this individual?

Effective psychosocial/psychological interventions and necessary collaboration with primary care physicians, nurses, dietitians, specialty care practitioners, etc.

4) Methodological considerations if conducting research with this population
5) Research agenda

This important book provides the multidimensional context and resulting difficulties of treating adolescents with chronic illnesses. As medical treatments for various chronic conditions improve, thus reducing mortality rates, and advanced technologies are developed to assist those with chronic conditions, psychologists are presented with a unique opportunity to advance research agendas in a medical setting. Also, behavioral health interventions implemented in pediatric populations can potentially assist in saving billions of dollars in health care spending by using evidence-based approaches to prevent long-term medical complications in a significant number of individuals. Through a succinct presentation of issues surrounding the adolescent (i.e., family considerations, developmental changes, cultural considerations, potential for burnout), a clear review of empirical data on adolescents with a number of common chronic illness, and finally evidence-based guidelines to assist the practitioner in working within a medical setting, this book assists in this process by providing practitioners with the knowledge and the tools to continue to make significant contributions in improving the quality of life of adolescents with chronic illnesses.

Reference

Chesney, M. A., & Antoni, M. H. (2002). Introduction: Translating a decade of innovations into clinical practice. In M. A. Chesney & M. H. Antoni (Eds.), *Innovative approaches to health psychology*. Washington, D.C.: American Psychological Association.

An Introduction to Adolescent Development

Angela J. Huebner

It was the best of times, it was the worst of times; it was the age of wisdom, it was the age of foolishness . . . Charles Dickens (1859, p. 1), A Tale of Two Cities

Although this quote was not intended to describe the period of adolescence, it does bear some striking truths to the "revolution" that is occurring during this time. Adolescence is a particularly exciting and uniquely vulnerable period of development. Not since infancy has the individual undergone so many changes at such a high rate of speed (Carnegie Council on Adolescent Development, 1996). These changes are occurring across multiple developmental systems—physiological, cognitive, and psychosocial. Additionally, these changes are occurring in part in reaction to the individual's environment. That's right. While development in infancy could be considered "generic" such that the organism is at that time primed to adapt to any environment (e.g., aboriginal tribe or middle-class American—they all begin the same), development during adolescence is designed to fit the organism more efficiently into his or her environment or context. Thus, development during the period of adolescence reflects an active interplay between the organism and his or her context. Such contexts include the individual, family, friends, community, and culture.

The purpose of this chapter is to provide the reader with an overview of what most agree to be "normative" development among adolescents. Such a basic understanding is necessary before one can begin to consider the unique burden that chronic health conditions (CHC) adds to an already stressed system. To this end, the reader is first presented with a framework for organizing considerations about development. Second, descriptions of normative development are presented, followed by unique considerations that must be addressed given the additional condition of CHC. Finally, special treatment considerations for working with adolescents will be provided.

A.J. Huebner (✉)
Department of Human Development, Virginia Tech University, Falls Church, VA, USA
e-mail: ahuebner@vt.edu

Ecological Model of Development

Because of its usefulness as a framework for mapping the contexts of adolescents, the ecological model of development (Bronfenbrenner, 1979) will be used to organize this discussion of normative adolescent development. Briefly, the ecological model of development assumes that development occurs in context and that in each context a unique "transaction" between the individual and others occurs. In other words, development is considered to be a *joint* function of the individual and his or her environment (Bronfenbrenner, 1992). The ecological model is intended to describe development over the entire life course. However, for purposes of this chapter, its scope has been narrowed to focus only on adolescent development. In the following section, each ecological "level" will be described and the associated contextual issues of adolescent development highlighted.

W.T. O'Donohue, L.W. Tolle (eds.), *Behavioral Approaches to Chronic Disease in Adolescence*,
DOI 10.1007/978-0-387-87687-0_2,

Let's begin in the innermost circle, with the individual organism: the "youth." This circle represents what the individual organism brings to the context. This includes issues of temperament, physical health, capacity for learning, skills, and the like. These characteristics influence the types of interaction the young person will have with those in the second circle. In the ecological model, the second circle is called the "microsystem" and refers to those contexts or immediate settings in which the individual interacts as a direct participant. This includes, for example, the family, the peer group, youth groups, sports teams, religious groups, and even health care professionals. For adolescents, these microsystems are a crucial influence on development. They provide the context in which the adolescent is trying to fit his or her behavior, ideals, and identity; similarly the adolescent is shaping the context through what they bring to the interactions. Development results from the interaction of the two.

The third level maps the potential connections among those individuals who interact with the adolescent. These connections are referred to as the "mesosystem." Because each microsystem may include different expectations or norms, it is important to consider how much cross-communication is occurring between them. The double-headed arrows in Figure 1 suggest that mesosystems influence each other, such that what happens in one mesosystem informs what happens in another. The adolescent is not a direct participant in these interactions; rather, he or she is the focus of the connection. For example, does the parent communicate directly with the adolescent's teachers? Do the adolescent's teachers talk with the youth group leaders? Do parents talk with youth's friends? Does the health care team talk with the parent? Does the physician talk with the adolescent's siblings?

Level four, known as the "exosystem," includes more indirect influences on adolescents. The exosystem includes those systems, policies, or decisions that impact adolescents, even though there is not necessarily a direct relationship with the adolescent. For example, does mom's place of work allow her to use her sick leave if her son is ill? Do parents have family health insurance benefits? Did the school board vote to hire a full-time nurse for the school? Did citizens vote to raise taxes in order to open their own hospital?

Finally, level five is called the "macrosystem." The macrosystem refers to the broad patterns of a culture and society. These tend to be reflected in the norms and values supported (directly or indirectly) by those in the community. For example, how do people treat those who are different? Is there discrimination? Is bullying or violence tolerated? Do people genuinely look out for each other?

Development is enhanced when there is goodness of fit between the individual and his or her environment. This model suggests a way of thinking about that fit and the implications it has for supporting youth with chronic health

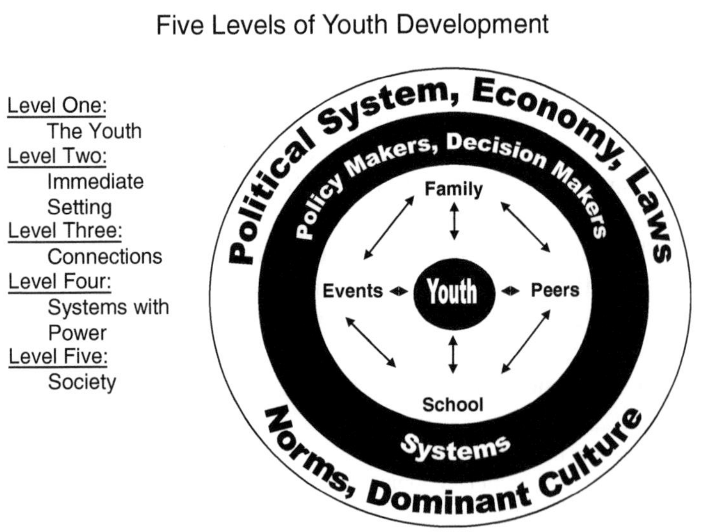

Fig. 1 Five levels of youth development

conditions. The next section focuses on issues of normative development at the individual (innermost circle) level.

Normative Adolescent Development

As part of this overview of "normative" adolescent development, physical development, cognitive development, and psychosocial development will all be briefly explored. As you read the following information, keep in mind that while adolescents develop in each of these areas, they do not all necessarily follow the same time line.

Physical Development

During the teen years, adolescents experience changes in their physical development at a rate of speed unparalleled since infancy. Physical development includes rapid gains in height and weight, development of secondary sex characteristics, and continued brain development (Archibald, Graber, & Brooks-Gunn, 2006). With respect to physical development, during a 1-year growth spurt, boys and girls can gain an average of 4.1 and 3.5 inches in height, respectively (Steinberg, 2007). This spurt typically occurs 2 years earlier for girls than for boys. Weight gain results from increased muscle development in boys and body fat in girls. During puberty, changing hormonal levels play a role in activating the development of secondary sex characteristics. These include (1) growth of pubic hair; (2) menarche (first period for girls) or penis growth (for boys); (3) voice changes (for boys); (4) growth of underarm hair; (5) facial hair growth (for boys); and (6) increased production of oil, increased sweat gland activity, and the beginning of acne.

Additionally, recent research suggests that regions of the adolescent brain are not completely developed or integrated. Of specific interest is the frontal cortex region of the brain. This region of the brain is responsible for impulse control, decision-making skills, and affect regulation. Research suggests that while neuron proliferation is expanding during the 0- to 3-year-old time frame, a process of "synaptic pruning" is occurring during adolescence, the suspected effect of which is to more efficiently "fit" the organism to his or her environment (Blakemore & Choudhury, 2006). Such "pruning" actually increases the speed of information processing. The individual is becoming specialized or refined to respond more efficiently to the type of stimuli presented in his or her particular context. It is important to note, however, the behaviors that occur during this pruning process (i.e., learning about impulse control, affect regulation, decision making) will most likely be inconsistent or spotty at best. It has been compared to the period of early development when a toddler is first learning to walk (Baird, 2008). For toddlers, walking doesn't happen right away, instead it occurs in steps with many starts and stops and much falling down in between. Adults are much better able to allow for this development in children (i.e., not punishing them for falling down) than they are in adolescents, probably in part because toddlers don't look as much like adults as do adolescents. This yet unfinished process of "pruning" and rewiring is thought to explain why some adolescents seem to be inconsistent in controlling their emotions, impulses, and judgments (Dahl, 2004).

How do these physical changes affect adolescents and their interactions with others?

Adolescents frequently sleep longer. Research suggests that adolescents' actually need more sleep to allow their bodies to conduct the internal work required for such rapid growth. On average, adolescents need about 9 ½ hours of sleep a night (Steinberg, 2007). This increased need for sleep is often at odds with conventional school day schedules and may become a source of conflict between parents and teens. It is important to recognize that medications involved in the treatment of CHC may interfere with sleep—either reducing or increasing the need impacting the adolescent's readiness and ability to interact with others or to perform well in school.

Adolescents may be more clumsy or overly sensitive about weight. Words like "gangly," awkward," and "gawky" are all great descriptions of the condition of the adolescent body. During this phase of development, body parts don't all grow at the same rate. Previous bodily mastery may have to be relearned as adolescents try to cope with limbs that seem to have grown overnight. This new awkwardness may contribute to teens becoming more sensitive about their looks and their physical abilities (Archibald et al., 2006). Previously active youth may hesitate to become involved in sports. Additionally, teenage girls may become overly sensitive about their weight. This concern arises because of the rapid weight gain associated with puberty. In a recent national survey, 62% of adolescent girls reported that they were trying to lose weight (Center for Disease Control, 2005). A small percentage of adolescent girls (1–3%) become so obsessed with their weight that they develop severe eating disorders such as anorexia nervosa or bulimia. These concerns about weight may influence their mealtime and activity choices. Again, the use of medications to control CHC may contribute to inflammation or "puffiness" that further increases self-consciousness about weight and appearance.

Adolescents may be concerned because they are not physically developing at the same rate as their peers. Adolescents may be more developed ("early maturers") or less developed ("late maturers") than their peers. Being out of developmental "step" with peers is concerning to adolescents because most just want to fit in. Early maturation affects boys and girls differently (for review see Archibald et al., 2006). Research suggests that early-maturing boys tend to be more popular with peers and hold more leadership positions. Adults often assume that early-maturing boys are cognitively mature as well. This assumption can lead to false expectations about a young person's ability to take on increased responsibility. Because of their physical appearance, early-maturing girls are more likely to experience pressure to become involved in dating relationships with older boys before they are emotionally ready. Early-maturing girls tend to suffer more from depression, eating disorders, and anxiety (Ge, Conger, & Elder, 2001). Medications or treatments related to CHC or the CHC itself may interfere with pubertal development, exacerbating off-time development with an adolescent and his or her peer group.

Cognitive Development

Most adults recognize that adolescents have better thinking skills than do younger youth. These advances in thinking skills tend to center around advanced reasoning skills, ability to abstract, and meta-cognitions (Byrnes, 2006). Advanced reasoning skills include the ability to think about multiple options and possibilities. It includes a more logical thought process and the ability to think about things hypothetically. It involves asking and answering the question of "what if…?." For example, What if I don't take my medicine on time? or What if I decide to skip this meal? or What if I decide to eat this cake? Advanced reasoning also includes the concept of abstract thinking. Abstract thinking means thinking about things that cannot be seen, heard, or touched. Examples include things like faith, trust, beliefs, and spirituality. Adolescents may begin to challenge parents or adults about what they believe, all in an effort to develop their own system of beliefs. Topics like faith and spirituality may take on new meaning for a young person with CHC, as they may have to come to terms with the possibility of a diminished quality of life or life span.

Finally, adolescents are developing the ability to think about thinking in a process known as "metacognition." Meta-cognition allows individuals to think about how they feel and what they are thinking. It involves being able to think about how one is perceived by others. It can be used to develop strategies for improving learning. The ability to think about one's thoughts also has implications for managing stress or for pain management (e.g., mindfulness meditation).

How do these cognitive changes affect adolescents and their interactions with others?

Adolescents demonstrate a heightened level of self-consciousness. Adolescents tend to believe that everyone is as concerned with their thoughts and behaviors as they are. This leads the teen to believe that they have an "imaginary audience" of people that are always watching them (Elkind, 1967). This may be especially true if they have an illness that is physically apparent (e.g., hair loss due to chemotherapy).

Adolescents tend to believe that no one else has ever experienced similar feelings and emotions (Elkind, 1967). They may become overly dramatic in describing things that are upsetting to them. They may say things like "You'll never understand," or "My life is ruined!" These feelings may be exacerbated for young people experiencing a chronic health condition. In some cases, their experience is truly unique as others really may not have experienced the same pain, frustrations, or stresses that they have.

Adolescents tend to exhibit the "it can't happen to me" syndrome, also known as a "personal fable" (Elkind, 1967). This belief may cause adolescents to take unnecessary risks like drinking and driving ("I won't crash this car"), having unprotected sex ("I can't possibly get pregnant"), or smoking ("I can't possibly get cancer") (Greene, Krcmar, Walters, Rubin, & Hale, 2000). Translated to the adolescent with CHC, this "personal fable" may facilitate lack of treatment adherence with respect to diet or behavioral restrictions—especially if the consequences of treatment non-compliance aren't immediate.

Adolescents tend to become very cause oriented. Their activism is related to the ability to think about abstract concepts. After reading about cruelty to animals a teen may become a vegetarian and a member of "People for the Ethical Treatment of Animals" (PETA). Another teen may become active in "Green Peace" or "Save the Whales" campaign. Similarly, they may begin to exhibit very strong opinions about the medications, treatments, or diets to which they are willing to adhere.

Adolescents tend to exhibit a "justice" orientation (Kohlberg, 1984). They are quick to point out inconsistencies between adults' words and their actions. They have difficulty seeing shades of gray. They see little room for error. They may ask questions like "What did I do to deserve this?" or believe that life is not fair. They may also have difficulty accepting non-definitive answers to questions related to their condition.

Psychosocial Development

There are five recognized psychosocial issues that adolescents deal with during their adolescent years. Essentially these issues all center around the interaction between self and others. "Who am I?" and "How am I perceived by others?" Specific tasks include establishing an identity, autonomy, intimacy, comfort with one's sexuality, and achievement.

Establishing an identity. This has been called one of the most important tasks of adolescents [see Kroger (2006) for review]. The question of "who am I" is not one that adolescents think about at a conscious level. Instead, over the course of the adolescent years, adolescents begin to integrate the opinions of influential others (e.g., parents, friends, other caring adults) into their own likes and dislikes. The eventual outcome is people who have a clear sense of their values and beliefs, occupational goals, and relationship expectations. People with secure identities know where they fit (or where they don't want to fit) in their world. CHC add another layer to the quest of identity development. Do I define myself as my illness? (e.g., "I am a diabetic") or do I define myself as a person with an illness ("I am Katie and I have diabetes"). How do others define me?

Establishing autonomy. Some people assume that autonomy refers to becoming completely independent from others. They equate it with teen "rebellion." Rather than severing relationships, however, establishing autonomy during the teen years really means becoming an independent and self-governing person *within* relationships (Allen & Land, 1999). Autonomous adolescents have gained the ability to make and follow through with their own decisions, live by their own set of principles of right and wrong, and have become less emotionally dependent on parents (Zimmer-Gembeck & Collins, 2006). Autonomy is a necessary achievement if the teen is to become self-sufficient in society. The experience of the CHC may complicate the task of establishing identity. Depending on the condition, parents or other adults may hesitate to allow the young person to be responsible for treatment adherence; similarly, young people may not be willing to give up support in this area.

Achievement. Our society tends to foster and value attitudes of competition and success. Because of cognitive advances, the teen years are a time when young people can begin to see the relationship between their current abilities and plans and their future vocational aspirations. They need to figure out what their achievement preferences are—what they are currently good at and areas in which they are willing to strive for success. CHC may limit the development or exploration of some skills and abilities. Such youth may need additional guidance and support in figuring out how to match their interests with their abilities.

Establishing intimacy. Many people, including adolescents, equate intimacy with sex. In fact intimacy and sex are not the same. Intimacy is usually first learned within the context of same-sex friendships and then utilized in romantic relationships. Intimacy refers to close relationships in which people are open, honest, caring, and trusting. Friendships provide the first setting in which young people can practice their social skills with those who are their equals. It is with friends that adolescents learn how to begin, maintain, and terminate relationships, practice social skills, and to become intimate. Adolescents with CHC may be hesitant to explore intimacy with their peers, in part because they may not feel as though they are really "equal."

How do these psychosocial changes affect adolescents and their interactions with others?

Adolescents begin to spend more time with their friends than their families. It is within friendship groups that adolescents can develop and practice social skills (Brown & Klute, 2006). Adolescents are quick to point out to each other which behaviors are acceptable and which are not. It is important to remember that even though adolescents are spending increased amounts of time with their friends, they still tend to conform to parental ideals when it comes to decisions about values, education, and long-term plans.

Adolescents may become elusive about where they are going or with whom. When asked what they'll be doing for the evening, adolescents typically reply with "nothing" or "hanging out." When asked whom they'll be with, adolescents reply "just some friends." They are spending increasing amounts of time in context with peers rather than with adults (Brown & Klute, 2006).

Adolescents may begin to interact with parents and other adults as people. Even though they may not want to be seen with parents in public, adolescents may begin to view parents more as people. They may ask more questions about how a parent was when he or she was a teen. They may attempt to interact with adults more as equals (Granic, Dishion, & Hollenstein, 2006). Along with this newfound "equality" adults may find that adolescents become more argumentative (Granic et al., 2006). Adolescents may question adults' values and judgments. When adolescents don't get their way, they may say "you just don't understand." This inconsistency in responses (i.e., sometimes acting as a adult, sometimes acting as a child) is a normal part of development.

Special Considerations

The previous discussion highlighted the major normative developmental tasks of adolescents and how this development changes or influences their interaction with others. It also highlighted the additional issues and complexity that arises when one adds a chronic health condition to this already highly transitional time. This section highlights issues unique to those with CHC. These include the therapeutic alliance and issues of treatment compliance as well as the recognition of the comorbidity of mental health issues with CHC.

Therapeutic Alliance and Treatment Compliance

Therapeutic alliance refers to the relationship between the health care team and the adolescent. The notion of therapeutic alliance has traditionally been relegated to the psychotherapy arena but its relational aspects are an important consideration in other health care contexts. A "good" therapeutic alliance suggests that the patient and health care provider(s) have a mutual understanding and agreement upon the treatment goals and tasks required to meet the goals (Bordin, 1979). Much research has demonstrated a positive relationship between therapeutic alliance and treatment compliance among adults (e.g., Martin, Garske, & Davies, 2000); that is, the more positive the therapeutic relationship, the more likely it is that compliance with treatment will occur.

Less empirical research has explored the therapeutic relationship for adolescents. This is unfortunate given the finding that about half of adolescents with chronic health conditions do not adhere to treatment recommendations (Kyngas, Kroll, & Duffy, 2000). Related research on communication between physicians and their adolescent patients is informative. For example, in their study of doctor–adolescent communication, Beresford and Sloper's (2003) findings suggest that three areas were important for facilitating effective physician–patient communication: adolescent choice about who they are engaging with; a sense of equality, or being treated as an individual rather than a "condition"; and continuity of contact with the same treating physician. Other researchers suggested that adolescents with CHC rated physician honesty, attention to pain, and physician expertise with their respective chronic illness as the most important aspects of care (Britto et al., 2007).

Sound familiar? All three of these areas are manifestations of developmental tasks that are occurring. Adolescents are beginning to experiment with their independence and autonomy. This means that formation of a mutually respectful relationship with their health care providers is important. Not only does it make the interaction less stressful, it may also facilitate honest communication about treatment compliance, including issues of risk behavior that may hinder CDC management. For example, Does the young person feel comfortable enough to reveal alcohol or drug use? Can they talk about sexual activity? By being intentional about fostering good communication with their adolescent patients, physicians and other health care providers can honor and facilitate normative development and identity potential issues related to treatment compliance. If a positive therapeutic alliance doesn't exist, it is much less likely that risk behaviors will be revealed (Beresford & Sloper, 2003).

The ecological model framework illustrates the important role that other microsystems have on adolescents. Given that adolescents are greatly influenced by their family, friends, and popular culture, it is important for the health care providers to be able to discuss those influences on the adolescent—both in terms of how they view their illness and their lives as well as in terms of how others influence their desire or ability to comply with treatment. How supportive are parents of the treatment method? How does the treatment affect the adolescent's interaction with friends? How aware of and supportive of are friends to necessary behavioral or dietary modifications?

Comorbidity with Mental Health

The final consideration that must be raised when working with adolescents having a CHC is that of the potential for comorbidity with mental health issues. It is important for health care providers to recognize that between 20 and 50% of "normal" adolescents self-report depressive symptoms (Kessler, Avenevoli, & Merikangas, 2001). This percentage is significant given that those experiencing depressive symptoms in adolescents are more likely than those who do not to develop depression during adulthood (Pine, Cohen, Cohen, & Brook, 1999). Additionally, researchers have demonstrated that adolescent depression often co-occurs with other internalizing (e.g., anxiety) or externalizing (e.g., aggression, risky behaviors) problems (Compas, Connor, & Hinden, 1998). Not surprisingly, the experience of CHC has been demonstrated to be a risk factor for adolescent depression (e.g., Hankin, 2006).

References

Allen, J., & Land, D. (1999). Attachment in adolescence. In J. Cassidy & P. Shaver (Eds.), *Handbook of attachment: Theory, research, and clinical application* (pp. 319–335). New York: The Guildford Press.

Archibald, A., Graber, J., & Brooks-Gunn, J. (2006). Pubertal processes and physiological growth in adolescence. In G. Adams & M. Berzonsky (Eds.), *Blackwell handbook of adolescence* (pp. 24-48). Malden, MA: Blackwell Publishing.

Baird, A. (May 8, 2008). *Whatever: Turning on the teen brain.* Research presentation presented at the 2008 Children, Youth, and Families at Risk Conference San Antonio, TX.

Beresford, B., & Sloper P. (2003). Chronically ill adolescents' experience of communicating with doctors: A qualitative study. *Journal of Adolescent Health, 33*, 172–179.

Blakemore, S-J., & Choudhury, S. (2006). Development of the adolescent brain: Implications for executive function and social cognition. *Journal of Child Psychology and Psychiatry, 47*(3–4), 296–312.

Bordin, E. (1979). The generalized ability of the psychoanalytic concept of the working alliance. *Psychotherapy Theory, Research & Practice, 16*, 252–260.

Britto, M., Slap, G., DeVellis, R., Hornung, R., Atheton, H, Knopf, J., et al. (2007). Specialists understanding of the health care preferences of chronically ill adolescents. *Journal of Adolescent Health, 40*(4), 334–341.

Bronfenbrenner, U. (1992). Ecological systems theory. In R. Vasta (Ed.), *Six theories of child development: Revised formulations and current issues* (pp. 187–249). London: Jessica Kingsley.

Bronfenbrenner, U. (1979). *The ecology of human development: Experiments by nature and design.* Cambridge, MA: Harvard University Press.

Brown, B., & Klute, C. (2006). Friendships, cliques, and crowds. In G. Adams & M. Berzonsky (Eds.), *Blackwell handbook of adolescence* (pp. 330–348). Malden, MA: Blackwell Publishing.

Byrnes, J. (2006). Cognitive development during adolescence. In G. Adams & M. Berzonsky (Eds.), *Blackwell Handbook of Adolescence* (pp. 227–246). Malden, MA: Blackwell Publishing.

Carnegie Council on Adolescent Development. (1996). *Great transitions: Preparing adolescents for a new century.* New York: Carnegie Corporation.

Center for Disease Control. (2005). *Youth Risk Behavior Survey.* Atlanta, GA: CDC.

Compas, B., Connor, J., & Hinden, B. (1998). New perspectives on depression during adolescence. In R. Jessor (Ed.),

New perspectives on adolescent risk behavior (pp. 319–362). New York: Cambridge University Press.

Dahl, R. (2004). Adolescent brain development: A period of vulnerabilities and opportunities. *Annals of the New York Academy of Sciences, 1021*, 1–22.

Dickens, C. (1859/1997). *A tale of two cities*. New York Signet Classic Printing.

Elkind, D. (1967). Egocentrism in adolescence. *Child Development, 38*(4), 1025–1034.

Ge, X., Conger, R., & Elder, G. (2001). Pubertal transition, stressful life events, and the emergence of gender differences in adolescent depressive symptoms. *Developmental Psychology, 37*(3), 404–417.

Granic, I., Dishion, T., & Hollenstein, T. (2006). The family ecology of adolescence: A dynamic systems perspective on normative development. In G. Adams & M. Berzonsky (Eds.), *Blackwell handbook of adolescence* (pp. 60–91). Malden, MA: Blackwell Publishing.

Greene, K., Krcmar, M., Walters, L, Rubin, D., & Hale J. (2000). Targeting adolescent risk-taking behaviors: The contribution of ego-centrism and sensation seeking. *Journal of Adolescence, 23*(4), 439–461.

Hankin, B., (2006). Adolescent depression: Description, causes, and interventions, *Epilepsy & Behavior, 8*, 102–114.

Kessler, R., Avenevoli, S., & Merikangas, K. (2001). Mood disorders in children and adolescents: An epidemiologic perspective. *Biological Psychiatry, 49*, 1002–1014.

Kohlberg, L. (1984). *Essays on moral development: Vol 2: The psychology of moral development*. San Francisco: Harper & Row.

Kroger, J. (2006). Identity development during adolescence. In G. Adams & M. Berzonsky (Eds.), *Blackwell handbook of adolescence* (pp. 205–226). Malden, MA: Blackwell Publishing.

Kyngas, H., Kroll, T., & Duffy, M. (2000). Compliance in adolescents with chronic diseases: A review. *Journal of Adolescent Health, 26*, 379–388.

Martin, D., Garske, J., & Davies, M. (2000). Relation of therapeutic alliance with outcome and other variables: A meta-analytic review. *Journal of Consulting and Clinical Psychology, 68*, 438–450.

Pine, D., Cohen, E., Cohen, P., & Brook, J. (1999). Adolescent depressive symptoms as predictors of adult depression: Moodiness or mood disorder? *American Journal of Psychiatry, 156*, 133–135.

Steinberg, L. (2007). *Adolescence*(8th ed.). New York: McGraw-Hill.

Zimmer-Gembeck, M., & Collins, A. (2006). Autonomy development during adolescence. In G. Adams & M. Berzonsky (Eds.), *Blackwell handbook of adolescence* (pp. 175–204). Malden, MA: Blackwell Publishing.

Unique Considerations when Treating Adolescents with Chronic Illness

Dorothy E. Warner and Stuart T. Hauser

Introduction

Adolescence is marked by significant developmental changes in virtually all aspects of life, encompassing major transformations as individuals move from childhood to adulthood. Changes associated with this era include significant *internal* processes (ego and identity development, changing self and body image, onset of and continued pubertal changes) and *psychosocial* influences (peer and family relationships, new romantic/sexual relationships). These salient developmental issues, as well as the overarching challenges represented by strivings for independence and future-oriented goals, *can* be made more complicated and stressful by the presence of a chronic illness – although this is not always the case.

Some researchers have suggested that the diagnosis of a chronic illness becomes a "biographical disruption" that makes the development of a sense of self more difficult than for adolescents who do not have a chronic illness (Schur, Gamsu, & Barley, 1999, p. 227). In addition to stressors that are directly related to living with a chronic illness, such a condition may increase individuals' vulnerability to stressors of daily life (Grey, Lipman, Cameron, & Thurber, 1997). To be sure, the type and degree of stress varies greatly among individuals, as does the availability and use of coping resources. Together these variables influence the developmental pathway for each individual (Seiffge-Krenke, 1995).

The physiological changes that occur during adolescence can make many chronic illnesses (e.g., asthma, diabetes, cystic fibrosis) particularly difficult to manage – for example, the influences of pubertal hormone fluctuations on metabolic control in adolescents with diabetes (Christian & D'Auria, 2006; Salonius-Pasternak, 2004; Williams, Holmbeck, & Greenley, 2002). In turn, chronic illness can influence the timing and pace of pubertal development (e.g., pubertal delays in adolescents with Crohn's disease, cystic fibrosis, and spina bifida; Blum, 1992). Adolescents with chronic illness also tend to experience greater distress in response to the physical changes that occur during puberty – for example, higher levels of anxiety in response to changes in weight and the presence of acne (Wallander & Varni, 1995).

Within these fundamental themes of adolescence and chronic illness, each separate illness has its own particular characteristics of diagnosis, symptoms, treatment, and prognosis – with unique implications in individuals' lives during and after adolescence. The symptoms, treatment, and prognosis of a chronic illness vary not only across different illnesses but also across individuals with the same illness. The experience of chronicity itself can vary, due to differences in frequency and severity of acute episodes (e.g., hypoglycemia, asthma attacks).

Dr. Hauser passed away during the final stages of our writing this chapter. He was significantly involved in the conceptualization and writing processes, and even after his death, his influence continued to shape the chapter's final form. The concepts explored in this chapter had been central foci in the relationship of its authors.

D.E. Warner (✉)
Harvard Medical School, Judge Baker Children's Center, Boston, MA, USA
e-mail: dwarner@jbcc.harvard.edu

W.T. O'Donohue, L.W. Tolle (eds.), *Behavioral Approaches to Chronic Disease in Adolescence*,
DOI 10.1007/978-0-387-87687-0_3, © Springer Science+Business Media, LLC 2009

Consequently, when considering adolescents with chronic illnesses, we must attend to the specific details of the illness in question, as well as individual differences among particular adolescents and their families.

The developmental issues that adolescents with chronic illnesses encounter occur within the ecological–transactional context of family environment, family and peer relationships, school and community environments, culture, and ontogenetic development. Consequently, it is not useful to simply consider one issue without taking into account the dynamic, multilevel, reciprocal nature of the relations among all relevant issues (Cicchetti, 2002).

Together, these issues present an enormous array of questions to be considered when treating adolescents with chronic illness. To lay a framework for exploring these questions, we apply a biopsychosocial approach – considering characteristics of biological, cognitive, and socioemotional development in the context of family, peers, school, and community settings. We discuss normative aspects of adolescent development that are especially relevant in the context of chronic illness – including the initial processes of diagnosis and adjustment, the maintenance or "long-haul" period of adherence to medical regimens (Rolland, 1994), and the development of autonomy in the context of chronic illness. Finally, we will discuss important considerations for treating adolescents with chronic illness – through interventions targeting adolescents and families, in the contexts of primary and specialty care, as well as schools and communities.

Normative Aspects of Adolescence

At the beginning of the twentieth century, when adolescence was first considered as a period of development worthy of social scientific inquiry, it was viewed as a time of *storm and stress* (Hall, 1904). According to Anna Freud, "to be normal during the adolescent period is by itself abnormal" (Freud, 1958, p. 275). Adolescence was characterized as a time of intrapsychic and interpersonal distress, manifesting in extreme mood swings and emotional upheaval, familial conflict, drama-laden peer relationships, and trouble with authority. Although this idea of adolescence is often perpetuated by media representations of this period in development even today, empirical evidence has refuted this characterization. Research has shown that adolescence is not ordinarily or necessarily marked by clinically significant turmoil (Powers, Hauser, & Kilner, 1989).

Certainly, adolescence is a period of significant change, second in magnitude only to that of infancy (Williams et al., 2002). Adolescence encompasses two major transitions – from childhood to adolescence and from adolescence to adulthood – and this level of change may exacerbate any problematic issues in individual development and the family, even in a normative context. No doubt, this period of development can be a challenging time for adolescents and their families – but only a small percentage experience clinically significant disturbances (Powers et al., 1989).

During adolescence, changes in cognitive, emotional, and social development contribute to identity development, the changing social landscape of familial and peer relationships, and emerging autonomy and individuation. Adolescents' increasing cognitive and neurological development facilitates their abilities for abstract thought, perspective taking, and the exploration of hypothetical ideals. As these new competencies develop, however, adolescents' self-perceptions and thought processes can be skewed in potentially maladaptive ways. Adolescents are often preoccupied with social norms and others' perceptions of them, believing that others form an *imaginary audience* that constantly attends to minute details of their appearance, actions, etc. (Elkind, 1998). Adolescents also tend to have difficulty anticipating the consequences of their actions, believing that they are somehow magically protected from anything negative; Elkind (1998) refers to this perceived sense of invulnerability as the *personal fable*.

Characteristics of Pubertal Changes

Over the past century, our definitions of adolescence have evolved – due to changes in the social context as well as a greater understanding of and ability to identify the aspects of biological maturation associated with puberty. Currently, the World

Health Organization defines adolescence as the period of development between 10 and 19 years of age (World Health Organization, 2008). Increasingly, however, researchers are turning away from age-based markers of adolescence toward more individually based indicators of biological, cognitive, and social maturation.

Some aspects of pubertal processes (e.g., increase in adrenal androgens) can emerge as early as 6–9 years of age, whereas some of the cognitive and social aspects of maturation (e.g., self-regulatory skills) continue to develop into the twenties. The timing of pubertal development (e.g., age of menarche) varies across cultures as well (Powers et al., 1989). Research has consistently demonstrated that "early" versus "late" onset of puberty, especially evident physical maturation, influences adolescents' self-image, socioemotional functioning, behavior, and academic achievement (Brooks-Gunn, Petersen, & Eichorn, 1985; Dorn, Dahl, Woodward, & Biro, 2006; Powers et al., 1989). Consequently, it is important to attend to individual indicators of development, rather than age alone – especially since the timing and rate of maturation during this period can influence psychosocial adjustment and developmental outcomes (Dorn et al., 2006).

Identity and Ego Development

Although identity development is a dynamic process that engages individuals throughout the life span, Erikson posited that overcoming the crisis of *identity versus role confusion* is the primary psychosocial task of adolescent development (Erikson, 1968). Other identity theorists have agreed that identity development is a salient process during adolescence but have considered other aspects of how this process unfolds. Marcia (1993) considered the ways in which adolescents engage in exploration and commitment of roles and activities and conceptualized the following four statuses of identity development: Identity achievement, in which the adolescent has made a commitment to roles and activities after exploration; moratorium, in which exploration is ongoing with commitments in the process of being established; foreclosure, in which the adolescent has made commitments without exploration; and identity diffusion, in which exploration may or may not be present, with no commitments. More recently, researchers have questioned the universality that exists in Erikson's and Marcia's theories of identity development, which emphasize a Western, individualistic orientation. Identity theorists now place increasing emphasis on the role of person–context transactions, gender, and acculturation (Schwartz & Montgomery, 2002; Beyers & Çok, 2008).

Ego development is intertwined with identity development, encompassing aspects of relationships, impulse control, and cognitive and moral development – all of which are particular foci in the period of adolescence, as individuals move toward higher levels of complexity, differentiation, and refinement, as well as increased coordination and integration (Hauser, 1976, 1991; Loevinger, 1976; Ryan, Deci, & Grolnick, 1995). Individual differences abound in ego development, which can take several paths, moving more quickly or slowly through stages, remaining at a particular stage for an extended period of time, or regressing to previous stages (Loevinger, 1976). Family and peer relations are important contexts for identity and ego development.

Family and Peer Relations

Although clinically significant levels of conflict are far less common during adolescence than originally thought, some amount of conflict in familial relations remain a normative aspect of this phase of development. Pubertal changes have been associated with transiently increasing conflict between adolescents and parents, particularly mothers (Powers et al., 1989). Conflicts tend to occur around differences regarding curfews, chores, dating, school work, and personal appearance – seemingly mundane issues that are often evidence of adolescents' exploration of identity, intimacy, and autonomy. Adolescent children often begin to assert their personal choice in these areas before their parents are ready to grant them such jurisdiction (Powers et al., 1989; Smetana, 1988).

Research shows that ego development plays a role in the family context. Higher levels of ego development in adolescents and their parents have been associated with more adaptive, enabling, communication strategies (e.g., problem solving, empathy), whereas lower levels have been associated with maladaptive, constraining, strategies (e.g., devaluing, withholding; Hauser, Powers, et al., 1984). Adolescents' engagement in higher levels of identity exploration (including aspects of perspective taking) is associated with parents' emphasizing mutuality and separateness, as well as their having a clear sense of boundaries between them and their children (Grotevant & Cooper, 1986).

Family relations in adolescence are particularly interesting in the context of attachment theory, which posits that attachment in infancy – an enduring emotional bond established between children and their primary caregivers – serves as a relatively stable model of what to expect in relationships over the life course (see Cassidy & Shaver, 1999). Children with a secure attachment status seek out their primary caregivers during times of stress and rely on them as a secure base of exploration. During adolescence, individuals tend to display the opposite of what is expected when the attachment system is aroused – in times of stress, rather than turn toward their parents, adolescents may turn away from their parents (Allen & Land, 1999). At the same time, adolescents' increases in social awareness and reflection may contribute to higher levels of understanding in their relationships with their parents. In this way, normative aspects of adolescent development can lead to their moving both toward and away from their parents in new ways (Hauser, Borman, Powers, Jacobson, & Noam, 1990).

Although parents remain important figures during adolescence, peer relations increase in salience during this phase of development. Adolescents become less dependent on their parents for emotional support and more dependent on their peers for guidance and security (East, Hess, & Lerner, 1987). Peer relations and identity development are interwoven during adolescence, as individuals refine their sense of self in the context of their friendships and comparisons with their peers. Anxiety may make some adolescents more likely to conform with peers who engage in risky behaviors, whereas adolescents who have made more solid identity commitments are likely to follow their own values when they conflict with those of peers (Elkind, 1998).

Autonomy

One of the unique qualities of adolescence is the presence of increasing competence in the face of social and legal prohibitions against exercising these emerging abilities (Orukibich, Nassaw, & Mori, 2005). As adolescents seek autonomy and demonstrate their increasing capabilities, their parents, in turn, must begin to gradually reduce their caregiving responsibility – although ongoing close engagement has been recognized as an often healthy component of adolescents' relations with their parents into adulthood. Adolescents' emerging competence in multiple arenas (e.g., cognitively, socially) can lead to their having higher perceptions of their capabilities than are realistically warranted, and strivings for autonomy can increase risk-taking behavior (Spear & Kulbok, 2004). Parents are often more aware of the consequences of adolescents' risk-taking behavior and may be less interested in promoting their autonomy in the face of these possibilities (Orukibich, Kenta, & Kazuo, 2005).

Establishing a balance among these at times conflicting perspectives, and making appropriate adjustments as needed, can facilitate adolescents' developing autonomy while maintaining familial relationships (Smetana, 1988). In the context of a supportive and nurturing environment, adolescents' autonomy development can be more adaptive – whereas in a more negative environment, adolescents may be at greater risk for impulsivity and risk-taking behavior (Baumrind, 1987; Eccles et al., 1991). A supportive family environment can facilitate adolescents' adaptively moving toward their achievement of autonomy in the context of their own needs and those of family, friends, and society (Spear & Kulbok, 2004).

Presence of Chronic Illness

The presence of a chronic illness in adolescence may complicate the changes and transitions that occur during this period of development. Chronic illness is defined as a medical condition that interferes with daily life over a sustained period of time (Pless & Pinkerton, 1975). Statistics and definitions vary but indicate that between 10 and 20% of adolescents in the United States are currently diagnosed with at least one type of chronic illness (van der Lee, Mokkink, Grootenhuis, Heymans, & Offringa, 2007; Williams et al., 2002; Newacheck, McManus, & Fox, 1991). Some examples of chronic illness experienced by adolescents include asthma, Crohn's disease, cystic fibrosis, diabetes [including insulin-dependent diabetes mellitus (IDDM) and non-insulin-dependent diabetes mellitus (NIDDM)], and spina bifida. Increasingly, advances in treatment have improved the quality of life and life expectancy for adolescents with a chronic illness (Boice, 1998). Individuals with cystic fibrosis (CF) currently have a life expectancy into the mid- to late thirties, which has nearly doubled over the past three decades (Berge, Patterson, Goetz, & Milla, 2007; Cystic Fibrosis Foundation, 2006). This growing number of individuals requiring ongoing treatment for a chronic illness warrants our attention–especially during adolescence, when critical patterns of health behaviors emerge (Williams et al., 2002). We consider the initial phases of diagnosis and adjustment, the maintenance or "long-haul" phase that follows unique aspects of autonomy in the context of chronic illness, and ways of coping.

Diagnosis and Initial Adjustment

The processes of diagnosis and initial adjustment to a chronic illness are phenomena that can vary dramatically not only across conditions but also across families facing the same illness. Symptoms may present themselves gradually without acute episodes or they may result in hospitalization at the beginning of, or throughout, the diagnostic process. Adolescents and families will also vary in their levels of prior exposure to illness, the health care system in general, and particular characteristics of the symptoms, treatment, and resulting implications they now face. Illnesses vary in their heritability, such that an adolescent with IDDM may be more likely to have a parent or other family member with the same condition than an adolescent with cystinosis (Spilkin & Ballantyne, 2007). The familiarity that accompanies prior exposure to a newly diagnosed chronic illness can improve illness adjustment (Warner & Hauser, 2005; Salonius-Pasternak, 2004).

The diagnosis of a chronic illness can be considered an ambiguous loss – there is often ambiguity prior to the diagnosis, in parents' wondering what might be wrong with their child; immediately following the diagnosis, when the parents and child do not yet understand the prognosis; throughout the family's adjusting to the illness, in their efforts to make sense of how the illness affects their lives; and as the adolescent determines how the illness fits into his or her sense of self – who he or she is and what he or she may or may not be able to do because of this illness. This ambiguity can make individuals feel helpless, promoting depression, anxiety, and relationship conflicts.

According to Boss and Couden (2002), the effects of an ambiguous loss in the context of chronic illness occur in five ways: (1) the confusion resulting from the ambiguity can make it difficult for families to make decisions about how they should respond to the diagnosis; (2) the ambiguity may prevent family members from adapting their roles, rules, and rituals in response to the illness; (3) without visible signs or markers of loss, individuals have trouble validating their distress within or outside the family; (4) the ambiguity can alter individuals' views of the world, making it seem unfair or unjust; and (5) as the duration of ambiguity increases, families can become physically and psychologically exhausted. In the face of this uncertainty, families who are able to engage in making meaning of the illness experience – individually and collectively – may be able to provide more understanding, and consequently diminish confusion, for themselves and each other in ways that might mitigate the distress caused by the ambiguity.

As adolescents and their families adjust to life with a chronic illness, their experiences shape their attitudes and actions pertaining to aspects of managing the condition and its impact on family and peer relationships, body image, and school adjustment (Sullivan, 1979). Illness adjustment has potential to influence physiological outcomes both directly, through stress-related hormonal activity, and indirectly, through its impact on aspects of adherence (Sullivan, 1979; Bradley, 1994; Aalto, 1999; Hanson, De Guire, Schinkel, Henggeler, & Burghen, 1992; Jacobson et al., 1994; Kager & Holden, 1992; La Greca et al., 1995; Welch, Dunn, & Beeney, 1994). Illness adjustment can also influence broader understandings of health that will shape self-care behavior in adulthood (Williams et al., 2002).

Perceptions of control during the initial illness experience may promote or inhibit adaptation following the subsequent illness experience. According to the theory of *learned helplessness* (Seligman & Maier, 1967), if an initial aversive experience is perceived as uncontrollable, individuals are more likely to develop learned helplessness, which can result in associative, motivational, and emotional deficits, as well as difficulty in responding to future aversive experiences. On the other hand, if the initial aversive experience is perceived as controllable, this is considered to serve as *immunization* for future aversive experiences, so that individuals are more likely to respond adaptively in the future. Further research has also explored the concept of *learned optimism* (Kamen & Seligman, 1987; Maier, Peterson, & Schwartz, 2000; Reivich & Gillham, 2003; Scheier & Carver, 1987) – over time, individuals who view the world with optimism are more likely to respond optimistically to aversive experiences that they encounter.

It is also helpful to consider the role of personal agency (Bandura, 2001) in the context of illness adjustment. Individuals who respond actively to the circumstances of living with a chronic illness, through their own personal agency or through collective agency as a family system, are more likely not only to be more actively promoting their desired outcomes but also to perceive themselves in this way – leading to their continuing to respond with agency in future experiences.

Adherence and the "Long Haul"

Typically, having a chronic illness requires that adolescents adhere to a medical regimen. The regimen may involve administering medication, orally, inhaled, or through injections; and/or following a special diet, often with requirements not only for what is consumed but also the timing. Physical activity is often a component of the medical regimen, as a way to facilitate adherence (e.g., exercise improving metabolic control in adolescents with IDDM or NIDDM) or something to monitor carefully due to its potential to induce acute episodes (e.g., aerobic exercise impeding lung functioning in asthma).

Adhering to a medical regimen involves ongoing communication with, and oversight by, a medical care team – which includes primary care physicians, endocrinologists, pulmonary specialists, physical or occupational therapists, psychologists, social workers, or many others – depending on the nature of the illness. Adolescents and their families may need to meet with the medical care team a couple of times a year or a couple of times a month. In between appointments, record keeping is often used to track important data patterns over time (e.g., blood glucose levels in IDDM).

Nearly every facet of daily life can have an effect on illness management, and it is difficult to be completely prepared at all times. Activity level, sleep quality and duration, timing and frequency of meals, stress, and acute illness are examples of significant factors that have an impact on illness management and that cannot always be controlled in individuals' lives. Coordinating all of the facets of adhering to a medical regimen can be stressful for adolescents and their families, in the context of what is often known as "the rest of life" – for adolescents, homework, after-school activities, spending time with friends and for parents, the marital relationship, the care of other children, other familial and peer relationships, work schedules and demands, financial concerns, and, not to mention, spending time together as a family. These demands may lead to increases in social isolation, due to parents' spending less time with friends or choosing to not work outside the home (Boice, 1998; Blum, 1992). From a systems perspective, some families may focus their conflicts on the illness as a "scapegoat," leaving other conflicts unexamined (Warner & Hauser, 2005).

Normative social preoccupations in adolescence – including group membership and social acceptability – can conflict with the reality of the medical regimen prescribed for adolescents with a chronic illness. Many adolescents with a chronic illness feel that disclosing details about their condition could jeopardize peer acceptance by bringing attention to the ways in which they are different from their peers, especially regarding their physical selves, a central focus of self-consciousness in adolescence (Berge et al., 2007). As the salience of peers increases during adolescence, not disclosing this important aspect of their lives to friends can place adolescents with chronic illnesses at great risk for not adhering to the medical care plan recommended to them. A lack of illness visibility, regardless of intentions, has been associated with poorer psychosocial adjustment (Thompson & Gustafson, 1996).

Typical adolescent behaviors such as an erratic diet and sleep schedule may, for the most part, be innocuous for adolescents without a chronic medical condition. Yet these uneven lifestyles can seriously jeopardize the health and even lives of adolescents who do have a chronic illness. Conflicts over acceptance, leading to masking their underlying and attention-demanding illness and inhibiting key health-related behaviors, can interfere with an individual's differentiation, refinement, coordination, integration of the self, and the deepening of friendships (Hauser, 1991).

Autonomy in the Context of a Chronic Illness

For adolescents with a chronic illness and their parents, autonomy can be further complicated. Research has shown that parents' remaining involved in illness-specific care can improve adherence-related outcomes, although adolescents must increasingly begin to take on more responsibility in adhering to their medical regimen (Botello-Harbaum, Nansel, Haynie, Iannotti, & Simons-Morton, 2008; Modi, Marciel, Slater, Drotar, & Quittner, 2008).

The attachment status of adolescents with a chronic illness can serve as yet another complexity affecting the dynamic of seeking support and separation from caregivers simultaneously. Attachment status can also influence adolescents' relationships with their medical team, particularly with intensive care requiring frequent appointments or hospitalization (Ciechanowski, Katon, Russo, & Walker, 2001; Hunter & Maunder, 2001). Adolescents with a chronic illness who have an insecure-avoidant attachment status may be more likely to resent and avoid close monitoring of their condition by either parents or physicians, disavowing the possibility of illness-related complications, and not adhering to their regimen. Depending on the particular dynamics of the family, an adolescent's attempts to resist or avoid parental caregiving could result in either increased conflict or, if avoidance is especially successful, a result could be promulgation of the illusion that the adolescent is adhering to his or her prescribed medical care plan when, in fact, this is not the case.

Coping in the Context of a Chronic Illness

Although the presence of a chronic illness can increase the number of challenges that adolescents face, this is not to say that *all* adolescents with a chronic illness will experience greater developmental difficulty than their non-affected peers. Great variation in developmental pathways exists among adolescents who do and do not have a chronic illness (Hauser, DiPlacido, Jacobson, Willett, & Cole, 1993). Gore and Eckenrode (1996) point out that "within any group of persons considered at risk, there will be variability in their exposure to stressors that are the more proximal causes of disorder" (p. 22). There will also be variability in how they cope with such stressors. Depending in part on how they view the illness, some adolescents and families may find greater levels of closeness in response to the stressors they face (Eiser, 1993; Hauser, DiPlacido, Jacobson, Paul, et al., 1993).

It is outside the parameters of this chapter to provide a comprehensive review of coping; and so we will consider examples of coping strategies in the context of chronic illness in the following three conceptual areas: appraisal focused, problem focused, and emotion management. *Appraisal-focused* coping strategies are those that involve the adolescent's or family's evaluation or interpretation of the experience, including characteristics of the stressor as well as available resources. *Problem-focused* coping strategies are oriented to planning and behavioral efforts to address aspects of the stressor. *Emotion management* strategies include efforts to express, contain, or regulate their emotional responses to the stressor. Within these conceptual areas, coping strategies may or may not be adaptive. A rigid, opinionated style of appraising a stressor, for example, could devalue other family members' perspectives – whereas a hopeful outlook could engender more positive interactions in the context of the stressor (Hauser, DiPlacido, Jacobson, Paul, et al., 1993).

Meaning-making is an example of an appraisal-focused coping strategy that also includes aspects of emotion management. Meaning-making of the illness experience refers to how individuals perceive the role or roles that illness plays in their lives and how those perceptions change over time, as well as how individuals develop, maintain, and change their responses to the illness. Cohler (1991) explains the importance of "managing the meaning of misfortune" by saying that "the experience of adversity may be used either as a means for understanding problems in realizing personal goals or in justifying self-defeating intentions" (p. 191). This attention to the meanings that people make of their experience can be traced back to Freud, who said that "...the symptom carries a meaning and is connected with the experience of the patient" (Freud, 1920, p. 221).

Illness appraisal is, as its name suggests, another example of an appraisal-focused coping strategy. It refers to how the individual assesses or evaluates the impact of the illness – including the degree to which it can be a positive or negative influence and the strength of the influence – and how these evaluations change over time. Adolescents' appraisals of chronic illness as a stressor can vary between a small annoyance to a source of significant disturbances in their lives. Depending on the nature of the illness and facets of their illness adjustment, some adolescents may appraise chronic illness as a minor hassle, or a habit that they have integrated into their lives, whereas others may view it as limiting their freedom, making them different from their peers, or seriously compromising their health. In a study of adolescents' appraisals of IDDM, some adolescents could not verbalize their description of the illness and instead drew pictures of a prison, a devil, coffins, and a cemetery. One adolescent said, "I could not describe my diabetes and I could not draw it. You know it is very difficult to draw death. How do you draw it?" (Kyngas & Barlow, 1995, p. 943). Given the heritability of CF and its effects on physical and sexual development, adolescents with this illness have also expressed concerns regarding their sexuality and reproductive potential (Krementz, 1989).

Likewise, in a study of adolescents' appraisal of adherence to their medical regimens, some adolescents with IDDM saw adherence as a way to ensure their health both now and in the future; some as something they were obligated or forced to do by their parents and doctors, resulting in stress, fatigue, guilt, restrictions, and limited freedom; and some as something about which they felt passive and indifferent, recognizing the consequences of non-adherence but prioritizing spending time with friends, which they saw as incompatible with the seeming excessively high goals of their medical regimen (Kyngas & Hentinen, 1995). Other themes in adolescents' illness appraisal include its potential to undermine their control and efficacy, on a practical level regarding the time and hassles involved in the self-care regimen, as well as on a more general level regarding feeling overwhelmed by fear and vulnerability associated with having a life-threatening illness (Schur et al., 1999).

Social support encompasses problem-focused and emotion management coping strategies. Research has shown that seeking social support in familial and peer relations plays a crucial role in the development of adolescents with chronic illnesses (Aalto, Uutela, & Aro, 1997; Skinner & Hampson, 1998; Hanson et al., 1992). Families tend to provide more problem-focused support than peers in the context of adherence behaviors, whereas peers tend to provide more emotional support (La Greca et al., 1995). Family cohesion also contributes to overall psychological adjustment (Hanson et al., 1992; Wysocki, 1993). Some studies suggest that its role may gradually decrease between childhood and late adolescence (Safyer et al., 1993; Varni, Babani, Wallander, Roe, & Frasier, 1989), whereas peer social support appears to remain a consistent predictor of psychological adjustment throughout childhood and adolescence (Varni et al., 1989). Adolescents with chronic illness can benefit from social support from similarly affected peers as well as from "typical" children (Varni, La Greca, & Spirito, 2000).

Treatment Considerations

Treatment for adolescents with a chronic illness may occur in a variety of formats and contexts, with different types of care providers. We explore perspectives on care and characteristics of interventions designed to serve adolescents and their families in a multiple settings, including medical and mental health clinics, schools, and community organizations.

Due to discrepancies among the realities of chronic illness and the general assumptions underlying health care relationships, there are three contradictions in care perspectives that affect both families and clinicians: (1) as families become more familiar and adept at managing the illness, clinicians' expertise often falls below that of the family; (2) Western clinicians tend to focus on more immediate aspects of decision making and outcomes, whereas families living with a chronic illness are typically more focused on long-term outcomes and reducing their use of clinical services over time; and (3) two idealized qualities in health care, compliance and self-reliance, can be viewed as mutually exclusive (Thorne, Nyhlin, & Paterson, 2000). Even the more person-focused concept of adherence and self-reliance have some opposite qualities, since many individuals living with a chronic illness are not involved in the development of their prescribed medical regimen (Clay & Hopps, 2003).

Considerations for Adolescent-Focused Interventions

Researchers are studying the design and outcome of interventions specifically targeted to serve adolescents with chronic illness. Interventions designed for adults are often not appropriate for adolescents, since they tend not to address some of the unique aspects of adolescent development that we have discussed in this chapter. The creation and implementation of effective interventions for adolescents with chronic illness can facilitate improved health outcomes not only during adolescence but also during and after the transition to adulthood – since the nature of their involvement in their care may have implications for health care throughout their lives (Williams et al., 2002).

Health-based interventions for adolescents can include health behavior and risk reduction, psychosomatics, and the management of medical illness. Goals of such interventions may be the prevention of disease (primary prevention), early identification and treatment before significant progression has occurred (secondary prevention), or ongoing treatment of conditions that may have long-lasting effects (tertiary prevention). Interventions for adolescents with chronic illness can incorporate one or more types of prevention and may focus on adherence to the medical regimen, preparation for medical procedures, stress management, family relationships, quality of life, or overall psychosocial adjustment (Williams et al., 2002). Intervention efforts to increase adolescents' illness-specific knowledge can also be helpful, since such knowledge is a predictor of adaptation during the transition to adulthood (Berge et al., 2007).

A biopsychosocial approach to health interventions is recommended, especially given the transactional relationships among a variety of psychosocial and physiological outcomes and their often-shared risk and protective factors. Regardless of the specific focus of a particular intervention, attention to the multiple contexts of adolescent development (e.g., individual characteristics, social relationships, home and school environments) can make interventions more effective. For example, research has shown that positive aspects of parental and peer relationships (e.g., connectedness, prosocial behavior) are associated with lower levels of risk-taking behavior and better health-related outcomes (Williams et al., 2002). And so interventions addressing risk-taking behaviors, such as substance use and precocious sexual relations, should take parental and peer relationships into account.

In the context of medical treatment provided by practitioners focused primarily on physiological aspects of illness management, adolescents' voices and perspectives are often given less attention than those of their parents (Jolly, Weiss, & Liehr, 2007; Beresford & Sloper, 2003). Adolescents tend to be reluctant to ask sensitive questions or reveal information that indicates non-adherence to the medical regimen (Beresford & Sloper, 2003). Engaging in non-judgmental dialogue with adolescents regarding their illness experiences may enhance their participation in their health care and empower them as they continue to move toward assuming responsibility for their self-care (Jolly, Weiss, & Liehr, 2007). In a study of adolescents' perspectives regarding their relationships with their doctors, they expressed preferences for consistently seeing the same doctor without residents or other professionals in the room, having time to talk without their parents in the room, and having their doctors speak directly to them even when their parents were in the room (Beresford & Sloper, 2003).

Considerations for Family-Focused Interventions

When treating adolescents with chronic illness, families are always involved. It is crucial to develop a treatment plan that is designed to fit among other demands of families' lives (Clay & Hopps, 2003). *Treatment accommodation* is "the extent to which a standardized treatment approach can accommodate to the complex and unique demands of patients' lives" (Clay, 2000, p.54). Collaborating with adolescents and their families when developing medical regimens can facilitate higher levels of treatment accommodation. Family characteristics, including structure and number of children, ethnicity, religious beliefs, education levels, socioeconomic status, and proximity to health care facilities, must be taken into account when establishing treatment regimens.

Clinicians should consider treatment accommodation and include families' perspectives in the initial and ongoing development of the prescribed medical regimen. By consistently involving families in developing and making adjustments to the regimen, including addressing how well the regimen does or does not fit into the family context, clinicians would be better able to not only assess a family's ability to adhere to the regimen but also to develop a regimen that is more likely to enable them to do so.

Adolescents and families benefit being able to apply appropriate levels of flexibility in managing illness-specific care in the context of life in general, in ways that promote general and illness-specific functioning (Salonius-Pasternak, 2004). For example, in some cases it may be possible to occasionally delay medication administration for an hour without any negative health effects – and that occasional extra "give" in the medication administration schedule may facilitate adolescents and their families engaging in meaningful non-illness activities, such as social events or sports practices. In addition, families' abilities to be flexible in the face of the changing illness-specific and developmental needs of the adolescent can also promote healthier outcomes (Spilkin & Ballantyne, 2007). Developing a method of assessing a family's ability to apply appropriate flexibility to illness management and other aspects of life could enable health care teams to better identify and address particular areas of difficulty in this area. Although some aspects of the medical regimen may be less affected by occasional schedule changes, others may be more time sensitive – and it is necessary for adolescents and families to know the difference. Assessing families' application of flexibility would enable clinicians to more effectively address the issue and intervene when appropriate.

Demands of the chronic illness that are placed on adolescents and families – including aspects of symptoms, treatment, and prognosis – will influence the efficacy of different coping strategies for adolescents and their families. In turn, coping effectively with the stressors involved in managing a chronic illness can facilitate better adherence to the medical regimen and improved psychosocial adaptation. However, coping and other aspects of mental health are often seen as secondary to medical outcomes (Spilkin & Ballantyne, 2007).

Assessing family coping strategies is an important aspect of treatment. Higher severity and frequency of acute episodes can make stronger family cohesion a more relevant protective factor (Hauser, DiPlacido, Jacobson, Willett, et al., 1993). The efficacy of coping strategies may also vary within families over the course of adolescence (Boice, 1998). Ongoing discussion regarding the efficacy of coping strategies may help adolescents and families to navigate through the bumps in the road and to learn to anticipate them, so that they can respond more effectively. Providing opportunities for family coping discussions can also provide further opportunities for exploring meaning-making and illness appraisal.

Considerations for Interventions in Schools and Other Community Settings

Schools are often appropriate intervention settings for adolescents with chronic illness, in countries in which the majority of adolescents attend school full time. Interventions can be designed to address the particular needs of adolescents with chronic illness as well as the general health concerns for individuals during this period of development (Williams et al., 2002). Given the increased salience of peers during adolescence, their participation in interventions may increase motivation and attendance.

Collaborative relationships among adolescents, parents, school professionals, and the medical treatment team may facilitate adolescents receiving comprehensive and coordinated care that reduces the potential for illness-related effects on learning and development in the school environment. Depending on the illness and its symptom presentation, adolescents may need to engage in self-care practices (e.g., blood glucose testing, taking medication) during the school day. School districts in the United States vary in their policies regarding such practices – for example, whether adolescents with a chronic illness are required to go to the nurse for guidance or oversight on occasions when portions of the medical regimen are implemented at school. And in the case of achievement or learning difficulties, it is important for teachers and other school professionals (e.g., psychologist, occupational therapist) to not dismiss an adolescent's difficulties solely as symptoms of a chronic illness and subsequently not warranting their attention (Spilkin & Ballantyne, 2007). Open communication among all involved parties may help to avoid miscommunication and address any issues that arise.

Just as adolescents and families need to balance illness-specific concerns within the context of the normative aspects of daily life, it may be helpful for intervention curriculum to do the same. Interventions that include recreation activities, e.g., after-school programs and summer camps, can be especially helpful when adolescents with chronic illness exhibit externalizing behavior (Floyd & Gallagher, 1997).

Contextual and cultural factors in the community may exacerbate or ease the limitations faced by adolescents with chronic illness and their families (Blum, 1992). This includes facility- or organization-specific characteristics, such as the presence or lack of wheelchair ramps or accommodations in the workplace for parents who need to shuttle adolescents to medical appointments, as well as broader cultural perspectives regarding chronic illness (e.g., stigma, beliefs surrounding the origin of illness). Community-based intervention efforts to increase awareness of chronic illnesses may help to reduce any stigma that may exist and may also help to increase the consideration of adolescents' and families' needs in policy making.

Conclusions

When treating adolescents with a chronic illness, applying a biopsychosocial approach helps to highlight relevant aspects of developmental and contextual influences. The presence of a chronic illness can complicate normative developmental processes, depending on characteristics of illness-related stressors and available coping resources. Attending to individual differences inherent in adolescents and families, as well as unique characteristics of the particular illnesses they face, can guide practitioners to develop more effective interventions. Treatment can be effective when targeted to adolescents and families in health care, school, and other community settings.

Acknowledgments The authors wish to thank Judith Crowell, MD, Luisa Ribeiro, Ph.D., and Ann Rifkin, Ph.D., for their assistance in reviewing the chapter at various stages in the process.

References

Aalto, A.-M. (1999). *Diabetes cognitions and social support in the management of diabetes: A cross-sectional study on social psychological determinants of health-related quality of life and self-care among adults with type I diabetes*. Jyväskylä, Finland: Gummerus Printing.

Aalto, A.-M., Uutela, A., & Aro, A. R. (1997). Health related quality of life among insulin-dependent diabetics: Disease-related and psychosocial correlates. *Patient Education and Counseling, 30*, 215–225.

Allen, J. P., & Land, D. (1999). Attachment in adolescence. In J. Cassidy & P. R. Shaver (Eds.), *Handbook of attachment: Theory, research, and clinical applications* (pp. 319–335). New York: Guilford Press.

Bandura, A. (2001). Social cognitive theory: An agentic perspective. *Annual Review of Psychology, 52*, 1–26.

Baumrind, D. (1987). A developmental perspective on adolescent risk taking in contemporary America. *New Directions for Child Development, 37*, 93–125.

Beresford, B. A., & Sloper, P. (2003). Chronically ill adolescents' experiences of communicating with doctors: A qualitative study. *Journal of Adolescent Health, 33*(3), 172–179.

Berge, J. M., Patterson, J. M., Goetz, D., & Milla, C. (2007). Gender differences in young adults' perceptions of living with cystic fibrosis during the transition to adulthood: A qualitative investigation. *Families, Systems, & Health, 25*(2), 190–203.

Beyers, W., & Çok, F. (2008). Adolescent self and identity development in context (editorial). *Journal of Adolescence, 31*, 147–150.

Blum, R. W. (1992). Chronic illness and disability in adolescence. *Journal of Adolescent Health, 13*, 364–368.

Boice, M. M. (1998). Chronic illness in adolescence. *Adolescence, 33*(132), 927–939.

Boss, P., & Couden, B. A. (2002). Ambiguous loss from chronic physical illness: Clinical interventions with individuals, couples, and families. *Psychotherapy in Practice, 58*(11), 1351–1360.

Botello-Harbaum, M., Nansel, T., Haynie, D. L., Iannotti, R. J., & Simons-Morton, B. (2008). Responsive parenting is associated with improved type 1 diabetes-related quality of life. *Child: Care, Health, and Development, 34*(5), 675–681.

Bradley, C. (1994). *Handbook of psychology and diabetes.* Amsterdam: Harwood Academic Publishers GmbH.

Brooks-Gunn, J., Petersen, A. C., & Eichorn, D. (1985). Time of maturation and psychosocial functioning in adolescence. *Journal of Youth and Adolescence, 14*, 149–264.

Cassidy, J., & Shaver, P. R. (1999). *Handbook of attachment: Theory, research, and clinical applications.* New York: Guilford Press.

Christian, B. J., & D'Auria, J. P. (2006). Building life skills for children with cystic fibrosis: Effectiveness of an intervention. *Nursing Research, 55*(5), 300–307.

Cicchetti, D. (2002). *Against all odds: Pathways to resilient adaptation in maltreated children.* Presentation given at the dedication of the Donald J. Cohen Auditorium, Yale University, Yale Child Study Center, June 19, 2002.

Ciechanowski, P. S., Katon, W. J., Russo, J. E., & Walker, E. A. (2001). The patient-provider relationship: Attachment theory and adherence to treatment in diabetes. *The American Journal of Psychiatry, 158*(1), 29–35.

Clay, D. L. (2000). Commentary: Rethinking our interventions in pediatric chronic pain and treatment research. *Journal of Pediatric Psychology, 25*, 52–55.

Clay, D. L., & Hopps, J. A. (2003). Treatment adherence in rehabilitation: The role of treatment accommodation. *Rehabilitation Psychology, 48*(3), 215–219.

Cohler, B. J. (1991). The life story and the study of resilience and response to adversity. *Journal of Narrative and Life History, 1*(2&3), 169–200.

Cystic Fibrosis Foundation. (2006). *New statistics show CF patients living longer.* Retrieved September 1, 2008, from http://www.cff.org/aboutCFFoundation/NewsEvents/2006NewsArchive/index.cfm?ID=2711&TYPE=1132.

Dorn, L. D., Dahl, R. E., Woodward, H. R., & Biro, F. (2006). Defining the boundaries of early adolescence: A user's guide to assessing pubertal status and pubertal timing in research with adolescents. *Applied Developmental Science, 10*(1), 30–56.

East, P. L., Hess, L. E., & Lerner, R. M. (1987). Peer social support and adjustment of early adolescent peer groups. *Journal of Early Adolescence, 7*(2), 153–163.

Eccles, J. S., Buchanan, C. M., Flanagan, C., Fuligni, A., Midgley, C., & Yee, D. (1991). Control versus autonomy during early adolescence. *Journal of Social Issues, 47*(4), 53–68.

Eiser, C. (1993). *Growing up with a chronic disease: The impact on children and their families.* London: Kingsley.

Elkind, D. (1998). *All grown up and no place to go: Teenagers in crisis.* Cambridge, MA: Perseus Books.

Erikson, E. H. (1968). *Identity: Youth and crisis.* New York: W.W. Norton & Company.

Floyd, F. J., & Gallagher, E. M. (1997). Parental stress, care demands, and use of support services for school-age children with disabilities and behavior problems. *Family Relations, 46*, 359–371.

Freud, A. (1958). Adolescence. *The Psychoanalytic Study of the Child, 13*, 255–278.

Freud, S. (1920). *A general introduction to psychoanalysis.* New York: Horace Liveright.

Gore, S., & Eckenrode, J. (1996). Context and process in research on risk and resilience. In R. J. Haggerty, L. R. Sherrod, N. Garmezy, & M. Rutter (Eds.), *Stress, Risk, and Resilience in Children and Adolescents: Processes, Mechanisms, and Interventions* (pp. 19–63). New York, NY; Cambridge University Press.

Grey, M., Lipman, T., Cameron, M. E., & Thurber, F. W. (1997). Coping behaviors at diagnosis and in adjustment one year later in children with diabetes. *Nursing Research, 46*(6), 312–317.

Grotevant, H. D., & Cooper, C. R. (1986). Individuation in family relationships: A perspective on individual differences in the development of identity and role-taking skill in adolescence. *Human Development, 29*(2), 82–100.

Hall, G. S. (1904). *Adolescence: Its psychology and its relations to physiology, anthropology, sociology, sex, crime, religion, and education.* New York: D. Appleton & Company.

Hanson, C. L., De Guire, M. J., Schinkel, A. M., Henggeler, S. W., & Burghen, G. A. (1992). Comparing social learning and family systems correlates of adaptation in youths with IDDM. *Journal of Pediatric Psychology, 17*(5), 555–572.

Hauser, S. T. (1976). Loevinger's model and measure of ego development: A critical review. *Psychological Bulletin, 83*(5), 928–955.

Hauser, S. T. (1991). Adolescents and their families: Paths of ego development. New York, NY: Free Press.

Hauser, S. T., Borman, E. H., Powers, S. I., Jacobson, A. M., & Noam, G. G. (1990). Paths of adolescent ego development: Links with family life and individual adjustment. *Psychiatric Clinics of North America, 13*(3), 489–510.

Hauser, S. T., DiPlacido, J., Jacobson, A. M., Paul, E., Bliss, R., Milley, J., et al. (1993). The family and the onset of its youngster's insulin-dependent diabetes: Ways of coping. In R. E. Cole & D. Reiss (Eds.), *How do families cope with chronic illness?* (pp. 25–55). Hillsdale, NJ: Lawrence Erlbaum Associates.

Hauser, S. T., DiPlacido, J., Jacobson, A. M., Willett, J., & Cole, C. (1993). Family coping with an adolescent's chronic illness: An approach and three studies. *Journal of Adolescence, 16*, 305–329.

Hauser, S. T., Powers, S. I., Noam, G. G., Jacobson, A. M., Weiss, B., & Folansbee, D. J. (1984). Familial contexts of adolescent ego development. *Child Development, 55*, 195–213.

Hunter, J. J., & Maunder, R. G. (2001). Using attachment theory to understand illness behavior. *General Hospital Psychiatry, 23*, 177–182.

Jacobson, A. M., Hauser, S. T., Lavori, P., Willett, J. B., Cole, C. F., Wolfsdorf, J. I., et al.(1994). Family environment and glycemic control: A four-year prospective study of children and adolescents with IDDM. *Psychosomatic Medicine, 56*, 401–409.

Jolly, K., Weiss, J. A., & Liehr, P. (2007). Understanding adolescent voice as a guide for nursing practice and research. *Issues in Comprehensive Pediatric Nursing, 30*, 3–13.

Kager, V. A., & Holden, E. W. (1992). Preliminary investigation of the direct and moderating effects of family and individual variables on the adjustment of children and adolescents with diabetes. *Journal of Pediatric Psychology, 17*(4), 491–502.

Kamen, L. P., & Seligman, M. E. (1987). Explanatory style and health. *Current Psychological Research & Reviews, 6*(3), 207–218.

Krementz, J. (1989). *How it feels to fight for your life*. Boston: Little, Brown.

Kyngas, H., & Barlow, J. (1995). Diabetes: An adolescent's perspective. *Journal of Advanced Nursing, 22*, 941–947.

Kyngas, H., & Hentinen, M. (1995). Meaning attached to compliance with self-care, and conditions for compliance among young diabetics. *Journal of Advanced Nursing, 21*, 729–736.

La Greca, A. M., Auslander, W. F., Greco, P., Spetter, D., Fisher, Jr., E. B., & Santiago, J. V. (1995). I get by with a little help from my friends: Adolescents' support for diabetes care. *Journal of Pediatric Psychology, 20*(4), 449–476.

Loevinger, J. (1976). *Ego development: Conceptions and theories*. San Francisco: Jossey-Bass Publishers.

Maier, S. F., Peterson, C., & Schwartz, B. (2000). From helplessness to hope: The seminal career of Martin Seligman. In J. E. Gillham (Ed.), *The science of optimism and hope: Research essays in honor of Martin E.P. Seligman. Laws of life symposia series* (pp. 11–37) Philadelphia: Templeton Foundation Press.

Marcia, J. E. (1993). The relational roots of identity. In J. Kroger (Ed.), *Discussions on ego identity* (pp. 101–120). Hillsdale, NJ: Lawrence Erlbaum Associates, Inc.

Modi, A. C., Marciel, K. K., Slater, S. K., Drotar, D., & Quittner, A. L. (2008). The influence of parental supervision on medical adherence in adolescents with cystic fibrosis: Developmental shifts from pre to late adolescence. *Children's Health Care, 37*(1), 78–82.

Newacheck, P. W., McManus, M. A., & Fox, H. B. (1991). Prevalence and impact of chronic illness among adolescents. *American Journal of Diseases of Children, 145*, 1367–1373.

Orukibich, J., Nassaw, K., & Mori, K. (2005). Comments on defining adolescence. *Psychological Reports, 97*(3), 737–738.

Pless, I. B., & Pinkerton, P. (1975). *Chronic childhood disorder: Promoting patterns of adjustment*. London: Kimpton Publishers.

Powers, S. I., Hauser, S. T., & Kilner, L. A. (1989). Adolescent mental health. *American Psychologist, 44*(2), 200–208.

Reivich, K., & Gillham, J. (2003). Learned optimism: The measurement of explanatory style. In S. J. Lopez & C. R. Snyder (Eds.), *Positive psychological assessment: A handbook of models and measures* (pp. 57–74). Washington, DC: American Psychological Association.

Rolland, J. S. (1994). *Families, illness, and disability: An integrative treatment model*. New York: Basic Books.

Ryan, R. M., Deci, E. L., & Grolnick, W. S. (1995). Autonomy, relatedness, and the self: Their relation to development and psychopathology. In D. Cicchetti & D. J. Cohen (Eds.), *Developmental psychopathology, volume II: Theory and methods* (pp. 618–655). New Jersey: John Wiley & Sons.

Safyer, A. W., Hauser, S. T., Jacobson, A. M., Bliss, R., Herskowitz, R. D., Wolfsdorf, J. I. et al. (1993). The impact of the family on diabetes adjustment: A developmental perspective. *Child and Adolescent Social Work Journal, 10*(2), 123–140.

Salonius-Pasternak, D. E. (2004). Developmental precursors of resilient outcomes in young adults with insulin-dependent diabetes mellitus. (Doctoral dissertation, Tufts University, 2004). *Dissertation Abstracts International, 65*(3-B), 1581.

Scheier, M. F., & Carver, C. S. (1987). Dispositional optimism and physical well-being: The influence of generalized outcome expectancies on health. *Journal of Personality, 55*(2), 169–210.

Schur, H. V., Gamsu, D. S., & Barley, V. M. (1999). The young person's perspective on living and coping with diabetes. *Journal of Health Psychology, 4*(2), 223–236.

Schwartz, S. J., & Montgomery, M. J. (2002). Similarities or differences in identity development? The impact of acculturation and gender on identity process and outcome. *Journal of Youth and Adolescence, 31*(5), 359–372.

Seiffge-Krenke, I. (1995). Ways of coping with everyday problems and minor events. In I. Seiffge-Krenke (Ed.), *Stress, coping, and relationships in adolescence* (pp. 94–129). New Jersey: Lawrence Erlbaum Associates, Inc.

Seligman, M., & Darling, R. B. (1993). *Ordinary families, special children*. New York: Guilford Press.

Seligman, M. E. P., & Maier, S. (1967). Failure to escape traumatic shock. *Journal of Experimental Psychology, 74*, 1–9.

Skinner, T. C., & Hampson, S. E. (1998). Social support and personal models of diabetes in relation to self-care and well-being in adolescents with type I diabetes mellitus. *Journal of Adolescence, 21*(6), 703–715.

Smetana, J. G. (1988). Adolescents' and parents' conceptions of parental authority. *Child Development, 59*, 321–335.

Spear, H. J., & Kulbok, P. (2004). Autonomy and adolescence: A concept analysis. *Public Health Nursing, 21*(2), 144–152.

Spilkin, A., & Ballantyne, A. (2007). Behavior in children with a chronic illness: A descriptive study of child characteristics, family adjustment, and school issues in

children with cystinosis. *Families, Systems, & Health, 25*(1), 68–84.
Sullivan, B.-J. (1979). Adjustment in diabetic adolescent girls: I. Development of the diabetic adjustment scale. *Psychosomatic Medicine, 42*(2), 119–125.
Thompson, R. J., & Gustafson, K. E. (1996). *Adaptation to chronic childhood illness*. Washington, DC: American Psychological Association.
Thorne, S. E., Nyhlin, K. T., & Paterson, B. L. (2000). Attitudes toward patient expertise in chronic illness. *International Journal of Nursing Studies, 37*, 303–311.
van der Lee, J. H., Mokkink, L. B., Grootenhuis, M. A., Heymans, H. S., & Offringa, M. (2007). Definitions and measurements of chronic health conditions in childhood. *Journal of the American Medical Association, 297*(24), 2741–2751.
Varni, J. W., Babani, L., Wallander, J. L., Roe, T. F., & Frasier, S. D. (1989). Social support and self-esteem effects on psychological adjustment in children and adolescents with insulin-dependent diabetes mellitus. *Child and Family Behavior Therapy, 11*(1), 1–16.
Varni, J. W., La Greca, A. M., & Spirito, A. (2000). Cognitive-behavioral interventions for children with chronic health conditions. In P. C. Kendall (Ed.), *Child and adolescent therapy: Cognitive behavioral procedures* (2nd ed., pp. 291–333). New York: Guilford Press.
Wallander, J. L., & Varni, J. W. (1995). Appraisal, coping, and adjustment in adolescents with a physical disability. In J. L. Wallander & L. J. Siegel (Eds.), *Adolescent health problems* (pp. 209–231). New York: Guilford Press.
Warner, D. E., & Hauser, S. T. (April, 2005). *Developmental precursors of resilient outcomes in young adults with insulin-dependent diabetes mellitus*. Poster session presented at the biennial meeting of the Society for Research in Child Development, Atlanta, Georgia, USA.
Welch, G., Dunn, S. M., & Beeney, L. J. (1994). The ATT39: A measure of psychological adjustment to diabetes. In C. Bradley (Ed.), *Handbook of psychology and diabetes: A guide to psychological measurement in diabetes research and practice* (pp. 223–245). Amsterdam: Harwood Academic Publishers GmbH.
Williams, P. G., Holmbeck, G. N., & Greenley, R. N. (2002). Adolescent health psychology. *Journal of Consulting and Clinical Psychology, 70*(3), 828–842.
World Health Organization. (2008). *Adolescent health*. Retrieved September 1, 2008, from http://www.who.int/topics/adolescent_health/en
Wysocki, T. (1993). Associations among teen-parent relationships, metabolic control, and adjustment to diabetes in adolescents. *Journal of Pediatric Psychology, 18*(4), 441–452.

Adolescent Physiology

Kathryn L. Eckert, Vincent A. Loffredo, and Kathleen O'Connor

Adolescence is a time of many changes anatomically, physiologically, neurologically, and behaviorally. The age of adolescence is considered to be between 10 and 21 years. However, great variability exists in terms of the chronologic age at which complete adult maturity is achieved in any given individual. Additionally, the anatomic and physiologic portions of adolescence may be earlier to mature than the neurological and behavioral aspects. This discordance in development may lead to difficulties in the adolescent including promiscuity, risk-taking behaviors, and adolescents being treated according to their physical, not neurological, development. An adolescent who develops earlier or later than his or her peers also may experience teasing about one's height and sexual development (or lack thereof). This chapter will discuss adolescent physiology with emphasis on the endocrine (hormonal) physiology and brain physiology. Case studies with examples of chronic disease in adolescents will also be presented.

The Endocrine System

The endocrine system is divided into three main parts: the hypothalamus, the pituitary gland, and the end organs (ovaries, testes, adrenal glands, thyroid gland). The hypothalamus controls the pituitary gland which in turn regulates the rest of the endocrine system. The pituitary gland is divided into the anterior and posterior lobes. The anterior pituitary hormones include luteinizing hormone, follicle-stimulating hormone, thyroid-stimulating hormone, growth hormone, prolactin and adrenocorticotropic hormone. The posterior pituitary gland contains oxytocin and antidiuretic hormone. Oxytocin is involved in parturition and antidiuretic hormone (ADH) is involved with regulation of salt and water balance. The anterior pituitary gland is regulated by the hypothalamus which secretes a stimulatory or inhibitory hormone, in turn causing the release or inhibition of the corresponding pituitary gland hormone. Luteinizing hormone (LH) is responsible for stimulating the ovaries and testicles to produce estrogen and testosterone, respectively. Follicle-stimulating hormone (FSH) stimulates the gonadal cells in ovaries and testicles to produce mature eggs and sperm, respectively. Adrenocorticotropic hormone (ACTH) stimulates the adrenal gland to produce androgens (male hormones) including testosterone and androstenedione, as well as cortisol. Androgens are responsible for hair growth in the pubic and axillary regions in females as well as acne production. In males, the testicles and adrenal glands work together to produce a high level of androgens resulting in facial hair, chest and back hair as well as pubic and axillary hair. Cortisol is a stress hormone responsible for maintenance of blood sugar and blood pressure.

Growth hormone levels increase dramatically during puberty and are produced in a cyclic fashion. Growth hormone releasing hormone (GHRH) from the hypothalamus is the stimulus for the pituitary gland to produce growth hormone. GHRH production and release is affected by many factors such as stress, sleep, food, medications, and chronic disease. Chronic sleep deprivation or disordered sleep patterns

K.L. Eckert (✉)
Department of Pediatrics, University of Nevada School of Medicine, Reno, NV, USA
e-mail: kathryneck@aol.com

W.T. O'Donohue, L.W. Tolle (eds.), *Behavioral Approaches to Chronic Disease in Adolescence*,
DOI 10.1007/978-0-387-87687-0_4, © Springer Science+Business Media, LLC 2009

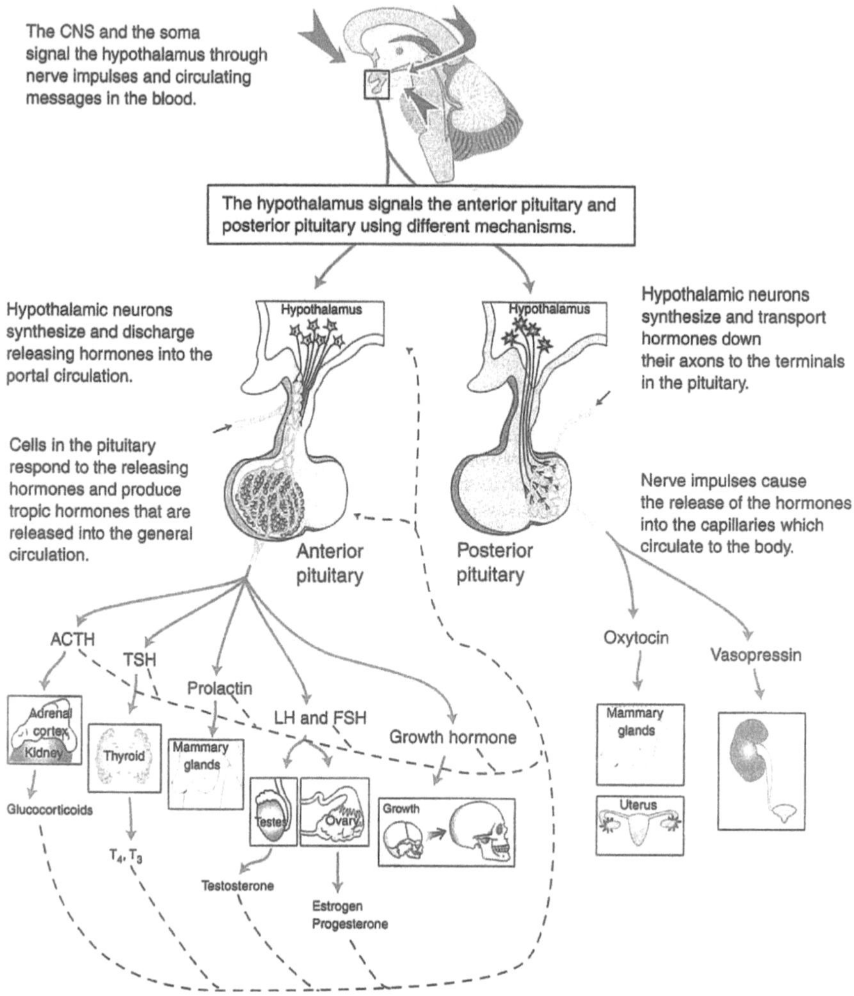

Fig. 1 Information from the cerebral cortex and blood stream converges on the hypothalamus, which instigates a cascade of actions and in turn responds to feedback from the target organs. CNS, central nervous system; ACTH, adrenocorticotropic hormone; TSH, thyroid-stimulating hormone; T_4, tetraiodothronine; T_3, triiodothyronine; LH, Luteinizing hormone; FSH fllicle-stimulating hormone Reprinted (permission pending) from Higgins and George (2007)

may have a large impact on growth hormone secretion and, in turn, result in abnormal growth. Growth hormone has some direct effect on growth of the long bones; however, most of the effect is mediated through insulin-like growth factors which are produced in the liver. These growth factors are carried in the blood to their target, the growth plates of long bones, where their action is then completed.

Puberty hormones and growth hormones generally increase together and are responsible for the tremendous skeletal growth and sexual maturation seen in pubertal children. Females and males undergo a dramatic growth acceleration throughout puberty with the peak occurring approximately 75% of the way through pubertal progression. This significant increase in height may cause turmoil in the adolescent, particularly when it is much earlier or later than the rest of one's peers.

The interactions between the hypothalamus, pituitary, and end organs are quite complex with both negative and positive feedback signals from the endocrine system as well as the skeleton, brain, and exogenous factors – see Fig. 1.

Puberty

It is little wonder that adolescence is a confusing period of time in most young people's lives. The changes occurring in the anatomy and physiology of the body are dramatic and occur over a relatively short period of time, generally 2–3 years in females and 4–5 years in males. During this time a transformation and maturation of the external genitalia takes place along with the many hormonal changes causing internal changes in emotions and brain function.

Puberty is a part of adolescence defining primarily the physical and hormonal changes associated with it. This stage of development includes the transition from sexually immature to sexually mature including the presence of secondary sexual characteristics (breast development, pubic and axillary hair, phallic growth and maturation, and testicular enlargement). Over the last several decades we have seen a slight decline in the age of onset of puberty, particularly in females. The average age of onset of puberty in females is 10 years with a range of 8–13 years. Generally, breast budding is the first manifestation of puberty with axillary and pubic hair following shortly behind. The average age of menarche is 12.5 years of age. The average age of pubertal onset for males is 12 years with pubertal progression continuing for approximately 4–5 years. In males, the first sign of puberty is usually testicular enlargement, which may be very subtle in appearance. The classification of sex maturity stages in girls and boys is shown in Tables 1 and 2.

Internal triggers, including skeletal maturation, body fat, genetic and ethnic factors, and biochemical markers initiate the process of puberty. There are also external factors which regulate the onset and tempo of puberty including stress, malnutrition or eating disorders, chronic disease, and medications. The normal sequence of pubertal, growth, and maturational events in males and females is shown in Figs. 2 and 3.

Table 1 Classification of sex maturity stages in girls

SMR stage	Pubic hair	Breasts
1	Preadolescent	Preadolescent
2	Sparse, lightly pigmented, straight, medial border of labia	Breast and papilla elevated as small mound; areolar diameter increases
3	Darker, beginning to curl, increased amount	Breast and areola enlarged, no contour separation
4	Coarse, curly, abundant but amount less than in adult	Areola and papilla form secondary mound
5	Adult feminine triangle, spreads to medial surface of thighs	Mature, nipple projects, areola part of general breast contour

SMR = sexual maturity rating.
Adapted (permission pending) from Nelson Textbook of Pediatrics 17th edition, 2004.

Table 2 Classification of sex maturity stages in boys

SMR stage	Pubic hair	Peni	Testes
1	Preadolescent	Preadolescent	Preadolescent
2	Scanty, long, slightly pigmented	Slight enlargement	Enlarged scrotum, pink texture altered
3	Darker, starts to curl small amount	Longer	Larger
4	Resembles adult type but less in quantity; coarse curly	Larger; glans and breadth increase in size	Larger, scrotum dark
5	Adult distribution, spreads to medial surface of thighs	Adult size	Adult size

SMR = sexual maturity rating.
Adapted (permission pending) from Nelson Textbook of Pediatrics 17th edition, 2004.

Abnormalities in Pubertal Hormones

Not infrequently, females may be noted to have the first signs of puberty (breast buds) at 8 or 9 years of age. The etiology of early puberty is not completely clear and is not seen in all populations. African-Americans and Hispanic females generally mature physically earlier than their counterparts. A rising incidence of obesity, which in turn may trigger the endocrine system to initiate pubertal changes, has been implicated. Food sources containing estrogens or phytoestrogens have also been implicated but no prevailing evidence for this is available. In females with very early pubertal maturation (<7 years) a causative factor is more likely to be found. Hydrocephalus, structural brain abnormalities, traumatic brain injury, and central nervous system tumors may cause precocious puberty. Males with early puberty are much more likely to have an organic or medical cause than females. Earlier age of onset of puberty may lead to an even greater disparity between the

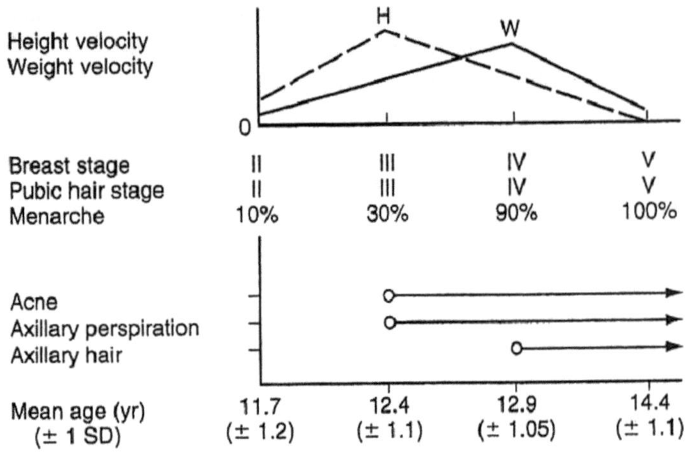

Fig. 2 Sequence of maturational events in females (Adapted from Marshall & Tanner 1969) Reprinted (permission pending) from *Nelson Textbook of Pediatrics* 17th edition 2004.

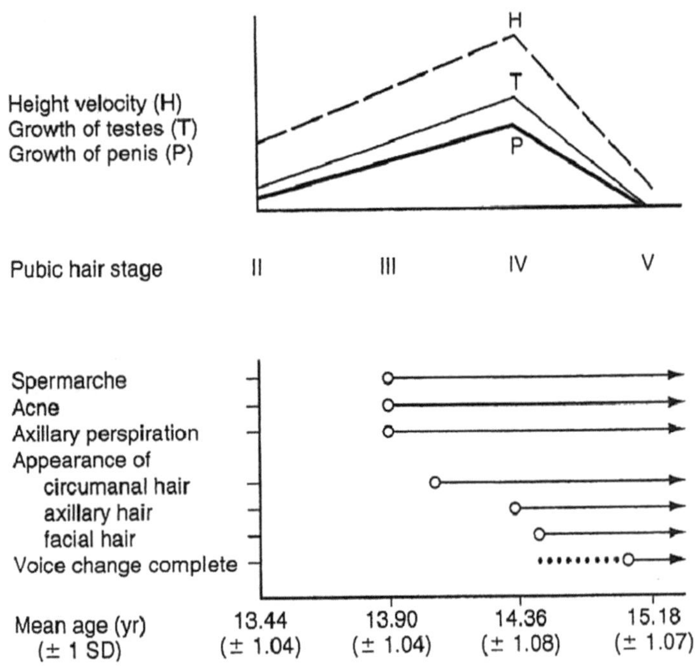

Fig.3 Sequence of maturatinal events in males (Adapted from Marshall & Tanner 1970) Reprinted (permission pending) from *Nelson Textbook of Pediatrics* 17th edition 2004.

anatomic and physiologic maturity as compared with the maturation of the central nervous system, lending itself to issues with early sexuality, difficulty in peer interactions, and school issues.

Pubertal delay is defined as no signs of puberty in a female by 13 years of age and in a male by 14 years of age. Delayed puberty more often occurs in males although referral bias may play a role in the reporting of this. A delay in puberty may have significant psychosocial consequences particularly when short stature also occurs. Genetic factors may predispose one to having a later puberty (i.e., a parent having delayed puberty increases the likelihood of offspring being delayed). Infrequently, a hormonal deficiency or anatomic abnormality may be the cause of the delay in puberty and require further evaluation and treatment. Medical therapy can hasten the onset of puberty in cases where this is indicated.

Hormonal abnormalities in females may result in altered secretion of LH, FSH, and androgens which can lead to irregularities or absence of menstruation, excessive hair growth on the face, chest, abdomen, and severe acne. Many factors can lead to these hormonal abnormalities including genetics, lifestyle issues such as weight gain, medications, and illness. Early in puberty, males may have a mild imbalance in their male and female hormone production which can lead to enlargement of the nipples and breast tissue termed gynecomastia. Typically this resolves during the first 1–2 years of puberty as the testosterone levels rise (Behrman, Kliegman, & Jenson, 2004; Kappy, Allen, & Geffner, 2005; Sperling, 2008; Porterfield, 1997).

Endocrine Abnormalities in Chronic Disease

Abnormalities in endocrine function are often seen in the presence of a chronic disease such as anorexia nervosa, poorly controlled diabetes mellitus, cystic fibrosis, asthma, and cancer. Some of this dysfunction may be due to the treatment of these illnesses; however, the physiology of the disease itself may impact the balance of hormones.

Asthma

Asthma is considered to be the most common chronic disease of childhood. Fortunately, the last decade has brought to use many new medications for the treatment of asthma. However, steroids are still used frequently to treat the inflammation associated with asthma. This form of medication may have a profound effect on many systems in the body, particularly the skeletal and endocrine systems. In the skeletal system steroids over time decrease the bone mineral present in the skeleton. Ultimately, this may lead to a higher incidence of osteoporosis. Additionally, steroid use may alter the function of the adrenal glands and the natural secretion of their hormones. Chronic, severe asthma may result in delayed puberty and growth due to the issues associated with steroids and other medications used for treatment, as well as the chronic hypoxia and inflammation associated with this disorder.

Diabetes

Type I diabetes mellitus (juvenile diabetes or insulin-dependent mellitus) affects approximately 0.3% of the population and is one of the most common chronic medical problems in children. This chronic disorder may be difficult for the adolescent to manage well because of the many invasive measures one must take to treat it well including multiple insulin injections each day, finger pricking for blood sugar monitoring four to eight times each day, and monitoring food intake. As blood sugars rise and remain chronically high, many other physiologic functions may become altered. These include abnormalities in growth hormone and pubertal hormone secretion which may result in poor growth and delayed puberty. The insulin-like growth factors that are involved with linear growth and other functions may be impaired in children with diabetes due to their likeness with insulin used for treating diabetes. In most patients this does not result in clinically abnormal growth; however, in patients with poor diabetes control a decline in growth velocity is not uncommon. Uncontrolled diabetes results in chronically high blood sugars. When blood sugars are >180 mg/dl (normal, non-diabetic blood sugar range = 70–100 mg/dl) the kidneys are unable to reabsorb the sugar. At this point the kidneys pull more fluid from the body along with the sugar, resulting in large volumes of urine. Since a significant amount of sugar is being lost through the kidneys this implies that many calories are lost as well. This may lead to significant weight loss and relative malnutrition. Adolescents, particularly females, may purposely forego insulin in the face of large amounts of food in order to keep weight gain to a minimum. This has been termed diabulimia or renal bulimiaand is a form of disordered eating. Eating disorders are most likely higher in the population affected by diabetes, but statistics vary among different studies. Some studies suggest that as many as 30% of females with diabetes engage in disordered eating behaviors (Crow, Keel, & Kendall, 1998; Herpertz, von Blume, & Senf, 1995; Takii et al., 1999; Herpertz et al., 1998).

Research has shown that cognitive functioning may also be significantly impaired in children and adolescents with diabetes mellitus. Some studies suggest that earlier age of onset and frequency and severity of hypoglycemia has an impact on functioning. Research in adults with diabetes suggests that hyperglycemia is associated with slowing of all cognitive performance tests. These abnormalities have significant implications for children and adolescents in their abilities to learn information, problem solve, and mature cognitively. (Cox et al., 2005; Brans, Biessels, de Haan, Kappelle, & Kessels, 2005; Northam et al., 2001; Northam, Bowden, Anderson, & Court, 1992; Naguib, Kulinskaya, Lomax, & Garralda, 2008; Kaufman, Epport, Engilman, & Halvorson, 1999).

Cancer

Survivors of childhood cancers are now more common that in the past; however, the treatment modalities used often result in long-term morbidities in several of the body's systems. Many commonly used chemotherapeutic agents used in the treatment of childhood cancers are toxic to the ovaries and testes. This may result in infertility as well as failure of the gonads to produce the hormones estrogen and testosterone, thereby causing the adolescent to fail to progress through puberty. Radiation therapy is also commonly used in the treatment of childhood cancers. Depending on the location and amount of radiation used, hypothalamic and pituitary hormone deficiencies may result. Growth hormone, LH, FSH, thyroid-stimulating hormone, and ACTH deficiencies commonly occur and result in poor growth, lack of puberty, fatigue, and other symptoms. Additionally, the neurological and cognitive issues associated with directed central nervous system radiation therapy for brain tumors and leukemias with central nervous system involvement have been shown to be quite significant, particularly in patients who are young at the time of treatment.

Eating Disorders

Anorexia nervosa and other eating disorders, as well as chronic malnutrition for any reason, are associated with significant dysfunction of the endocrine system. As the hypothalamus and pituitary are quite sensitive to stressors, parts or all of this system may be impaired. In this state, the hormones involved in puberty, menses, and fertility are not being produced in appropriate amounts and are not cycling normally. The thyroid hormone generally is suppressed as well in an attempt to slow the metabolism down in an undernourished state. The ACTH–cortisol pathway is also impaired although typically high levels of cortisol are noted in this high stress state. Adolescents with eating disorders or significant malnutrition may not reach their full height potential due to the disturbance of the normal puberty and growth phases during this period of time. This group of adolescents also has a greater risk of poor bone density as adolescents and ultimately are at higher risk of developing osteoporosis as an adult because of the poor bone mineral accretion associated with these endocrine abnormalities (Lawson & Klibanski, 2008; Licinio, Wong, & Gold, 1996; Connan et al., 2007).

Cystic Fibrosis

Cystic fibrosis is an autosomal recessive disorder affecting 1/3,000 babies born in the United States annually. This disorder affects the pulmonary system and the gastrointestinal system including the pancreas. Because of the progressive nature of this disorder, death typically occurs by the third decade of life. This disorder is associated with significant pulmonary impairment resulting in hypoxia. Frequently patients also develop diabetes mellitus as well. The function of the endocrine system may be significantly impaired because of the disease but also due to the treatments, particularly high-dose steroids that are given for long periods of time. As in other chronic disorders mentioned, growth and puberty may be significantly delayed as the hypothalamic and pituitary axis may be suppressed due to the chronic stress of this disease. Final adult height may be significantly impaired and pubertal progression may be limited until control of the pulmonary aspects of the disease improve. Malnutrition is also associated with this disorder due to the high caloric demands of the respiratory system. Additionally, poorly controlled diabetes associated with cystic fibrosis as well as malabsorption of nutrients in the gastrointestinal tract further impacts the nutrition status. Osteoporosis has also been associated with this disorder, most likely due to the use of steroids for treatment as well as chronic nutrition and vitamin deficiencies.

As has been discussed, the endocrine system may be disrupted by a variety of chronic disease states commonly seen in adolescents. The severity of the disease as well as the treatment modalities influence the short- and long-term aspects of growth and puberty. Significant delay or advancement in these areas may add considerable angst to an adolescent who is already dealing with the effects of his/her disease and should be addressed from a medical and psychological standpoint as early as possible.

Adolescent Brain Physiology

It was once thought that the human brain was completely developed by adolescence. Newer research has refuted that idea. Cognitive changes are actually occurring during a time of structural change and development inside the human brain, primarily in the cerebral cortex. These changes are influenced by our environment, our experiences, hormones, drugs, and alcohol.

Overview of Cortical Development

The cerebral cortex is composed of gray matter and white matter. The gray matter is where nerve cells (neurons) and their connections (filamentous projections called axons) reside. The white matter is primarily myelinated axons transporting impulses between the gray matter and lower brain structures. Myelin in an insulating sheath formed by supporting brain cells. The connection between an axon and another cell is a synapse (Higgins & George, 2007; Young, Young, & Tolbert, 2008; Purves et al., 2004). Figure 4 depicts the gray and white matter and their layers.

It was once thought that you were born with all the neurons you were going to have. It has now been proved that humans do continue to make new nerve cells (neurogenesis) into adulthood, albeit at a much slower pace. The primary time for creating new nerve cells is probably in the prenatal period. When a human is born there are about 100 billion neurons with 100 trillion connections. This process is largely genetically driven. Adults have had new neurons detected in only two areas: the dentate gyrus of the hippocampus and the olfactory bulb. Non-neuronal brain cells continue to form until about age 5 years (Higgins & George, 2007).

Another way the nervous system develops is by cell expansion: the branching of axons (filamentous projections away from a nerve cell) and dendrites (filamentous projections that receive signals from other cells) to make new connections. Researchers have discovered that human brains tend to have a preponderance of this process up to about age 5 years. Specific areas of the brain do this first, i.e., the visual centers have peaked before age 1 year. Synaptic density was first determined in postmortem studies and was later confirmed with studies of glucose utilization by PET scan (Windle et al., 2008).

A third way we see the nervous system develop is the process of connection refinement. This is the elimination of excessive branching and synapse connections. Again different regions of the brain undergo this at different times. Sensory and motor areas of the brain go through this first followed by areas of executive function. Remarkably the prefrontal cortex, which is the site of most executive functions, goes through significant pruning and reduction in size during middle and late adolescence.

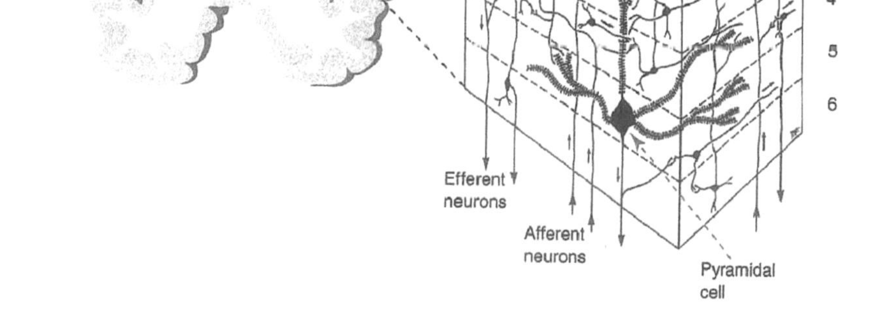

Fig. 4 The six layers of the neocortex, from the pial surface above layer 1 to the white matter below layer 6 (Adapted from Bear, Connors, & Paradiso, 2007; Snell, 2001)

MRI studies of the maturation of the human cortex generally show increases in gray matter density at early ages and loss of gray matter starting around puberty. This reduction in gray matter is assumed to be related to synaptic pruning, but could be related to other factors as well. Cell shrinkage and vascular changes are also theorized as possible contributors (Giedd et al., 1999; Gogtay et al., 2004). Recent studies on the development of the adolescent brain have shown that between the ages of 12–16 years maturation of the parietal cortex occurs. The parietal lobe tends to be concerned with somatosensory input including the processing of visual and tactile information, taste, and spatial relationships. Young adults show maturation of the prefrontal cortex and lenticular nuclei, a collection of neurons concerned with voluntary movement (Gotay et al., 2004; Sowell, Thompson, Holmes, Jernigan, & Toga, 1999).

Other studies have shown an increase in myelination well into the third decade of life. Myelination is the process of covering an axon with a protective coat made by a supporting cell in the brain. It occurs in sequence from inferior to superior and from posterior to anterior; i.e., the brainstem and cerebellar regions are first, the cerebral hemispheres later, and the frontal lobes myelinate last (Sowell et al., 1999). With myelination the neural signals transmit more rapidly. With myelination the white matter also increases in density, organization, and integration of neural pathways. It is the changes in white matter that have allowed more complex and higher order reasoning. So, the maturing of the human brain during adolescence is actually a refinement and reduction of gray matter in the prefrontal cortex. The brain is assumed to be developing by making better connections and not just by making more connections or more neurons (Higgins & George, 2007; Brown et al., 2008).

The Prefrontal Cortex

The prefrontal cortex is almost one-fourth the size of the entire cerebral cortex. It is sometimes called the frontal association cortex. It functions in social behavior, concentration, conceptualizing, planning, judgment, and problem solving. Patients without a prefrontal cortex lose initiative and ambition and show cognitive dysfunction; they are concrete and inflexible and have diminished sense of responsibility, judgment, and foresight. They are easily distracted, careless in their appearance, and lose the sense of acceptable behavior. They are often impulsive and inappropriate and can have explosive outbursts due to less inhibition of aggression (Young et al., 2008).

We have obtained insight into the function of the prefrontal cortex through an historical accident. In the mid-1800s a railroad construction foreman, Phineas Gage, suffered a prefrontal lobotomy when a dynamite tamping rod was blown through the front of his head. The prefrontal lobes were damaged and the resulting clinical picture helped delineate the function of that specific area. Before the accident Gage was punctual, hardworking, and highly respectable. Afterward, he lost all sense of responsibility; he became impulsive, irascible, profane, and drifted aimlessly the rest of his life.

An example of how the lack of development of the prefrontal cortex may explain interactions with our patients involves adolescents with asthma who are typically prescribed one or two inhalers. One inhaler, albuterol, is for rescue (i.e., immediate use) when they have an acute asthma attack; the other, an anti-inflammatory, is to be used daily for prevention of asthma attacks. Many physicians have trouble getting adolescents to use their preventative inhaler and this results in periodic flare-ups that sometimes put them in the hospital. We tend to call this noncompliance, but it may actually be developmentally appropriate. The early adolescent does not yet have a brain that can look to the future and plan with good decisions. Their cognitive skills are still very concrete, meaning they live in the here and now. Taking medicine when "I feel bad" is concrete and immediate. When we point out to them that they ended up in the hospital because they did not use their preventative inhaler, we may be helping them make cognitive connections between cause and effect. They may or may not make better choices the next time (Ginsburg & Jablow, 2002).

The Limbic Lobe

The pattern of brain maturation seems to be that evolutionarily older areas of the brain mature first. Indeed, we have spent a great deal of time talking about the development of the prefrontal cortex, but functional MRI studies also demonstrate deeper and older areas of the brain maturing in early adolescence, i.e., areas key to the limbic system (Gogtay et al., 2004). The limbic system consists essentially of the hippocampus and amygdala. The hippocampus is a section of the cerebral cortex folded in deep to the temporal lobe. It is the most primitive part of the cerebral cortex (Steinberg, 2008). It is essential to the development of memories. It is also one of the few locations in the adult brain where stem cells reside. Stem cells are primitive cells that can divide and make new neurons (Higgins & George, 2007). Lesions of the hippocampus produce a profound loss of short-term memory and significantly impair the ability to learn. The amygdala is a cluster of neurons within the temporal lobe of the brain, just anterior to the hippocampus. The amygdala associates experiences with consequences and then programs the appropriate emotional and behavioral responses. Lesions of the amygdala produce a profound loss of fear, placid behavior, and decreased emotional excitability. These two structures have rich connections to many parts of the brain including the hypothalamus (the master coordinator), autonomic structures in the brainstem, the prefrontal cortex, the nucleus accumbens (the major structure in the reward pathways of the brain), and the olfactory lobe (Young et al., 2008) (Fig. 5).

Environmental Influence

So what determines which synapses get pruned and which get to stay? This process is largely activity driven. It is the interaction with our environment that shapes our brain. Neuronal activity over certain pathways will stabilize those circuits rather than allow elimination through pruning. Cognition can be loosely defined as the ability to attend to stimuli, identify their significance, and respond appropriately. So our brains receive sensory input, complex processing then takes place in the brain, and subsequently, we show a response or action. As we experience, we learn. Our brains are molded by our environment through adolescence and into early adulthood (Chugani, 1998a).

The importance of the role of our environment on shaping our brains is probably most evident in the early stages of brain development. During the time of cellular expansion the environmental input is so crucial to determining the structure of the brain

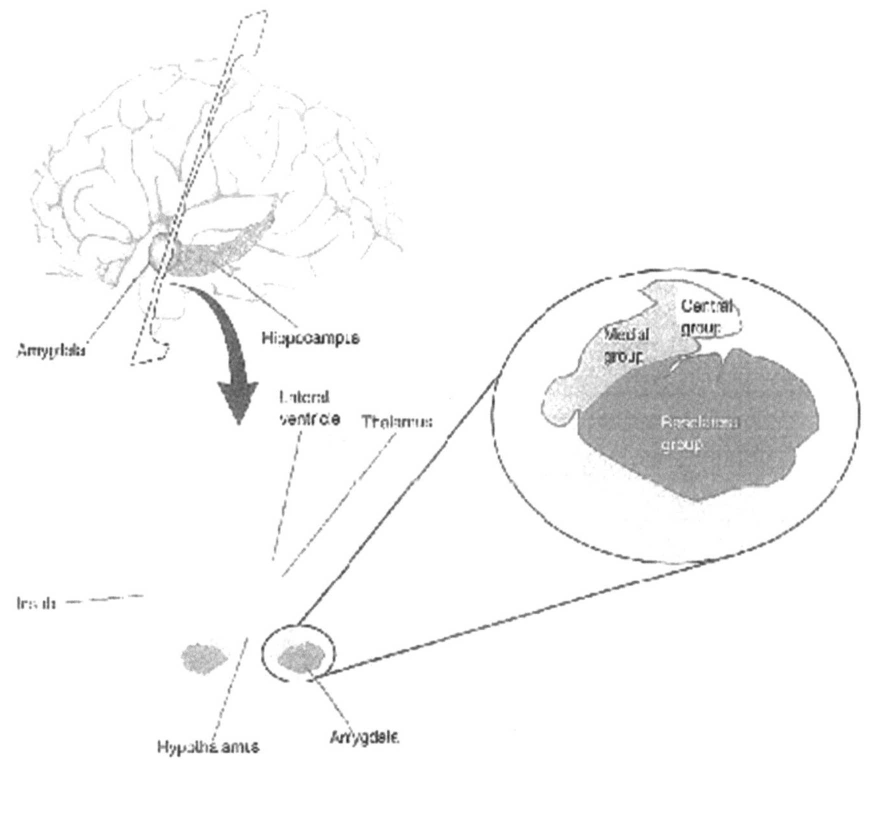

Fig. 5 The location and groups often called nuclear of the amygdala Reprinted (permission pending) from Higgins and George (2007)

we term these times critical periods. An example is the development of language acquisition. Early exposure to native sounds has a lasting impact on speech. Studies have shown that subjects who are exposed to another language before age 7 years had equivalent fluency to native speakers. There was a linear decline in the performance of language grammar until puberty if the individual was exposed to the new language after age 7 years. The critical period for vision extends out to about 5 or 6 years. Congenital cataracts must be repaired quickly in newborns to preserve vision (before 4 months), but adults regain their preexisting visual acuity because their visual cortex is already intact. Children with a lazy eye, or strabismus, see double due to the misalignment of the two eyes. This condition is usually repaired by age 7 years to protect vision. The brain will not tolerate seeing double and will turn off one of the eyes, leading to cortical blindness termed amblyopia (Chugani, 1998a). We do not know if there are any critical periods of development during the adolescent years but it is important to recognize that this is the time period where important new behaviors begin: social development and intimate relationships, decision making, and the ability to self-regulate and delay gratification.

Chemical Effects on Development

Communication at synapses is usually through the use of substances called neurotransmitters. Neurotransmitters are small, easily recyclable chemicals. They are stored in the terminal end of an axon, then released and taken up by specific receptors on dendritic connections. Some of the common neurotransmitters are GABA, dopamine, norepinephrine, and serotonin. Specific neurotransmitters and receptors are associated with certain neural pathways. For example, GABA (gamma-aminobutyric acid) is an inhibitory transmitter present in 25% of cortical neurons; it puts the brakes on the brain. Dopamine is utilized in pathways of movement and reward. Norepinephrine is involved in systems of stimulation and arousal. Serotonin has a major role in depression and anxiety. Neurons also receive signals through the bloodstream via hormones.

The dopaminergic activity in the prefrontal cortex increases significantly during early adolescence; indeed, it actually peaks at this time. Remodeling occurs in the form of increases, decreases, and redistribution of dopamine receptors, especially in the projections from the limbic lobe. As stated above, dopamine pathways play a critical role in the reward circuitry of the brain. This remodeling is thought to have implications for the reward seeking/risk-taking behavior seen in early adolescence. The dopaminergic pathway is also implicated in diverse aspects of social processing; for example, the recognition of socially relevant stimuli, social judgments, and social reasoning. In addition, adolescents seem to have greater activation in brain regions implicated in reward salience when peer acceptance is involved. The overlap between the neural circuits that process social information and reward may help explain adolescent behavior. Social acceptance by peers may be processed in ways similar to other sorts of rewards (Steinberg, 2008).

The importance of social and emotional factors in adolescent thinking is only now being appreciated. Cognitive evaluations of adolescents show that they are no worse than adults at perceiving risk or estimating vulnerability. It appears that the decision to take risks is heavily influenced by social and emotional factors. This helps explain why educational interventions to reduce risk like the DARE program and abstinence programs have been largely ineffective at actually changing behavior. The importance of social factors also helps explain why so much risk taking occurs in the presence of the peer group. Indeed, the strongest predictor of whether an adolescent will use alcohol or drugs is the use of those substances in the peer group.

Certainly, the physical changes of puberty are obvious, such as the development of secondary sex characteristics due to the action of the sex hormones peripherally. But the brain also is a target for estrogen and testosterone. There are receptors for testosterone and estrogen in various parts of the brain; there are high densities in the amygdala, hippocampus, and nucleus accumbens. The gonadal steroids exert strong influence on memory for social information and social bonding. This helps explain why early adolescence is a time of heightened awareness of others' opinions. One can surmise that changes in the amygdala (which is active when people are anxious or angry and plays the role of choosing an appropriate emotional response) play an important role in the intensity of emotions that we see in early adolescence (Windle et al., 2008; Sowell et al., 1999).

The sex hormones are lipophilic (fat soluble) and can pass through the cell wall and bind to receptors inside the cytoplasm. This steroid–receptor combination then couples with the cell DNA and initiates protein synthesis which then triggers change. Steroids and other hormones generally affect behavior and physiology over days and weeks. Of note, the steroid hormones also influence the receptor for GABA and have modulatory effects on the dopaminergic and serotonergic systems.

Many hormones are secreted cyclically in a circadian rhythm and may be affected by the changing sleep cycle of adolescents. Preteens have sleep requirements that fluctuate but adolescents generally need 8.5–9.25 h each day. There is a delay in the intrinsic sleep phase, meaning they often do not feel physiologically tired until close to midnight with the need then to sleep later in the morning (Higgins & George, 2007; Brown et al., 2008).

The Effects of Alcohol

As noted, adolescence is a time of maturation and neuroplasticity (capable of being formed or molded) of the brain especially in areas of self-regulation, emotional tone and reactivity, and higher level cognitive function. So with this new understanding, it is worth reexamining what exposure to alcohol does to the adolescent brain. We know from adult alcoholics that alcohol is a neurotoxin; we also see the effects of alcohol from in utero exposure, i.e., fetal alcohol syndrome. Most research on the neurotoxic effects of alcohol on the adolescent brain were done in adolescent rodents (Brown et al., 2008).

In adolescent rats, the hippocampus appears especially sensitive to the neurotoxic effects of both acute and chronic exposure. Memory formation is inhibited and there is cognitive impairment. The adolescent rats seem unusually sensitive to the cognitive ability impairment, and with chronic exposure the impairments are long term. Periods of heavy drinking followed by withdrawal, the equivalent of human binge drinking, seemed particularly more damaging. Chronic intermittent ethanol exposure was associated with damage to the frontal association cortex and other frontal regions in adolescents but not adult rats. It was also associated with reduced neurogenesis in the hippocampus and long-term alteration of the serotonergic pathways. In contrast to the heightened sensitivity to cognitive ability impairment, adolescent rats are less sensitive to the motor impairing effects and sedating effects of alcohol (Brown et al., 2008).

In humans, adolescents seem to show heightened sensitivity to the cognitive ability-impairing effects of alcohol and reduced sensitivity to other effects like motor function impairment and sedation. In humans the reduced sensitivity to motor function impairment and aversive effects of alcohol is a potent risk factor for the development of alcoholism. Consequently adolescent drinking is worrisome because some brain regions such as the hippocampus and prefrontal cortex are especially vulnerable to the direct neurotoxic effects of alcohol. Second, adolescent exposure may lead to long-term reduction in sensitivity to the cues that typically moderate consumption such as sedation and motor impairment. Lastly, both of these effects are amplified by the typical drinking pattern of youth (binge drinking).

The Effects of Antidepressants

It is not just with alcohol that we see adolescent physiology resulting in different effects from exposure – we also see this in the response to medications. For many years, there was difficulty proving the efficacy of antidepressants in children and adolescents. Their use in children and adolescents was largely assumed based on studies in adults. Recently, however, efficacy was proved in the class of antidepressants collectively termed SSRIs (the selective serotonin reuptake inhibitors) (Bylund & Reed, 2007). Studies that look at brain development have begun to shed light on possible explanations for this. Animal studies in rats and monkeys show that the neural circuits that involve serotonin develop early in life and the circuits involving norepinephrine mature later. Specifically, the rat's norepinephrine system develops at about 5 weeks of age, which is the age of sexual maturity; the serotonin system reaches adult levels 2–3 weeks earlier. In the monkey, whose brain at birth is similar to that of a human at 10–15 years of age, serotonin systems reach adult levels at 2 and 8 weeks and norepinephrine systems mature at about 2 years of age. In these animals, SSRIs do seem effective in behavioral models for depression. However, antidepressants such as desipramine, which also block norepinephrine uptake, are ineffective. In humans, serotonin is detected by 5 weeks gestation and increases to 12 weeks. Levels of serotonin are significantly higher than norepinephrine, except in the medulla oblongata. The synthesis of serotonin in humans is highest between the ages of 2 and 5 years (twice the level of adults) and then it declines to adult levels by age 11 years. It is by deduction from other mammal studies that we assume that the development of the norepinephrine system in humans also occurs later. This earlier maturation of the serotonin pathways would explain why SSRIs are effective in younger children and adolescents – the beneficial effects of antidepressants are seemingly only realized when they act on mature neurotransmitter systems (Bylund & Reed, 2007; Murrin, Sanders, & Bylund, 2007).

In summary, we are now seeing the period of adolescence as one of neurologic plasticity and vulnerability. Animal studies in rats give rise to both hope and caution. Animals raised in an enriched environment during puberty have been able to mitigate the influences of perinatal and postnatal stress (Romeo & McEwen, 2006). The period of adolescent plasticity may serve as a time of opportunity for the developing brain. More worrisome though is that studies on the use of norepinephrine uptake inhibitors in adolescent rats show not only poor efficacy but brain effects that were actually the opposite of those seen in adults. Receptor density was upregulated instead of downregulated. The developing brain also showed differences in the regulation of some gene expression by norepinephrine (Murrin et al., 2007). We have begun to appreciate how the environment plays a role in the structural development of the brain. It is quite possible that the use of centrally acting medications on the immature brain is having more of an effect than we previously realized. In light of this, it would be prudent to use centrally acting medications sparingly and with great caution in children and adolescents.

Adolescent physiology encompasses a multitude of complex changes. This chapter illustrates those changes on a physical, hormonal, and neurological level. It is a testament to the wonders of the human body that a child transforms into an adult in only 5–10 years. As previously discussed there is great variability in the maturation process, which makes the medical and/or psychological care of the adolescent so daunting. Whether the health care team encounters physical differences such as the "early bloomer" or "late bloomer", or faces the mysterious nature of the prefrontal cortex, it is critical to approach each and every teenager as an individual. When chronic illness is injected into the picture, this combination unleashes a torrent of unpredictable behaviors that cannot be ignored. The best way to confront chronic disease in the adolescent is to be educated in basic pathophysiology and at the same time understand the dynamic nature in which the brain and body metamorphosize into a healthy adult. As medical professionals we must realize that genuine concern and compassion will always be the foundation of quality care for the adolescent.

The following are three case studies involving adolescents with chronic disease and the behavioral and management issues associated with these disorders. It is our intent for these cases to help clarify some of the complexities that have been identified in this chapter.

Case 1

Arnie

Arnie is a 15-year-old male who has been successfully cured of acute lymphocytic leukemia (ALL), a type of cancer that affects the white blood cells. Patients may experience anemia, impaired clotting function which leads to easy bruising or bleeding, and a weakened immune system. Arnie was diagnosed at the age of 12 years and has spent many years coping with multiple treatment regimens. The diagnosis of leukemia initiates a cascade of scheduled interventions that take place over several months. The need for compliance is of paramount importance and, due to the nature of being a child, much of the burden rests upon family and care providers. Arnie has dutifully attended all the required doctor visits and his parents have helped him through the painful blood draws, days spent in the hospital, and the side effects of treatment. His immune system is compromised and therefore, each sniffle or fever invokes anxiety within the family and a prompt call to the doctor is made.

Once Arnie was admitted to the hospital because he was experiencing fatigue and bleeding from the gums. His laboratory studies showed extremely low platelet and red blood cell counts. Platelets initiate healing processes which allow insults to the body to be repaired. Without the proper number of platelets, our bodies can weaken, bruise, and even bleed into the intestines, mouth, nose, and joint spaces. Not only did Arnie experience bleeding, but his admission to the hospital was necessitated by fatigue and weakness due to anemia. Red blood cells are responsible for carrying oxygen from the lungs to the body where it is used to create energy. When someone is anemic, the energy production is compromised which leads to generalized fatigue. Unknown to Arnie and his family at the time of admission to the hospital, the leukemia, which was thought to have been eradicated in the prior year by chemotherapy, had returned. Most patients with leukemia are treated for approximately 3 years, and parents are reminded that a relapse can occur at any time. Quite understandably, families are under constant fear of this and the pressures of maintaining compliance with treatment can be burdensome. Arnie endures another intensive course of chemotherapy in hopes of keeping the cancer at bay. Most of the chemotherapeutic agents target the ability of the cancerous white blood cells to replicate. Unfortunately, the chemotherapeutic agents affect normal cells of the body as well. The symptoms of nausea, hair loss, and serious infection are a direct result of the healthy cells being destroyed. The endocrine system can also be affected by chemotherapy thereby leading to hormone deficiencies and impaired development. Time passes and Arnie's leukemia is back in remission. He returns to school and normal activities. Over the next year he begins to notice that his friends were growing a lot bigger and taller than he was. Many excelled in sports and some were even going on dates. Although Arnie had spent many years battling his disease and undoubtedly matured more so than his peers through emotional and cognitive obstacles placed upon him, his physical development had been inhibited. Arnie has been labeled as the "shrimp" and, in some circumstances, a social outcast. He desperately seeks acceptance and begins to feel more alienated. Slowly, Arnie finds a new peer group of friends that engage in more risky behaviors. His anger and frustration coupled with the burdens of surviving leukemia has sent him on a path filled with poor decision making, threatening the healthy transition into adulthood. This example demonstrates how a chronic illness, such as cancer, can compound the normal physiologic hurdles found in the maturing adolescent brain.

Marie

Marie is a 15-year-old female with a history of type I diabetes mellitus. She presents to the emergency room with the complaint of vomiting, extreme thirst, copious urination, and weight loss. The young adolescent states that she has been feeling very tired for the past week and has missed several days of school. She is accompanied by her mother who works the swing shift and reports nothing out of the ordinary at home. In fact, when questioned further about her daughter's symptoms, she believed Marie was "just being a teenager" in regard to her "excessive laziness" and sleeping patterns. Routine blood tests reveal that Marie is dehydrated, has a blood sugar of 640, and large amounts of ketones in her urine. The physician on call examines her and diagnoses her with diabetic ketoacidosis.

DKA (diabetic ketoacidosis) is a medical condition that occurs when the body lacks sufficient insulin. One of the most important functions of insulin is to utilize glucose, or sugar, to provide energy to the body. When the body cannot utilize the glucose, it builds up in the blood stream and can cause a myriad of problems including thirst and increased urine production, both of which Marie experienced prior to her trip to the emergency room. When there is inadequate energy production from glucose, the body looks elsewhere for the energy needed to maintain life. In response to this requirement adipose tissues, or fat cells, are broken down which release the much needed energy. However, the breakdown of adipose cells releases chemicals known as free fatty acids which are converted eventually into ketoacids or ketones and spilled into the blood stream. These substances are found at low levels normally, but when they build up it can cause the blood to become more acidic. The acidic nature of the body makes one feel fatigued, nauseated, and quite often vomiting will occur. When the acids build up significantly, lethargy, loss of consciousness, and death may result.

Marie's situation is a common problem for those with type I diabetes mellitus; however, during adolescence this condition tends to be more severe and frequent due to the fact that proper management of this chronic disease requires planning, good judgment, and discipline. Many adolescents lack these skills and are not always equipped to face the challenges that every person with diabetes encounters on a daily basis.

Marie is admitted to the hospital and receives intravenous fluids and insulin. She quickly recovers overnight and is feeling much better the next morning. Upon further review of her recent management at home, Marie states that she has been checking her blood glucose levels "once or twice" a day and "usually" remembers to give herself insulin injections but sometimes forgets the evening dose which normally should be taken before dinner. Recently her mother lost her job and had to find a new one with different hours. Marie and her mother have had fewer conversations and most of their communication takes place in the morning before school and sometimes late at night when she gets home. When probed further about the relationship between mother and daughter, Marie declares that her mother has been more critical and "nagging" when the topics of insulin injections and blood glucose monitoring are discussed. At her bedside in the hospital, Marie becomes more tearful and declares that she understands how important it is to take control of her diabetes but wishes it would just go away and does not want to worry about it anymore.

This scenario outlines another important aspect of diabetes and how it affects adolescents. For children with this chronic disease, the management rests almost entirely with the adult care provider, but as the child grows into the transitional period of adolescence more and more responsibility must be transferred to the individual. Some adolescents make this transition with little difficulty and suffer only minor setbacks, but some such as Marie require more patience and continuous supervision. Marie's social support system has changed dramatically and this has likely led to her recent medical problems.

Over the next few weeks, things improve for Marie, and she is feeling much better. Her daily blood glucose records show good control and the physician believes the supervision at home has become more adequate. Three months after her admission to the hospital, routine laboratory studies are done and Marie comes into the office for another visit. Much to the physician's surprise, the hemoglobin A1C is 13.5 which is an alarmingly high number. Hemoglobin A1C is a blood test that is used to measure the degree of control a person has with diabetes. While the blood tests obtained from a simple finger prick done several times a day show the level of glucose at that moment in time, the hemoglobin A1C gives an average glucose measurement over several weeks. The question that must be answered in the case of Marie is why her daily records show good control, whereas her hemoglobin A1C shows poor control. The answer is another common theme encountered while caring for people with diabetes mellitus. Many times patients (especially adolescents) will falsify their daily records in order to appease those involved in their medical management. There is a certain expectation to play the "good patient" role and when coupled with the challenges of transitioning from child to adult, the teenager is particularly vulnerable to these behaviors.

After some counseling in the office, the rest of Marie's medical records are reviewed. Since her admission to the hospital some 3 months ago, there has been a 20 lb weight loss. Once again Marie is questioned about this finding and despite many attempts to downplay the weight loss, she finally opens up. Her friends at school have been talking about weight and how the boys are more interested in the thinner girls. Although Marie is not overweight, she wants to look more like the women on television and decided to lose a few pounds. The easiest way to do this for a patient with diabetes is quite simple: take less insulin or skip injections completely. The body is unable to use the glucose from food for energy without the insulin and it is eliminated through the urine instead. Also, the adipose tissue gets consumed as described earlier and over time can lead to significant weight loss. Adolescents are constantly aware of the many social expectations placed upon them from peers and the media. Although their chronic illness can manifest itself in a life-threatening and acute medical emergency, there are more insidious aspects to diabetes that the health care team must be made aware of.

Tim

Tim is a 14-year-old male with mild persistent asthma. He is on a regimen of inhaled steroids to be taken twice a day. In the last 2 years he has been compliant with his routine maintenance medications and has enjoyed good health. Tim has always been interested in organized sports and decides to try out for freshman football this year. Much to his delight, he makes the team and starts to participate in the required practices.

In the locker room, Tim's friends notice that he is using an inhaler before they start practicing. Some comments are made and although Tim knows that his fellow teammates are just joking around with him, he feels awkward and a bit out of place. After all, "fitting in" is an important goal of every adolescent especially one who is on the football team. Over the next few weeks he stops taking his routine inhaled steroids and starts to rely heavily on the use of his quick-acting emergency medication inhaler (albuterol). He hides the use of the albuterol from his friends when experiencing chest tightness and shortness of breath. His asthma is giving him problems, but football is so much fun and Tim likes being part of a team and "one of the guys".

Asthma is the most common chronic illness found in the adolescent age group. It is also the most common cause of hospitalization for children in the United States. It can be defined simply as a chronic inflammatory disorder of the airways leading to periodic episodes of airway constriction, thereby causing impaired lung function. The lungs are comprised of thousands of airways and they must stay open in order for the body to receive the necessary oxygen to function properly. Also, the airways serve as a conduit for carbon dioxide to leave the body. Lastly, these airways are wrapped with special muscles that contract or relax in response to the demands of air exchange. People with asthma have chronic inflammation of the airways, and therefore, more mucus is present inside these tubes which leads to a compromise in the ability to move air in and out of the lungs. The contraction of the muscles surrounding the airways can be triggered by a variety of events such as exercise, allergies, or even emotional states which can lead to the classic "asthma attack". Asthma can be mild, moderate, or severe and the various treatment modalities will vary depending on the degree of illness. In general, there are two basic concepts to understand when dealing with the treatments used for asthma. First, medications such as inhaled steroids target the inflammation present in the lungs and only work if they are taken on a daily basis in order to reduce the amount of mucus generated by the disease process. Second, there are medications such as albuterol which work by relaxing the muscles encompassing the airways and are taken in an emergency situation when one cannot get enough air into and out of the lungs.

One day, during a football game, Tim begins to experience chest pain and wheezing. His albuterol inhaler is in a duffle bag on the sidelines but he figures he can "play through" the symptoms. As the game progresses Tim starts to feel a little dizzy and is much slower getting back to the huddle for the next play. He decides that perhaps a break would make him feel better and heads over to talk to the coach. Tim tells the coach that he does not feel well and is having a hard time catching his breath. His coach listens attentively but tells him to get back on the field and play ball. He grabs his albuterol inhaler which provides some relief but Tim is feeling anxious and a little scared. Obediently he returns to play and on the second snap of the football, he collapses. The game takes a pause while staff members and fellow players kneel over Tim. He struggles to get up. The air is difficult to take into his lungs and slowly he loses consciousness. The ambulance is called and Tim is taken to the local hospital where he is admitted for intensive treatment. After 5 days in the hospital, he is discharged to his family in stable condition much to the relief of everyone involved in his care.

This case report represents many common issues involved with adolescents with asthma. The chronic nature of the disease demands constant attention. The lapse in judgment which led to discontinuing daily inhaled steroids was a direct result of multiple factors. Adolescents, especially males, can be particularly vulnerable in conforming to established codes of conduct. While sports may be an innocent endeavor to many youth, those with chronic diseases such as asthma sometimes pay the heaviest price of participation. The ignorance of Tim's coach and the fear of "being different" proved to be a dangerous combination for the well-being of this teenager.

References

Bear, M. F., Connors, B. W., & Paradiso, M. A. (Eds.). (2007). *Neuroscience: Exploring the brain* (3rd ed.). Baltimore: Lippincott Williams & Wilkins

Behrman, R. E., Kliegman, R. M., & Jenson, H. B. (2004). *Nelson textbook of pediatrics* (17th ed.). Philadelphia: Saunders.

Brans, A. M., Biessels, G. J., deHaan, E. H., Kappelle, L. J., & Kessels, R. P. (March, 2005). The effects of type 1 diabetes on cognitive performance: a meta-analysis. *Diabetes Care, 28*(3), 726–735.

Brown, S. A., McGue, M., Maggs, J., Schulenberg, J., Hingson, R., Swartzwelder, S., et al. (April, 2008). A developmental perspective on alcohol and youths 16 to 20 years of age. *Pediatrics, 121* Suppl 4, S290–S310.

Bylund, D. B., & Reed, A. L. (October, 2007). Childhood and adolescent depression: Why do children and adults respond differently to antidepressant drugs? *Neurochemistry International, 51*(5), 246–253.

Chugani, H. T. (November, 1998a). Biological basis of emotions: Brain systems and brain development. *Pediatrics, 102*(5 Suppl E), 1225–1229.

Chugani, H. T. (March–April, 1998b). A critical period of brain development: Studies of cerebral glucose utilization with PET. *Preventive Medicine, 27*(2), 184–188.

Connan, F., Lightman, S. L., Landau, S., Wheeler, M., Treasure, J., & Campbell, I. C. (January-February, 2007). An investigation of hypothalamic-pituitary-adrenal axis hyperactivity in anorexia nervosa: The role of CRH and AVP. *Journal of Psychiatric Research, 41*(1–2), 131–143.

Cox, D. J., Kovatchev, B. P., Gonder-Frederick, L. A., Summers, K. H., McCall, A., Grimm, K. J., et al. (January, 2005). Relationships between hyperglycemia and cognitive performance among adults with type 1 and type 2 diabetes. *Diabetes Care, 28*(1), 71–77.

Crow, S. J., Keel, P. K., & Kendall, D. (1998). Eating disorders and insulin-dependent diabetes mellitus. *Psychosomatics, 39*(3), 233–243.

Giedd, J. N., Blumenthal, J., Jeffries, N. O., Castellanos, F. X., Liu, H., Zijdenbos, A., et al. (1999) *Brain development during childhood and adolescence: A longitudinal MRI study*. New York: Nature America Inc.

Ginsburg, K., & Jablow, M. M. (2002). *But I'm almost 13! An action plan for raising a responsible adolescent*. New York: Contemporary Books.

Gogtay, N., Giedd, J. N., Lusk, L., Hayashi, K. M., Greenstein, D., Vaituzis, A. C., et al. (May 25, 2004) Dynamic mapping of human cortical development during childhood through early adulthood. *Proceedings of the National Academy of Sciences of the United States of America, 101*(21), 8174–8179.

Herpertz, S., Albus, C., Wagener, R., Kocnar, M., Wagner, R., Henning, A., et al. (July, 1998). Comorbidity of diabetes and eating disorders. Does diabetes control reflect disturbed eating behavior? *Diabetes Care, 21*(7), 1110–1116.

Herpertz, S., von Blume, B., & Senf, W. (1995). Eating disorders and diabetes mellitus. *Z Psychosom Med Psychoanal, 41*(4), 329–343.

Higgins, E. S., & George, M. S. (2007). *The neuroscience of clinical psychiatry, the pathophysiology of behavior and mental illness*. Philadelphia: Lippincott Williams & Wilkins.

Kappy, M. S., Allen, D. B., & Geffner, M. E. (2005). *Principles and practice of pediatric endocrinology*. Springfield, IL: Charles C Thomas Publisher.

Kaufman, F. R., Epport, K., Engilman, R., & Halvorson, M. (January–February, 1999). Neurocognitive functioning in children diagnosed with diabetes before age 10 years. *Journal of Diabetes and Its Complications, 13*(1), 31–38.

Lawson, E. A., & Klibanski, A. (July, 2008). Endocrine abnormalities in anorexia nervosa. *Nature Clinical Practice. Endocrinology & Metabolism, 4*(7), 407–414.

Licinio, J., Wong, M. L., & Gold, P. W. (April 16, 1996). The hypothalamic-pituitary-adrenal axis in anorexia nervosa. *Psychiatry Research, 62*(1), 75–83.

Marshall, W. A., & Tanner, J. M. (1969). Variations in pattern of pubertal changes in girls. *Archives of Disease in Childhood, 44*, 291.

Marshall, W. A., & Tanner, J. M. (1970). Variations in pattern of pubertal changes in boys. *Archives of Disease in Childhood, 45*, 13

Murrin, L. C., Sanders, J. D., & Bylund, D. B. (2007). Comparison of the maturation of the adrenergic and serotonergic neurotransmitter systems in the brain: Implications for differential drug effects on juveniles and adults. *Biochemical Pharmacology, 73*(8):1225–1236. (PMID: 17316571).

Naguib, J. M., Kulinskaya, E., Lomax, C. L., & Garralda, M. E. (July 17, 2008). Neuro-cognitive performance in children with type I diabetes-a meta-analysis. *Journal of Pediatric Psychology*.

Northam, E., Bowden, S., Anderson, V., & Court, J. (November, 1992). Neuropsychological functioning in adolescents with diabetes. *Journal of Clinical and Experimental Neuropsychology, 14*(6), 884–900.

Northam, E. A., Anderson, P. J., Jacobs, R., Hughes, M., Warne, G. L., & Werther, G. A. (September, 2001). Neuropsychological profiles of children with type 1 diabetes 6 years after disease onset. *Diabetes Care, 24*(9), 1541–1546.

Porterfield, S. P. (1997). *Endocrine physiology*. St. Louis, MO: Mosby-Year Book, Inc.

Purves, D., Augustine, G. J., Fitzpatrick, D., Hall, W. C., LaMantia, A-S., McNamara, J. O., et al. (2004). *Neuroscience* (3rd ed.). Sunderland, MA: Sinauer Associates Inc.

Romeo, R. D., & McEwen, B. S. (December, 2006). Stress and the adolescent brain. *Annals of the New York Academy of Sciences, 1094*, 226–234.

Snell, R. S. (2001). *Clinical neuroanatomy: A illustrated review with questions and explanations* (3rd ed.). Philadelphia: Lippincott Williams & Wilkins.

Sowell, E. R., Thompson, P. M., Holmes, C. J., Jernigan, T. L., & Toga, A. W. (1999). *In vivo evidence for post-adolescent brain maturation in frontal and striatal regions.* New York: Nature America Inc.

Sperling, M. A. (2008). *Pediatric endocrinology* (3rd ed.). Philadelphia: Saunders Elsevier.

Steinberg, L. (March, 2008). A social neuroscience perspective on adolescent risk-taking. *Developmental Review, 28*(1), 78–106.

Takii, M., Komaki, G., Uchigata, Y., Maeda, M., Omori, Y., & Kubo, C. (September, 1999). Differences between bulimia nervosa and binge-eating disorder in females with type 1 diabetes: The important role of insulin omission. *Journal of Psychosomatic Research, 47*(3), 221–231.

Windle, M., Spear, L. P., Fuligni, A. J., Angold, A., Brown, J. D., Pine, D., et al. (2008). Transitions into underage and problem drinking: Developmental processes and mechanisms between 10 and 15 years of age. *Pediatrics, 121*, S273–S289.

Young, P. A., Young, P. H., & Tolbert, D. L. (2008). *Clinical neuroscience* (2nd ed.). Philadelphia: Lippincott Williams & Wilkins.

Family Influence on Adolescent Treatment Outcomes

Clint Field and Rachel Duchoslav

Family Influence on Adolescent Treatment Outcomes

Social ecological models have often been utilized as a framework in which the level of function and recovery of health-impaired children may be considered in relation to environmental settings and associated variables (Bronfenbrenner, 1979; Brown, 2002; Kazak, 1989). In graphical representations of such models, the child is typically conceptualized as the central element within a series of circles of increasing size. Each circle represents an additional "layer" of the model with larger circles representing distal social variables that may influence child functioning, even if indirectly. From a behavioral theoretical perspective, the strengths of such models lay in organizing potential classes of pertinent variables to loosely illustrate context.

The primary function of this chapter is to provide the reader with an overview of the empirical findings describing reliable relations among the two innermost circles of the model, those representing the child and the immediate family. Of particular interest is the impact of familial variables on the daily functioning and outcomes of adolescent youth with a chronic health condition. Outcome variables that have received consistent attention within the empirical literature base include child emotional or physical well-being, treatment and medication adherence, and adjustment. Thus, it is the impact of familial variables on these outcomes, in particular, that comprises the primary focus of this chapter.

The relationship between family variables and adolescent chronic illness should be conceptualized as reciprocal in nature. Family factors may have a significant effect on the course of illness, and an adolescent's illness may impact family functioning. To date, however, the effects of adolescent illness on family functioning are better established than the impact of family on the course of illness or recovery (Finkelstein, 1993). Nonetheless, there have been consistent findings that suggest that at least three domains of family factors are influential: family functioning (i.e., conflict, cohesion, relationships, expressiveness), family response to treatment (i.e., illness appraisal/representation, available family resources, family coping strategies), and parental factors (i.e., maternal adjustment/distress, parental overprotection).

Generally, there are a few characteristics of this body of research that should not be overlooked. First, it should be noted that the majority of research available for review has been conducted with children rather than adolescents. All too often adolescents have been entirely excluded from recruited research samples. Undoubtedly, there are a myriad of reasons that could account for this circumstance; regardless, it can be viewed as a significant weakness of this research domain. Research reviewed in this chapter has been limited to that which included samples of children and adolescents or was conducted solely with adolescents. This limitation is important given the developmental context that is unique to, yet common among, chronically ill adolescents.

C. Field (✉)
Department of Psychology, Utah State University, Logan, UT, USA
e-mail: clint.field@usu.edu

W.T. O'Donohue, L.W. Tolle (eds.), *Behavioral Approaches to Chronic Disease in Adolescence*,
DOI 10.1007/978-0-387-87687-0_5,

A second characteristic of this research that is important to consider is the impact of theoretical traditions that have guided this work. Theoretical perspective often permeates research methods and may influence the development of hypotheses, selection of target variables, methods utilized, strategies for analysis of results, and conclusions drawn. A variety of theoretical influences may be discerned within the literature; however, behavioral theory and associated empirical methods are underrepresented in this area of research. The reasons for this are not entirely clear. On the surface, it may seem that this type of research, targeting loosely defined family variables and course of recovery, does not align well with traditional practices of behavioral investigation which tend to emphasize experimental control over well-operationalized variables and clear explication of controlling influences. Yet, behavioral theory has contributed in many ways in the effective research and practice of pediatric psychology and there is no reason to believe that a similar contribution could not occur in this domain of research. At present, however, most of the findings that will be reviewed here reflect a bias in the direction of identifying variables that share an association rather than establishing controlling influences.

As referenced previously, adolescents share some unique developmental characteristics that must be considered in the context of chronic illness and family interaction. A brief discussion of such characteristics follows. Subsequently, research findings describing the relationship between adolescent outcomes and factors associated with family functioning, family response to treatment, and parental factors will be reviewed. In conclusion, treatment implications associated with these findings and apparent limitations present in this domain of research will be considered.

Adolescent Development

The stage of development associated with adolescence is unique and often described by parents as a challenging period of time for the youth and family. Chronic illness within a family system can be devastating, regardless of which member of the family is ill. Perhaps not surprisingly, research has suggested that the combination of these circumstances requires special consideration as all members of the family attempt to strike a precarious balance between managing developmentally typical challenges, facilitating important developmental processes, and being responsive to needs associated with chronic illness.

Adolescence may be thought of as a developmental stage during which youth experience increased yearning for independence and autonomy. Such needs are often expressed socially, suggesting a significant degree of dependence on context that involves rapidly changing relations within peer and family group settings. It has been hypothesized that alterations in these social contexts may jeopardize developmental processes as a result of altered social experiences and unpredictable role shifts among family members (Kazak, Rourke, & Crump, 2003). Additionally, the likelihood of parent–child conflict increases as the adolescent strives for increased autonomy and yet discovers a pragmatic dependence on parents or caregivers for medical care, transportation, and adherence to treatment regimens (Brown, Boeving, LaRosa, & Carpenter, 2006).

Chronic illness in adolescence is often associated with increased responsibility in caring for oneself. However, attending medical appointments, adhering to treatment protocols, learning to cope with pain or discomfort, and making lifestyle adjustments are examples of responsibilities that are qualitatively juxtaposed to that which developing adolescents crave. Compounding the scenario further, adolescents may experience a significant loss of or failure to obtain desired privileges as a result of a chronic illness. Consider the example of an adolescent with end-stage renal disease described by Finkelstein (1993). This particular adolescent required 4 hours of hemodialysis, 3 days a week, and was responsible for managing much of his own treatment. This case illustrated how increased health-related responsibility (i.e., health management, treatment adherence) and associated physical restrictions may be accompanied by a significant decrease in privileges, autonomy, or independence (i.e., time away from friends, school, social activities). Such alterations in typical or expected functioning may be experienced as aversive and may disrupt developmental processes linked to social context (Eiser & Berrenberg, 1995).

The implications of chronic illness on developmental concerns such as these have not been adequately explored or delineated. Additionally, the probability of long-term survival has never been greater as a result of significant advances in medical science and technology. Further study of interactions among developmental, family, and illness factors will be necessary before an accurate understanding of longitudinal effects may be developed.

Family Functioning

A variety of factors associated with the level of family functioning have been found to impact outcomes among chronically ill children. Such factors may be generally placed in domains that emphasize conflict, cohesion, relationships, and expressiveness. Among these, a high degree of cohesion and quality family relationships have been consistently linked to effective adjustment and child adaptation. General findings associated with each of these domains are reviewed in this section.

Family Conflict

Family conflict (FC) may be conceptualized as a variety of processes that are related and can be characterized as negative or ineffective interaction among family members. Overt family discord, poor communication, and ineffective interpersonal styles may be examples of conflict behavior. The presence of FC has been consistently identified as a risk factor for negative treatment outcomes among chronically ill adolescents. Among adolescents, FC has been linked to the display of internalizing behaviors, poor adjustment over time, and less adaptive functioning and appears to be most detrimental when present at time of diagnosis (Hoffman, Rodriguez, Andres, & Novak, 1995). FC has also been linked to the display of behavioral problems and disruptions in general psychological functioning (Drotar, 1997), as well as the experience of stress in chronically ill adolescents, which may mediate additional negative outcomes related to adherence, and well-being (Drotar, 2006).

Family Cohesion

Family cohesion (C) may be the most commonly cited protective factor for chronically ill adolescents in the literature. C has traditionally been conceptualized as appropriate, healthy, and positive interactions within the family system. That C is an important factor impacting the functioning of the chronically ill adolescent is not surprising given that C is a major predictor of optimal family functioning overall (Brown et al., 2006). However, research findings have also suggested that adolescent perception of C may actually be more crucial to the adolescent's adjustment to illness and overall well-being than parent perception of C (Salewski, 2003). High levels of C have also been linked to decreased displays of behavioral problems and healthy psychological functioning, such as self-esteem (Drotar, 1997).

An important age effect has been found in the study of C with chronically ill adolescents. In short, the age of the ill adolescent significantly affects C within the family; as age increases, C has been found to decrease (Holden, Chmielewski, Nelson, & Kager, 1997; Northam, Anderson, Adler, Werther, & Warne, 1996). These data have suggested that optimal C is less likely in older adolescents and that family conflict may be more of a risk factor for this population (Barakat & Kazak, 1999). C has also been shown to impact healthy siblings and is predictive of healthy adjustment and adaptation of other children or adolescents in the family (Kazak et al., 2003).

Family Relationships

Family relationships (FR) have been conceptualized as either protective or risk factors among adolescents with chronic illness. FR can be variously defined, and is best viewed, as a heterogeneous construct reflecting many combinations of multiple family member systems or dyads. However, the most commonly researched family relationship has been the parent–child relationship. Unfortunately, most of the research in the literature has focused solely on mother–child relationships; this has significantly limited understanding of the father's effect on illness outcomes.

The quality of FR has been referenced as a critical protective factor and a predictor of adaptive responses (e.g., effective coping, stress management, adjustment) to adolescent chronic illness (Carlson, Kubiszyn, & Guli, 2004). Positive parent–child relationships characterized by warmth, authoritative parenting style, and positive support (Kazak et al., 2003), especially in combination with child diligence and self-reliance (Barakat & Kazak, 1999; Eiser & Berrenberg, 1995), have been associated with improved treatment outcomes, effective adjustment, and enhanced treatment adherence in chronically ill adolescents.

Unfortunately, FR also functions as a risk factor for the treatment outcomes of chronically ill adolescents. For example, an age effect, similar to that reported for family cohesion, has been described in the context of research examining outcomes and FR. As age of the chronically ill adolescent increases, FR has been predicted to decline in quality and may be predictive of poor treatment adherence (Hanson, Henggeler, & Burghen, 1987). These data have drawn speculation that FR may be more important for younger adolescents than older adolescents.

FR also functions as a risk factor when it is characterized by neglect, physical, sexual, or emotional abuse within the family. Under these circumstances, FR may decrease the adolescent's capacity to cope with a variety of life stressors (Lewis & Vitulano, 2003). Research has yet to be conducted examining the effect of child abuse on treatment outcomes among chronically ill adolescents. However, data have indicated that within this population, significant stress is predictive of poor psychological adjustment to illness (Drotar, 2006).

Expressiveness

Expressiveness (E) within the family also functions as a protective factor for chronically ill adolescent youth. E has typically been operationalized in terms of emotional expression or display and can be conceptualized as falling along a positive–negative continuum that characterizes the emotional climate of the family. E has been identified as a predictor of optimal family functioning and effective functioning of the chronically ill adolescent (Brown et al., 2006). Specifically, positive E has been linked with better adjustment following illness and overall functioning of the chronically ill adolescent (Barakat & Kazak, 1999) as well as improved treatment adherence (Drotar, 2006). Finally, there are many ways that a family may express E; it has been reported that families who promote family recreation to achieve bonding and attachment have observed decreased treatment adherence in their chronically ill adolescent (Drotar, 2006). This finding suggests that a need for further research exists in this domain as characteristics of E, beyond perceived positive and negative dimensions, may yield varied influences on adolescent function.

Family Response to Treatment

In addition to the aspects of family functioning described previously, the manner in which a family responds to treatment, immediately and across time, can influence a range of child responses such as perception, experience of distress, adjustment, and adherence. Illness appraisal, family resources, and coping strategies represent three general categories of family responding that have been identified as impacting adolescent outcomes

Parent–Child Illness Appraisal

Both parent and child appraisals of illness have been found to significantly influence treatment outcomes among chronically ill adolescents. Illness appraisal (IA), also known as illness representation, refers to the personal conceptualization of a disease, including its perceived severity, as well as individual attitudes and ideas related to the experience of the illness. IA is well represented in the professional literature and has consistently been identified as a factor effecting treatment outcomes. The size of the effect of IA has been debated and remains unclear; yet, findings have revealed that general positive outcomes are associated with mild perceptions of severity, a high degree of self-efficacy, and expectations related to positive outcome.

Adolescents' beliefs about their illness may have a greater impact on treatment outcome than the objective severity of their illness and have also been utilized as a predictor of psychological distress and post-traumatic stress disorder symptomatology (Kazak et al., 2003). IA has been established as influential in relation to family system adjustment, as well as individual parent, sibling, and adolescent adjustment to illness (Barakat & Kazak, 1999). Mother IA, in particular, has been demonstrated to have an effect on treatment outcome (Barakat & Kazak, 1999; Brown et al., 2006; Salewski, 2003), and parent IA has shown promise as the overall best predictor of treatment adherence and use of medical services (Brown et al., 2006). However, in certain cases, IA may function as a risk factor for adolescents with chronic illness. For example, the presence of a large disparity between the illness representations of parents, and their chronically ill adolescent, has been found to be predictive of poor treatment adherence (Kazak et al., 2004).

Available Family Resources

Family resources (R) may be variably defined, but generally have been used as a reference for the availability of social support networks, financial resources, and other practical resources (e.g., transportation, location, access to hospital personnel). When available, the presence of R has been shown to impact treatment outcomes for chronically ill adolescents with greater amounts of resources being linked to improved outcomes.

Social support has been found to be a key R in the literature of chronically ill adolescents. Low social support (as well as low perceived social support) can make adaptation to an adolescent's chronic illness more difficult. Low levels of social isolation, high social support, and high satisfaction related to social support have yielded correlations with improved levels of adjustment to adolescent illness. Also, significant maternal social support has been linked to effective family expressiveness which, as mentioned previously, functions as a protective factor (Barakat & Kazak, 1999) and can also affect the adjustment and adaptation of healthy siblings in the family system in a positive way (Kazak et al., 2003).

The presence of adequate financial resources functions as a protective factor for adjustment to adolescent chronic illness (Barakat & Kazak, 1999) and may be indirectly linked to a variety of other factors that promote positive outcomes. Similarly, practical resources available in the family promote the social competence of chronically ill adolescents (Drotar, 2006), although the exact mechanisms of function related to practical resources have not been delineated and likely vary with context. Given the critical nature of social competence and the hypothesized influence of social contexts on adolescent youth, the nature of this effect warrants additional exploration. In sum, families with greater R are more likely to experience resiliency in the presence of most life stressors. The available evidence base has suggested that this relationship also applies to the chronic illness of an adolescent.

Family Coping Strategies

Family coping strategies also impact treatment outcomes of chronically ill adolescents. Effective coping has often been conceptualized as communication about concerns and information sharing about the illness within the family, appropriate stress management, open communication with medical staff, and maintenance of family structure in the presence of stressors.

A relationship between effective coping techniques and family adjustment has been consistently observed in the literature. Specifically for mothers, open communication with medical staff and a high degree of family structure and integration has been shown to promote family cohesion, which is predictive of overall positive treatment outcomes (McCubbin et al., 1983). Families who develop and maintain family tradition and related rituals or structured daily routines (i.e., consistent religious activities, household chore consistency, consistent daily schedules) are more likely to exhibit treatment adherence and appear to elicit more effective treatment management practices in their chronically ill adolescent (Kazak et al., 2003). Generally, families who employ effective, positive, and healthy coping strategies are more likely to adjust well to an adolescent's chronic illness and function positively as a family system (Drotar, 2006).

Parental Factors

Overall family functioning and positive family responding to illness have been demonstrated to promote a variety of positive outcomes among adolescents. However, the family may be further parsed into subunits (e.g., parental alliance, parent–child dyad, sibling constellations), and certain parent variables have been examined in relation to their impact on the child with chronic health concerns. Maternal psychological functioning and parental overprotection are two categories of parent variables that are reviewed here.

Maternal Psychological Adjustment and Distress

Maternal psychological adjustment and maternal distress refer to the emotional and psychological state of the mother of the chronically ill adolescent and have been shown to have an effect on treatment outcomes. Specifically, mood state and the degree of emotional distress of the mother has been observed to positively and negatively affect the adjustment, functioning, and adaptation of all children in the family, including healthy siblings (Kazak et al., 2003). Further, it has been observed that chronically ill adolescents who are maladjusted to their illness are more likely to have mothers with poor psychological adjustment than adolescents who are well adjusted to their illness (Drotar, 1997); however, the direction of this effect has not been established. Overall, knowledge regarding the influence of parental psychological adjustment and experience of distress on adolescent responding is quite limited and almost entirely based on research conducted with mothers, which highlights a serious shortcoming of this research domain.

Parental Overprotection

Parental overprotection (PO) of chronically ill adolescents has also been observed to impact treatment outcomes. PO can be conceptualized as high parental investment or involvement in the well-being of the adolescent and is often operationalized as overmonitoring. PO may also be termed miscarried helping. High rates of PO have been associated with family conflict (Anderson & Coyne, 1991). As previously discussed, family conflict may be highly detrimental to chronically ill adolescent adjustment as it may place additional stress on the adolescent during the illness (Barakat & Kazak, 1999; Drotar, 2006). High levels of paternal PO, in particular, are concerning as this has been described as a significant predictor of perceived loss of self-control among adolescents (Mayes, Handford, Kowalski, & Schaefer, 1988) and, as mentioned previously, such perceptions have been associated with concerns regarding treatment adherence.

Conclusions and Future Directions

Investigation of family factors that influence outcomes among adolescents with chronic illness has clearly increased over the past few decades. Yet, this remains a domain of research in need, a point that is punctuated by at least three factors. First, adolescent youth have often been excluded from studies examining the impact of family factors on treatment outcome. Future research should aim to better clarify the risk and protective factors, specifically for families with chronically ill adolescents (Kazak et al., 2003). Second, the period of adolescence is developmentally unique, which raises questions about the degree to which child and adult findings may generalize to this clinical population. Finally, with advances in medical science, survivorship has greatly increased among children with chronic illness, making it more important to understand the long-term of factors that could influence treatment outcomes and developmental processes during adolescence.

To date, much of the research conducted in this domain may be best characterized as exploratory in nature. While awareness of specific variables that are reliably associated with certain outcomes has improved, attempts to operationalize, isolate, and control pertinent variables have rarely been undertaken. Investigations of the impact of specific family factors on treatment outcome have yielded beneficial findings although conclusions regarding several factors may be best construed as preliminary at this time. Emerging from past investigation has been increased awareness that observed effects may be context specific and that impact on outcome may vary in magnitude and direction depending on certain factors, such as age. The sheer number of family variables that may impact outcomes, when combined with the context-specific factors that may yield meaningful interactions and differential outcomes, yields a daunting amount of investigatory work that appears to remain.

Nonetheless, there are some very specific areas of research that must be addressed, several of which have been previously identified. As previously discussed, fathers are largely ignored in the literature, with almost all parental research focusing solely on mothers (Kazak et al., 2003). There are few longitudinal studies investigating the effect of family factors on treatment outcomes over time (Barakat & Kazak, 1999), and there is little known about how family factors effect treatment outcomes during illness change or transitions (i.e., severity increase or treatment change; Drotar, 1997). A common practice in the field of pediatric psychology has been to examine outcomes in relation to specific illnesses and while such research is certainly beneficial, this condition carries with it challenges in generalizing effects across illnesses (i.e., family influence on cancer vs. sickle cell disease vs. cystic fibrosis). More research is needed examining how research conclusions may apply to multiple adolescent diagnoses.

Implications for Treatment

The primary value of this research largely resides in applied domains. Promotion of adjustment, level of functioning over time, adherence, and psychological well-being is often the focus of clinical work and the family factors that have been reviewed have been shown to reliably influence these outcomes. At a minimum, advances in our understanding of these family factors should influence case conceptualization, treatment access points, and the degree to which family may be involved in or even targeted by treatment. It might be argued that assessment and treatment have historically attempted to focus on the "context-less child". However, children function within contexts and interact with influential others; these factors should be fully incorporated in our clinical work. Within the practice of pediatric psychology, social ecological perspectives have been helpful in emphasizing the child within the systems that they operate. However, there is limited evidence that prevention and intervention efforts have fully incorporated these factors. As a broader profession, we continue to move in the direction of embracing and promoting evidence-based practices which have at their essence an integrated emphasis on effective practice and sensitivity in understanding the patient in their unique context. In addition to the basic research being conducted, there is an evident need to begin critically examining how family factors may best be targeted in the context of prevention and intervention.

References

Anderson, B. J., & Coyne, J. C. (1991). "Miscarried helping" in the families of children and adolescents with chronic disease. In J. H. Johnson & S. B. Johnson (Eds.), *Advances in child health psychology* (pp. 166–177). Gainesville: University of Florida Press.

Barakat, L. P., & Kazak A. E. (1999). Family issues. In R. T. Brown (Ed.), *Cognitive aspects of chronic illness in children* (pp. 333–354). New York: Guilford.

Bronfenbrenner, U. (1979). *The ecology of human development*. Cambridge, MA: Harvard University Press.

Brown, R. T. (2002). Society of pediatric psychology presidential address: Toward a social ecology of pediatric psychology. *Journal of Pediatric Psychology, 27*, 191–201.

Brown, R. T., Boeving, A., LaRosa, A., & Carpenter, L. A. (2006). Health and chronic illness. In D. A. Wolfe & E. J. Mash (Eds.), *Behavioral and emotional disorders in adolescents: Nature, assessment, and treatment* (pp. 505–531). New York: Guilford Press.

Carlson, C., Kubiszyn, T., & Guli, L. (2004). Consultation with caregivers and families. In R. T. Brown & N. J. Mahwah (Eds.). *Handbook of pediatric psychology in school settings* (pp. 617–635). New Jersey: Lawrence Erlbaum.

Drotar, D. (1997). Relating parent and family functioning to the psychological adjustment of children with chronic health conditions: What have we learned? What do we need to know? *Journal of Pediatric Psychology, 22*, 149–165.

Drotar, D. (2006). Theoretical models and frameworks for psychological intervention. In D. Drotar (Ed.), *Psychological interventions in childhood chronic illness* (pp. 33–55). Washington, DC: American Psychological Association.

Eiser, C., & Berrenberg, J. L. (1995). Assessing the impact of chronic disease on the relationship between parents and their adolescents. *Journal of Psychosomatic Research, 39*, 109–114.

Finkelstein, J. W. (1993). Familial influences on adolescent health. In R. M. Lerner (Ed.), *Early adolescence: Perspective on research, policy, and intervention* (pp. 11–126). New Jersey: Lawrence Erlbaum.

Hanson, C. L., Henggeler, S. W., & Burghen, G. A. (1987). Model of associations between psychological variables and health outcome measures of adolescents with IDDM. *Diabetes Care, 10*, 752–758.

Hoffman, R. G., Rodriguez, J. R., Andres, J. M., & Novak, D. A. (1995). Moderating effects of family functioning on the social adjustment of children with liver disease. *Children's Health Care, 24*, 107–117.

Holden, E., Chmielewski, D., Nelson, C., & Kager, V. (1997). Controlling for general and disease-effects in child and family adjustments to chronic illness. *Journal of Pediatric Psychology, 22*, 15–27.

Kazak, A. (1989). Families of chronically ill children: A systems and social ecological model of adaptation and challenge. *Journal of Consulting and Clinical Psychology, 57*, 25–30.

Kazak, A. E., McClure, K. S., Alderfer, M. A., Hwang, W. T., Crump, T. A., Le, L. T., et al. (2004). Cancer-related parental beliefs: The Family Illness Beliefs Inventory (FIBI). *Journal of Pediatric Psychology, 29*, 531–542.

Kazak, A. E., Rourke, M. T., & Crump, T. A. (2003). Families and other systems in pediatric psychology. In M. C. Roberts (Ed.), *Handbook of pediatric psychology* (3rd ed., pp. 159–175). New York: Guilford Press.

Lewis, M., & Vitulano, L. A. (2003). Biopsychosocial issues and risk factors in the family when the child has a chronic illness. *Child and Adolescent Psychiatric Clinics of North America, 12*, 398–399.

Mayes, S. D., Handford, H. A., Kowalski, C., & Schaefer, J. H. (1988). Parent attitudes and child personality traits in hemophilia: A six-year longitudinal study. *International Journal of Psychiatry in Medicine, 18*, 339–355.

McCubbin, H. I., McCubbin, M. A., Patterson, J. M., Cauble, A. E., Wilson, L. R., & Warwick, W. (1983). CHIP – Coping Health Inventory for Parents: An assessment of parental coping patterns in the care of the chronically ill child. *Journal of Marriage and the Family, 45*, 359–370.

Northam, E., Anderson, P., Adler, R., Werther, G., & Warne, G. (1996). Psychosocial and family functioning in children with insulin-dependent diabetes at diagnosis and one year later. *Journal of Pediatric Psychology, 21*, 699–717.

Salewski, C. (2003). Illness representations in families with a chronically ill adolescent: Differences between family members and impact on patients' outcome variables. *Journal of Health Psychology, 8*, 587–598.

Ethics and the Teen Patients

Michael Lavin

Psychologists treating sick teenagers must decide how they should behave toward them. The question has a technical and a moral dimension. First, the psychologist must decide whether he has the competencies required to provide good enough assessment or care to the child. Second, there are a number of moral difficulties that rarely occur in the treatment of adults that are routine in the assessment and treatment of adolescents. For example, when treating adults, psychologists do not have to obtain permission of the parents to proceed or expect to have contact with the parents as treatment progresses. Adults entitled to a level of privacy in their treatment that minors do not enjoy. Law and custom have created a set of expectation and practices that limit the ability of minors to decide matters relating to their treatment. At the extreme, adults may deny that a teen has the capacity to consent to treatment or non-treatment, though teen may have ability to assent to them. The reason is that consent, especially once conjoined to the idea of being informed, requires that an informed consenter have had (a) an adequate comprehension of (b) what is conveyed about a proposed treatment, and that he (c) willingly and (d) without coercion (e) authorize treatment or reject it (Beauchamp & Childress, 2008). Adults and therapists are often skeptical of a teen's ability to meet these five conditions. When teens are sick, especially if their infirmity is grave and chronic, adults tend to gravitate to an even deeper skepticism about their decisional capacity. Furthering the tradition of skepticism about teens having what it takes to guide their own treatment is the economics of treatment. In the archetypical case, teens depend on their parents to pay for treatment.

Developmental facts reinforce skepticism about the possibility of treating teens as mini adults. Sick adults may retreat to earlier developmental levels when challenged by unpleasant experiences, including illness. Teens may do the same; however, the adult, at least if mentally healthy, has attained levels of mature personality organization that most teens lack. Psychologists can rely on this reservoir of adult strength during their treatment. An adult tends to have more "observing ego" to rely on than an ordinary teen. This is a defeasible claim. Foolish adults may have less maturity than wise teens; however, the ordinary presumption is that adults have a greater capacity for autonomous choices than teens.

To repeat, a familiar clinical observations support the view that teens lack something that adults have when it comes to personality organization. First, as Freud noticed, children, teens, and adults, when faced with life's stresses, rely on coping strategies that Freud re-conceptualized as defenses. Some defenses arise at earlier developmental stages than others. So, an infant may have little to rely on other than tears to get its way when anxious. A teen might assault somebody. An anxious adult might anticipate a crisis or make jokes about it. If environmental challenges are great enough, teens and adults may "regress" to earlier stages of maturity and rely on defenses typical of earlier developmental stages, as when they become immobile and tearful. Second, authors of organized psychiatry's Diagnostic and Statistical Manual of Mental Disorders (DSM-TR)

M. Lavin (✉)
Private Practice, Washington, DC, USA
e-mail: mlavin1952@earthlink.net

W.T. O'Donohue, L.W. Tolle (eds.), *Behavioral Approaches to Chronic Disease in Adolescence*,
DOI 10.1007/978-0-387-87687-0_6, © Springer Science+Business Media, LLC 2009

(American Psychiatric Association, 2000) have cautioned against over diagnosing personality disorders in children and teens, in part because neither children nor teens have attained stable personality organizations. What it comes to in practice, for the working psychologists, is that children, including teens, are not mini adults. Teens are presumed to lack characteristics that make typical adults sovereigns of their own treatment. At the same time, wise psychologists know that teens are not docile children. They are old enough to have strong preferences about their treatment and to care about their privacy. They may also have the capacity to make wise decisions about their own treatment, whatever their guardians or courts may think. As with adults the forging of a good therapeutic alliance is an element of effective treatment. Protecting teens from too much adult intrusion into their therapy is a therapist's among routine clinical tasks.

The Ethics of Treating Teens

Many psychologists look to the American Psychological Association's Ethics Code (American Psychological Association [APA], 2002) to guide them on matters of professional ethics, as if compliance with it settles whether they have behaved decently. The Code has a prominent place in the moral deliberations of psychologists for at least two reasons.

First, if they are members of the American Psychological Association (hereafter APA), they have specific demands placed on their professional conduct by the Code (APA, 2002). The Code specifies that, for example, psychologists must obtain informed consent from patients to treat them. Failure to meet a standard places a psychologist in violation of the Code and subject to discipline by the APA. The Code also continues "aspirational" principles that are to guide psychologists in their professional conduct.

Second, even when psychologists are not a member s of the APA, perhaps because they wisely affiliated with the American Psychological Society instead, Boards of Psychological Examiners may rely on the Code to assess the professional conduct of psychologists licensed in their jurisdiction. Courts may also look to the Code for information on the professions conduct.

In addition to its Code, the APA also publishes guidelines for psychologists that advocate for particular forms of conduct toward particular classes of patients or in relation to grave matters like pronoun choice. And of course the references to the APA's Code and guidelines are merely illustrative. Physicians, nurses, psychoanalysts, and social workers all have ethics Codes of their own that replicate the previous points about professional conduct. Given the state of the helping professions, Codes and guidelines are prone to encumber moral deliberations of any professionals trying to decide how to conduct themselves.

Despite the utility of Codes for membership associations, licensing boards, and courts, they have limited use when a psychologist seeks, for example, to determine how to be with a particular patient. Moral life is vast. Much of what matters in moral and professional life has no codified answer, though the impulse to create codified answers is perennial. Examples abound. The APA's Council of Representatives (2006) has adopted an official ban on psychologists helping to torture prisoners. The absence of an explicit proscription in the Code pains them. Council members wished to have and campaigned to have the APA on record as opposed to its members helping to torture people because the behavior of several psychologists during the interrogation s of prisoners held by the US military enflamed them. These alleged rogue psychologists are also military officers. It seemed to distress enraged members of the council that the current ethics Code does not permit the excommunication of torturers. But, then, why should it? The Code does not have among its standards a prohibition on members shooting dead their patients, or even worse, fellow members. But murder and torture are crimes. They are also grave moral wrongs. In some religious traditions, they are also mortal sins. Members are prohibited from torturing, for example, not because it is wrong for psychologists to torture but because it is wrong for anybody to torture. A Code is not intended to be an inventory of the moral wrongs that professionals might commit while doing their work.

In any event, Codes have numerous limitations that will make them of limited use in guiding clinicians in their work with sick teens. Perhaps the best way to use the Code is as a compliance check. After moral deliberation or assessment, psychologists can refer to the Codes and relevant guidelines to determine whether their conclusions conform to the Code. If what they believe is permissible or a duty is at odds with the Code, they then can rethink the matter to decide whether they or the Code is wrong.

If Codes and guidelines provide limited guidance to clinicians, what is the alternative? To begin, nothing equals having a virtuous character. As Aristotle noticed, people trained to be virtuous, conduct themselves than people without a sound upbringing. Second, steeping oneself in the world's great literary, philosophical, and religious traditions helps. Great literatures make available a range of cases that exceeds anything a single person can experience. Third, thinking about cases with an eye to moral details helps. Focus on a case will be the procedure in this chapter. It will be a literary case.

Peter Shaffer's *Equus*(1977) is an apt heuristic for coming to terms with the moral complexities of treating teens. For readers unfamiliar with the plot the action unfolds as a psychiatrist, Martin Dysart, seeks to understand why a 17-year –old teen, named Allan Strang, committed a crime of hideous violence. While in a stable at night, Strang had used a hoof pick to blind six horses. There is no doubt that the boy did blind the horses. Although he is in his late teens, the court did not try him as an adult. Instead, an aid of the court managed to convince the judge to turn him over to Dr. Dysart for assessment and treatment. The psychiatrist is middle-aged, with difficulties of his own. His approach to the boy is psychodynamic. He does not make a sharp separation between assessment and treatment, but like Winnicott (Phillips, 1989) proceeds as if psychotherapy is an extended anamnesis.

As often happens with very sick patients, the boy's psychological distress interferes with his forming a relationship with Dysart. When Dysart first meets Strang, the boy is speaking gibberish sprinkled with jingles from commercial jingles. His initial presentation has a psychotic quality prevents Dysart from doing a routine intake interview. Although Dysart does inform the boy of his most immediate plan of placing him in a private room and asks him to visit with him again the next day, he also makes his first therapeutic intervention. As a parting observation, he asks Strang which of his parents, if not both, refuses to let him watch television. There is no clear basis for this intervention. At least it is mysterious how the boy can understand what has led Dysart to ask his question. As it turns out, the boy's father does forbid him to watch television.

This Beginning

In this initial meeting between Dysart and Strang, three ethical challenges have already made an appearance. First, although no mention of it, there is a question of whose agent Dysart is. Second, although the boy's condition makes getting his assent to his assessment and treatment impossible, he never explicitly assents to treatment. Third, aside from technical considerations, the morality of Dysart's intervention is at least suspect.

For whom does Dysart work? During the play, although Strang is never told so, Dysart has qualms about what he is doing. An officer of the court had approached him with a plea to help the boy. If he declines to help, the boy may well go to prison. The magistrate hopes that treatment will avoid that outcome. The implicit goal, that Dysart laments, is that Strang become "normal." Strang's current orientation to the world will not do. He is to become more like the rest of the human herd. Strang never identifies being normal as among his goals. Nor does he even assent to a plan of treatment, though readers are free to imagine that a nurse or some other backstage artiste arranged for him to sign some forms. Still, the relationship of a patient to what society's agents wish is perilous. The alcoholic may like his drinking. The blind or deaf child may be content enough to stay that way or his parents may believe that cochlear or retinal implants will destroy his special qualities or subvert their relationship with their child. Perhaps it would be better for the therapist to glide by these matters in silence. The boy's treatment is a Hobson's choice. He can accept the goal of the court or be punished. And even if the coercive dimensions of a sick child entering treatment are brushed aside, how is a child, or anybody else, to appraise a treatment that aims to change his total experience of the world?

Nor are the problems of agency limited to treatment goals. The state is paying for treatment. At one point, Strang becomes enraged at Dysart for having ended a session early. The boy complains that Dysart gets good money to treat him. With an adult patient, if the therapist ends an hour early because the patient is refusing to cooperate, the patient may refuse to pay for the hour. In fact, adult patients may withhold payment. The child is denied this recourse. He is also at the mercy of his insurers or his parents, if they stop paying for treatment the child likes.

Because the parents pay or must provide proxy consent to treatment, they have a larger role than would be typical in the treatment of adults. If a court has involved itself, the judge or officers of the court may wish to receive reports on the patient's "progress." Again, the interests of the child may or may not be served. It may be sanctimoniously proclaimed that the child's proxies have an obligation to decide in the child's "best interest," but the idea of a child's best interests a cipher for all manner of reasons. In the best case, the child and proxy may agree on what they think is best for the child. Their agreement does not prevent them from being wrong. The best interest standard may also be obnoxiously tyrannical. By what right does a sick child's interests make a bonfire of all other interests in even so negligible a unit as a nuclear family? Do a sick child's interests entitle him to transplants from brothers and sisters, or do *their* best interests place limits on what others owe a child? Airy talk about interests ignores the grim truth that interests collide. They compete. Loving parents know full well that they must balance interests within a family. Parents may *sacrifice* to make a happy child's life better, but, aside from the guilt besotted parent, nobody believes that every bottle of Beefeaters must be forsaken to put a few dollars more into their children's college funds. When all is said and done, what parents, proxies, and therapist owe a child is good enough care. It is unfortunate that even determining what is good enough verges on being impossible in complicated clinical work. And without reliance on force, there may be no solutions in complicated cases

I, for example, am willing to overrule the objections of a young Jehovah's Witness to being transfused. I am not sure I wish courts to side with me, even if I go to court to force a transfusion. And why? It is because I believe the opposition to blood transfusions is an ignorant, lethal superstition. However, my opposition hinges on skepticism to supernaturalism that neither the child nor its parents in these cases shares. If they are right and I am wrong, it is I, not they, who is pressing for a treatment contrary to the child's good enough interests. Within time limits of a hard case, Fabian hopes of a happy accommodation are seldom satisfied. Anybody seeking more information on the topic of deciding for others is well served to read Buchanan and Brock (1990).

These difficulties over agency permeate the consent and assent process as well in hard cases. According to the standard lore, clinicians obtain a competent patient's informed consent by providing him or his proxies with a diagnosis and a description of the proposed treatment, along with its probable benefits and risk. The alternatives, including their risks and benefits, are canvassed as well (Beauchamp & Childress, 2008; see also Brock, 1993, especially Chaps. 1 and 2). Clinicians also invite the patient to ask questions, if they have any. They finally obtain authorization to proceed with their proposed treatment or to rely on one of the alternatives that may include doing nothing.

In the case of minors, the law ordinarily rejects contention that minors are competent to give informed consent. So, as already mentioned, a proxy gives it for them. For many chronic illnesses that afflict teens, clinicians can enact the consent scenario. The teen has a chronic condition, for example, asthma or diabetes, whose physiopathology understood. Well articulated and studies treatments exist. Even if the treatments do no more than manage a chronic condition, clinicians have a treasure house of information about many chronic diseases and their treatments. Despite the vicissitudes of the orthodox consent process, it makes sense in these routine medical contexts.

Matters are less happy in regard to psychopathology. It is instructive that the dominant diagnostic system proclaims itself to etiologically neutral. One of the central premises of medicine, the junction to treat causes not symptoms, is difficult to nail down because it is so difficult to get anybody to agree on what a cause in mental illness is. I can think of no instance in psychopathology, for example, that comes close to the knowledge that exists in cardiology. Cardiologists know how much blood a heart squirts out of it and how inflow of blood it receives. If there is a measurable discrepancy between the two, cardiologist can tell what constellation of symptoms the patients will develop. If the problem is uncorrected, he will develop congestive heart failure. Understanding the underlying problem allows the cardiologist to identify treatments that ought to work and even what the best treatment would be, that is, something that restored the normal balance between inflow and outflow of blood in a patient's heart.

Causal understanding of mechanisms is conspicuously absent in the study of psychopathology, and it can make the consent process in the cases like the one in *Equus* jejune. Similar problems can arise in medical cases where the patient's constellation of signs and symptoms confronts his doctors with a medical novelty. In the case of Strang, what is the patient being treated for? Years ago, Jerome Frank (Frank & Frank, 1993) proposed that patients fall into five overlapping groups: the psychotic, the neurotic, the shattered, the misbehaving, and the seekers. The patient has come to Dysart's office because of a spectacular, singular instance of misbehavior. He has gouged out the eyes of horses. He is not the routine, drug-addled juvenile delinquent. Even if Dysart were treating a teen with a chronic drug problem, clinicians, even lacking causal understanding of drug addiction, know enough about an array of correlations to enable them to fashion a set of familiar interventions aimed at getting the teen to stop using drugs. The consent process has a way of proceeding down familiar channels.

Strang's case is a singular one. One might attempt to assimilate it to familiar categories by pretending the main problem is that he had a psychotic break or even that he is shattered after committing a sequence of horrific deeds while psychotic, the best diagnosis when all the facts come in. In truth, whatever the correct diagnosis, and even in the record of the play, Dysart sees the boy because he has, to put it gently, misbehaved. What is the treatment for this misbehavior? What is its goal? What are its risks and benefits? What are the alternatives? It seems plain that nobody knows the answers to these questions. Control agents have a simple enough project. They wish the psychiatrist to intervene to learn if he is likely to do anything like he did in the future (whatever that might mean) and whether he can be treated to make it very unlikely he will do anything like he did in the future. Given the circumstances, it seems impossible for anything like an *informed* consent to take place, unless one makes the gamey move of pretending that informing the patient of the absence of scientific knowledge in cases like his counts giving the patient the information he needs. If a therapist wishes to engage in the pretense of obtaining the patient's assent and the patient's proxy's assent, so be it. The legal ritual may be unavoidable, but let nobody be confused about what a hallow sham of the orthodox process this is.

At least one other moral question arises in the initial interchange between Dysart and his patient. He asks, as gifted clinician's have a gift for doing, a prescient question. In response to the patients avalanche of telly jingles to ward off Dysart's queries, Dysart asks which parent or both denied him permission to watch television. The boy latter confesses that his father forbid TV, though his mother colluded with the boy to get around the proscription. Perhaps most people will view this intervention as morally indifferent. Whether it is a good intervention hinges on non-moral, technical considerations. So, if other psychologists disliked this intervention, they might complain that Dysart made inadequate preparation. He gave the patient no way to observe how his own mind works (Gray, 1994, especially Chaps. 1 and 3).

Although technical observations interventions have a central place in teaching clinicians, techniques often have unexamined moral implications. In the case of Dysart's intervention, and in subsequent interventions he makes as well, as in giving or withholding cigarettes or proclaiming what the consequences of an intervention will be, he is wielding power. From the perspective of power, Strang also uses power. His jingles are defense that also defeat efforts by Dysart to pierce his privacy. Brody (1993) canvasses vagaries of the ethics of power, including taxonomy of power as aimed, owned, and shared. One problem with the initial interactions between Dysart and Strang has to do with an insufficiency of owned and shared power. As happens with patients in chronic care, clinicians and patients struggle with conflicting demands. Teens with PKU or diabetes may resist the dietary demands placed on them by powerful adults, with teens prone to value their autonomy interests over their welfare interests. When this happens, clinicians tend to evade the moral dimension of the battle by transforming it into a concern over treatment compliance, as if their own lack of compliance with the patient's desires posed no clinical or moral problems. The problem escalates when clinicians deform their practice by becoming more interested in technical problems of treating the condition than in treating the patient.

To sum up, the initial stage of a sick teens treatment routinely faces three problems. First, therapists face problems relating to whose agent they are. Second, they have to manage a consent process that involves them in obtaining a proxy's consent and, if things go well, the teen's assent. Third, therapists must manage power. They must do what they can to target their power well, to own that they have it, and to share it. Therapists must resolve other problems as well during, and even after, the initial stages of therapy, but these problems are subject to neglect.

The Middle Game

Sooner or later, psychologists treating teens are likely to meet parents. Fit parents love their children. They wish to assist in helping an ailing teen get well. If they are astute parents, they know facts about their teen that savvy psychologists know how to use. So it is in *Equus*. After establishing a therapeutic alliance with Strang — an alliance that arises in part from Dysart's suspect intervention of asking which parent had banned watching television – Dysart can begin to pierce Strang's character armor. Once Strang has begun to talk, Dysart discerns something about Strang's relationship to horses requires more knowledge than he can readily get from Strang alone. And of course the parents also wish to involve themselves in Strang's treatment. His blinding of the horses has inflicted a deep hurt on his parents. It is also during this period that the intensity of Dysart's countertransference becomes visible, as well as its hindrance of Dysart having a clear-cut commitment to making Strang "normal." In any case, Dysart does begin meeting informants.

Dysart meets Strang's mother on a Sunday. She is without the boy's father, who is at work as a printer. He learns the boy's father is a man hostile to religion. Despite the hostility of Strang's father to religion, his mother gives him religious training. Early on Strang developed a fascination with horses after his father made him a gift of a handsome calendar with a powerful white horse on it. It became a fixation point for the boy, a venerated object. Besides being a gift of his father, the horse became a vehicle of religious instruction, with the mother using it to teach the boy Bible verses that exalt the horse. The boy's experience of the horse appears to have led to an inner representation of the horse in which sexuality, power, and religious impulses fuse. The fusion includes a fusion of the horse with the crucified Christ. Oedipal themes are discernible as well. In fact, when Dysart does interview the father, he discovers the boy fashioned a bridle for himself. He places the bridle in his mouth while whipping himself during sessions of onanistic identification with his horse-gods.

The play's storyline's details matter less than the ethics of the interaction. Although Strang is the identified patient, his parents have entered into the therapeutic matrix. Psychologists, upon arrival of a teen's family, co-opted into the larger family struggles. They must consider how the mother and son collude against the father. They must consider the role of each member of the family and what, if anything, they will do to change it, even though (officially) only the teen is in treatment. Perhaps it is unsurprising that some doctors do call themselves Family Practitioners. Family practitioners tend to operate on the theory that the family is the unit of treatment, even if the law designates a particular member of the family as the patient. Family-systems therapists are also familiar with this idea of a corporate patient. All the same, as proxies consent to treatment for their teen children, legal and medical custom gravitates toward focusing on the treatment consequences to the young patient while ignoring the impact of treatment on the family, despite what family-systems clinicians may prefer.

Nothing Dysart does with Strang's family moves outside this familiar and dominant individualism. As Dysart comes into contact with a range of key people in his patient's life, his patient's concerns have a centrality that may be contrary to the interests and well being of these people, but nobody mentions this to them.

In fact, Dysart, as do many therapists, imposes his power to alter the distribution of power between parent and child. So, when Strang's mother slaps him for giving him a look she hates, Dysart banishes her from his ward. The enraged woman then observes how everything in therapy world is targeted on the "poor" boy. She savagely asks if she must blind animals to get any staff sympathy. When Dysart undertakes the predictable negation of her perception, she rejoins with a lengthy observation that the hospital staff has lost a moral perspective on her son's problems. They have buried any concern they might have felt for the boy's family in favor of him. She accuses the staff of robbing him of responsibility for his own actions. Although chronic illness in teens seldom has the clear moral dimensions of Strang's case, readers may do well to ask how often a child with a chronic illness becomes a resource hog in the family structure. Sick teens may leave their families weary and angry at the demands of the teen's condition. Blandishments by staff to families to understand the medical necessities may well seem to family members as driven by a crude utilitarian scheme of justice. The utilitarian calculus may permit therapists to feel they act justly when other people's trifling aspirations for benefits like guitar lessons are sacrificed to the teen's care, but a brother deprived of lessons by his sibling's medical necessity may favor a rather more complicated conception of justice than the crude utilitarianism invoked by therapists like Dysart or philosophers like Singer (1979). Engelhardt (1986) is forthright in his denial of this perspective, noting that much of what happens to sick people of all ages is a misfortune that may evoke acts of charity from others rather an injustice crying out for correction.

Dysart's own insecurities color his interpretation of Strang's predicament. Dysart believes he is too domesticated. The intensity of Strang's bestial passion stirs him as he compares it to his own normal life. Hostility to the Normal, coupled with a disdain for his own domesticated life, distort Dysart's response to his patient. For example, Dysart has a dream of being a High Priest sacrificing children by cutting out their entrails in conformance to local, ancient custom, but the job sickens him, as does his own excavation of the minds of troubled patients to restore them to normality. In an effort to secure Strang's cooperation, he recounts the dream to Strang. Although in the play, the intervention works, that success is the dramatist's decision. Many psychologists would be aghast at parleying self-disclosure for a patient's cooperation. Of course the difficulties of working with very ill patients encourage therapeutic departures from common practice. The departures may be presented as innovations, but from the moral point of view these departures may have less to do with pushing the frontiers of science than indulging the passions of a frustrated therapist.

Dysart, unlike the boy's parents, has an envious admiration for Strang's sex-suffused horse worship. He compares it with his own feeble devotion to unconstrained passions of Hellenic antiquity. Dysart has an admiration for a capacity to worship without the hesitation lost to him by too easy a familiarity with modern science. He contrasts his own well-scheduled excursions to Greece with Strang's riding a horses naked, then kissing the spit off slobbering equine faces. His taste for primitivism puts his inner life in turmoil over that taste's incompatibility with his state-financed mission of making sick people normal. During one soliloquy, he laments his work on behalf of Normality, ridiculing his successful cases for letting his work doom them to a drone's life of bread and circuses. Although the dramatist casts Dysart's cliché of whining highbrows in gorgeous language, the moral conflict between Dysart and representatives of the Ordinary is plain. He is not, in any ordinary sense, a man that parents would wish to have treating their children. All the same, the tension is familiar. Psychologists tend to belong to society's Brahmin classes. Parents may lack the sophistication to express this idea, but they do from time to time sense, it, as when Strang's mother observes how the hospital treats parents as pathogens. The moral is that psychologists do tend to ignore how their therapeutic goals tend to ride roughshod over family dynamics, though sometimes therapists do seek to deny the charge by contending that it is part of their creed to attend to "diversity, " a watery term that never seems ready to respect the desires of old-fashioned, conventional parents for their children. Unlike Dysart, Strang's parents exhibit no inhibitions about their son becoming a normal boy; however, great Dysart's reverence for the abnormal may be. It is not Dysart's son who will pay to price for having a stigma of what

Goffman (1963) characterizes as a spoiled identity. If made normal, Strang does have the hope that his stigma will lack visibility (Goffman, 1963, pp. 48–51). Unlike a boy with a cane, Strang's stigma of animal abuser and bestialist will be invisible, except to those in the know.

Neither of the moral problems under survey prevents Dysart from doing his job. What they may do is make him readier to criticize the parents and to exile a mother. They might make him harsher with a family whose damage to Strang was inadvertent.

One other difficulty emerges as the ring of Dysart's informants expands. It becomes more difficult to protect their confidentiality. In particular, Dysart learns of the existence of a girl whose attraction to the boy led to his blinding horses. As it turns out, Strang had taken a job at the stable, where he did outstanding work, despite his eccentricities like refusing to ride horses during the day at work. A girl at the stables, a bit older and more experienced than him, takes an interest in him. They go on a date. As it happens, they make the date risqué by going to an adult theatre. While there, they encounter Strang's father. It is manifest that his father is a customer, but he denies it. He orders the boy home. Strang ignores his father. Instead, he and the girl go to the stable where they attempt intercourse. Strang becomes fearful of being observed by the horses that he feels he is betraying by having sex with the girl. Fearful of equine judgment, he is unable to achieve an erection. The girl is a model of compassionate, understanding, but he imagines the horses have witnessed them. After ordering her to leave, he blinds the horses.

How is it possible for Dysart to use this information without damaging the relationship between the boy and the girl? How is he to use the information without a non-psychotic patient knowing where it came from? In the play, no problem over this emerges. In life, it is a routine part of the interaction between professionals and sick teens. People do tell on teens. Their clandestine lives are unveiled, for informants or, from a different perspective, stooges reveal much about their own secret doings when speaking to the doctor. And how is a therapist like Dysart to sequester what he learns from informants to protect their privacy while serving his patient well. Small wonder many therapist have qualms about accepting friends of patients or more than one family member into individual psychotherapy. Small wonder too the interplay of secrets and privacy has drawn sustained philosophical interest, as in Bok's fine book (Bok, 1989). Psychologists seeking guidance on how to manage the concealment, privacy, and secrets, and revelation during a therapy will look to the APA Code (2002) in vain, if they seek intelligent guidance. Section four of the Code is about "Privacy and Confidentiality," but is legalistic, being focused on the legal obligations of the psychologist. The word "lying" does not appear in the APA Code. There is a contrast between lying and sex in the Code. The Code lavishes detail on sexual misconduct. The Code's precise prohibitions on sexual relations with clients and their relatives, both competent and incompetent, including a minimum 2-year-post-therapy limit on sexual relations with former clients, might lead those unfamiliar with life on this planet to believe psychologist are likelier to have sex with their patients than to lie to them. Of course absence from the Code has no bearing on whether an act is immoral. As previously noted, the absence of a prohibition on torturing patients does not show torture is morally permissible. The absence does show the need to think about what one is doing, beyond the mere technical questions, when dealing with patients and informants.

End Game

Strang's symptoms that include a constellation of symptoms that fall within the trauma spectrum—nightmares, avoidance of thoughts about the trauma, avoidant defenses—seem in the context of the play to yield to Dysart's therapeutic challenge of them. In the play, Dysart induces an old-fashioned abreaction that leads to relief of Strang's symptoms. Psychologists without a psychodynamic bent may prefer to view Dysart's intervention as a variant of exposure techniques (Cooper & Glum, 1989). Whatever the success, which after is theatrical, of what Dysart does, his technique has suspect dimensions to it.

In particular, Dysart embraces a temptation that all therapists face. He promises big. From the birth of psychodynamic therapy, the irresistible temptation of therapists to make big promises has existed

(Ellenberger, 1981, especially Chaps. 4 and 5). As he presses and succeeds in getting his patient to relive the nigh he blinded horses, he ultimately promises his patient that his reliving the events will free him of his symptoms.

With the exception of the almighty, no mere therapist, however, shrewd, can know a patient will cease to have symptoms after a psychotherapeutic intervention. What a psychotherapist may know (Frank & Frank, 1993; Lambert, 2003) is that certain interventions may work and that belief in a therapy's power is crucial to its working. However, nobody can make an honest claim that a therapy will work, even though it may help a patient if the therapist exudes confidence.

Dysart's misleading his patient does nowise settle the either the rightness or the wrongness of his act of the praiseworthiness or blameworthiness of it, either. Moralists who make a fetish of honesty may think the matter closed from the beginning, since they proscribe even benevolent lies, even if known to be beneficial (Kant, 1797). Few go that far. Bok (1999), who has also written on secrecy, surveys the terrain of lying. Therapists, if honest, live uneasy lives as they balance candor with a patient's welfare interests. And those with an extreme distaste for lying may wish to recall a line from Blake's "Auguries of Innocence"

> A Truth that's told with bad intent/
> Beats all the Lies you can invent (Blake, 1789).

For all his hubris, for all the moral difficulties that sneak into *Equus*, Dysart is presented as a master therapist. If one accepts the play, one cannot reject its finale. It is Dysart's triumph in his role as therapist. Dysart's victory over Strang's lunacy is a secular apotheosis.

Denouement

Psychologists working with sick teens have numerous moral perplexities awaiting them, as do all therapists. Professional Codes provide scant guidance for many of the salient moral problems. Several factors complicate the work with teens. In particular teens are not adults. Adults provide proxy consents that may or may not match a teens preferences or interests. Often psychologists disrupt family dynamics, replacing parental authority with their own. In many instances, psychologists may have values that run contrary to conventional values of families. Implicit therapeutic values, such as consulting the "best" interests of the teen patient, may threaten to devour other family interests. Therapists may also become involved in "outing" wayward behaviors of the teen and others. Quandaries regarding multiple agency, confidentiality, secrecy, complicity, privacy, and honesty abound. Therapeutic goals of good outcome expectancy and self-efficacy, palliation, and cure may collide with the plain truth.

Equus has served as an heuristic for brining these and related moral difficulties into relief. The purpose in this essay has been modest. Instead of arguing for specific lines of moral decision, I have opted to engage in the moral equivalent of motivational interviewing (Miller & Rollnick, 2002). Consciousness raising is my goal. Once therapists begin to notice how moral considerations suffuse the treatment of teens, they can begin to work out for themselves how to come to terms with the problems they encounter. If they had loving and good parents from infancy through their teens, they may even have emerged virtuous enough to do discover answers they can live with.

References

American Psychiatric Association. (2000). *Diagnostic and statistical manual of mental disorders* (4th ed.) (Text Revision). Washington, DC: Author.

American Psychological Association. (2002). *Ethical principles of psychologists and code of conduct.* Washington, DC: Author.

Beauchamp, T. L., & Childress, J. F. (2008). *Principles of biomedical ethics* (6th ed.) New York: Oxford University Press.

Blake, W. (1789). *Auguries of Innocence.* In *The complete poetry and prose of William Blake, Revised Edition.* (1997). Ed. David V. Erdman with commentary by Harold Bloom. New York: Anchor Books.

Bok, S. (1989). *Secrets: On the ethics of concealment and revelation.* New York: Vintage.

Bok, S. (1999). *Lying: Moral choice in public and private life* (updated ed.). New York: Vintage.

Brock, D. W. (1993). *Life and death: Philosophical essays in biomedical ethics.* Cambridge: University of Cambridge.

Brody, H. (1993). *The healer's power.* New Haven, CT: Yale.

Buchanan, A. E., & Brock, D. W. (1990). *Deciding for others: The ethics of surrogate decision making.* Cambridge: Cambridge University Press.

Cooper, N. A., & Glum, G. A. (1989). Imaginal flooding as a supplementary treatment for PTSD in combat veterans: A controlled study. *Behavior Therapy, 20*, 381-391.

Council of Representatives of the American Psychological Association. (2006). *Resolution against torture and other cruel, inhuman, and degrading treatment or punishment*. Washington, DC: Author.

Ellenberger, H. F. (1981). *The discovery of the unconscious: A history of psychodynamic psychiatry*. New York: Basic Books.

Engelhardt, H. T. (1986). *Foundations of bioethics*. Oxford: Oxford University Press.

Frank, J. D., & Frank, J. B. (1993). *Persuasion and healing: a comparative study of psychotherapy* (3rd ed.). Baltimore: Johns Hopkins University Press.

Goffman, E. (1963). *Stigma: Notes on the management of spoiled identity*. Englewood Cliffs, NJ: Prentice Hall.

Gray, P. (1994). *The ego and analysis of defense*. Northvale, NJ: Jason Aronson.

Kant, I. (1797). On the supposed right to tell lies from benevolent motives. In James W. Ellington (Trans.) (1993). *Grounding for the metaphysics of morals: With on a supposed right to lie because of philanthropic concerns*. Indianapolis, IN: Hackett.

Lambert, M. (Ed.). (2003). *Bergin and Garfield's handbook of psychotherapy and behavior change* (5th ed.). New York: John Wiley & Sons.

Miller, W. R., & Rollnick, S. (2002). *Motivational interviewing: Preparing people to change*. New York: Guildford Press.

Phillips, A. (1989). *Winnicott*. Boston: Harvard University Press.

Shaffer, P. (1977). *Equus*. New York: Penguin.

Singer, P. (1979). *Practical ethics*. Cambridge: Cambridge University Press.

Overextending the Overextended: Burnout Potential in Health-Care Professionals, Psychologists, Patients, and Family Members

Lauren Woodward Tolle and Steve Graybar

- A nurse providing care on the intensive care unit for children complains of debilitating headaches and is becoming increasingly socially isolated and detached from others.
- A pediatrician is suffering from insomnia and days of vacation do not appear to alleviate symptoms of anxiety or sadness.
- A mother of a child who survived a brain tumor is experiencing problems in her marriage and fears that the tumor will come back. She frequently worries about her child's capacity to have meaningful relationships and a fulfilling career as an adult.
- An adolescent living with type 1 diabetes for 8 years has become lax in his diabetes management and feels hopeless about the future.
- A psychologist assisting families with chronically ill adolescents feels powerless to change behavior and improve outcomes outside of her control and frequently experiences intrusive thoughts about her patients.

Which of these individuals is at risk for experiencing burnout? Sadly, each one is. Burnout is a concept that many researchers have attempted to define, and many individuals have experienced. In their book, *Women's Burnout*, Freudenberger and North (1985) define burnout as "the point at which you exhaust your energies by overextending yourself; the result of your excessive intensity and conscientiousness to other people and situations; the consequence of denying yourself attention – pleasure, affiliation, intimacy; when motivation is lost due to overabundant responsiveness to your husband, lover, or job; waning enthusiasm, irritability, and feelings of disengagement caused by stress, pressure, and exhaustion". This comprehensive definition examines burnout by its etiology as well as its symptomatology. Burnout has also been conceptualized as consisting of three domains: (1) emotional exhaustion, characterized by feeling emotionally depleted or drained; (2) depersonalization, or treating people like they are impersonal objects (i.e., often characterized by calling patients by their diagnosis rather than their name), while growing more cynical or pessimistic; and (3) a reduced sense of personal and professional accomplishment (Maslach, 1982). Symptoms of burnout include somatic complaints (i.e., fatigue, sleep problems, headaches, colds, etc.), irritability, anxiety, depression, pessimism, substance abuse, and interpersonal problems (Kahill, 1988).

Many professions, largely helping professions, are at risk for developing burnout including elementary and secondary education teachers (Stoeber & Rennert, 2008), police officers (Martinussen, Richardsen, & Burke, 2007), prison personnel (Carlson & Thompson, 2006), hotel and restaurant personnel (Hayes & Weathington, 2007), bank employees (Allam & Ali, 2007), and even the clergy (Miner, 2007). The risk for burnout in medical professions is very high, especially for primary-care physicians (Vela-Bueno et al., 2008), pediatricians (Kushnir & Cohen, 2006), nurses (Maytum, Heiman, & Garwick, 2004), residents (Thomas, 2004), and medical students (Dyrbye et al., 2006). Much of the literature examining the potential for social workers and psychologists to experience

L.W. Tolle (✉)
Department of Psychology, University of Nevada, Reno, NV, USA
e-mail: ltolle@unr.nevada.edu

W.T. O'Donohue, L.W. Tolle (eds.), *Behavioral Approaches to Chronic Disease in Adolescence*,
DOI 10.1007/978-0-387-87687-0_7, © Springer Science+Business Media, LLC 2009

burnout focuses on working with child or adult victims of sexual or physical abuse (Conrad & Kellar-Guenther, 2006; Deighton, Gurris, & Traue, 2007; Sprang, Clark, & Whitt-Woosley, 2007). Given the relative infancy of integrated care with psychologists and other mental health professionals being a fixture in medical settings, there is little research regarding the likelihood of burnout of these professionals working in this setting.

While burnout is often described as being something that an individual experiences with regard to their job, it has also been purported as being caused by long-term stress regardless of where it originates (Swedish National Board of Health and Welfare, 2003). The initial diagnosis of a chronic illness in children can be an extremely distressing event for parents (Kazak et al., 2004). After diagnosis, substantial changes in the family structure, roles, and responsibilities take place. It can be overwhelming to cope with hearing of one's child's diagnosis, seeing one's child in pain or distress, while at the same time attempting to be educated about the disease, its progression, potential complications, and treatment. Parents frequently take on responsibility for illness and treatment monitoring initially, thus adding to the demands of their schedule. This is all while attempting to maintain relationships, maintain financial stability to pay for costly treatments or medications, and maintain familial stability (Hauenstein, 1990). The chronic nature of the disease also contributes to risk of prolonged stress for parents of chronically ill children. Parents of children with chronic illness have been found to experience more symptoms of depression, anxiety, parenting stress, sleep disturbances, and poorer health than parents whose children are not chronically ill (Meltzer & Moore, 2008). Norberg (2007) examined the potential for burnout in parents whose child survived a brain tumor and found that mothers especially reported higher levels of burnout when compared to parents of children with no history of chronic disease. Other chronic conditions including autism and mental retardation in children have also been found to predict burnout in mothers (Weiss, 2002). These findings are consistent with extant literature that mothers frequently assume primary caregiving roles within the family, while also taking on multiple other roles, putting them at risk for chronic strain (Naerde, Tambs, Mathiesen, Dalgard, & Samuelsen, 2000; Norberg, 2007).

In addition to parents of children and adolescents with chronic illnesses being at risk for burnout, the chronically ill patients themselves are also at risk. An inherent part of experiencing something "chronic" is that it is unrelenting and has no clear end in sight. When this term is coupled with negative factors such as pain, vigilant adherence, limitation, or disability, it would only be natural to desire respite from this, to distance oneself from its certainty, its constancy. As this is rarely a possibility for those who endure chronic illness, it is clear that this would be a common pathway for experiencing burnout. Adolescents with chronic illness face many difficulties that accompany their diagnosis including fears about the future, a recurrent episode, surgery or procedure; limited social interaction with peers due to frequent school absences to attend medical appointments/procedures or not being able to engage in normal adolescent activities; social stigma related to their disease; coping emotionally with the disease and others' reactions to it (i.e., parents, teachers, peers, etc.) and depending on the type and severity of the condition, constant adherence and lifestyle modifications to successfully manage their disease (Erickson, Patterson, Wall, & Neumark-Sztainer, 2005). Erickson and colleagues (2005) surveyed 4,746 middle and high school students from ethnically diverse backgrounds about their physical health, mental health, and engagement in risky behaviors (i.e., use of tobacco, drugs, or alcohol). Students with chronic health conditions were found to be significantly more likely to experience depressive symptoms and low self-esteem; were twice as likely to consider suicide and three and a half times more likely to have attempted suicide and finally reported more cigarette, alcohol, and drug use than students without chronic health conditions.

Compassion Fatigue

In the context of professional burnout, researchers have termed a similar phenomenon, compassion fatigue, or what some have purported can lead to burnout (Conrad & Kellar-Guenther, 2006). Figley (1995) originally operationalized the construct of compassion fatigue upon examining the effects of working with trauma victims on trauma workers, police officers, first responders, and similar emergency responders and stated that it was "the natural behavior and emotion that arises from knowing about traumatizing events experienced by a significant other, and the stress resulting from helping or wanting to help a traumatized person" (p. 7). While burnout and compassion fatigue are similar in that they both can cause feelings of helplessness, anxiety, and depression, they are also thought to be dissimilar in a number of ways. Burnout is thought to be due to excessive and prolonged exposure to stress, while compassion fatigue can be experienced following an individual being exposed to as little as a single incident in which they experience sadness, anxiety, and grief from working with an individual with a traumatic history (Conrad & Kellar-Guenther, 2006).

Caring for patients with chronic illnesses with the realization that full recovery is rare can be extremely challenging for health providers (Figley, 1998). Research has demonstrated that nurses who work with chronically ill adolescents and children are at risk for compassion fatigue (Meadors & Lamson, 2008). Providers must be able to effectively care for and assist the family of a chronically ill or terminal patient, while also attempting to manage their own grief (Brosche, 2003). In their interviews of 20 experienced nurses who care for chronically ill children and their families, Maytum et al. (2004) identified several triggers of compassion fatigue and burnout that were separated into work-related triggers and personal triggers. Work-related triggers included being exposed to too many painful procedures being done to children, experiencing and observing too much sadness and death, interacting with angry families, non-compliant patients and families, staffing shortages, excessive paperwork, insurance frustrations, lack of time and feeling that the demands of work exceeded what they were capable of reasonably giving, and lack of support or feeling alone. Personal triggers that were identified included becoming overly involved with patients and their families or crossing professional boundaries, taking things personally, having too high of expectations for oneself, trying to get outside needs met at work, and family problems. Among psychologists, risk factors for developing compassion fatigue have been found to include a personal history of trauma, lower social support, being female and having a higher percentage of victims of sexual violence as clients (Adams, Boscarino, & Figley, 2006). It can be assumed that psychologists working in medical settings would likely encounter the same or similar triggers to compassion fatigue that nurses working with chronically ill children and their families reported previously.

Research has indicated that experiencing compassion fatigue or burnout may impact a practitioner's ability to provide effective services and maintain positive relationships both at work and outside of work (Collins & Long, 2003). Compassion fatigue in the workplace can also lead to reduced productivity, more work absenteeism, and higher turnover rates (Pfifferling & Gilley, 2000). Mental health professionals experiencing compassion fatigue are prone to making poor clinical judgments such as misdiagnosis, poor treatment planning, or even abuse of the client more so than professionals not experiencing compassion fatigue (Rudolf, Stamm, & Stamm, 1997, as cited in Collins & Long, 2003). Because there is potential for burnout in every member of an integrated care team, as well as for the patients and patients' family members, it is essential to help meet each individual's needs to treat compassion fatigue and prevent burnout from occurring.

Assessment of Burnout and Compassion Fatigue

One of the first steps in treating or preventing compassion fatigue that can lead to burnout in professionals is to be aware of its signs or symptoms as they occur (Bride, Radey, & Figley, 2007). Several measures have been developed to assess various aspects of compassion fatigue.

The *Compassion Fatigue Self-Test* (CFST; Figley, 1995) is a 40-item self-report measure designed to assess the risk for both compassion fatigue and burnout in clinicians. Respondents are asked to indicate the frequency with which they believe certain characteristics are true of themselves or their situation. Higher scores on the compassion fatigue and burnout subscales are indicative of higher risk for experiencing these stress responses. Internal consistency alphas reportedly range from 0.86 to 0.94 (Figley, 1995). Factor analysis suggests one stable factor characterized by depressed mood relative to work, feelings of disillusionment and worthlessness, and fatigue. Figley and Stamm (1996) report that the test is still being developed and that at that time there had been insufficient data to determine a second structure.

A revision of the CFST yielded the *Professional Quality of Life Scale* (ProQOL; Stamm, 2002), which is a 30-item self-report measure that assesses the risk of compassion fatigue, compassion satisfaction, and burnout. Compassion satisfaction (CS) has been defined as a sense of satisfaction from helping others and has been purported to mitigate the effects of compassion fatigue (Stamm, 2002). Respondents are asked to indicate on a 6-item Likert scale how frequently each item was experienced for the past 30 days. Higher scores on each of the three subscales indicate higher risk or more satisfaction (for the CS subscale). Alpha coefficients range from 0.72 (burnout) to 0.80 (compassion fatigue) and 0.87 (compassion satisfaction), demonstrating adequate internal consistency. Stamm reports discriminant and convergent validity, however, data is not reported (Bride et al., 2007).

The *Maslach Burnout Inventory* (MBI; Maslach & Jackson, 1986) is a 22-item, self-report questionnaire that consists of three subscales, designed to assess each area of burnout (i.e., emotional exhaustion, depersonalization, and low sense of personal accomplishment). High scores on the emotional exhaustion and depersonalization subscales are considered to be indicative of burnout (Dyrbye et al., 2006; Fahrenkopf et al., 2008). The MBI was originally constructed to be used in social service contexts and so further development of the instrument led to the MBI-General Survey, to be used across occupational groups (MBI-GS; Maslach et al., 1996). Numerous factor analytic studies have confirmed the three-factor structure comprising the construct burnout, and convergent and discriminant validity have been found to be moderate (Demerouti et al., 2003; Kitaoka-Higashiguchi et al., 2004; Langballe, Falkum, Innstrand & Aasland, 2006; Oh & Lee, 2009; Schutte, Toppinen, Kalimo, & Schaufeli, 2000; Storm & Rothmann, 2003).

Although there appear to be some psychometrically reliable instruments used to measure the risk of compassion fatigue and burnout in clinicians, a limitation in this area is that few have been developed for use across a wider population and for a wider variety of traumatic experiences (Motta, Chirichella, Maus, & Lombardo, 2004). The majority of measures have been tested on mental health professionals including therapists and social workers, not on nurses, physicians, patients, or caregivers who also experience these symptoms (Sabo, 2006). Additionally, the traumatic events intended to be captured in theses assessments may be guided by compassion fatigue literature regarding psychologists and social workers working with interpersonal trauma (i.e., sexual and/or physical abuse) and may not necessarily be tapping into the other unique factors associated with health-related traumas inherent to chronic illness (i.e., initial diagnosis, procedures and treatment, noncompliance issues, etc.).

Prevention of Burnout by Attending to Compassion Fatigue

Similar to the request on airplanes that it is important first to secure one's own oxygen mask before assisting others, treating one's own compassion fatigue and risk for burnout before assisting others with similar symptoms is vital, as a professional's ability to be effective in delivering interventions is compromised by compassion fatigue. Provided are strategies, guided by empirical literature, to assist professionals in preventing burnout by attending first to what some have termed, the inevitable symptoms of compassion fatigue (Figley, 1995).

Research on treating compassion fatigue indicates that adopting or returning to self-care strategies can mitigate the effects of stress (Maytum et al., 2004). When caring for one's self becomes eclipsed by caring for others, as is often the case with individuals in the helping professions, a significant drop-off in self-care behaviors is observed. While the authors were not able to find rigorous methodological outcome research for the following strategies in specifically treating compassion fatigue or preventing burnout, they have been frequently cited as being helpful in treating these clusters of symptoms.

Self-Care Strategies

Exercise

Regular physical activity has repeatedly been found to be efficacious in reducing anxiety and other stress-related symptoms (Berger & Motl, 2001; Sarafino, 2002) as well as improving mood and overall health.

Yoga, Tai Chi and Qigong have also been found to assist individuals coping with anxiety and depression and can lead to overall improved psychological well-being (Granath et al., 2006). Individuals who engage in regular fitness have also reported that their work performance and attitudes improved as a result and that they made fewer errors at work (Quick, Quick, Nelson, & Hurrell, 1997). In examining compassion fatigue among health-care providers at a children's hospital, Meadors and Lamson (2008) found that health-care workers in the low-stress group endorsed fewer compassion fatigue symptoms and exhibited more healthy behaviors including regular exercise. Exercise has also been recommended by other researchers examining the effects of compassion fatigue and burnout (Iliffe & Steed, 2000; Maytum et al., 2004).

Healthy Eating Behaviors

Research indicates that high levels of stress are associated with both increased and decreased food intake (Wardle, Steptoe, Oliver, & Lipsey, 2000). Stress is also associated with the food choices people make, in that under stress, individuals are more likely to choose foods high in fat and calories as well as more convenient foods such as fast food (Oliver, Wardle, & Gibson, 2000). Individuals with busy schedules and stressful lives engage in many other unhealthy eating behaviors, including skipping meals and consuming large quantities of caffeine, both of which can impact individuals' ability to concentrate, their level of anxiety, irritability, and also can contribute to feelings of shakiness. Nurses have noted that engaging in healthy eating habits has assisted them when feeling initial symptoms of compassion fatigue (Maytum et al., 2004). Healthy eating habits has also been linked to lower stress and lower risk for compassion fatigue in health-care workers (Meadors & Lamson, 2008).

Journaling

Journaling is a common strategy used for expressing strong emotion with the added benefits of doing so in a personal and confidential nature (Nazarian & Smyth, 2008). Journaling, or scriptotherapy, the process of writing one's emotions and thoughts regarding a stressful or traumatic event, has been empirically supported in providing benefits to one's somatic and psychological health (Smyth & Greenberg, 2000) and decreasing distress and symptoms of depression (Sloan & Marx, 2004). Alford, Malouff, and Osland (2005) evaluated the utility of journaling with child protective service workers in reducing stress reactions. Individuals in the intervention group were found to report significantly decreased distress levels and significantly greater job satisfaction than a control group who did not engage in the journaling intervention. Journaling has also been cited by nurses who work with children with chronic conditions and their families as a coping strategy employed to prevent compassion fatigue and burnout (Maytum et al., 2004).

Meditation/Mindfulness

Meditation and mindfulness practices have been increasingly used as part of a stress management treatment package, and increasingly, evidence points to the utility of meditation practice in improving health outcomes in clinical populations (Seeman, Dubin, & Seeman, 2003). Oman, Hedberg, and Thoresen (2006) examined the effectiveness of Passage Meditation for health-care professionals in reducing perceived job stress and burnout via a randomized, controlled trial. Passage Meditation, also called the Eight-Point Program (EPP), involves silent repetition in the mind of inspirational passages practiced for 30 min a day, followed by repetition of a single calming word throughout the day. Passage Meditation, as with other forms of meditation, also involves a slowing down and increasing awareness to the task at hand. It emphasizes putting others first and seeking out time for mutual support. Results indicated that at 19 weeks post-intervention, individuals in the meditation group expressed significantly lower levels of stress and improved mental health. Meditation has also been associated with lower stress levels and lower risk for compassion fatigue among nurses working in pediatric intensive care units (Meadors & Lamson, 2008).

Mindfulness Meditation involves the observation of one's thoughts and bodily sensations in a nonjudgmental manner. Frequently, mindfulness practice begins by noticing one's breath and focusing awareness to the sensations of breathing, without attempting to change or deepen the breath (Kushner & Marnocha, 2008). Galantino, Baime, Maguire, Szapary, and Farrar (2005) recruited health-care professionals to take part in a Mindfulness Meditation, 8-week program, and to test the intervention's impact on symptoms of stress and burnout. Upon completion of the program, participants reported significantly improved mood and scores on the emotional exhaustion subscale of the Maslach Burnout Inventory.

Other relaxation strategies are the hallmark of stress management programs. These include progressive muscle relaxation, autogenics training, guided visualization, and diaphragmatic breathing skills (Kaplan & Laygo, 2003). Bughi, Sumcad, and Bughu (2006) conducted a brief behavioral intervention program on stress management in medical students. Results of the intervention, which consisted of relaxation skills training (deep diaphragmatic breathing, self-control relaxation and meditation), indicated that stress levels decreased significantly.

Other Self-Care Strategies

The following are other strategies that have been cited in literature on stress management and improving mood (Linehan, 1993; McCrae, Nau, Taylor, & Lichstein, 2006; Martell, 2003):

- Elicit positive social support from friends and family members
- Engage in pleasurable, meaningful activities
- Engage in good sleep hygiene
- The use of humor can serve as a moderator of compassion fatigue (Moran, 2002)

Bibliotherapy and web sites that might also be helpful to clinicians, physicians, nurses, and other health-care professionals include:

- Kabat-Zinn, J. (1994). *Wherever you go, there you are: Mindfulness meditation in everyday life.* New York: Hyperion.
- Figley, C. (1995). *Compassion fatigue: Coping with secondary traumatic stress disorder in those who treat the traumatized.* New York: Brunner-Mazel.
- Davis, M., Eshelman, E. R., & McKay, M. (2000). *The relaxation and stress reduction workbook.* Oakland, CA: New Harbinger Publications Inc.
- Preventing Burnout: Signs, Symptoms and Strategies to Avoid it: http://www.helpguide.org/mental/burnout_signs_symptoms.htm
- Compassion Fatigue Awareness Project: http://www.compassionfatigue.org/

In addition to the self-care strategies that have been presented, other work-related strategies are important for reducing the effects of compassion fatigue and for preventing burnout. Several of these have been cited in the literature on compassion fatigue and burnout.

Work-Related Strategies

Work-related risk factors for compassion fatigue and burnout that have been cited in health-care literature include administrative duties (i.e., paperwork), inadequate staffing, lack of support or feeling alone, feeling unable to provide care given lack of time, working overtime frequently or working double shifts, becoming overinvolved or crossing therapeutic boundaries, and feeling pressured to commit to taking on additional tasks (Kushnir & Cohen, 2006; Maytum et al., 2004).

Factors associated with lower stress and lower risk for experiencing compassion fatigue among nurses included having adequate time away from work, focusing on self-assertive behaviors (i.e., saying "no" to taking on additional tasks), and setting limits at work concerning putting in overtime or agreeing to work double shifts (Meadors & Lamson, 2008). Some therapies are specifically designed with preventing burnout in mind. Specifically, Dialectical Behavior Therapy (DBT; Linehan, 1993) incorporates the use of peer supervision and consultation to prevent burnout in therapists working with a difficult population. By providing peer support to the therapist in a collaborative way, DBT uses the positive benefits of teamwork to provide supervision as well as mindfulness training for the therapist in order to better help them help their clients. DBT's use of mindfulness, previously mentioned as a self-care strategy for preventing burnout, is used in a group atmosphere to help prevent burnout. This team aspect also ensures that therapists do not feel isolated or on their own, which has also been cited as a risk for experiencing compassion fatigue and burnout.

It would seem then that integrated care teams would be set up to function similarly to consultation teams. Joint staff meetings between medical and behavioral health-care professionals to discuss coordination of separate but related care agendas for adolescents and their families would allow parties to discuss difficult cases and receive support and feedback (Chaffee, 2005). Being part of an integrated team would also provide health-care professionals with a sounding board to monitor their own burnout and compassion fatigue symptoms, as well as to note their level of involvement with a particular case (i.e., having peer consultation regarding crossing boundaries). In addition, psychologists have the unique ability to provide support to other health professionals regarding the effective management of difficult families, stressful professional-family interactions, burnout symptoms, and bereavement in integrated care settings (Spirito et al., 2003).

Assisting the Burned Out Adolescent and Family

Several models of adolescent adjustment to their chronic illness have been purported, and several of them involve the idea that parental adaptation and coping to a chronic illness diagnosis in their child influences the child's adaptation to their own diagnosis (Harbeck-Weber, Fisher, & Dittner, 2003). Parental coping has been purported to influence child coping by means of parents modeling coping behaviors, teaching children coping behaviors, or by creating a home environment that might be either destructive or conducive to effective and open communication (Kliewer, Sandler, & Wolchik, 1994).

Studies have confirmed that mothers of children with type 1 diabetes assume much of the responsibility for their child's diabetes management initially report more parenting stress than mothers of healthy children and also have a higher incidence of experiencing depression during the first year of their child's diagnosis (Wysocki, Greco, & Buckloh, 2003). Kovacs and colleagues (1990) followed children diagnosed with type 1 diabetes and their mothers for a period of 6 years to repeatedly assess adjustment to the chronic disease. Results indicated that though depression scores dropped after the first year of diagnosis, mothers' reported level of distress shortly following diagnosis were the strongest predictors of adjustment over time.

Adolescents with type 1 diabetes are at an increased risk for experiencing depression and anxiety (Kovacs et al., 1997), which is consistent with earlier reported estimates (Erickson et al., 2005). Stress management and coping skills training have been found to alleviate stress symptoms, and in addition, perceived social support may buffer the effects of stress in adolescents with type 1 diabetes. Social support has been found to be an important factor in reducing stress and enhancing coping strategies in adolescents when faced with stressful events (Hartup, 1993). Though the authors could not find empirical evidence testing interventions to decrease the risk of burnout in adolescents with chronic health conditions, it is reasonable to suggest that implementing stress management and coping skills training interventions could be efficacious in ameliorating some burnout symptoms. In addition, assisting adolescents and family members in soliciting social support is another potentially fruitful option (Harbeck-Weber et al., 2003). Accessing peer support online for adolescents with chronic health conditions has been another attempt made to assist adolescents in improving access to social support (Tichron & Shapiro, 2003). Chronically ill children and adolescents who engaged in accessing an online community to talk to other chronically ill children have reported less pain intensity, pain aversiveness, and anxiety than compared to controls who received standard care without access to online communities (Holden, Bearison, Rode, Kapliloff, & Rosenberg, 2000). Summer camp programs are another method used to provide chronically ill children with an opportunity to meet their social needs and improve attitudes toward their condition. Few studies examining the utility of summer camps have used rigorous methodological designs that allow for interpretation of the camps' effectiveness (Plante, Lobato, & Engel, 2001). More research is needed to examine what interventions are effective in treating burnout symptoms in adolescents with chronic health conditions.

Treatment of Burnout in Patients and Their Families – Case Example: Type 1 Diabetes

Sadly, stress, and burnout are relatively common occurrences among our diabetic patients and their caretakers. Chronic stress leads to an erosion of coping skills, interpersonal isolation, and if left untreated to burnout. We take burnout very seriously and view it as a first cousin of, and often a precursor to, major depression. Together, un-addressed stress and burnout can significantly interfere with a patient or family's interpersonal relationships, ability to engage in the daily self-care activities required to manage type I diabetes, and severely diminish the overall quality of their lives. The inability to follow a proscribed medical regimen can lead type I diabetics into immediate and long-term medical complications. The immediate complications often mimic depression by robbing the uncontrolled diabetic patient of the energy needed to think clearly, feel normally, and behave adaptively. The long-term complications of unmanaged diabetes are legend and can lead to catastrophic damage to nerves, eyes, kidneys, and heart.

In our work, burned out adolescents neglect and at times completely ignore self-care activities. Burned out parents often unconsciously collude with their teenager's self-neglect for they too share his/her anger, wish to be normal, desire to live a spontaneous life free of injections, finger sticks, carbohydrate counting, doctors, nurses, and more recently psychologists. Parents who are burned out have, "tried everything" to get their child to manage their diabetes. Often they present to our clinic angry, emotionally numb, defensively philosophical, or simply depressed. Like their diabetic child, these parents want to be done with this relentless and unforgiving disease. In the end stages of burnout, they allow most if not all of the disease management to fall to their adolescent son or daughter. These parents often rationalize this stance and explain it through a veil of anger or apathy. They view themselves as simply giving their teenager the responsibility he/she must soon bear as a young adult. We have found such a parental tack to be less a thoughtful parenting decision than a surrender to futility and feelings of failure, frustration, and fatigue.

We draw heavily from the work of Freudenberger and North (1985) to understand and intervene with stress and burnout among our diabetic patients and families. The diagnosis and management of type I diabetes for a child and his/her parents are incredibly stressful. For many of our families, the initial diagnosis of diabetes did not come easily. Parents and medical professionals alike often missed the diagnosis and incorrectly assumed the onset of the illness was a virus, cold, or flu bug. In such cases, the actual diagnosis was often made as the child's blood sugars swung wildly out of control and necessitated life-saving measures via our medical center's emergency room and intensive care unit. Whether or not the initial diagnosis was life threatening or traumatic, the diagnosis of diabetes mellitus is a shattering experience for the family. It brings an early and abrupt end to the innocence childhood and the sense of a safe, simple, and protected family life. Compounding the immediate shock of the initial diagnosis is the intensive disease management program that accompanies it. In the hospital, families are given a crash course in endocrinology and diabetes care. Often, within the span of 4–5 days, they are expected to function as the primary care provider for their diabetic child. This includes drawing and administering correct dosages of insulin four to five times daily, testing blood sugars five to six times per day, understanding the effects of diet, stress, illness and exercise on blood sugars as well as recognizing and responding to high and low blood sugars. Such demands place a heavy burden on the most well-adjusted families let alone those families struggling with social, emotional, or economic difficulties.

In the case study below, we include a brief discussion of burnout experienced to a greater and lesser extent by each member of a family seen in the University of Nevada School of Medicine's Pediatric Diabetes Program. The family's situation is a familiar one in our clinic and involves an all too frequent clinical scenario.

Beth," was a 16 year old, Caucasian, female who had been dealing with type I diabetes for almost 10 years. She was the youngest of three children and the only child still living at home with her parents. Beth's "control" had ebbed and flowed over the years but rarely entered dangerous or otherwise alarming levels. She was referred to family therapy with the second author after a recent clinic visit revealed that her blood sugars had become dangerously high over the past several months; so high that she was taken to a local emergency room following an acute hyperglycemic episode. These sessions lasted an hour and 15 min and except for the second session and a follow-up session were held 2 weeks apart.

Beth was accompanied to the first "family session" by her mother "Dana." It was not quite clear whether her father was not invited or interested in attending the meeting. (Beth's father, "Roger" was virtually unknown to clinic staff). In this first session, it was obvious that Beth and her mother were emotionally very close and that each was very concerned about the other. Despite their emotional closeness and concern, both Beth and Dana seemed genuinely surprised by Beth's latest HbA1c which indicated that she had not been taking all or even most of her prescribed insulin nor had she been testing her blood. The HbA1c is a simple blood test that yields invaluable information about a patient's mean blood sugar levels over the previous 2 to 3 months. While this test provides an extended or long-term picture of diabetes control, daily finger-pokes/blood testing would yield essentially the same information on a day-to-day basis. The first indication that Beth and Dana were burning out was the fact that neither was following Beth's diabetes on a regular basis. This initial session revealed that both mother and daughter were tired of the diabetes grind and while each felt guilty and ashamed, neither felt able to hold up their respective ends of diabetes care. In Beth's case this would involve testing regularly, taking her insulin, eating appropriately and covering with additional insulin meals or snacks that raised her blood sugars. On Dana's side, she needed to be more consistently involved in Beth's daily regimen without smothering, cajoling, nagging, or threatening (all easier said than done). One un-obtrusive way Dana would become more involved was to semi-regularly check Beth's blood sugar monitor to verify Beth's numbers and then generally reinforce, redirect, or support Beth in making appropriate adjustments in her diabetes care based on this information. In the first session, neither Beth nor her mother appeared willing or able to maintain this regimen.

Like many of our children and parents, Beth and Dana viewed the HbA1c as a characterological report card. To Beth, the test revealed to everyone who cared to see that she was a bad person and unworthy of the clinic staff's care or support. To Dana, the test seemed to underscore how bad and inadequate a parent she was. The looming thought of an HbA1c had led Dana to cancel, reschedule, and at times simply skip Beth's clinic appointments over the past year. The therapist offered, "It was no wonder that their quarterly clinic visits had decreased to once every six months. Who would want their entire existence reduced to a single number on a single blood test?" Further discussion revealed that despite having diabetes for nearly 10 years, Beth's father, had remained relatively uninvolved in her disease management. In addition, Beth and Dana described him as largely ignorant of her illness and completely in the dark about the emotional toll it was taking on his wife and daughter.

Rather than viewing this family as dysfunctional, non-compliant, or in, "denial," a straightforward approach to their emotional, mental, physical, and spiritual exhaustion was taken. An empathic, non-judgmental therapeutic stance allowed Beth and Dana to speak openly about their fatigue, frustration, resentment, and shame about failing to follow through on their treatment team's advice.

Genuine empathy was used to underscore how exposed and vulnerable they felt when coming to the clinic, and how resentful they must have felt when it seemed that all the team cared about was Beth's blood work. A good deal of time was spent validating their fears of judgment and the emotional and physical strain managing diabetes was taking on the two of them. After providing Beth and Dana with a good, "listening too" (which was the opposite of what each had expected), the therapist identified their depletion as a form of burnout and normalized burnout as a natural and normal response to the lifelong marathon of diabetes care. This psycho-education seemed to make sense to Beth and Dana, and softened some of their guilt and defensiveness. Last, the therapist requested that Roger be invited to the next session. This invitation seemed to trigger anxiety in Dana but curiosity and a subtle enthusiasm in Beth. Both seemed to agree with the therapist that Dad's involvement might be helpful to our overall success. The first session ended quite well. And though the therapist never asked, both Beth and Dana volunteered that they would both make more of an effort to, "get things" under control. Each seemed to have let go of a significant burden during the session. Beth came "clean" about being "sick" of her diabetes and some of her dishonesty around "blowing off her diabetes." Dana admitted that she had let Beth carry the ball perhaps unfairly over that past several months.

Often, in the first session it is a good idea to ask about the child and family's illness story (Seaburn, 2001). In our clinic, the illness story gives everyone in the family a chance to speak to and describe the thoughts and feelings that surrounded the initial diagnosis and about the changes diabetes brought to the family since it was discovered. The illness story provides everyone an opportunity to discuss unspoken or unacknowledged emotions or experiences. It allows the therapist to join with the family and the family (often estranged from each other) a chance to join with each other by acknowledging what each member has been dealing with separately and together. Since "Roger," Beth's father and Dana's husband, was not present, the illness story was held back for the next family session.

The second session with Roger was a surprise to everyone including the therapist. Rather than being a brooding, silent, ogre, Roger was a shy, soft-spoken, passive, and anxious individual. After a brief welcoming period the therapist dove into the illness story by asking, "Who first noticed something was wrong with Beth nine years ago?" Dana erupted with her recollections and Beth chimed in all while Roger listened. After a lengthy and at times emotional discussion, Roger was invited into the conversation. Softly, but thoughtfully, Roger shared his recollections many of which seemed to take Dana and Beth by surprise. Not only did he have many clear memories but significant feelings about what took place before during and after Beth's initial hospitalization. Roger was able to add, clarify, and expand on some of Beth and Dana's memories. Later in the session, Roger tentatively mentioned that he had felt excluded from Beth's diabetes care since her initial diagnosis. He confessed that he had not challenged being moved to the side because of his own anxiety and self-doubt. Roger explained that at first he felt hurt but subsequently decided that his wife and daughter had a special relationship and a special insight and ability to deal with diabetes and that he did not want to, "get in the way." Despite his acquiescence and feelings of inadequacy, Roger elaborated on his feelings of sadness about being left out of important discussions and decisions regarding Beth and her health. Further, and over the course of several years, Roger expressed both guilt and regret about being excluded from other aspects of Beth's life as well. He stated that he felt like a third wheel in her life. Roger came to feel that his only value seemed to be in, "paying the bills."

With some prompting, Beth told Roger that she felt rejected by him. She told him that she thought he was afraid of her because of the diabetes and as a result she came to rely on Dana for advice, nurturing, support, direction, even discipline. Roger shook his head silently as he listened to Beth. While Beth felt her father's interest in her fade, Dana felt completely abandoned by her husband after Beth's diagnosis. Dana was more critical and decidedly harsher as she expressed how angry and resentful she had become with her husband. She also felt that his current explanation of his lack of involvement were just, "more excuses." Again, in an in impressive fashion, Roger shook his head and silently communicated that he understood how Dana could feel this way.

What triggered this interactive cycle was less important than acknowledging and correcting it. Everyone in the family felt misunderstood and unappreciated. Each felt burdened by their respective roles and worked hard not to burden the other two by complaining or asking for help. By silently accepting their roles Beth, Dana, and Roger were vulnerable to burning out, to dismissing their own needs, to disengaging from each other and suffering silently while smoldering with anger, hurt, and resentment. This second session ended with the therapist suggesting that everyone seemed to have powerful memories of the early days of Beth's diabetes and that everyone had felt varying degrees of hurt and disappointment since. Further, it seemed crucial that everyone participate in both therapy and Beth's diabetes if we were to, "turn things around." There was a general agreement with this sentiment but it seemed to fall short of Dana's emotional needs in the moment. The therapist acknowledged Dana's hesitation and suggested that there might be more for her to discuss next time.

The third session was used to backtrack some and provide Dana with a forum to express some of her unexpressed feelings. Dana's recollections of Beth's very first symptoms, doctor's visit's, stay in ICU, all combined to throw her into crisis mode. Since the first hours after Beth's diagnosis, Dana felt a compulsion to prove that she was a good, competent, and ubiquitously involved parent. She took on the role as primary caregiver with great intensity and anxiety. Her subtle and not so subtle deprivations were many and included not accepting help from anyone including family and friends. She under utilized her husband in Beth's care, ignored her own needs for sleep, nourishment, exercise, intimacy, and conflict resolution. She denied her fatigue, anger, and grief. Each time she experienced emotional upset or distress she did double time. Dan's anger and sadness about Beth's diabetes and Roger's lack of involvement pushed her to work faster and harder all in an effort to deny, distort, and upsetting feelings. By doing so she extended her stress and magnified her sense of isolation, depletion, and physical exhaustion. Dana's crisis mode moved her further from her husband and left her estranged from her family, friends, and her faith. Dana's burnout led her to experience huge losses in her life, robbed her of her dreams for her daughter, and even chipped away at her reality testing. By the time she presented for therapy her over-determined approach to her daughter's illness led to a martyred view of herself, a distrusting, and at times paranoid view of others. Dana's intense coping style left her alienated from her husband, family, and friends and included leaving her church because she had even lost her faith in God. What sealed her burnout was that Dana had lost almost everything including her sense of self. She had lost who she was, what was important to her, and what else still mattered in her life.

In the same session, Beth began to share her feelings. As many active teenagers do, Beth grew tired and progressively annoyed about having to attend to her diabetes. She was tired of the shots, sick of the finger pokes, and simply refused to count carbs before she ate. By the time of her clinic visit, she was almost never testing, guessed at her insulin needs, and frequently ate anything and everything she wanted. Further, she had also become aware of her mother's decreasing involvement. Beth's diabetes had been a source of closeness and contact between herself and her mother. Lately, it had become a source of friction. As such, Beth simply began lying to her mother about her diabetes care and Dana simply accepted the lies all while Roger diligently worked at paying the bills.

At times during the third session, Dana and to a lesser extent Beth, both took passing shots at Roger. Again, he absorbed his wife's anger and his daughter's sadness about his lack of involvement. Instead of being defensive he let both his wife and daughter finish their thoughts and share their feelings. In response, he apologized again for leaving so much work and responsibility to Beth and Dana. At the same time, Roger spoke eloquently as he returned to his own feelings of being left out and rejected. He expressed how embarrassed he was that he knew so little about Beth's diabetes after so many years. He was brief, sincere, and genuine in his current desire to get more involved. Beth was appreciative of her father's offer, Dana remained wary. At the end of the third session, Roger agreed to observe in a supportive way Beth's supper time testing and injection as well as be present for her night time snack and long-acting insulin injection. Dana agreed to step up her involvement with Beth in the mornings and reach out to Beth's school nurse about her lunchtime regimen. For her part, Beth seemed relieved to see her parents working together again. She agreed to allow her parents to be present for her injections and check her meter on a regular basis.

Our fourth session addressed bumps in the road which were surprisingly few and big picture issues that we use in our clinic with all of our patients. These big picture issues are the need for agency, communion, and meaning (McDaniel, Hepworth, & Doherty, 1992). These three factors have been found to be critical to positive long-term outcomes for seriously, chronically, and terminally ill patients. It was explained to the family that Roger's enrollment in an upcoming diabetes class was a big first step toward increasing his sense of agency. Having Dana and Roger attend a monthly parents support group while Dana attended a diabetes teen group were two additional steps toward developing a sense of community and support. Such steps served to decrease Dana's sense of sole responsibility and added to her sense of community by meeting with other parents and families. No one can be provided a sense of meaning in the face of such personal difficulties and hardship. Yet, in a later session, the family was asked if anything positive had come from Beth's diabetes? Beth and Roger answered this question with a sense of optimism. They hoped that our recent discussions might bring them closer together as a family. Again, Dana demurred but acknowledged that she had learned a great deal medically, believed that Beth was quite mature for her age, and that everyone in the family was more health conscious because of Beth's diabetes. Answering this question affirmatively has been a consistently positive prognostic sign for our families.

Two weeks later, in our fifth session, Dana began the meeting by admitting that Roger had been following through with Beth and that Beth seemed to be following through with her own care. With Beth and Roger listening silently, Dana tearfully admitted that she had been so angry for so long that she was not sure how well she was following through herself. Both Roger and Beth were reassuring and supportive. Each in their own way let Dana off the hook. Each suggested that perhaps it was Dana's turn to take a break. It was a very powerful session where father and daughter aligned themselves together to support a beleaguered Mom. It was in this session that Dana was referred for her own individual therapy to address her own concerns. This idea was again supported by Roger and ultimately accepted by Dana.

Our sixth session took place 3 weeks later and included a second HbA1c. It had been just over 2 months since Beth's last test. Everyone including Beth's physician and school nurse were interested (but not consumed) in the results. The findings of the test indicated a significant positive change in Beth's blood sugars. Beth was extremely proud, as were both her parents. Dana seemed relieved and Roger, grasping for the first time what these numbers actually meant, was overjoyed. Not only did he participate in Beth's care he had become more involved with his wife and all while still paying the bills.

A sixth session 4 weeks later was scheduled to overlap with a clinic visit. The session was brief and very positive. Beth had continued to take her insulin and test her blood (less frequently than we would have liked but enough), Roger seemed to enjoy his expanded role in Beth's life and diabetes care and Dana was visibly stronger, more positive, and appreciative for her referral to individual therapy. In addition to her individual therapy, Dana was re-contacting family and friends and perhaps most important for her had resumed attending church with Roger.

This therapy took six sessions and occurred over a period of three and a half months. While Beth was clearly, "non-adherent" and Dana clearly suffering from burnout, such problems do not occur in isolation. We believe it would have been a mistake to simply see Beth or Dana in isolation or in individual therapy or to simply have her family physician prescribe Dana an anti-depressant. Their problems were family problems and needed to include the excluded Roger. Therefore the therapist resisted the temptation of providing individual therapy and addressed Beth's problems systemically. In fact, we believe like many other burned out patients and caregivers; had either Beth or Dana been initially referred for individual treatment, Beth would have passively or aggressively resisted it and Dana would have refused it. However, once the family was involved in treatment, Beth quickly warmed up to therapy and Dana, like many other burned out givers, could allow herself to receive help (as long as others were receiving help as well). Finally, while this is a familiar scenario in our clinic it is unfortunately not a frequent outcome. Roger like many fathers was under-involved in his child's care. However, unlike many father's, he was anxious to get involved and hurt that he was not. Many other factors worked in this family's favor and complicate the treatment of other families in our program. Many of our clinic's families present with more serious financial, educational, cultural, and language barriers as well as more serious behavioral problems. Of any possible treatment modality, we believe family therapy with the support and involvement of a committed and diverse medical team is the most effective way to engage and assist these burned out and struggling families. Finally, we ask clinicians to resist the comfort and familiarity of individual treatment when working in medical settings and encourage them to wade into the less familiar but often more fruitful waters of family therapy.

Conclusion

Dealing with menial, day-to-day administrative tasks are triggers for burnout in health-care professionals caring for adolescents with chronic health conditions. Health-care professionals who allow for adequate time away from work and take vacations to regroup and reflect may minimize the effects of these triggers. Adolescents with type 1 diabetes are required to continually monitor their blood glucose levels, administer appropriate insulin dosages, and calculate the content of the food they eat. These are menial, day-to-day tasks, though they are vitally important to improved long-term health trajectory. Adolescents with type 1 diabetes may feel the effects of burnout from constant attention given to their disease management and from pressure from others to monitor their blood glucose, or cover their meals appropriately. Adolescents with type 1 diabetes do not have the luxury of taking a vacation from their disease; it is a constant, Sisyphean task. Parents, caregivers, siblings, and close friends can help ease the burden of this. Though much literature has spoken to the importance and need to successfully transition disease management responsibilities to adolescents and that adolescents often want to exert autonomy in taking over control, occasionally offering to allow the adolescent to take a diabetes vacation, or manage it for them on a day that they seem particularly burned out, will provide them with some respite from these menial but vital daily tasks.

The majority of literature on distress and risk for burnout in parents of chronically ill children and adolescents reports on the psychological well-being of mothers. Mothers of chronically ill children report less opportunity to engage in community or other outside activities which was associated with more frustration and distress (Brown et al., 2008). Mothers also have less socially diverse support networks than mothers of healthy children and this has been associated with greater distress (Kazak & Wilcox, 1984). Mothers also frequently handle monitoring the disease, making medical appointments, administering medications, and treatments, while also maintaining the household, cooking, cleaning, and taking care of other family members. This phenomenon has been termed the "burden of care" and has been found to be stable across the course of the illness (Steele, Long, Reddy, Luhr, & Phipps, 2003). Mothers may feel that they are not allowed to take breaks from this, resulting eventually in exhaustion and a sense of depletion of one's resources (Brown et al., 2008; Coffey, 2006). This sense of exhaustion from overextending oneself to care for others fits perfectly with Freudenberger and North's definition of burnout (1985).

Psychologists working with families of chronically ill adolescents need to assess and treat burnout in primary caregivers, who may be taking on all of the responsibilities of the disease, as well as numerous other roles within the family. Helping the parent employ some of the self-care strategies mentioned previously will assist the parent in making time for caring for themselves. In addition, assisting parents in receiving effective social support online support forums, support groups, or through other mediums may be helpful in decreasing the risk for burnout in parents of adolescents with chronic illness.

It is clear that burnout is a large problem in the medical community that can lead to job dissatisfaction, increased turnover, work absenteeism, more work errors, and pessimistic, emotionally exhausted health-care professionals. Chronic illness may also lead to exhaustion and burnout in patients and family members of patients. Individuals who make the career choice to assist children and their families who are suffering with chronic, and in some cases, fatal diseases should be applauded and supported for their efforts. It takes much strength and compassion to walk through pain and uncertainty with others, though with this ability comes the risk of giving too much of one's self away and losing sight of how this impacts one's own health. Utilizing self-care strategies and work-related strategies can mitigate the effects of compassion fatigue and prevent burnout, allowing mental health professionals the ability to continue managing patients' and families' risk for burnout.

Continued research in the areas of assessing and treating compassion fatigue and burnout is necessary to address the specific needs of integrated care teams, and in individuals working with chronically ill adolescents and their families. More attention is also needed to address the prevalence of burnout in adolescents with chronic illness and various correlates of burnout that might be targeted and intervened upon. Until cures for some of these chronic conditions are found, practitioners' efforts can continue to examine how to further advance treatments and improve the quality of life in adolescents and their families, though only after first remembering to secure their own oxygen mask.

References

Adams, R. E., Boscarino, J. A. & Figley, C. R. (2006). Compassion fatigue and psychological distress among social workers: A validation study. *American Journal of Orthopsychiatry 76*(1), 103–108.

Alford, W. K., Malouff, J. M., & Osland, K. S. (2005). Written emotional expression as a coping method in child protective services officers. *International Journal of Stress Management, 12*(2), 177–187.

Allam, Z., & Ali, N. (2007). Job involvement, job anxiety and job burnout: A comparative study of bank employees. *Social Science International, 23*(1), 104–113.

Berger, B. G., & Motl, R. (2001). Physical activity and quality of life. In R. N. Singer, H. A. Hausenblas, & C. M. Janelle (Eds.) *Handbook of Sports Psychology*. New York: Wiley.

Bride, B. E., Radey, M., & Figley, C. R. (2007). Measuring compassion fatigue. *Clinical Social Work Journal, 35*, 155–163.

Brosche, T. (2003). Death, dying and the ICU nurse. *Dimensions of Critical Care Nursing, 22*, 173–179.

Brown, R. T., Wiener, L., Kupst, M. J., Brennan, T., Behrman, R., Compas, B. E., et al. (2008). Single parents of children with chronic illness: An understudied phenomenon. *Journal of Pediatric Psychology, 33*(4), 408–421.

Bughi, S. A., Sumcad, J., & Bughu, S. (2006). Effect of brief behavioral intervention program in managing stress in medical students from two Southern California universities. *Medical Education Online 11*, 1–8.

Carlson, J. R., & Thomas, G. (2006). Burnout among prison caseworkers and correction officers. *Journal of Offender Rehabilitation, 43*(3), 19–34.

Chaffee, B. (2005). Implementing integrated behavioral health care in TRICARE. In N. A Cummings, W. T. O'Donohue, & M. A. Cucciare (Eds.). *Universal healthcare: Readings for mental health professionals*. Reno, NV: Context Press.

Coffey, J. S. (2006). Parenting a child with chronic illness: A metasynthesis. *Pediatric Nursing, 32*, 51–59.

Collins, S., & Long, A. (2003). Working with the psychological effects of trauma: Consequences for mental health professionals, a literature review. *Journal of Psychiatric and Mental Health Nursing, 10*, 417–424.

Conrad, D., & Kellar-Guenther, Y. (2006). Compassion fatigue, burnout, and compassion satisfaction among Colorado child protection workers. *Child Abuse & Neglect, 30*, 1071–1080.

Deighton, R. M., Gurris, N., & Traue, H. (2007). Factors affecting burnout and compassion fatigue in psychotherapists treating torture survivors: Is the therapist's attitude to working through trauma relevant? *Journal of Traumatic Stress, 20*(1), 63–75.

Demerouti, E., Bakker, A. B., Vardakou, I., & Kantas, A. (2003). The convergent validity of two burnout instruments: A multitrait-multimethod analysis. *European Journal of Psychological Assessment, 19*, 12–23.

Dyrbye, L. N., Thomas, M. R., Huntington, J. L., Lawson, K. L., Novotny, P. J., Sloan, J. A., et al. (2006). Personal life events and medical student burnout: A multicenter study. *Academic Medicine, 81*(4), 374–384.

Erickson, J. D., Patterson, J. M., Wall, M., & Neumark-Sztainer, D. (2005). Risk behaviors and emotional well-being in youth with chronic health conditions. *Children's Health Care, 34*(3), 181–192.

Fahrenkopf, A. M., Sectish, T. C., Barger, L. K., Sharek, P. J., Lewin, D., Chiang, V. W., et al. (2008). Rates of medication errors among depressed and burnt out residents: A prospective cohort study. *British Medical Journal, 336*, 488–491.

Figley, C. R. (1995). *Compassion fatigue: Secondary traumatic stress*. New York: Bruner/Mazel.

Figley, C. R. (1998). *Burnout in families: The cost of caring*. Boca Raton, FL: CRC Press.

Figley, C. R., & Stamm, B. H. (1996). Psychometric Review of Compassion Fatigue Self Test. In B. H. Stamm (Ed), *Measurement of Stress, Trauma and Adaptation*. Lutherville, MD: Sidran Press.

Freudenberger, H. J., & North, G. (1985). *Women's burnout: How to spot it, how to reverse it, and how to prevent it*. Garden City, NY: Doubleday & Company, Inc.

Galantino, M. L., Baime, M., Maguire, M., Szapary, P. O., & Farrar, J. T. (2005). Short communication: Association of psychological and physiological measures of stress in health-care professionals during an 8-week mindfulness meditation program: Mindfulness in practice. *Stress and Health, 21*, 255–261.

Granath, J., Ingvarsson, S., von Thiele, U., & Lundberg, U. (2006). Stress management: A randomized study of cognitive behavioral therapy and yoga. *Cognitive Behavior Therapy 35*(1), 3–10.

Harbeck-Weber, C., Fisher, J. L., & Dittner, C. A. (2003). Promoting coping and enhancing adaptation to illness. In M. C. Roberts (Ed.). *Handbook of pediatric psychology* (3rd Ed.). New York: Guilford Press.

Hartup, W. W. (1993). Adolescents and their friends. In B. Laursen (Ed.) *Close friendships in adolescence*. (pp. 3–22). San Francisco, CA: Jossey-Bass.

Hauenstein, E. (1990). The experience of distress in chronically ill children: Potential or likely outcome? *Journal of Clinical Child Psychology, 19*, 356–364.

Hayes, C. T., & Weathington, B. L. (2007). Optimism, stress, life satisfaction and job burnout in restaurant managers. *Journal of Psychology: Interdisciplinary and Applied, 141*(6), 565–579.

Holden, G., Bearison, D. J., Rode, D. C., Kapiloff, M. F., & Rosenberg, G. (2000). The effects of a computer network on pediatric pain and anxiety. *Journal of Technology in Human Services 17*(1), 27–47.

Iliffe, G., & Steed, L. G. (2000). Exploring the counselor's experience of working with perpetrators and survivors of domestic violence. *Journal of Interpersonal Violence 15*(4), 393–412.

Kahill, S. (1988). Symptoms of professional burnout: A review of the empirical evidence. *Canadian Psychology, 29*, 284–297.

Kaplan, A., & Laygo, R. (2003). Stress management. In W. O'Donohue, J. E. Fisher, & S. C. Hayes (Eds.). *Cognitive behavior therapy: Applying empirically supported techniques in your practice*. Hoboken, NJ: John Wiley & Sons, Inc.

Kazak, A. E., Alderfer, M., Rourke, M. T., Simms, S., Streisand, R., & Grossman, J. R. (2004). Posttraumatic stress disorder (PTSD) and posttraumatic stress symptoms (PTSS) in families of adolescent childhood cancer survivors. *Journal of Pediatric Psychology, 29*, 211–219.

Kazak, A. E., & Wilcox, B. (1984). The structure and function of social support networks in families with a handicapped child. *American Journal of Community Psychology, 12*, 645–661.

Kitaoka-Higashiguchi, K., Nakagawa, H., Morikawa, Y., Ishizaki, M., Miura, K., Naruse, Y., et al. (2004). *Construct validity of the Maslach Burnout Inventory-General Survey*. New York: John Wiley.

Kliewer, W., Sandler, I., & Wolchik, S. (1994). Family socialization of threat appraisal and coping: Coaching, modeling and family context. In F. Nestmann and K. Hurrelmann (Eds.) *Social networks and social support in childhood and adolescence*. (pp. 271–291). Oxford, England: Walter De Gruyter.

Kovacs, M., Goldstein, D., Obrosky, D. S., & Bonar, L. K. (1997). Psychiatric disorders in youths with IDDM: Rates and risk factors. *Diabetes Care 20*, 36–44..

Kovacs, M., Iyengar, S., Goldston, D., Obrosky, D. S., Stweart, J., & Marsh, J. (1990). Psychological functioning among mothers of children with insulin dependent diabetes: A longitudinal study. *Journal of Consulting and Clinical Psychology, 58*(2), 189–195.

Kushner, K., & Marnocha, M. (2008). Meditation and relaxation. In W. T. O'Donohue & N. A. Cummings (Eds.). *Evidence-based adjunctive treatments*. Burlington, MA: Academic Press.

Kushnir, T., & Cohen, A. H. (2006). Job structure and burnout among primary care pediatricians. *Work, 27*, 67–74.

Langballe, E. M., Falkum, E., Innstrand, S. T., & Aasland, O. G. (2006). The factorial validity of the Maslach Burnout Inventory-General Survey in representative samples of eight different occupational groups. *Journal of Career Assessment 14*(3), 370–384.

Linehan, M. (1993). *Cognitive-behavioral treatment of borderline personality disorder*. New York: Guilford Press.

Martell, C. R. (2003). Behavioral activation treatment for depression. In W. O'Donohue, J. E. Fisher, & S. C. Hayes (Eds.). *Cognitive behavior therapy: Applying empirically supported techniques in your practice*. Hoboken, NJ: John Wiley & Sons, Inc.

Martinussen, M., Richardsen, A. M., & Burke, R. J. (2007). Job demands, job resources and burnout among police officers. *Journal of Criminal Justice, 35*(3), 239–249.

Maslach, C. (1982). *Burnout: The cost of caring*. Englewood Cliffs, NJ: Prentice Hall.

Maslach, C., & Jackson, S. E. (1986). *The Maslach Burnout Inventory Manual* (2nd ed.). Palo Alto: Consulting Psychologists Press.

Maslach, C., Jackson, S. E., & Leiter, M. P. (1996). *The Maslach Burnout Inventory* (3rd ed.). Palo Alto, CA: Consulting Psychologists Press.

Maytum, J. C., Heiman, M. B., & Garwick, A. W. (2004). Compassion fatigue and burnout in nurses who work with children with chronic conditions and their families. *Journal of Pediatric Health Care, 18*, 171–179.

McCrae, C. S., Nau, S. D., Taylor, D. J., & Lichstein, K. L. (2006). Insomnia. In J. E. Fisher & W. O'Donohue (Eds.). *Practitioner's guide to evidence-based psychotherapy*. New York: Springer.

McDaniel, S. H., Hepworth, J., & Doherty, W. J. (1992). *Medical family therapy: A biopsychosocial approach to families with health problems*. New York: Basic Books.

Meadors, P., & Lamson, A. (2008). Compassion fatigue and secondary traumatization: Provider self care on intensive care units for children. *Journal of Pediatric Health Care, 22*(1), 24–34.

Meltzer, L. J., & Moore, M. (2008). Sleep disruptions in parents of children and adolescents with chronic illness: Prevalence, causes and consequences. *Journal of Pediatric Psychology 33*(3), 279–291.

Miner, M. (2007). Burnout in the first year of ministry: Personality and belief style as important predictors. *Mental Health, Religion & Culture, 10*(1), 17–29.

Moran, C. C. (2002). Humor as a moderator of compassion fatigue. In C. R. Figley (Ed.). *Treating compassion fatigue*. New York: Brunner-Routledge.

Motta, R. W., Chirichella, D. M., Maus, M. K., & Lombardo, M. T. (2004). Assessing secondary trauma. *The Behavior Therapist, 27*, 54–57.

Naerde, A., Tambs, K., Mathiesen, K. S., Dalgard, O. S., & Samuelsen, S. O. (2000). Symptoms of anxiety and depression among mothers of preschool children: Effect of chronic strain related to children and child care-taking. *Journal of Affective Disorders, 58*, 181–199.

Nazarian, D., & Smyth, J. (2008). Expressive writing. In W. T. O'Donohue & N. A. Cummings (Eds.). *Evidence-based adjunctive treatments*. Burlington, MA: Academic Press.

Norberg, A. L. (2007). Burnout in mothers and fathers of children surviving brain tumor. *Journal of Clinical Psychology in Medical Settings, 14*, 130–137.

Oh, S. H., & Lee, M. (2009). Examining the psychometric properties of the Maslach Burnout Inventory with a sample of child protective service workers in Korea. *Children and Youth Services Review 31*(2), 206–210.

Oliver, G., Wardle, J., & Gibson, L. (2000). Stress and food choice: A laboratory study. *Psychosomatic Medicine 62*(6), 853–865.

Oman, D., Hedberg, J., & Thoresen, C. E. (2006). Passage meditation reduces perceived stress in health professionals: A randomized controlled trial. *Journal of Consulting and Clinical Psychology, 74*(4), 714–719.

Pfifferling, J., & Gilley, K. (2000). Overcoming compassion fatigue. *Family Practice Management, 7*, 39–45.

Plante, W. A., Lobato, D., & Engel, R. (2001). Review of group interventions pediatric chronic conditions. *Journal of Pediatric Psychology, 26*(7), 435–453.

Quick, J. C., Quick, J. D., Nelson, D. L., & Hurrell, J. J. (1997). *Preventive stress management in organizations*. Washington D.C.: American Psychological Association.

Rudolf, J. M., Stamm, B. H., & Stamm, H. E. (1997). *Compassion fatigue, a concern for mental health policy, providers and administration*. Poster presented at the 13th annual meeting of the International Society for Traumatic Stress Studies, Montreal.

Sabo, B. M. (2006). Compassion fatigue and nursing work: Can we accurately capture the consequences of caring work? *International Journal of Nursing Practice, 12*, 136–142.

Sarafino, E. P. (2002). *Health psychology: Biopsychosocial interactions*. New York: John Wiley & Sons, Inc.

Schutte, N., Toppinen, S., Kalimo, R., & Schaufeli, W. (2000). The factorial validity of the Maslach Burnout Inventory-General Survey (MBI-GS) across occupational groups and nations. *Journal of Occupational and Organizational Psychology, 73*, 53–66.

Seaburn, D. A. (2001). Chronic illness. *The American Association for Marriage and Family Therapy: Clinical Update, 3*(4), 1–6.

Seeman, T. E., Dubin, L. F., & Seeman, M. (2003). Religiosity, spirituality and health: A critical review for the evidence of biological pathways. *American Psychologist, 58*, 53–63.

Sloan, D. M., & Marx, B. P. (2004) A closer examination of the structured written disclosure procedure. *Journal of Consulting and Clinical Psychology, 72*, 165–175.

Smyth, J. M., & Greenberg, M. A. (2000). Scriptotherapy: The effects of writing about traumatic events. In P. R. Duberstein and J. M. Masling (Eds.). *Psychodynamic perspectives on sickness and health*. (pp. 121–160). Washington D.C.: American Psychological Association.

Spirito, A., Brown, R. T., D'Angelo, E. J., Delamater, A. M., Rodrigue, J. R., & Siegel, L. J. (2003). Training pediatric psychologists for the 21st century. In M. C. Roberts (Ed.).

Handbook of pediatric psychology (3rd ed.). New York: Guilford Press.

Sprang,G., Clark, J. J., & Whitt-Woosley, A. (2007). Compassion fatigue, compassion satisfaction, and burnout: Factors impacting a professionals quality of life. *Journal of Loss & Trauma, 12*(3), 259–280.

Stamm, B. H. (2002). Measuring Compassion Satisfaction as Well as Fatigue: Developmental History of the Compassion Fatigue and Satisfaction Test. In C. R. Figley (Ed.), 107–119. *Treating Compassion Fatigue*. New York: Brunner Mazel.

Steele, R., Long, A., Reddy, K., Luhr, M., & Phipps, S. (2003). Changes in maternal distress and child-rearing strategies across treatment for pediatric cancer. *Journal of Pediatric Psychology, 28*, 447–452.

Stoeber, J., & Renner, D. (2008). Perfectionism in school teachers: Relations with stress appraisals, coping styles and burnout. *Anxiety, Stress & Coping: An International Journal, 21*(1), 37–53.

Storm, K., & Rothmann, S. (2003). A psychometric analysis of the Maslach Burnout Inventory-General Survey in the South African police service. *South African Journal of Psychology, 33*, 219–226

Swedish National Board of Health and Welfare. (2003). *Syndrome of exhaustion. Stress-related psychological ill health.* Swedish 123(18), Stockholm: Author

Tichron, J. G.,& Shapiro, M. (2003). With a little help from my friends: Children, the internet and social support. *Journal of Technology in Human Services, 21*(4), 73–92.

Thomas, N. (2004). Resident burnout. *Journal of the American Medical Association, 292*(23), 2880–2889.

Vela-Bueno, A., Moreno-Jimenez, B., Rodriguez-Munoz, A., Olavarrieta-Bernadino, S., Fernandez-Mendoza, J., De La Cruz-Troca, J. J., et al. (2008). Insomnia and sleep quality among primary care physicians with low and high burnout levels. *Journal of Psychosomatic Research, 64*(4), 435–442.

Wardle, J., Steptoe, A., Oliver G., & Lipsey, Z. (2000). Stress, dietary restraint and food intake. *Journal of Psychosomatic Research 48*(2), 195–202.

Weiss, M. J. (2002). Hardiness and social support as predictors of stress in mothers of typical children, children with autism, and children with mental retardation. *Autism, 6*(1), 115–130.

Wysocki, T., Greco, P., & Buckloh, L. M. (2003). Childhood diabetes in psychological context. In M. C. Roberts (Ed.) Handbook of Pediatric Psychology 3rd ed. New York, NY: Guilford.

Part II
Integrated Care Practice Guidelines

Type 1 Diabetes Mellitus

Annette M. La Greca and Eleanor R. Mackey

Description of Type 1 Diabetes Among Adolescents

Type 1 (formerly insulin-dependent or juvenile-onset) diabetes mellitus is a complex, chronic disease. The management of type 1 diabetes melliltus (T1DM) is especially challenging for adolescents, who consistently have been found to have problems with adherence and metabolic control (e.g., Anderson, Auslander, Jung, Miller, & Santiago, 1990; La Greca, Follansbee, & Skyler, 1990; La Greca, Auslander, et al., 1995).

Because the treatment regimen for T1DM is intensive and requires substantial self-monitoring and complex lifestyle choices, it is a critical area for the involvement of behavioral health-care providers. Efforts to promote treatment adherence and metabolic control among adolescents are of utmost importance, given that poor disease control is associated with serious health complications, such as renal disease and retinopathy (Diabetes Control and Complications Trial Research Group, 1994). This chapter provides an overview of T1DM in adolescents and related behavioral health issues.

Epidemiology

T1DM typically has its onset during childhood and is the major form of diabetes diagnosed in children under 10 years of age (International Society for Pediatric and Adolescent Diabetes [ISPAD], 2007). However, the incidence of type 2 (non-insulin-dependent or adult-onset) diabetes is increasing among youth around the world and has complicated the picture of "childhood" diabetes (ISPAD, 2007; also see "Non-Insulin Dependent Diabetes Mellitus", this volume).

Because the typical age of onset for T1DM is prior to 14 years of age, estimates of prevalence and incidence of this disease track children between birth and 14 years of age. According to the International Diabetes Federation (IDF), in 2003 there were 49,200 cases of T1DM among US children aged 0–14 years, with an estimated incidence of 13.2 cases per 100,000 population per year (www.eatlas.idf.org/incidence). In 2006, the IDF estimated that there were approximately 440,000 cases of T1DM worldwide in youth under the age of 15 years, with 70,000 newly diagnosed cases per year (ISPAD, 2007). Currently, in the United States, approximately 176,500 individuals under 20 years of age have diabetes and approximately 1 in every 400–600 children has T1DM (National Institute of Diabetes and Digestive and Kidney Diseases [NIDDK], 2007). Recent data from the United States and abroad indicate that the incidence of T1DM in children and adolescents is rising, especially among children less than 5 years of age (e.g., Chong et al., 2007; Vehik et al., 2007).

Diagnosis and Symptoms

T1DM is an autoimmune disease characterized by the destruction of the pancreatic beta cells that produce insulin (see NIDDK, 2007). Without insulin, the

A.M. La Greca (✉)
Department of Psychology, University of Miami, Coral Gables, FL, USA
e-mail: alagreca@miami.edu

W.T. O'Donohue, L.W. Tolle (eds.), *Behavioral Approaches to Chronic Disease in Adolescence*,
DOI 10.1007/978-0-387-87687-0_8, © Springer Science+Business Media, LLC 2009

body is unable to process glucose effectively, which is essential for survival. Although there are various stages of prediabetes (Atkinson & Eisenbarth, 2001), the clinical onset of the disease is typically manifested by hyperglycemia (high glucose levels, due to insulin deficiency) and is associated with several classic symptoms: weight loss, excessive thirst, frequent urination, and fatigue. Although rare, death at the time of onset may occur, and it is likely to be associated with a delayed diagnosis (Atkinson & Eisenbarth, 2001).

Once diagnosed with T1DM, youngsters begin a complicated, life-long treatment regimen (see below) that includes daily exogenous insulin administration. Following the clinical onset of diabetes, many individuals experience a "honeymoon" period for the first few months or year after diagnosis, during which their glucose levels may be well controlled (due to some residual insulin-producing beta cells). However, this effect is short lived, and most individuals struggle with a challenging treatment regimen in order to achieve good metabolic control.

Research efforts have been directed toward finding a cure (e.g., via islet cell transplantation) and also toward preventing diabetes (see NIDDK, 2006). However, at the present time there is no cure for T1DM, and no known means of preventing the disease. Nevertheless, with proper disease management and glucose control, most individuals with T1DM lead normal lives.

Progression and Prognosis

The key to diabetes management is maintaining near normal (if possible) *levels* of metabolic control. This is typically evaluated with a glycosylated hemoglobin assay (HbA_{1c}) that estimates average glucose levels over the prior 4- to 6-week period. The Diabetes Control and Complications Trial (1994) clearly demonstrated the importance of strict metabolic control for the prevention and delay of serious and common health complications. Complications include renal disease (including renal failure leading to dialysis treatment), cardiovascular disease (including stroke and congestive heart failure), retinopathy (blindness), symptomatic neuropathy, and foot ulcers (e.g., Coffey et al., 2002; NIDDK, 2007). In fact, very early stages of disease complications may be detected as soon as 2–5 years after disease diagnosis (Sochett & Daneman, 1999) and bear monitoring, even among adolescents.

Maintaining good metabolic control is especially challenging during periods of stress, illness, and rapid physical or metabolic changes. Adolescence, in particular, is a remarkably challenging developmental period for the management of this disease (La Greca & Skyler, 1991) and metabolic control often deteriorates during this developmental period (e.g., Greening, Stoppelbein, Konishi, Jordan, & Moll, 2007). Increased insulin resistance that accompanies puberty (e.g., Bloch, Clemons, & Sperling, 1987; Goran & Gower, 2001) may contribute to problems with metabolic control among adolescents and necessitate substantial adjustment in insulin requirements to achieve acceptable levels of glycemia. Moreover, given adolescents' "present orientation," concerns about future health complications are typically insufficient to motivate them to maintain good metabolic control. In fact, adolescents' levels of treatment adherence are typically poorer than those for younger children or for adults (e.g., Greening et al., 2007; La Greca et al., 1990).

Despite the challenges of maintaining good metabolic control, many individuals with this disease have close to a normal life expectancy and a quality of life that is comparable to that of healthy adolescents (Hoey et al., 2001; Wagner, Muller-Godeffroy, von Sengbusch, Hager, & Thyen, 2005). At the same time, quality of life has been associated with metabolic control and disease progression. Specifically, adolescents with T1DM who have better metabolic control also report a better quality of life (e.g., Hoey et al., 2001; Wagner et al., 2005). Moreover, among adults with T1DM, serious health complications, such as neuropathy, retinopathy, and macrovascular disease, are associated with a significantly lower quality of life (e.g., Coffey et al., 2002) and greater depression (e.g., de Groot, Anderson, Freedland, Clause, & Lustman, 2001). Depression also has been associated with poor levels of metabolic control (Lustman et al., 2000).

Treatment Regimen

The treatment regimen for T1DM is complicated and involves multiple daily insulin injections (or insulin delivery via a pump); frequent daily monitoring of blood glucose levels; major lifestyle adjustments, such as regulating the timing, amount, and content of meals; planning regular exercise; and understanding how to make adjustments in insulin dosage or meals in order to accommodate illness, stress, or inevitable disruptions or variations in daily life activities. Because the Diabetes Complications and Control Trial (1994) found that lower blood glucose levels were clearly associated with a reduction in morbidity and with the prevention or delay of serious health complications associated with T1DM, efforts to promote better glycemic control have become an important aspect of treatment. Over the past decade, this has led to the intensification of the daily diabetes treatment regimen, by prescribing more frequent insulin injections and monitoring of blood glucose levels (more than 3 times a day) so that better glycemic control can be achieved.

In general, the treatment regimen for type 1 diabetes requires exogenous insulin administration, monitoring blood glucose levels, and regulating meals and exercise. Nevertheless, there are variations in this basic overall treatment approach (see Mortensen et al., 1998). For example, some adolescents are on "conventional" regimens (insulin administered twice daily), some are on intensified regimens (insulin administered more than three times a day), and some receive insulin through a pump that administers a steady stream of low-dose insulin with additional insulin units administered when meals are eaten (e.g., Wagner et al., 2005). In addition, there are variations on the recommended diet, with some adolescents following a meal plan that balances amounts and types of foods (e.g., protein, carbohydrates, fats) consumed at each meal, whereas other adolescents use a system of "counting carbohydrates." These variations are useful in adapting the treatment regimen to individual adolescents' lifestyles. In general, however, the more flexible variations of the treatment regimen are associated with greater demands for monitoring blood glucose levels and making frequent adjustments in food or insulin intake on a daily basis.

Glycemic Control and Short- and Long-Term Complications

Despite their importance, treatment adherence and proper glycemic control are serious problems for many adolescents. Numerous investigations have found that adolescents with T1DM have poorer levels of treatment adherence than younger children (e.g., Anderson et al., 1990; La Greca et al., 1990; La Greca, Auslander et al., 1995). Adolescents with diabetes also have poorer levels of glycemic control than younger children or adults, which puts adolescents at risk for developing short- and long-term disease complications (Diabetes Complications and Control Trial Research Group, 1994).

On a daily basis, one of the many challenges of managing diabetes is striking the right balance between administering enough insulin to metabolize food and keep blood glucose levels in the normal range. *Hypoglycemia* or "insulin reactions" occur when blood glucose levels fall below the normal range and can result if too much insulin is administered, not enough food is consumed, if meals are delayed, or if the adolescent engaged in sustained and hard exercise (without corresponding alterations in insulin or food levels). Symptoms of hypoglycemia include feeling shaky, lightheaded, or faint; extreme hypoglycemia can lead to loss of consciousness or even coma. Treatment typically involves the ingestion of a fast-acting source of sugar (e.g., soda, orange juice, glucose tablets) to quickly raise blood glucose levels.

In contrast, *hyperglycemia*, or higher than normal levels of blood glucose, occurs when insulin levels are too low or too much food has been ingested. Illness and stress may also contribute to hyperglycemia. At least at mild levels, there may be no symptoms associated with hyperglycemia, so it can be difficult for adolescents to know that their blood glucose levels are elevated without checking their blood glucose levels directly (i.e., via blood testing and glucose monitoring devices). Moderate to very high levels of hyperglycemia may be associated with the classic symptoms of the disease; that is, frequent urination, thirst, weight loss, and fatigue. If left untreated, extremely high levels of blood glucose can lead to diabetic ketoacidosis, which requires hospitalization/medical treatment and can be life threatening.

Aside from the symptoms associated with hyper- or hypoglycemia, there are no obvious symptoms or visible features that are associated with T1DM. The absence of direct symptoms, however, may contribute to the challenges of adhering to the complex treatment regimen that T1DM demands (La Greca & Bearman, 2003).

Cost of Treatment

The cost of routine diabetes management and treatment is difficult to estimate, but as of 2007, the total annual cost of diabetes management and treatment in the United States was determined to be $174 billion (NIDDK, 2007). Specifically, the cost of medical care is 2.3 times higher over a lifetime for people with diabetes compared to those without diabetes, even when controlling for age, gender, and ethnicity. In short, diabetes is a very costly disease.

For many (but not all) adolescents, the cost of insulin, glucose monitors and testing supplies, and regular medical visits to an appropriate health-care provider (e.g., pediatrician, pediatric endocrinologist) in order to monitor their treatment and course of the disease (3–4 times a year) may be covered by health-care insurance or by Medicaid (for low income adolescents). However, consultations with a diabetes educator, nutritionist, psychologist, or social worker, or other health-care professionals that provide valuable services for diabetes management, may or may not be covered by medical insurance.

Common Problems Associated with Type 1 Diabetes Among Adolescents

Developmental Issues

For most adolescents, diabetes presents a challenge in terms of its potential interference with development. Adolescents' strivings for autonomy and independence may create conflict when family members (especially parents) try to remain interested and involved in their youngster's disease management (see Follansbee, 1989; La Greca et al., 1990). In addition, adolescents' concerns about peer relations, friendships, and acceptance by peers may lead them to minimize their disease or fail to adhere to all aspects of treatment management in order to "fit in" with peers or feel accepted (La Greca, Auslander et al., 1995). Concerns about romantic appeal might also inhibit adolescents' from disclosing their disease condition to dating partners or from adhering to their treatment regimen while on a date (La Greca, 1990).

Perhaps the biggest developmental transition that occurs during adolescence is the shift in *responsibility for disease management*. During childhood and preadolescence, typically parents are primarily responsible for their youngsters' diabetes care, although adolescents begin to take on increasing levels of responsibility over time until they assume full responsibility for disease management (Anderson et al., 1990; Follansbee, 1989; La Greca et al., 1990; La Greca, 1998). Further, most youngsters begin to assume responsibility for insulin injections and blood glucose testing before assuming responsibility for some of the lifestyle aspects of management, such as meal planning, dietary management, and exercise schedules (e.g., La Greca et al., 1990). Youngsters who assume independent responsibility for diabetes management too soon have been found to be in poorer glycemic control than those whose families remain actively involved in treatment management (e.g., La Greca et al., 1990; Wysocki et al., 2006). The developmental challenge is for families to encourage their adolescents to assume increasing responsibility for their own self-care while family members continue to remain involved and supportive (La Greca, Auslander et al., 1995).

The tremendous changes in physical development that accompany adolescence also have an impact on diabetes care. T1DM is more difficult to manage and control during periods of rapid growth and metabolic fluctuation, such as puberty (e.g., Bloch et al., 1987; Goran & Gower, 2001). Because of these physical changes and metabolic disruptions, adolescents need to become skilled in understanding how to make adjustments in their daily treatment regimen.

Further complicating disease management for T1DM is the common adolescent experimentation with alcohol, drugs, and tobacco, as these substances can have a much greater adverse physical impact on an individual with diabetes. For example, adolescence is a time that many teens experiment with cigarette smoking (e.g., Prinstein & La Greca, in press); yet, cigarette smoking is a major risk factor for long-term health complications of diabetes (Gallego, Wiltshire, & Donaghue, 2007).

In general, several key issues are important for disease management during adolescence. Specifically, it is important to (a) keep families interested and involved in adolescents' diabetes management and promote family communication regarding diabetes management issues; (b) encourage adolescents to assume increasing responsibility for their disease management while ensuring that adolescents have the proper skills to management their disease successfully; and (c) help adolescents negotiate the normal social and emotional challenges of this developmental period without either compromising their disease management or interfering with the development of friendships and romantic relationships or with strivings for autonomy and identity.

Comorbid Psychological Problems

Although for the most part, adolescents with T1DM do not differ from healthy adolescents in terms of psychosocial functioning or levels of psychopathology (see Helgeson, Snyder, Escobar, Siminerio, & Becker, 2007), there are some areas of vulnerability or risk that have been identified. In particular, some evidence suggests that adolescents with T1DM may be at risk for developing depressive symptoms and disordered eating behaviors, as discussed below.

Depression. Research among adults provides strong evidence that T1DM is associated with depression and depressive symptoms (Lustman et al., 2000). Among adolescents, however, the findings are less robust. Some studies find elevated rates of depression among adolescents with diabetes (Hassan, Loar, Anderson, & Heptulla, 2006), although other studies, especially those focusing on adolescents under 16 years of age, indicate that prevalence rates of depressive symptoms among adolescents with diabetes are similar those without diabetes (e.g., de Wit et al., 2007; Helgeson et al., 2007; Lawrence et al., 2006). However, consistent with findings for adolescents in general, rates of depression and depressive symptoms do appear to be higher among adolescent girls with diabetes than among boys (de Wit et al., 2007; Helgeson et al., 2007; La Greca, Swales, Klemp, Madigan, & Skyler, 1995).

Regardless of whether prevalence rates for depression are elevated, the presence of depressive symptoms among adolescents with diabetes remains an area of concern. Consistently, studies have found that symptoms of depression among adolescents with diabetes are associated with indicators of poor diabetes control, such as elevated HbA_{1c} levels and emergency room visits (e.g., Helgeson et al., 2007; La Greca, Swales et al., 1995; Lawrence et al., 2006). Thus, health-care providers might consider screening adolescents with T1DM for depressed mood, especially those with poor glycemic control (Lawrence et al., 2006).

Body Image and Eating Disorders. Adolescents with T1DM are at risk for eating disorders, such as anorexia and bulimia, due in part to the dietary restraint that accompanies the treatment regimen (Marcus & Wing, 1990), as well as to the typical weight gain that accompanies the onset of diabetes or the intensification of the treatment regimen (Diabetes Control and Complications Trial Research Group, 1988). Although overt eating disorders are not more prevalent among adolescents with T1DM than in the general population, milder forms of disordered eating behaviors are common and contribute to problems with disease management and control (e.g., Bryden et al., 1999).

For adolescents with T1DM (especially girls) who are struggling with body image issues or their weight, it may be tempting to skip an insulin injection or to reduce the amount of insulin taken as an easy way to lose weight (Rubin & Peyrot, 1992). Although such weight loss is easy, the manipulation or omission of insulin is associated with poor glycemic control, greater diabetes-related hospitalizations, and higher rates of retinopathy and neuropathy (e.g., Bryden et al., 1999; Polonsky et al., 1994). In fact, among adolescents and adults (especially women) with T1DM, eating disorders and disturbed eating behaviors (e.g., symptoms of bulimia) are associated with poor levels of metabolic control (e.g., Jones, Lawson, Daneman, Olmstead, & Rodin, 2000; Meltzer et al., 2001; Polonsky et al., 1994).

Given the above concerns, it has been recommended that health-care providers screen for disturbed eating patterns among adolescents with T1DM, especially adolescent girls. In particular, screening for those who are very dissatisfied with their weight and/or who report bulimic behaviors would help to identify adolescents who are at high risk for poor glycemic control as a result of disordered eating behaviors (Meltzer et al., 2001).

Social Support: Family Members and Friends

Social support is extremely important for the management of chronic disease conditions such as T1DM (Burroughs, Harris, Pontious, & Santiago, 1997). Parents, in particular, represent a primary source of support for adolescents with diabetes (Hanson, De Guire, Schinkel, Henggeler, & Burghen, 1992; La Greca, Auslander et al., 1995). Most often, parental support focuses on providing tangible assistance (e.g., buying insulin and testing supplies), preparing meals, and providing emotional support (La Greca, Auslander et al., 1995).

Adolescents who receive high levels of diabetes-specific support from family members have better treatment adherence than adolescents who received less family support for their diabetes care (Hanson et al., 1992). La Greca, Auslander, and colleagues (1995) assessed the specific types of support adolescents received from family members for five diabetes management tasks: administering insulin, blood glucose (BG) monitoring, eating properly, exercising, and "feeling good about diabetes." Family members provided significant levels of support for the three daily aspects of diabetes management – administering insulin, BG monitoring, and eating properly. Furthermore, regardless of the youngster's age, higher levels of family support for these diabetes tasks were related to better treatment adherence.

Although these findings underscore the importance of family support for diabetes, one of the challenges parents face is finding ways to remain supportive and involved in their adolescent's diabetes management, while at the same time allowing adolescents to assume increasing responsibility for their own health care (Follansbee, 1989; La Greca, 1998). Thus, a critical aspect of managing diabetes is finding ways for parents and family members to remain *involved and supportive*, but not intrusive, in their youngsters' diabetes care.

In addition to family members, peers (especially close friends) are another key source of support for adolescents with diabetes. In fact, close friends rank second only to parents in terms of the emotional support they provide during adolescence (Cauce, Reid, Landesman, & Gonzalez, 1990). Despite their importance, the role of close friends in the management of diabetes has not been well studied.

Available findings indicate that adolescents' close friends provide support for diabetes care that is distinct from, yet complimentary to family members' support (La Greca & Bearman, 2002). For example, La Greca, Auslander, and colleagues (1995) interviewed adolescents regarding the social support provided by friends for key diabetes management tasks, finding that friends provided more emotional support for diabetes than family members (especially for "feeling accepted" by others); friends also provided high levels of support for some of the lifestyle aspects of diabetes care (e.g., exercising with them). Based on these findings, Greco, Pendley, McDonell, and Reeves (2001) conducted a group intervention for adolescents with diabetes and their best friends, finding that the intervention was successful in increasing positive peer involvement in adolescents' diabetes care. Specifically, the intervention led to increases in adolescents' and their friends' knowledge of diabetes and in social support and to decreases in parent-reported diabetes-related conflict. All together, findings suggest that social support from friends may facilitate adolescents' adjustment, disease adaptation, and adherence to lifestyle aspects of the diabetes treatment regimen.

Family Conflict

Although family support is beneficial, problems with adherence or disease control are almost certain to emerge when a high degree of family conflict is present (Anderson et al., 2002; Hauser et al., 1990). Although it is not always possible to elucidate whether family conflict is a cause or consequence of poor diabetes management, both pathways are plausible. For example, given the complexities of diabetes management, it is easy to see how family conflict could undermine treatment (Hauser et al., 1990). On the other hand, diabetes management also might contribute to family stress, as the complex regimen may disrupt the family's routine and lifestyle (La Greca, 1998) and elicit substantial parental concern if the adolescent is nonadherent.

Regardless of the pathway, efforts to reduce family conflict around diabetes management issues have been an important focus of interventions for adolescents with T1DM. For example, Satin, La Greca, Zigo, and Skyler (1989) examined the effects of a 6-week multifamily intervention for adolescents with T1DM that focused on reducing family conflict and improving family communication and support. Multifamily sessions stressed communication around diabetes-specific situations, problem-solving strategies for diabetes management, and family support for self-care. Adolescents who participated in the multifamily groups demonstrated significant improvements in self-care and metabolic control six months post-treatment relative to control youngsters.

As another example, Wysocki and colleagues (2006, 2008) conducted randomized, controlled trials of Behavioral Family Systems Therapy for Diabetes (BFST-D), with families of adolescents with diabetes. This intervention was intended to improve family relationships (increase family communication and support; reduce family conflict) in order to improve adolescents' treatment adherence and glycemic control. Recent findings revealed that BFST-D resulted in significant and positive changes in metabolic control and adherence, as well as reductions in family conflict, compared to standard care or an educational control condition (Wysocki et al., 2006, 2008).

In general, it would be useful for health-care providers to identify and closely monitor adolescents whose families are conflictual as these adolescents are at considerable risk for problems with diabetes management and control. In fact, diabetes-specific conflict that emerges early on in the course of T1DM (i.e., within 6 months–6 years after clinical onset) is strongly and significantly related to poor metabolic control in youth (Anderson et al., 2002). Interventions such as BFST-D, that address diabetes-related family conflict directly, may be indicated for teens from conflictual families who evidence problematic adherence or control.

Cultural and Other Considerations

Various sociodemographic characteristics, such as ethnicity and parents' marital status, have been associated with problems in adherence or glycemic control among youth with T1DM. For instance, adolescents who reside in single-parent families are more likely to have problems with treatment adherence and/or metabolic control than those who come from two-parent families (e.g., Auslander, Thompson, Dreitzer, White, & Santiago, 1997; de Wit et al., 2007).

In terms of ethnicity, both Hispanic and African-American youth have been found to have poorer metabolic control than white non-Hispanic youth with T1DM (e.g., Auslander et al., 1997; Delamater, Albrecht, Postellon, & Gutai, 1991; Gallegos-Macias, Macias, Kaufman, Skipper, & Kalishman, 2003). In particular, the discrepancy in metabolic control between ethnic minority youth with T1DM and their white counterparts is greater for Black and African-American youth (e.g., 1.5% difference in HbA1c: Auslander et al., 1997) than for Hispanic youth (e.g., .42% difference in HbA1c; Gallegos-Macias et al., 2003; also see Delamater et al., 1991).

Understanding the *reasons underlying* such large (and unfavorable) discrepancies in the metabolic control of minority youth is an important issue. In this regard, Gallegos-Macia et al. (2003) found that Hispanic youths with T1DM (under 21 years of age) not only had poorer metabolic control than white non-Hispanic youth but also came from families that had lower income, lower rates of health insurance, and lower levels of parental educational attainment, all of which were associated with poorer metabolic control, regardless of ethnicity. Such findings suggest that ethnic minority youth may be at risk for greater problems with metabolic control, at least in part, because of lower socioeconomic status and more restricted access to health care.

However, it is likely that other factors, such as health literacy and acculturation, also play a role. Hsin, La Greca, Valenzuela, Delamater, and Moine (2008) recently reported that Hispanic adolescents with T1DM whose parents (mothers) had higher educational attainment also had better treatment adherence and metabolic control, possibly because the more educated mothers had a better under standing of the diabetes regimen (i.e., better health literacy). In addition, Hispanic adolescents who had more recently immigrated to the United States had better adherence than those whose families had been in the United States for more generations (Hsin et al., 2008), raising the interesting possibility that as adolescents become more acculturated in the

United States they may also adopt less healthy lifestyles (e.g., eat fast foods, engage in sedentary activities) that could interfere with diabetes management and control. Future studies that address some of the *underlying mechanisms* that can explain the associations between demographic and cultural variables and adolescents' problems with treatment adherence or metabolic control would be important and desirable.

Working with Adolescents with Type 1 Diabetes

Role of the Behavioral Health Clinician

The role of the behavioral health clinician (hereafter referred to as "clinician") is multifaceted and flexible within an integrated, multidisciplinary team. Most diabetes teams are composed of endocrinologists, nurses, certified diabetes educators, social workers, nutritionists, and psychologists (American Diabetes Association [ADA], 2005). In the role of behavioral health specialist, a clinician must thoroughly assess adolescents diagnosed with T1DM and their parents, provide effective treatment, and consult with and give feedback to the health-care team so as to provide appropriate and comprehensive care.

The clinician's role is to *provide support for adolescents and families, as well as for the interdisciplinary team.* This role includes providing referrals for youth and families who have mental health concerns. Adolescents with diabetes, like the general population of adolescents, may experience problems ranging from anxiety and depression to conduct problems and learning disabilities. As noted earlier, psychosocial difficulties may contribute to problems with treatment adherence or glycemic control; therefore, it is essential that clinicians both assess youth for psychosocial concerns and provide appropriate psychological/behavioral treatment, or referrals for treatment, as indicated.

More specifically related to diabetes management, adolescents and families often have difficulties with specific aspects of the regimen and may need assistance with problem solving, encouraging parents to remain involved and supportive with their adolescent's diabetes care, and counseling for family conflict that occurs around diabetes management issues (e.g., ADA, 2005). Further, clinicians can enhance communication between families and health-care team members, ensuring that adolescents and their parents understand medical recommendations and also helping to convey families' concerns and questions to the medical team. The clinician should also be available to the health-care team for consultation on specific concerns that may be affecting an adolescent's diabetes management.

Another area in which clinicians play a role is in *assessing and preparing adolescents for transitions in their treatment regimen.* Changing insulin regimens, for example, from conventional regimens to intensified regimens (with multiple daily injections), can be complex and require adolescents to be proficient with carbohydrate counting, diligent about blood glucose checks, and prepared for accompanying lifestyle changes. Therefore, it is important for the clinician to assess adolescents and their families as they prepare for a change in regimen, to ensure that they are equipped for the transition and prepared for challenges they might encounter. This is a crucial role for the clinician, as blood glucose levels frequently become less stable as adolescents adapt to a new insulin regimen (Gonder-Frederick, Cox, & Ritterband, 2002).

Best Practices for Assessment

At the time of diagnosis and throughout the course of treatment for T1DM, a thorough assessment is critical in order for the clinician to identify areas of strength and weakness and to provide appropriate treatment and referrals for families. Below we discuss important areas to assess initially and throughout treatment.

Initial Assessment

The initial assessment often begins shortly after an adolescent's diagnosis of T1DM, either when the adolescent is still hospitalized or shortly after release. This interview should be comprehensive and in depth and should assess the individual, family, peer, school, and environmental factors that are related to an adolescent's adjustment to diagnosis and adherence to diabetes treatment regimen.

At the time of diagnosis, it is particularly important to assess both parents' and adolescents' *emotional response to the diabetes diagnosis.* Parents and youth often experience a response akin to posttraumatic stress (Landolt et al., 2002), and a large number of parents report symptoms of anxiety and depression following a child's diagnosis (Kovacs et al., 1985). It is important that clinicians recognize the difficulties that families encounter upon diagnosis. A clinician should be equipped to provide advice for parents and adolescents experiencing symptoms of extreme distress, to normalize their psychosocial responses, and to recognize when additional professional assistance or referrals are needed.

Individual ("adolescent") factors such as school performance, intellectual functioning, learning disabilities, and comorbid psychological concerns play a large role in diabetes management (ADA, 2005) and should also be part of a comprehensive initial evaluation. If an adolescent has a learning disability in math, for example, it will be important to let the medical team know not to expect independent carbohydrate counting or dosing of insulin and that these tasks should be carefully monitored by a parent. Additionally, comorbid psychological problems such as attention deficits, depression, or eating disorders, may affect regimen adherence, as an adolescent may forget elements of his/her regimen, omit or alter insulin needs, or decide to not adhere to the regimen as a form of self-harm (ADA, 2005; La Greca, Swales, et al., 1995).

Family structure, family conflict, and parenting stress also are related to adolescents' adherence to their diabetes regimen and should be assessed in an initial interview (ADA, 2005; Grey & Tamborlane, 2003). In particular, as noted earlier, adolescents who come from single-parent homes, and homes where there is a high level of family conflict, are at risk for having difficulties with diabetes management (e.g., Streisand, Swift, Wickmark, Chen, & Holmes, 2005). In these cases, additional monitoring and support from the health-care team may be important to ensure that the adolescent and family members have the knowledge, resources, and support to manage the disease. Clinician's might use a family-based intervention, such as Behavioral Family Systems Therapy for Diabetes (Wysocki et al., 2008), or make appropriate referrals for family treatment when high levels of conflict and stress are present in the family.

Environmental and social support are also strongly related to adherence (Glasgow & Anderson, 1995; La Greca & Bearman, 2002), so it is important to assess for support from close friends (e.g., Does the adolescent have close friends? What are the friends like? Is the adolescent comfortable with sharing/discussing diabetes with a friend?), the nature of the school context (e.g., Is there a school nurse? Are teachers supportive? Are there others with diabetes in the school?), as well as family conflict and support. Areas of support or challenge should be communicated to the health-care team so that all can be aware of areas of strength and difficulty when providing treatment recommendations.

Assessment Throughout Treatment

Assessment should occur not only at the time of diagnosis but also during important life transitions. Many adolescents were diagnosed with diabetes earlier in childhood and may not have had a comprehensive assessment in many years. Thus, it is important to assess youth in a comprehensive manner as they make the important transition into adolescence and begin to take on increased responsibility for their self-care. Many of the issues described above would be appropriate to assess at this important life transition.

In addition, families and children who appear to be at risk for specific difficulties in the initial interview should be monitored throughout treatment. Specifically, for youth identified as "at risk," a clinician should ensure that referrals have been pursued and that families are receiving appropriate support and treatment; the clinician should also be available to provide any additional services required. The health-care team should be made aware of any specific concerns so that adolescents can be monitored at regular medical appointments, and any medical recommendations can take these individual needs into account.

As noted earlier, adolescents with T1DM often have poor levels of treatment adherence (e.g., Anderson et al., 1990). Thus, this developmental period is a key time for clinicians to monitor adolescents who are having trouble maintaining adequate glycemic control or adhering to their regimen. Important areas to assess include (a) motivation for adhering to medical recommendations, (b) comprehension of medical recommendations, (c) knowledge of diabetes management tasks and problem-solving skills, and (d) barriers to adherence. It also is very important to help parents remain involved (Follansbee, 1989; La Greca, Auslander et al., 1995), to encourage youth to obtain support for their diabetes care from close friends (La Greca et al., 1995; La Greca & Bearman, 2002), and to help youth problem solve with regards to barriers to adherence (Hill-Briggs & Gemmell, 2007). Finally, because parents and youth who share responsibility for diabetes management have better metabolic control (e.g., Anderson et al., 1990), the clinician should regularly *assess and clarify* the division of responsibility for diabetes management tasks in adolescents and their parents.

Effective Psychosocial/Psychological Interventions

Several psychosocial and psychological interventions have been identified for improving adherence and psychosocial functioning, and several randomized clinical trials are underway to evaluate other treatment approaches for adolescents with T1DM. These interventions can be conducted in various formats, including individual, family, and group therapy.

Individual Therapy

Individual therapies that have been shown to be effective for improving adolescents' treatment adherence include coping skills training (Boardway, Delamater, Tomakowsky, & Gutai, 1993; Grey et al., 1998), motivational interviewing (Channon et al., 2007), problem solving (Hill-Briggs & Gemmell, 2007), and behavioral therapies (Wysocki, Green, & Huxtable, 1989). Many individual interventions help adolescents identify barriers to adherence, make changes in their behaviors, learn how to cope with disease challenges, and problem solve new ways of approaching their treatment. Clinicians can use these methods through brief, focused counseling or through more intensive interventions over several weeks or months.

Family Therapy

Although adolescents often resist parental involvement, it is crucial that parents remain involved and supportive in order to promote adolescents' diabetes care. In fact, parental involvement is one of the key factors that help youth adolescents stay on track with their diabetes management (Follansbee, 1989; La Greca, Auslander et al., 1995).

Several interventions have focused on the parent–child relationship in order to promote good adherence, such as through reducing family conflict (Anderson, Brackett, Ho, & Laffel, 1999; Wysocki et al., 2006), maintaining parental involvement (Anderson et al., 1999), and teaching parents and teens problem solving and coping skills that can be applied to diabetes management (Satin et al., 1989). In particular, Behavioral Family Systems Therapy for Diabetes (Wysocki et al., 2006, 2008), described earlier in this chapter, may be especially useful for helping families and adolescents deal effectively with problematic diabetes management issues.

Group Therapy

Finally, evidence suggests that group therapy for adolescents with T1DM, such as coping skills training (Grey, Boland, Davidson, Li, & Tamborlane, 2000), may be effective in promoting diabetes management. Further, providing support networks for teens and their parents is an important aspect of care, as youth frequently feel "alone" or feel that others do not understand the burden of diabetes management. Support groups can provide emotional and tangible support and allow adolescents to teach each other strategies for managing diabetes and related stress.

Group interventions have also provided education and support to adolescents with T1DM and their best friend (Greco et al., 2001). These interventions have improved adolescents' and friends' knowledge about diabetes, increased the proportion of support adolescents' receive from their friends as compared to family members, and reduced family conflict around diabetes (Greco et al., 2001).

Collaboration with an Integrated Health Care Team

In order to be maximally effective, a clinician must be well integrated and collaborate with other members of the health-care team. There are multiple models of collaboration (Drotar, 1995); the most basic and common is *consultation*, in which a physician requests feedback about a specific concern from the behavioral health clinician. Important issues involved in this type of collaboration include clarifying the role of the clinician, ensuring that the referral questions are specific and can be addressed by the clinician, and making sure that the requesting physician receives timely and appropriate feedback on the issue.

A more integrated form of collaboration, however, involves a *systems approach* that emphasizes regular and ongoing interactions among all members of the health-care team. In this approach, each team member has a role to fill that is clear and specific and the roles of the team members complement one another. An example of this is when a physician recommends dietary change in order to improve an adolescent's glycemic control; the dietitian then provides specific recommendations with regards to changes in food intake; and the behavioral health clinician helps the family and adolescent decide how to implement the changes. This type of collaboration fosters comprehensive care by integrating the mental health clinician into the system of care and reduces the potential stigma associated with involving a mental health professional in treatment.

Regardless of the type of collaboration, it is always necessary to maintain boundaries between the roles (i.e., not to practice outside one's area of expertise), to define expertise clearly to other team members and to families, and to facilitate communication among team members and with families. Further, providing timely feedback and recommendations to collaborators and giving suggestions on how to integrate those recommendations into diabetes care are crucial in order for the collaborative relationships to be effective and translate into good patient care.

Methodological Considerations When Conducting Research

When conducting research with adolescents with T1DM, the goal of research is frequently to improve treatment adherence, glycemic control, or psychosocial functioning. Hence, adherence, glycemic control, and psychosocial functioning are the outcomes most frequently studied in research with adolescents with T1DM. However, there are a number of challenges involved in measuring these outcomes and determining which measurements to use in research. The next section will touch briefly upon some of these challenges and some of the most commonly used research measures.

Measuring Glycemic Control and Treatment Adherence

With diabetes, there are biological indicators to signify an adolescent's health status. Namely, hemoglobin A_{1c} (HbA_{1c}) is an indicator of an adolescent's average blood glucose level over the previous 3 months and is frequently used by health-care providers and researchers to evaluate glycemic control. However, research suggests that there is not a strong correlation between HbA_{1c} levels and adolescents' adherence to the prescribed regimen (Johnson, Freund, Silverstein, Hansen, & Malone, 1990). The modest strength of this relationship is partly due to differences in the way treatment adherence and HbA_{1c} are measured, but also because a number of variables, such as behavioral, psychological, and other medical conditions, also affect adolescents' glycemic control (Wysocki, Greco, & Buckloh, 2003).

Therefore, in addition to measuring biological indicators of glycemic control (such as HbA_{1c}), researchers often measure treatment adherence, which is difficult to capture and operationalize (La Greca & Bearman, 2003; Quittner, Modi, Lemanek, Ievers-Landis, & Rapoff, 2007). There are several strategies for measuring adherence, such as using 24 h recall interviews (Freund, Johnson, Silverstein, & Thomas, 1991); self-reports, including the *Self Care Inventory* (La Greca, Swales, Klemp, & Madigan, 1988), and the *Diabetes Regimen Adherence Questionnaire* (Brownlee-Duffeck et al., 1987); reports by health-care providers (e.g., La Greca et al., 1990); and information that is downloaded from blood glucose monitor readings (Wilson & Endres, 1986). Although important for measuring adherence, each of these methods has the possibility of bias due to reporting errors, social desirability, and/or technological errors (La Greca & Bearman, 2003; Quittner et al., 2007). In particular, adolescents and parents have been found to overestimate adherence, and health-care providers' ratings of adherence can be unduly influenced by adolescents' glycemic control (La Greca & Bearman, 2003).

To reduce the possibility of error in measuring treatment adherence, it is recommended that researchers use multiple methods and multiple sources of information in order to assess adolescents' adherence to a diabetes regimen. Further, asking about recent time frames, such as in a 24 h recall interview, and asking detailed, measurable questions reduces error and bias in reporting on adherence (La Greca & Bearman, 2003).

Psychosocial Functioning

Measures of psychosocial functioning frequently have been used in diabetes research. Widely used self-report measures of psychological and behavioral functioning include behavior inventories, depression and anxiety inventories, and family functioning scales, to name a few.

There have also been a number of diabetes-specific measures developed to assess constructs such as responsibility for diabetes management (*Diabetes Family Responsibility Questionnaire*; Anderson et al., 1990), diabetes-specific family conflict (*Diabetes Family and Conflict Scale*; Rubin, Young-Hyman, & Peyrot, 1989), health-related quality of life (*PedsQL*; Varni et al., 2003), diabetes-specific social support (*Diabetes Social Support Questionnaire;Diabetes Social Support Interview*; see La Greca, Auslander et al., 1995; La Greca & Bearman, 2002), and parental monitoring of diabetes care (*Parental Monitoring of Diabetes Scale*; Ellis et al., 2007). These are important aspects of psychosocial functioning and diabetes care that researchers have used to evaluate intervention programs and risk factors for problems with treatment adherence, glycemic control, or other outcomes.

Summary

In sum, although assessment of adolescents with T1DM can be challenging, there are a number of instruments that have been developed and have proven to be useful in evaluating important constructs. It is important for researchers to use assessment methods that are applicable to all adolescents (e.g., measures of general depression) as well as those that are disease specific (e.g., measures of diabetes-specific support). When possible, constructs should be measured using multiple methods (e.g., blood glucose monitoring, HbA_{1c}, self-report, and 24 h recall interview) and multiple informants (e.g., child, parent, and health care provider) (see also La Greca & Lemanek, 1996). Whenever possible, advanced statistical tools, such as structural equation modeling (e.g., Quittner et al., 2007), which allow for the combination of information from a variety of reporting sources and methods (Kline, 2005), should be employed.

Research Agenda and Chapter Summary

As noted throughout this chapter, adolescents with diabetes and their families are responsible for managing a challenging and multidimensional treatment regimen. It is not surprising, then, that high rates of nonadherence (as high as 50% or more) have been reported (Drotar, 2000). In fact, with such a complex disease, along with the challenges of normal adolescent development, behavioral clinicians and other health providers should *expect adolescents to be nonadherent*, at least some of the time, and do whatever possible to reinforce, promote, and encourage adequate levels of adherence.

Critical issues for further research include how *best to promote* adequate treatment adherence among adolescents (even before problems arise) as well as *how to intervene*, and *how to match the intervention approach* to the specific needs of adolescents who display problems with adherence or metabolic control. Although several treatment studies were described briefly in this chapter, such as Behavioral Family Systems Therapy for Diabetes (Wysocki et al., 2008) and peer group interventions involving adolescents' best friends (Greco et al., 2001), there is a critical need for further development in this important area of research and practice.

A recent meta-analysis of psychological interventions to promote adherence to chronic pediatric health conditions (Kahana, Drotar, & Frazier, 2008), including diabetes, found that behavioral and multicomponent interventions were relatively potent in terms of promoting adherence to chronic disease regimens (also see La Greca & Bearman, 2003); psychosocial interventions and educational/instructional interventions fared less well overall (with negligible changes in adherence). Also noteworthy were findings that effect sizes for interventions to improve adherence among youth with diabetes were in the small to medium range and that the few studies providing follow-up data suggest that intervention effects weaken over time (Kahana et al., 2008). Such findings underscore the need for additional intervention research that examines the effective components of multidimensional treatments and that evaluates mediators and moderators of treatment effects, so that interventions could be better matched to the specific needs of adolescents who are having problems with diabetes management. Studies that evaluate *preventive* intervention strategies, by assisting adolescents on an ongoing basis (e.g., during routine care), are also needed to prevent the typical erosion of adherence and metabolic control that occurs during adolescence.

Another an important area for research is the development of evidence-based assessment instruments (or batteries of instruments) that could help identify adolescents, early on, who are at high risk for developing problems with adherence or glycemic control. Throughout this chapter, a number of factors were described that contribute to adolescents' risk for problems with diabetes management, including demographics (e.g., single-parent family, ethnic minority background), family variables (e.g., high levels of family conflict, low levels of parental/family involvement and support for diabetes care), knowledge of the treatment regimen, biological considerations (e.g., puberty), and comorbid psychological difficulties (e.g., depressive symptoms, disordered eating behaviors), among others. Yet, there is no comprehensive tool (or standardized battery of measures) available to evaluate adolescents' risk for problems; measurement development in this area might help to screen adolescents who are having problems early on, and direct them (and their families) to effective intervention approaches.

Finally, as noted earlier in this chapter, youth with diabetes who come from minority ethnic and cultural backgrounds appear to be at risk for problems with adherence or metabolic control. Gaining a better understanding of the underlying reasons for these health disparities would contribute valuable information that could be translated into the development of effective prevention and intervention strategies for promoting adherence, glycemic control, and quality of life among minority youth with T1DM.

In conclusion, adolescence is a particularly challenging time for diabetes management. Efforts to develop better strategies for managing this chronic condition and promoting treatment adherence and metabolic control will go a long way toward improving adolescents' quality of life and reducing subsequent adult morbidity and mortality associated with this complex disease.

References

American Diabetes Association. (2005). Standards of medical care in diabetes. *Diabetes Care, 28*(S1), S4–S36.

Anderson, B. J., Auslander, W. F., Jung, K. C., Miller, J. P., & Santiago, J. V. (1990). Assessing family sharing of diabetes responsibilities. *Journal of Pediatric Psychology, 15*, 477–491.

Anderson, B. J., Brackett, J., Ho, J., & Laffel, L. M. B. (1999). An office-based intervention to maintain parent-adolescent teamwork in diabetes management: Impact on parent involvement, family conflict, and subsequent glycemic control. *Diabetes Care, 22*, 713–721.

Anderson, B. J., Vangsness, L., Connell, A., Butler, D., Goebel-Fabbri, A., & Laffel, L. M. (2002). Family conflict, adherence, and glycemic control in youth with short duration Type 1 diabetes. *Diabetes Medicine, 19*, 635–642.

Atkinson, M. A., & Eisenbarth, G. S. (2001). Type 1 diabetes: New perspectives on disease pathogenesis and treatment. *The Lancet, 358*, 221–228.

Auslander, W. F., Thompson, S. J., Dreitzer, D., White, N. H., & Santiago, J. V. (1997). Disparity in glycemic control and adherence between African-American and Caucasian youths with diabetes. *Diabetes Care, 20*, 1569–1575.

Bloch, C. A., Clemons, P., & Sperling, M. A. (1987). Puberty decreases insulin sensitivity. *Journal of Pediatrics, 110*, 481–487.

Boardway, R. H., Delamater, A. M., Tomakowsky, J., & Gutai, J. P. (1993). Stress management training for adolescents with diabetes. *Journal of Pediatric Psychology, 18*, 29–45.

Brownlee-Duffeck, M., Peterson, L., Simonds, J. F., Goldstein, D., Kilo, C., & Hoette, S. (1987). The role of health beliefs in the regimen adherence and metabolic control of adolescents and adults with diabetes mellitus. *Journal of Consulting and Clinical Psychology, 55*, 139–144.

Bryden, K. S., Neil, A., Mayou, R. A., Peveler, R. C., Fairburn, C. G., & Dunger, D. B. (1999). Eating habits, body weight, and insulin misuse: A longitudinal study of teenagers and young adults with type 1 diabetes. *Diabetes Care, 22*, 1956–1960.

Burroughs, T. E., Harris, M. A., Pontious, S. L., & Santiago, J. V. (1997). Research on social support in adolescents with IDDM: A critical review. *The Diabetes Educator, 23*, 438–448.

Cauce, A. M., Reid, M., Landesman, S., & Gonzales, N. (1990). Social support in young children: Measurement, structure, and behavioral impact. In B. R. Sarason, I. G. Sarason, & G. R. Pierce (Eds.), *Social support: An interactional view* (pp. 64–94). New York: John Wiley.

Channon, S., Huws-Thomas, M. V., Rollncik, R., Hood, K., Cannings-John, R. L., Rogers, C., et al. (2007). A multicenter randomized controlled trial of motivational interviewing in teenagers with diabetes. *Diabetes Care, 30*(6), 1390–1395.

Chong, J. W., Craig, M. E., Cameron, F. H., Clarke, C. F., Rodda, C. P., Donath, S. M., et al. (2007). Marked increase in type 1 diabetes mellitus incidence in children aged 0–14 yr in Victoria, Australia, from 1999 to 2002. *Pediatric Diabetes, 8*, 67–73.

Coffey, J. T., Brandle, M., Zhou, H., Marriott, D, Burke, R., Tabael, B. P., et al. (2002). Valuing health-related quality of life in diabetes. *Diabetes Care, 25*, 2238–2243.

de Groot, M., Anderson, R., Freedland, K. E., Clause, R. E., & Lustman, P. J. (2001). Association of depression and diabetes complications: A meta-analysis. *Psychosomatic Medicine, 63*, 619–630.

Delamater, A. M., Albrecht, D. R., Postellon, D., & Gutai, J. (1991). Racial differences in metabolic control of children and adolescents with type 1 diabetes mellitus. *Diabetes Care, 14*, 20–25.

de Wit, M., Delemarre-Van de Waal, H. A., Bokma, J. A., Haasnoot, K., Houdijk, M. C., Gemke, R. J., et al. (2007). Self-report and parent-report of physical and psychosocial well-being in Dutch adolescents with type 1 diabetes in relation to glycemic control. *Health and Quality of Life Outcomes, 5*, 10–18.

Diabetes Control and Complications Trial Research Group. (1988). Weight gain associated with intensive therapy in the Diabetes Control and Complications Trial. *Diabetes Care, 11*, 567–573.

Diabetes Control and Complications Trial Research Group. (1994). Effect of intensive diabetes treatment on the development and progression of long-term complications in adolescents with insulin-dependent diabetes mellitus: Diabetes Control and Complications Trial. *Journal of Pediatrics, 125*, 177–188.

Drotar, D. (1995). *Consulting with pediatricians: Psychological perspectives.* New York: Plenum.

Drotar, D. (2000). *Promoting adherence to medical treatment in childhood chronic illness: Concepts, methods, and interventions.* Mahwah, NJ: Lawrence Erlbaum Associates.

Ellis, D. A., Podolski, C. L., Frey, M. A., Naar-King, S., Wang, B., & Moltz, K. (2007). The role of parental monitoring in adolescent health outcomes: Impact on regimen adherence in youth with type 1 diabetes. *Journal of Pediatric Psychology, 32*, 907–913.

Follansbee, D. S. (1989). Assuming responsibility for diabetes management: What age? What price? *The Diabetes Educator, 15*, 347–352.

Freund, A., Johnson, S., Silverstein, J., & Thomas, J. (1991). Assessing daily management of childhood diabetes using 24-hour recall interviews: Reliability and stability. *Health Psychology, 10*, 200–208.

Gallego, P. H., Wiltshire, E., & Donaghue, K. C. (2007). Identifying children at particular risk of long-term diabetes complications. *Pediatric Diabetes, 8*(S6), 40–48.

Gallegos-Macias, A. R., Macias, S. R., Kaufman, E., Skipper, B., & Kalishman, N. (2003). Relationship between glycemic control, ethnicity, and socioeconomic status in Hispanic and white non-Hispanic youths with type 1 diabetes mellitus. *Pediatric Diabetes, 4*, 19–23.

Glasgow, R. E., & Anderson, B. J. (1995). Future directions for research on pediatric chronic disease management: Lessons from diabetes. *Journal of Pediatric Psychology, 20*, 389–402.

Gonder-Frederick, L. A., Cox, D. J., & Ritterband, L. M. (2002). Diabetes and behavioral medicine: The second decade. *Journal of Consulting and Clinical Psychology, 70*(3), 611–625.

Goran, M. L., & Gower, B. A. (2001). Longitudinal study on pubertal insulin resistance. *Diabetes, 50*, 2444–2450.

Greco, P., Pendley, J. S., McDonell, K., & Reeves, G. (2001). A peer group intervention for adolescents with type 1 diabetes and their best friends. *Journal of Pediatric Psychology, 26*(8), 485–490.

Greening, L., Stoppelbein, L., Konishi, C., Jordan, S. S., & Moll, G. (2007). Child routines and youths' adherence to treatment for type 1 diabetes. *Journal of Pediatric Psychology, 32*, 437–447.

Grey, M., Boland, E. A., Davidson, M., Li, J., & Tamborlane, W. V. (2000). Coping skills training for youth with poorly controlled diabetes mellitus has long-lasting effects on metabolic control and quality of life. *Journal of Pediatrics, 137*, 107–113.

Grey, M., Boland, E. A., Davidson, M., Yu, C., Sullivan-Bolyai, S., & Tamborlane, W. V. (1998). Short-term effects of coping skills training as adjunct to intensive therapy in adolescents. *Diabetes Care, 21*, 902–908.

Grey, M., & Tamborlane, W. V. (2003). Teaching teens to cope. *Practical Diabetology, 22*, 26–29.

Hanson, C. L., De Guire, M. J., Schinkel, A. M., Henggeler, S. W., & Burghen, G. A. (1992). Comparing social learning and family systems correlates of adaptation in youth with IDDM. *Journal of Pediatric Psychology, 17*(5), 555–572.

Hassan, K., Loar, R. Anderson, B. J., & Heptulla, R. A. (2006). The role of socioeconomic status, depression, quality of life, and glycemic control in type 1 diabetes mellitus. *Journal of Pediatrics, 149*, 526–531.

Hauser, S. T., Jacobson, A. M., Lavori, P., Wolfsdorf, J. I., Herskowitz, R. D., Milley, J. E., et al. (1990). Adherence among children and adolescents with insulin-dependent diabetes mellitus over a four-year longitudinal follow-up: II. Immediate and long-term linkages with the family milieu. *Journal of Pediatric Psychology, 15*, 527–542.

Helgeson, V. S., Snyder, P. R., Escobar, O., Siminerio, L., & Becker, D. (2007). Comparison of adolescents with and without diabetes on indices of psychosocial functioning for three years. *Journal of Pediatric Psychology, 32*, 794–806.

Hill-Briggs, F., & Gemmell, L. (2007). Problem solving in diabetes self-management and control: A systematic review of the literature. *The Diabetes Educator, 33*(6), 1032–1050.

Hoey, H., Aanstoot, H. J., Chiarelli, F., Daneman, D., Danne, T., Dorchy, H., et al. (2001). Good metabolic control is associated with better quality of life in 2,101 adolescents with type 1 diabetes. *Diabetes Care, 24*, 1923–1928.

Hsin, O., La Greca, A. M., Valenzuela, J., Delamater, A. M., & Moine, C. T. (2008). Adherence and glycemic control among Hispanic youth the type 1 diabetes: Role of family involvement and acculturation. *Journal of Pediatric Psychology*, under review.

International Society for Pediatric and Adolescent Diabetes. (2007). Diabetes in children: Epidemiology. *Pediatric Diabetes, 8* (Suppl. 8), 10–18.

Johnson, S. B., Freund, A., Silverstein, J., Hansen, C., & Malone, J. (1990). Adherence-health status relationships in childhood diabetes. *Health Psychology, 9*, 606–631.

Jones, J. M., Lawson, M. L., Daneman, D., Olmstead, M. P., & Rodin, G. (2000). Eating disorders in adolescent females with and without type 1 diabetes: Cross sectional study. *British Medical Journal, 320*, 1563–1566.

Kahana, S., Drotar, D., & Frazier, T. (2008). Meta-analysis of psychological interventions to promote adherence to treatment in pediatric chronic conditions. *Journal of Pediatric Psychology, 33*, 590–611.

Kline, R. B. (2005). *Principles and practice of structural equation modeling* (2nd ed.). New York: Guilford Press.

Kovacs, M., Finkelstein, R., Feinberg, T. L., Crouse-Novak, M., Paulauskas, S., & Pollock, M. (1985). Initial psychologic responses of parents to the diagnosis of insulin-dependent diabetes mellitus in their children. *Diabetes Care, 8*(6), 568–575.

La Greca, A. M. (1990). Social consequences of pediatric conditions: Fertile area for future investigation and intervention? *Journal of Pediatric Psychology, 15*, 285–308.

La Greca, A. M. (1998). It's "All in the Family": Responsibility for diabetes care. *Journal of Pediatric Endocrinology & Metabolism, 11*, 379–385.

La Greca, A. M., Auslander, W. F., Greco, P., Spetter, D., Fisher, E. B. & Santiago, J. V. (1995). I get by with a little help from my family and friends: Adolescents' support for diabetes care. *Journal of Pediatric Psychology, 20*, 449–476.

La Greca, A. M., & Bearman, K. J. (2002). The diabetes social support questionnaire – family version: Evaluating adolescents' diabetes-specific support from family members. *Journal of Pediatric Psychology, 27*, 665–676.

La Greca, A. M., & Bearman, K. J. (2003). Adherence to pediatric regimens. In M. C. Roberts (Ed.), *Handbook of pediatric psychology* (3rd ed.). New York: Guilford.

La Greca, A. M., Follansbee, D. J., & Skyler, J. S. (1990). Developmental and behavioral aspects of diabetes in children and adolescents. *Children's Health Care, 19*, 132–139.

La Greca, A. M., & Lemanek, K. L. (1996). Assessment as a process in pediatric psychology. *Journal of Pediatric Psychology, 21*, 137–151.

La Greca, A. M., & Skyler, J. S. (1991). Psychosocial issues in IDDM: A multivariate framework. In P. McCabe, N. Schneiderman, T. Field, & J. S. Skyler (Eds.). *Stress, coping and disease*. Hillsdale, NJ: Erlbaum.

La Greca, A. M., Swales, T., Klemp, S., & Madigan, S. (1988). Self care behaviors among adolescents with diabetes. *Proceedings of the Ninth Annual Sessions of the Society of Behavioral Medicine*, Boston, A42.

La Greca, A. M., Swales, T., Klemp, S., Madigan, S., & Skyler, J. S. (1995). Adolescents with diabetes: Gender differences in psychosocial functioning and glycemic control. *Children's Health Care, 24*, 61–78.

Landolt, M. A., Ribi, K., Laimbacher, J., Vollrath, M., Gnehm, H. E., & Sennhauser, F. H. (2002). Incidence and associations of parental and child posttraumatic stress symptoms in pediatric patients. *Journal of Child Psychology and Psychiatry, 44*, 1199–1207.

Lawrence, J. M., Standiford, D. A., Loots, B., Klingensmith, G. J., Williams, D. E., Ruggiero, A., et al. (2006). Prevalence and correlates of depressed mood among youth with diabetes: The SEARCH for diabetes in youth study. *Pediatrics, 117*, 1348–1358.

Lustman, P. J., Anderson, R. J., Freedland, K. E., de Groot, M., Carney, R. M. & Clouse, R. E. (2000). Depression and poor glycemic control: A meta-analytic review of the literature. *Diabetes Care, 23*, 934–942.

Marcus, M. D., & Wing, R. R. (1990). Eating disorders and diabetes. In C. Holmes (Ed.), *Neuropsychological and behavioral aspects of diabetes* (pp. 102–121). New York: Springer.

Meltzer, J. J., Johnson, S. B., Prine, J. M., Banks, R. A., Desrosiers, P. M., & Silverstein, J. H. (2001). Disordered eating, body mass, and glycemic control in adolescents with type 1 diabetes. *Diabetes Care, 24*, 678–682.

Mortensen, H. B., Robertson, K. J., Aanstoot, H. J., Danne, T., Holl, R. W., Hougaard, P., et al. (1998). Insulin management and metabolic control of type 1 diabetes mellitus in childhood and adolescence in 18 countries. Hvidore Study Group on Childhood Diabetes. *Diabetes Medicine, 15*, 752–759.

National Institute of Diabetes and Digestive and Kidney Diseases. (2006). *Advances and emerging opportunities in type 1 diabetes research: A strategic plan (August 2006)*. Bethesda, MD: National Institutes of Health. Downloaded on September 23, 2008 from http://www2.niddk.nih.gov/AboutNIDDK/ResearchAndPlanning/Type1Diabetes/

National Institute of Diabetes and Digestive and Kidney Diseases. (2007). *National diabetes statistics, 2007*. Bethesda, MD: National Institutes of Health. Downloaded on September 23, 2008 from http://diabetes.niddk.nih.gov/dm/pubs/statistics/

Polonsky, W. H., Andeson, B. J., Lohrer, P. A., Aponte, J. E., Jacobson, A. M., & Cole, C. F. (1994). Insulin omission in women with IDDM. *Diabetes Care, 17*, 1178–1185.

Prinstein, M. J., & La Greca, A. M. (in press). Child depressive symptoms and adolescent cigarette use: A six-year longitudinal study controlling for peer relations correlated. *Health Psychology 28*.

Quittner, A. L., Modi, A. C., Lemanek, K. L., Ievers-Landis, C. E., & Rapoff, M. A. (2007). Evidence-based assessment of adherence to medical treatments in pediatric psychology. *Journal of Pediatric Psychology, 32*, 1–21.

Rubin, R. R., & Peyrot, M. (1992). Psychosocial problems and interventions in diabetes: A review of the literature. *Diabetes Care, 13*, 510–513.

Rubin, R., Young-Hyman, D., & Peyrot, M. (1989). Parent-child responsibility and conflict in diabetes care. *Diabetes, 38*(Suppl. 2), 28A

Satin, W., La Greca, A. M., Zigo, M., & Skyler, J. S. (1989). Diabetes in adolescence: Effects of multifamily group intervention on parent simulation of diabetes. *Journal of Pediatric Psychology, 14*, 259–275.

Sochett, E., & Daneman, D. (1999). Early diabetes-related complications in children and adolescents with type 1 diabetes: Implications for screening and intervention. *Endocrinology and Metabolism Clinics of North America, 28*(4), 865–862.

Streisand, R., Swift, E., Wickmark, T., Chen, R., & Holmes, C. S. (2005). Pediatric parenting stress among parents of children with type 1 diabetes: The role of self-efficacy, responsibility, and fear. *Journal of Pediatric Psychology, 30*(6), 513–521.

Varni, J. W., Burwinkle, T. M., Jacobs, J. R., Gottschalk, M., Kaufmann, F., & Jones, K. L. (2003). The PEDSQL (tm) in type 1 and type 2 diabetes. *Diabetes Care, 26*, 631–637.

Vehik, K., Hamman, R. F., Lezotte, D., Norris, J. M., Klingensmith, G., Bloch, C., et al. (2007). Increasing incidence of type 1 diabetes in 0- to 17-year old Colorado youth. *Diabetes Care, 30*, 503–509.

Wagner, V. M., Muller-Godeffroy, E., von Sengbusch, S., Hager, S., & Thyen, U. (2005). Age, metabolic control and type of insulin regimen influences health-related quality of life in children and adolescents with type 1 diabetes. *European Journal of Pediatrics, 164*, 491–496.

Wilson, D. P., & Endres, R. K. (1986). Compliance with blood glucose monitoring in children with type 1 diabetes mellitus. *The Journal of Pediatrics, 108*, 1022–1024.

Wysocki, T., Greco, P., & Buckloh, L. M. (2003). Childhood diabetes in psychological context. In M. C. Roberts (Ed.), *Handbook of pediatric psychology* (3rd ed., pp. 304–320). New York: Guilford Press.

Wysocki, T., Green, L., & Huxtable, K. (1989). Blood glucose monitoring by diabetic adolescents: Compliance and metabolic control. *Health Psychology, 8*, 267–284.

Wysocki, T., Harris, M. A., Buckloh, L. M., Mertlich, D., Lochrie, S., Taylor, A., et al. (2006). Effects of behavioral family systems therapy for diabetes on adolescents' family relationships, treatment adherence, and metabolic control. *Journal of Pediatric Psychology, 31*, 928–938.

Wysocki, T., Harris, M. A., Buckloh, L. M., Mertlich, D., Lochrie, A. S., & Taylor, A. (2008). Randomized, controlled trial of behavioral family systems therapy for diabetes: Maintenance and generalization of effects on parent-adolescent communication. *Behavior Therapy, 39*, 33–46.

Type 2 Diabetes in Youth

Alan M. Delamater, Farrah Jacquez, and Anna Maria Patino-Fernandez

This chapter first describes type 2 diabetes in youth including symptoms and the treatment regimen and reviews studies concerning its epidemiology. Common problems, co-morbidities, and cultural issues are then considered. The role of the behavioral health clinician is discussed next, followed by consideration of methodological issues and future research.

Description

There are several types of disorders characterized by high blood glucose, including type 1 diabetes mellitus, type 2 diabetes mellitus (T2DM), gestational diabetes mellitus, and diabetes secondary to other conditions. In type 1 diabetes, an autoimmune process results in destruction of the insulin-producing beta cells resulting eventually in an absolute deficiency of insulin production. Insulin is a hormone that regulates the blood glucose level by allowing glucose into cells where it can be used for energy. In contrast, in T2DM, high blood glucose (or hyperglycemia) is the result of the pancreas producing insufficient quantities of insulin due to beta-cell dysfunction, as well as insulin resistance.

Peripheral insulin resistance, in which cells resist the action of insulin at the receptor level, occurs early in the disease course. Initially this is compensated for by increased production of insulin, or hyperinsulinemia. Over time, however, insulin secretion declines and hyperglycemia results. There is no single cause of T2DM, although it is generally accepted to be the result of genetic, physiologic, and lifestyle factors, including obesity and physical inactivity.

Epidemiology. Type 2 diabetes among youth has increased dramatically in recent years. Studies indicate that the average age of onset of type 2 diabetes in youth is about 13 years of age (American Diabetes Association [ADA], 2000; Neufeld Raffel, Landon, Chen, & Vadheim, 1998; Pinhas-Hamiel et al., 1996; Rosenbloom & Silverstein, 2003). Before the mid-1990s, only 1–2% of children with diabetes were classified as having type 2 diabetes. However, according to the American Diabetes Association, this incidence has more recently increased to approximately 8–45% of all youth diagnosed with diabetes (ADA, 2000). In a study conducted in Ohio, the number of patients in the age range of 10–19 years who were diagnosed with type 2 diabetes increased ten-fold between 1982 and 1995 and accounted for 33% of all newly diagnosed cases (Pinhas-Hamiel et al., 1996). Obesity was prominent in these patients, and first-degree relatives with type 2 diabetes were noted in 65% of these cases. In a study conducted in California, the medical records of all Mexican American youth diagnosed with diabetes during the period of 1990–1994 revealed that 45% of all new cases were type 2 (Neufeld et al., 1998), with all of the youth being obese and 75% having a positive family history of type 2 diabetes.

In addition to studies reporting increases in Ohio and California, the American Diabetes Association

A.M. Delamater (✉)
Department of Pediatrics, University of Miami Leonard M. Miller School of Medicine, Miami, FL, USA
e-mail: adelamater@med.miami.edu

W.T. O'Donohue, L.W. Tolle (eds.), *Behavioral Approaches to Chronic Disease in Adolescence*,
DOI 10.1007/978-0-387-87687-0_9, © Springer Science+Business Media, LLC 2009

(ADA) reported increases in the incidence of youth with T2DM in Pennsylvania and Chicago, Tokyo, Bangladesh, Libya, and in specific aboriginal populations in Australia and Canada, as well as among the Pima Indians, where the prevalence was highest (ADA, 2000). Epidemiologic studies suggest that T2DM in children has an incidence of 1–50/1000, depending upon the ethnic group surveyed (Fagot-Campagna et al. 2000). For example, among 15- to 19-year-old North American Indians, the prevalence per 1000 has been estimated as 51 for Pima Indians, 4.5 for all US American Indians, and 2.3 for Canadian Indians. From 1967–1976 to 1987–1996, the prevalence of type 2 diabetes increased six-fold for Pima Indian adolescents (Fagot-Campagna et al., 2000).

A recent study in the United Kingdom found that of all cases of non-type 1 diabetes during 2004–2005, 40% were considered as type 2, with an estimated annual incidence of 0.5/100,000/year (Haines, Wan, Lynn, Barrett, & Shield, 2007). Ethnic minorities (primarily Black and South Asian) were over-represented, and 95% of these youth were overweight, with 84% having a family history of T2DM. While still less common than type 1 diabetes in the United Kingdom, these data indicate that T2DM in youth is increasing in prevalence. The prevalence of T2DM among youth in India is reported to be rapidly increasing over the past decade as obesity rates have also increased (Mohan, Jaydip, & Deepa, 2007).

In summary, although epidemiological data are still fairly limited, it is clear that T2DM is being increasingly diagnosed in older children and young adolescents (Shaw, 2007). There is a wide range of prevalence and incidence reported in the literature, with higher rates among youth of minority ethnicities such as black, Hispanic, Native American Indian, and southern Asian. While still relatively uncommon in Europe, it is nonetheless increasing in prevalence there. Risk factors for T2DM include obesity and family history of T2DM, as well as in utero exposure to hyperglycemia (Shaw, 2007).

Symptoms. The symptoms of type 2 diabetes include high blood glucose (hyperglycemia) and associated excessive thirst, urination, and hunger. Hyperglycemia may occur every day, and individuals may feel fatigued or have difficulty concentrating as a result. Over time, patients may become used to feeling hyperglycemic as normal. For most patients with type 2 diabetes, however, hyperglycemia usually does not progress to ketoacidosis, a very serious complication of hyperglycemia that may result in coma and death if untreated. However, diabetic ketoacidosis may occur at diagnosis (Pozzilli, Guglielmi, Pronina, & Petraikina, 2007; Pinhas-Hamiel & Zeitler, 2007). It is clear that sustained hyperglycemia does eventually result in serious health complications, including cardiovascular disease, retinopathy, neuropathy, and nephropathy. The long-term prognosis of youth with T2DM is not known, but it can be expected that many will eventually suffer from these health complications, depending on their level of glycemic control. It is documented that many youth with T2DM already have hypertension, dyslipidemia, fatty liver, and the beginning of microvascular complications related to kidney, eye, and nerve disease (Dean & Sellers, 2007). Unlike those with type 1 diabetes, youth with T2DM are unlikely to experience hypoglycemia, unless they are also taking insulin injections as part of their treatment regimen.

Treatment Regimen. The goal of treatment is to maintain blood glucose as close to the normal range as possible. In order to achieve this, daily monitoring of blood glucose is prescribed, usually one or two times per day, as well as daily medications; patient and family education and lifestyle modification are also important components of treatment (Pinhas-Hamiel & Zeitler, 2007). The most common medication prescribed for the treatment of T2DM in youth is an oral medication, Metformin, that is prescribed twice daily, in the morning and at night. Metformin, an insulin sensitizer, was shown in a double-blind placebo-controlled study with eighty-two 10- to 16-year-old patients with T2DM to significantly improve glycemic control (Jones, Arslanian, Peterokova, Park, & Tomlinson, 2002). Other medications can be used in the treatment of T2DM, but Metformin is the only one that is approved for use in adolescents. Some patients are also prescribed insulin injections. The International Society of Pediatric and Adolescent Diabetes (ISPAD) recently published consensus clinical practice guidelines for treatment of T2DM in children and adolescents (Rosenbloom, Silverstein, Amemiya, Zeitler, & Klingensmith, 2008), although it should be noted that the evidence base needs additional controlled research for the selection and initiation of specific pharmacologic agents and insulin (Pinhas-Hamiel & Zeitler, 2007).

In addition, because almost all youth with T2DM are overweight, another part of the treatment regimen is to lose weight by improving lifestyle habits, focusing on increasing healthful dietary intake, increasing physical activity, and decreasing sedentary behaviors. Interventions with youth who have type 2 diabetes must also involve the entire family, as family influences are significant in this patient population.

Youth with T2DM are typically seen by pediatric endocrinologists and are generally followed as outpatients every 3–4 months. The primary laboratory test used to measure their glycemic control is the hemoglobin A1c test, which assesses the average blood glucose level over the preceding 2- to 3-month period. Weight and height, used to determine body mass index, and blood pressure and blood lipids are also typically measured because obesity, high blood pressure, and high cholesterol are often seen in youth with T2DM.

Common Problems Seen in Adolescents with T2DM

Obesity. The diagnosis most often comorbid with T2DM in youth is obesity (Fagot-Campagna et al., 2000; Pinhas-Hamiel et al., 1996; Rosenbloom & Silverstein, 2003). The growing incidence of T2DM among children and adolescents has mirrored the increasing rates of obesity in youth in the United States (Arslanian, 2000; Fagot-Campagna, 2000). Similar parallels between growing rates of obesity and T2DM have been observed in Japan, China, the United Kingdom, and Australia (Shaw, 2007).

Obesity is a well-known correlate of type 2 diabetes, with over 85% of children with type 2 diabetes being either overweight or obese at diagnosis. A study that compared characteristics of type 1 diabetes to type 2 diabetes found 96% of children with type 2 diabetes were overweight or obese as opposed to only 24% of children with type 1 diabetes (Scott, Smith, Michaeleen, & Pihoker, 1997). Research findings also show that obese children are at high risk for having impaired glucose tolerance, a metabolic precursor to type 2 diabetes. In a study of 167 obese children and adolescents referred for obesity treatment, oral glucose tolerance tests revealed that 25% of obese children and 21% of obese adolescents had impaired glucose tolerance, with an additional 4% having type 2 diabetes (Sinha et al., 2002).

Overweight adolescents are more likely to have unhealthy dietary habits and less physical activity and engage in more sedentary behaviors than non-overweight peers. Although research with youth diagnosed with T2DM is quite limited, existing studies have shown similar findings. For example, one study found that both adolescents with T2DM and their family members had high fat intake, low fiber intake, and no regular physical activity (Pinhas-Hamiel et al., 1999). In a study of over 100 teens with T2DM, adolescents reported poor diet (frequent episodes of overeating, drinking sugary drinks, and eating fast food) and high rates of sedentary activity (Rothman et al., 2008). Another recent study found that youth with T2DM reported less physical activity and had lower levels of cardiorespiratory fitness than youth without diabetes who were matched for age and BMI (Shaibi, Faulknere, Wegensberg, Fritschi, & Goran, 2008).

In addition to obesity, family history of diabetes is also strongly associated with T2DM in youth (ADA, 2000). As such, many adolescents with T2DM live with an adult who shares the diagnosis and an even higher percentage live with an adult who is overweight (Pinhas-Hamiel et al., 1999). The shared family experience of diabetes can have both positive and negative consequences. In a qualitative study of parents of children with T2DM, parents reported ambivalence about the role of other family members in their child's diabetes management (Mulvaney et al., 2006). Parents acknowledged the unique opportunity for family members with T2DM to provide support and guidance and to serve as positive role models; however, they also reported difficulty promoting good diet and exercise behaviors when they were not using these behaviors themselves. Having multiple family members with T2DM may also have a negative impact on adolescents through family acceptance of diabetes complications. When older family members have experienced consequences from sustained hyperglycemia such as poor eyesight, organ failure, and even premature death, adolescents may see these complications as part of the regular course of the disease (Jones, 1998).

Adherence Issues. T2DM has specific physical, developmental, and psychosocial dynamics that distinguish it from type 1 diabetes and other chronic diseases in youth. Perhaps as a result of these factors, rates of non-adherence among T2DM are very high. Researchers have discussed the high rates of non-adherence to diet and exercise recommendations as well as to medical treatment among adolescents with T2DM, noting that many patients remain overweight with poor glycemic control or drop out of treatment (Kawahara et al., 1994; Owada, Nitadori, & Kitagawa, 1998; Pihoker, Scott, Lensing, Cradock, & Smith, 1998; Rosenbloom, Joe, Young, & Winter, 1999). Longitudinal studies of self-management have reported low follow-up rates. In a study of German and Austrian adolescents diagnosed with T2DM, 60% of participants dropped out of care after a mean of 7.1 months (Reinehr, Schober, Roth, Wiegand, & Holl, 2008). In a sample of African- and Caribbean-American youth in New York, 39% of participants dropped out of care by 2 years and 78% after 5 years (Grinstein, et al., 2003).

In order to understand the low rates of adherence, it is necessary to understand the factors that distinguish T2DM from other childhood chronic diseases. Physically, there is often a disconnect between what is happening in the body and the adolescent's physical experience; youth with T2DM most often do not feel sick. Unlike adolescents with T1DM, who may be motivated to adhere to their medical regimen by uncomfortable physical consequences of poor self-management such as hypoglycemia (loss of consciousness, seizures) and hyperglycemia (vomiting, ketoacidosis), adolescents with T2DM do not feel immediate consequences if they do not check blood glucose or take medication. The lack of connection between treatment recommendations and physical experience may contribute to the high rates of non-adherence often observed among adolescents with T2DM.

T2DM also differs from most childhood chronic diseases because it is diagnosed in early adolescence, a time in which youth are transitioning from dependence to autonomy. Non-adherence is an issue for all adolescents with chronic disease, in part because most adolescents do not relate unhealthy behaviors with negative health outcomes (Gochman, 1971; Radius, Dillman, Becker, Rosenstock, & Horvath, 1980). Whereas children with T1DM, asthma, rheumatoid arthritis, and other chronic childhood diseases are typically diagnosed at younger ages when parents are primarily in charge of illness management tasks, youth with T2DM are diagnosed as young teenagers and are expected to pick up management tasks more independently. In addition, the unhealthy lifestyle behaviors that contribute to obesity and the development of T2DM have already been established by the time an adolescent is diagnosed. Whereas parents can take charge of feeding, physical activity, and sedentary activity in younger children, adolescents have more autonomy and must be motivated to make these changes on their own. Finally, many adolescents are focused on fitting in with peers and are reluctant to behave in ways that will distinguish them in any way. As a result, they may be reticent to administer blood glucose checks, to eat differently, or to take medication in front of other adolescents.

In qualitative studies with parents of youth with T2DM, parents report that typical adolescent behavior, like the tendency for immediate gratification, amplified the effects of living with diabetes (Mulvaney et al., 2006). They also identified several other characteristics of adolescence, such as the role of peers, limited awareness of long-term consequences of diabetes, conflict, and deception, which made diabetes management more difficult. Another qualitative study examined the accuracy of perceptions of overweight status among 104 adolescents with T2DM and their parents (Skinner, Weinberger, Mulvaney, Schlundt, & Rothman, 2008). Both the parents and the adolescents perceived weight issues as being less severe than it actually was. Only 41% of parents and 35% of adolescents considered the adolescent to be overweight, whereas 87% were actually obese. The failure to recognize weight problems was associated with poorer dietary habits, less physical activity, and more barriers to a healthy lifestyle.

Few studies are available concerning the role of psychological disorders in relation to management of T2DM in youth. In a study of newly diagnosed youth with T2DM, nearly 20% were found to have pre-existing psychiatric disorders, including depression, attention deficit disorder, schizophrenia, and bipolar disorder (Levitt Katz et al., 2005). One recent study found that youth with type 2 diabetes, especially boys, were much more likely to report depressed mood than youth with type 1 diabetes

(Lawrence et al., 2006). In this study which included 371 youth with T2DM and 2,266 youth with type 1 diabetes, boys with T2DM were 3.48 times more likely to report moderately to severely depressed mood than boys with type 1 diabetes. In addition, depressed mood was associated with poorer glycemic control and more emergency department visits.

Cultural Considerations. Minority children, especially African-Americans, Latinos, and Native Americans, are disproportionately affected by T2DM in the United States (ADA, 2000; Fagot-Campagna, et al., 2000; Kaufman, 2002). Research does indicate that minority groups are at increased risk for developing type 2 diabetes. An Ohio study found that 69% of youth with type 2 diabetes were African-American (Pinhas-Hamiel et al., 1996). A study from Arkansas investigated differences in children with type 1 versus type 2 diabetes and found that 74% of children with type 2 diabetes were African-American, as opposed to only 18% of children with type 1 (Scott et al., 1997). Racial differences in correlates of type 2 diabetes have also been demonstrated in non-diabetic children, with African-American children demonstrating lower insulin sensitivity and higher insulin secretion, after controlling for body mass index and/or visceral fat accumulation (Arslaian & Suprasongsin, 1996).

Hispanic youth are another minority group with increased risk for T2DM, as indicated by a study finding that 45% of newly diagnosed Mexican-American diabetic children had T2DM (Neufeld et al., 1998). This increased risk in Mexican-American children may be related to behavioral factors. Studies have shown that Mexican-American children consume a higher percent of calories from fat and saturated fat, have lower consumption of fruits and vegetables, increased body fat, lower physical fitness, and sedentary lifestyle (Trevino, Marshall, Hale, Rodriguez, Baker, & Gomez, 1999). Another study demonstrated increased body mass index, insulin, glucose, triglycerides, and systolic blood pressure, as well as lower HDL cholesterol, all consistent with early appearance of the metabolic syndrome in Mexican-American children (Cruz et al., 2004). Mexican-Americans may be more "Westernized" than Hispanics from other Latin American countries.

Although socioeconomic (SES) data of adolescents with T2DM are not available, it is probable that youth with T2DM are also more likely to be from lower SES environments because T2DM disproportionately affects adults with lower SES (Tang, Chen, & Krewski, 2003). The racial and economic disparities in T2DM in youth are associated with the disparities in the childhood obesity epidemic. Minority children and low-income children are more likely to be obese than White, middle class youth (Delva, O'Malley, & Johnston, 2006).

Ethnic and socioeconomic disparities in obesity rates are influenced by differences in physical activity and inactivity. Overall, minority students get less physical activity and have higher rates of sedentary activity than White students in the United States (Troiano, 2002; Gordon-Larsen, McMurray, & Popkin, 2000). Individuals living in low-income neighborhoods get less physical activity and are more inactive (Black & Macinko, 2008). Low rates of physical activity among minority and low SES children are partly attributable to environmental characteristics of urban and low-income neighborhoods.

Recent research has focused on the degree to which physical activity is influenced by the "built environment": neighborhood characteristics like residential/commercial land use, transportation systems, green space, and degree of urbanization (Poortinga, 2006). Minority youth have reported fewer safe facilities (parks, schoolyards, community centers, etc.) convenient to them (Romero, 2005). Low-income neighborhoods are often characterized by a lack of sidewalks and unsafe neighborhoods and these factors are associated with higher rates of obesity (Frank, Andreson, & Schmid, 2004).

School environments also influence physical activity in adolescents. Research has shown that children in high SES schools are more likely to participate in regular physical education classes than children from low SES schools (Sallis, Zakarian, Hovell, & Hofstetter, 1996). In struggling schools, many children are not scoring at adequate levels on standardized achievement tests. Thus, many schools have removed physical education from students' schedules altogether in order to spend more time on test preparation.

Minority and/or low-income students also face barriers to a healthy diet. Families living in low SES neighborhoods are less likely to have convenient access to supermarkets and to healthy foods like fresh fruits and vegetables, low-fat milk, and high-fiber bread

(Black & Macinko, 2008). Instead of going to supermarkets, families must rely on convenience stores or bodegas, which have a higher concentration of high-sodium, high-fat, and processed foods. Whereas supermarkets are less available, fast food restaurants are more prevalent in low-income and high-minority neighborhoods (Baker, Schootman, Barnidge, & Kelly, 2006). In addition to availability barriers, the low cost of unhealthy foods may be a barrier to healthy eating. Many poor parents question the financial viability of eating fresh fruits and vegetables and other healthy foods when feeding a family fast food is so much more affordable.

Behavioral Health Specialists

Collaboration among physicians, nurses, dieticians, and mental and behavioral health professionals is crucial in helping youth with T2DM and is recommended by various national and international organizations (such as the ADA and the ISPAD) dedicated to understanding type 2 diabetes in youth (Rosenbloom et al., 2008). As put forth in clinical practice guidelines, a behavioral health specialist should be part of every interdisciplinary team working with children with diabetes. The behavioral health specialist can offer the medical team suggestions for adjusting treatment approaches based on the specific needs of the family and patient, attend to psychiatric diagnoses that are interfering with disease management, and provide problem-focused assistance for specific difficulties. In addition, the behavioral health specialist can help to monitor the patient in between medical visits and design tailored psychological interventions to assist the family as they consider changes in their lifestyle.

It can be assumed that enhancing treatment recommendations may lead to a reduction in long-term complications. Unfortunately adherence is poor and long-term success modest. This is attributed to numerous barriers that patients present with, as well as difficulties designing effective interventions for this group of individuals. The treatment of type 2 diabetes in adolescent youth is further complicated, as adolescence is known to be associated with decreased adherence to medical regimens and increases in risk-taking behaviors.

However, little is known about how to effectively intervene with youth who have T2DM. In developing a treatment plan, consideration should be given to the patient's age, school conditions, physical activity, eating patterns, social and economic circumstances, cultural and parenting factors, and the presence of complications of diabetes or other medical conditions (ADA, 2000, 2007). Because lifestyle changes of decreasing energy intake and increasing energy expenditure via a balanced diet and exercise program remain the cornerstone of the treatment for obesity, weight management programs focusing on lifestyle modifications and changes are indicated for most youth with T2DM. Thus, one of the goals of treatment of T2DM is for the individual to acquire and integrate healthful behaviors in nutrition, exercise, and weight management.

Best Practices for Assessment and Treatment. There are a number of issues that are important to consider in the treatment of T2DM in youth. These include dealing with obesity and weight loss, the high-risk lifestyles of family members, reduced patient motivation, psychological denial, the presence of behavioral and emotional disorders such as binge eating and depression, the lack of attention to and awareness of short-term health complications, and the cultural issues of working with ethnic minority and low-income families.

The goal of psychosocial interventions should be to identify, support, and provide tools for positive behavior change through assessment of families and the individual, fostering healthy peer activities, and increasing peer and family support and involvement. Before planning a weight management program, a comprehensive psychosocial assessment should be conducted to determine a patient's attitudes about diabetes, expectations for medical management, current behaviors, mood, goals for the future, and motivation and confidence with respect to specific treatment goals and regimen behaviors.

Because depression, other mood disorders, and eating disorders are common in patients with obesity, the initial assessment should include a screening for symptoms of depression, low self-esteem, anxiety, and eating disorders. Overweight children may be teased and harassed, resulting in reduced self-esteem and body image concerns, possibly leading to clinical depression. The presence of mood disorders may adversely affect adherence to weight management interventions; thus, treating the mood disorder in conjunction with the lifestyle changes is indicated in these cases.

Psychosocial assessment should also include an assessment of the patient's readiness to change, barriers to weight loss, current physical activity levels, dietary habits, and sedentary behaviors (including screen time). One of the most important aspects of treatment, and one that is often overlooked, is the teen and family's readiness to change. That is, how important is weight management to the patient and family and what is their level of motivation to commit to a plan to change their current behavior in order to achieve a goal. In addition, it should not be forgotten that family conflict during adolescence is typical. However, family conflict around diabetes management may interfere with treatment outcomes. Therefore, this should be addressed during the assessment and intervention phases of treatment.

Role of the Behavioral Health Clinician. The behavioral health clinician has many roles in the interdisciplinary treatment of T2DM in youth. Primary among these are the assessment of psychosocial and behavioral issues and development and implementation of psychosocial and behavioral interventions. These interventions can include behavior modification and cognitive behavioral therapy, as well as psychotherapy to address additional mood and/or anxiety symptoms, and family therapy to deal with communication problems, conflict, or lack of parental involvement. The behavioral clinician can also consult with other team members to assist them in providing effective interventions. The behavioral health clinician may help the patient initiate the recommendations made by the physician, monitor the patient's status, and provide ongoing support and positive reinforcement so that the patient maintains the dietary and lifestyle changes over time, as well as adheres to their glucose monitoring and medication regimens. It may be easy for patients to deny their disease and not follow recommendations for monitoring blood glucose and taking prescribed medications. The behavioral health clinician should take an active role in assessing psychological factors like denial and depression that may inhibit appropriate self-care behaviors.

Effective Interventions. The overall goal for managing T2DM in youth is controlling blood glucose by improved adherence to medications and by implementing behavioral lifestyle changes. Weight control or weight reduction, along with maintenance of emotional well-being, must be an integral part of treatment. Interventions with youth who have type 2 diabetes must involve the entire family, as parental involvement is crucial to support any intervention effort and behavior change on the part of the youth. Although effective family-based, behavioral interventions exist for the treatment of obesity in children, these interventions have not yet been reported to be successful with youth who have type 2 diabetes.

An individualized, comprehensive lifestyle modification program can help individuals achieve realistic weight loss or weight maintenance goals. Most successful weight management programs focus on behavior change rather than weight loss as an outcome. Weight management programs are typically comprised of various components, such as nutrition therapy, physical activity, reducing screen time, and cognitive behavior therapy. With youth as patients, this also means involving parents, particularly for their own weight loss efforts as well as supporting their children. Studies have shown that one of the best predictors of success for children in weight loss is the weight loss of their parents (Wrotniak, Epstein, Paluch, & Roemmich, 2004). Emphasis on the short-term benefits of physical activity and healthy eating is recommended rather than the long-term benefits, as the latter often are not salient to youth.

In the beginning, the behavioral health clinician can help the family choose a few specific behavior change goals to work toward. Having the child and family choose their own goals will likely contribute to better adherence as well as provide the family a sense of control. Adolescents and their families must be encouraged to consistently make better food choices. This includes helping parents determine what foods to bring into the home, how to plan and prepare snacks and meals, and discussing the importance of family meals and mealtime behaviors. An important component of an effective long-term weight control program is to help youth recognize cues of satiety and hunger.

The behavioral health clinician and dietician can work closely together to help the family set small, achievable goals for reducing calories, replacing empty calories with healthy foods, limiting high-density carbohydrate foods and drinks, and increasing intake of foods with high fiber. Goals for physical activity change should also be gradual, so that the youth builds tolerance and develops a healthy pattern of physical activity and reduced sedentary behaviors. Adolescents are more likely to accept fitness goals when they are framed in terms of feeling better, looking better, or doing more (Teufel & Ritenbaugh, 1998). Having family members participate in physical activities and helping the family chose activities they enjoy is often helpful in the family adopting these changes. When making behavioral changes, simple, achievable goals promote efficacy.

Whether the adolescent participates in a weight management program or is only seen during regularly scheduled outpatient medical appointments, psychosocial status should continue to be assessed. This can be done during hospitalizations, at discovery of complications, or when problems with glucose control, adherence, and quality of life arise. If the patient is not participating in a weight management program and could benefit from this intervention, assessment of readiness to change and barriers as changes in health status arise is indicated, as these may make patients more receptive to making changes.

Methodological Considerations

In research with youth who have T2DM, one of the primary methodological issues concerns accurate diagnosis, as recent research suggests that differences between type 1 and type 2 diabetes are not always distinct, and many youth with T2DM present at diagnosis with ketoacidosis (Pozzilli et al., 2007). Studies show some youth exhibit features of both type 1 and type 2 diabetes, a "double diabetes," or "hybrid diabetes." Some youth may be obese and insulin resistant at diagnosis, yet also have autoantibodies to beta cells. Thus, it is critical in research on youth with T2DM to be certain they in fact have T2DM.

Other methodological issues concern sampling, standardization of measures, and controls for medical treatment. Because T2DM is still relatively uncommon, single site studies may be limited by potential bias in study samples, or findings which may have limited external validity. Many youth with T2DM drop out of treatment, so an important issue concerns recruitment and retention of the study sample. Because ethnic minority youth are over-represented in clinical samples of youth with T2DM, it is necessary to ensure that measures are culturally relevant for use in specific ethnic minority populations. In behavioral intervention research, it is necessary to control for changes that may be made to medical regimens, in order to isolate the effects of those behavioral interventions.

Research Agenda

More descriptive research is needed to document rates of adherence to the various components of the prescribed regimen, not only with blood glucose monitoring and medication taking but also with dietary and exercise prescriptions, weight loss efforts, and attendance at scheduled medical outpatient visits. In addition, such research should investigate the role of demographic and psychosocial factors as correlates or predictors of regimen adherence and glycemic control and identify factors that predict treatment dropout.

More research is needed that addresses psychosocial functioning and quality of life of youth with T2DM. Very few studies have been reported in this area, but there is already evidence that depression and other psychiatric disorders may be increased in these youth. How psychological and psychosocial functioning affects diabetes management and glycemic control is an important research issue. In addition, research should focus on interventions to treat psychological and psychosocial disorders such as depression and evaluate the effects not only on psychosocial functioning and quality of life but also on diabetes management.

Relatively little is known about how to effectively intervene with youth who have T2DM, but clearly weight control must be an integral part of treatment. Although efficacious family-based, behavioral interventions exist for the treatment of obesity in children, these interventions have not yet been conducted with youth who have type 2 diabetes. Because weight reduction is an essential aspect of treatment for type 2 diabetes, future studies should evaluate the effects of such interventions, or modifications of them, for type 2 diabetes in youth, as well as behavioral interventions, to enhance adherence to other aspects of the medical regimen.

Type 2 diabetes affects approximately 20 million adults in the United States and is a cause of significant morbidity and excess mortality, as well as health-care expenditures. More and more youth are being diagnosed with T2DM, and many will be expected to suffer significant health complications within 15 years of their diagnosis. This is a very serious public health issue. The health complications associated with poorly controlled diabetes, whether from type 1 or type 2 diabetes, include cardiovascular disease, renal disease, blindness, and limb amputations. Given the significant health risks associated with diabetes, programs should be developed to screen at-risk groups, for example, overweight children, ethnic minority youth, and especially overweight children who have a positive family history for type 2 diabetes. Secondary prevention efforts should be implemented, so that these high-risk children can receive weight control interventions that may reduce their risk for developing T2DM. More research addressing the prevention of type 2 diabetes, both in high-risk populations and in the general population, is urgently needed.

References

American Diabetes Association. (2000). Type 2 diabetes in children and adolescents. *Diabetes Care, 23*, 381–389.

American Diabetes Association. (2007). Standards of medical care in diabetes – 2007. *Diabetes Care, 30*(Supp.1), S4–S41.

Arslanian, S. A. (2000). Type 2 diabetes mellitus in children: Pathophysiology and risk factors. *Journal of Pediatric Endocrinology & Metabolism, 13*, 1385–1394.

Arslaian, S., & Suprasongsin, C. (1996). Differences in the vivo insulin secretion and sensitivity of healthy black versus white adolescents. *Journal of Pediatrics, 129*, 440–445.

Baker, E. A., Schootman, M., Barnidge, E., & Kelly, C. (2006). The role of race and poverty in access to foods that enable individuals to adhere to dietary guidelines. *Prevention of Chronic Disease, 3*, A76.

Black, J. L., & Macinko, J. (2008). Neighborhoods and obesity. *Nutrition Reviews, 66*, 2–20.

Cruz, M. L., Weigensberg, M. J., Huang, T. T., Ball, G., Shaibi, G. Q., & Goran, M. I. (2004). The metabolic syndrome in overweight Hispanic youth and the role of insulin sensitivity. *The Journal of Clinical Endocrinology & Metabolism, 89*, 108–113.

Dean, H. J., & Sellers, E. (2007). Comorbidities and microvascular complications of type 2 diabetes in children and adolescents. *Pediatric Diabetes, 8*(Suppl. 9), 35–41.

Delva, J., O'Malley, P. M., & Johnston, L. D. (2006). Racial/ethnic and socioeconomic status differences in overweight and health-related behaviors among American students: national trends 1986–2003. *Journal of Adolescent Health, 39*, 536–545.

Fagot-Campagna, A. (2000). Emergence of type 2 diabetes mellitus in children: epidemiological evidence. *Journal of Pediatric Endocrinology & Metabolism, 13*, 1395–1340.

Fagot-Campagna, A., Pettitt, D. J., Engelgau, M., Burrows, N. R., Geiss, L., Valdez, R., et al. (2000). Type 2 diabetes among North American children and adolescents: An epidemiologic review and a public health perspective. *Journal of Pediatrics, 136*, 664–672.

Frank, L. D., Andresen, M. A., & Schmid, T. L. (2004). Obesity relationships with community design, physical activity, and time spent in cars. *American Journal of Preventive Medicine, 27*, 87–96.

Gochman, D. (1971). Some correlates of children's health beliefs and potential health behaviour. *Journal of Health and Social Behavior, 12*, 148–154.

Gordon-Larsen, P., McMurray, R. G., & Popkin, B. M. (2000). Determinants of adolescent physical activity and inactivity patterns. *Pediatrics, 105*, e83–e90.

Grinstein, G., Muzumdar, R., Aponte, L., Vuguin, P., Saenger, P., & DiMartino-Nardi, J. (2003). Presentation and 5-year follow-up of type 2 diabetes mellitus in African-American and Caribbean-Hispanic adolescents. *Hormone Research, 60*, 121–126.

Haines, L., Wan, K. C., Lynn, R., Barrett, T. G., & Shield, J. (2007). Rising incidence of type 2 diabetes in children in the U.K. *Diabetes Care, 30*, 1097–1101.

Jones, K. L. (1998). Non insulin dependent diabetes in children and adolescents: The therapeutic challenge. *Clinical Pediatrics, 37*, 103–110.

Jones, K. L., Arslanian, S., Peterokova, V. A., Park, J., & Tomlinson, M. J. (2002). Effect of Metformin in pediatric patients with type 2 diabetes. *Diabetes Care, 25*, 89–94.

Kaufman, F. R. (2002). Type 2 diabetes mellitus in children and youth: A new epidemic. *Journal of Pediatric Endocrinology and Metabolism, 15*, 737–744.

Kawahara, R., Amemiya, T., Yoshino, M., Miyamae, M., Sasamoto, K., & Omori, Y. (1994). Dropout of young non-insulin-dependent diabetics from diabetic care. *Diabetes Research Clinical Practice, 24*, 181–185.

Lawrence, J. M., Standiford, D. A., Loots, B., Klingensmith, G. J., Williams, D. E., Ruggiero, A., et al. (2006). Prevalence and correlates of depressed mood among youth with diabetes: The SEARCH for diabetes in youth study. *Pediatrics, 117*, 1348–1358.

Levitt Katz, L. E., Swami, S., Abraham, M., Murphy, K. M., Jawad, A. F., McKnight-Menci, H., et al. (2005). Neuropsychiatric disorders at the presentation of type 2 diabetes mellitus in children. *Pediatric Diabetes, 6*, 84–89.

Mohan, V., Jaydip, R., & Deepa, R. (2007). Type 2 diabetes in Asian Indian youth. *Pediatric Diabetes, 8*(Suppl. 9), 28–34.

Mulvaney, S. A., Schlundt, D. G., Mudasiru, E., Fleming, M., Vander Woude, A. M., Russell, W. E., et al. (2006). Parent perceptions of caring for adolescents with type 2 diabetes. *Diabetes Care, 29*, 993–997.

Neufeld, N. D., Raffel, L. J., Landon, C., Chen, Y. D. I., Vadheim, C. M. (1998). Early presentation of type 2 diabetes in Mexican-American youth. *Diabetes Care, 21*, 80–86.

Owada, M., Nitadori, Y., & Kitagawa, T. (1998). Treatment of NIDDM in youth. *Clinical Pediatrics, 37*, 117–121.

Pihoker, C., Scott, C. R., Lensing, S. Y., Cradock, M. M., & Smith, J. (1998). Non-insulin dependent diabetes mellitus in African-American youths of Arkansas. *Clinical Pediatrics, 37*, 97–102.

Pinhas-Hamiel, O., Dolan, L. M., Daniels, S. R., Standiford, D., Khoury, P. R., & Zeitler, P. (1996). Increased incidence of non-insulin-dependent diabetes mellitus among adolescents. *Journal of Pediatrics, 128*, 608–615.

Pinhas-Hamiel, O., Standiford, D., Hamiel, D., Dolan, L. M., Cohen, R., & Zeitler, S. (1999). The type 2 family: a setting for development and treatment of adolescent type 2 diabetes. *Archives of Pediatrics and Adolescent Medicine, 153*, 1063–1067.

Pinhas-Hamiel, O., & Zeitler, P. (2007). Clinical presentation and treatment of type 2 diabetes in children. *Pediatric Diabetes, 8*(Suppl. 9), 16–27.

Poortinga, W. (2006). Perceptions of the environment, physical activity, and obesity. *Social Science and Medicine, 63*, 2835–2846.

Pozzilli, P., Guglielmi, C., Pronina, E., & Petraikina, E. (2007). Double or hybrid diabetes associated with an increase in type 1 and type 2 diabetes in children and youths. *Pediatric Diabetes, 8*(Suppl. 9), 88–95.

Radius, S. M., Dillman, T. E., Becker, M. H., Rosenstock, I. M., & Horvath, W. J. (1980). Adolescent perspectives on health and illness. *Adolescence, 15*, 375–384.

Reinehr, T., Schober, E., Roth, C. L., Wiegand, S., & Holl, R. (2008). Type 2 diabetes in children and adolescents in a 2 year follow up: insufficient adherence to diabetes centers. *Hormone Research, 69*, 107–113.

Romero, A. J. (2005). Low-income neighborhood barriers and resources for adolescents' physical activity. *Journal of Adolescent Health, 36*, 253–259.

Rosenbloom, A. L., Joe, J. R., Young, R. S., & Winter, W. E. (1999). Emerging epidemic of type 2 diabetes in youth. *Diabetes Care, 22*, 345–354.

Rosenbloom, A. L., & Silverstein, J. H. (2003). *Type 2 diabetes in children and adolescents: A guide to diagnosis, epidemiology, pathogenesis, prevention, and treatment.* Alexandria, VA: American Diabetes Association.

Rosenbloom, A. L., Silverstein, J. H., Amemiya, S., Zeitler, P., & Klingensmith, G. (2008). ISPAD Clinical Practice Consensus Guidelines 2007–2007. Type 2 diabetes mellitus in the child and adolescent. *Pediatric Diabetes, 9*, 512–526.

Rothman, R. L., Mulvaney, S., Elasy, T. A., VanderWoude, A., Gebretsadik, T., Shintani, A., et al. (2008). Self management behaviors, racial disparities, and glycemic control among adolescents with type 2 diabetes. *Pediatrics, 121*, e912–e919.

Sallis, J. F., Zakarian, J. M., Hovell, M. F., & Hofstetter, R. (1996). Ethnic, socioeconomic, and sex differences in physical activity among adolescents. *Journal of Clinical Epidemiology, 49*, 125–134.

Scott, C. R., Smith, J. M., Michaeleen, C., & Pihoker, C. (1997). Characteristics of youth-onset noninsulin-diabetes mellitus and insulin-dependent diabetes mellitus at diagnosis. *Pediatrics, 100*, 84–91.

Shaibi, G., Faulknere, M., Wegensberg, M., Fritschi, C., & Goran, M. (2008). Cardiorespiratory fitness and physical activity in youth with type 2 diabetes. *Pediatric Diabetes, 9*, 460–463.

Shaw, J. (2007). Epidemiology of childhood type 2 diabetes and obesity. *Pediatric Diabetes, 8*(Suppl. 9), 7–15.

Sinha, R., Fisch, G., Teague, B., Tamborlane, W., Banyas, B., Allen, K.et al. (2002). Prevalence of impaired glucose tolerance among children and adolescents with marked obesity. *New England Journal of Medicine, 346*, 802–810.

Skinner, A. C., Weinberger, M., Mulvaney, S., Schlundt, D., & Rothman, R. L. (2008). Accuracy of perceptions of overweight and relation to self-care behaviors among adolescents with type 2 diabetes and their parents. *Diabetes Care, 31*, 227–229.

Tang, M., Chen, Y., & Krewski, D. (2003). Gender-related differences in the association between socioeconomic status and self-reported diabetes. *International Journal of Epidemiology, 32*, 381–385.

Teufel, N. I., & Ritenbaugh, C. K. (1998). Development of a primary prevention program: Insight gained in the Zuni Diabetes Prevention Program. *Clinical Pediatrics, 37*, 131–141.

Trevino, R., Marshall, R., Hale, D., Rodriguez, R., Baker, G., & Gomez, J. (1999). Diabetes risk factors in low-income Mexican-American children. *Diabetes Care, 22*, 202–207.

Troiano, R. P. (2002). Physical inactivity among young people. *New England Journal of Medicine, 347*, 706–707.

Wrotniak, B. H., Epstein, L. H., Paluch, R. A., & Roemmich, J. N. (2004). Parent weight change as a predictor of child weight change in family-based behavioral obesity treatment. *Archives of Pediatrics and Adolescent Medicine, 158*, 342–347.

Integrated Care Practice Guidelines for Adolescents with Asthma

Anthony R. Cordaro, Jr. and Marianne Z. Wamboldt

What is Asthma?

Asthma is a complex disease process involving obstruction of the airway passages, which on occasion can lead to death. It is the most common chronic disease of childhood. The National Asthma Education and Prevention Program's Expert Panel Report-3 ("Expert Panel Report 3 (EPR-3): Guidelines for the Diagnosis and Management of Asthma-Summary Report 2007," 2007) more directly defines asthma as:

> a chronic inflammatory disorder of the airways in which many cells and cellular elements play a role: in particular, mast cells, eosinophils, neutrophils (especially in sudden onset, fatal exacerbations, occupational asthma, and patients who smoke), T lymphocytes, macrophages, and epithelial cells. In susceptible individuals, this inflammation causes recurrent episodes of coughing (particularly at night or early in the morning), wheezing, breathlessness, and chest tightness. These episodes are usually associated with widespread but variable airflow obstruction that is often reversible either spontaneously or with treatment.

The etiology of asthma involves both genetic predispositions and environmental inputs. While asthma is fairly heritable, as evidenced by the fact that the concordance between monzygotic (MZ) twins is higher than that between dizygotic (DZ) twins, the rates vary over age cohorts and countries. For example, a 1971 study of 7,000 same sex twins in Sweden established that the prevalence of asthma in that country was 3.8%, and the concordance for asthma in MZ twins was 19%, while in DZ twins only 4.8% (Edfors-Lubs, 1971). More recently, researchers (Duffy, Martin, Battistutta, Hopper, & Mathews, 1990) examined 3808 Australian twin pairs and found prevalence of asthma to be 13.2%, with MZ correlations of $r = 0.65$ and DZ correlations of $r = 0.25$. Clearly, while there is a genetic component to the disease, the low concordance rate in monozygotic twins indicates substantial environmental inputs, as does the variability between countries and age cohorts. The major genetic risk is for a propensity toward atopy, and most patients with asthma have a variety of allergies and may also have atopic dermatitis or allergic rhinitis (hay fever). There are also genetic risks for hyperresponsive airways (Amelung, Scott, & Bleecker, 1996) and genetic risk for dysregulation of the autonomic nervous system (Liggett, 1996).

Major environmental risk factors implicated in the development of asthma include infections with parainfluenza or respiratory syncytial viruses, parental smoking habits, and specific antigen exposure (Arshad & Hide, 1992; Horwood, Fergusson, & Shannon, 1985). Other environmental factors hypothesized to be important in the increased prevalence of asthma in developed countries include decreases in certain other infections (e.g., Hepatitis A virus and those averted by routine vaccinations), dietary alterations (e.g., "cleaner" food preparation and processed foods), subtle differences in intrauterine milieu, obesity, and the urban environment (with smaller families, pollution, and different fauna and flora exposures) (Morgan & Khan, 2003). Given these varying determinants of asthma, there are

A.R. Cordaro, Jr. (✉)
Department of Psychiatry, The Children's Hospital, University of Colorado at Denver and Health Sciences Center, Aurora, CO, USA
e-mail: anthony.cordaro@ucdenver.edu

W.T. O'Donohue, L.W. Tolle (ed.), *Behavioral Approaches to Chronic Disease in Adolescence*,
DOI 10.1007/978-0-387-87687-0_10,

different types of asthma, and the psychosocial correlates of each may vary. For example, children who either do not report clear allergic triggers for their asthma or report emotional and family stress triggers appear to have higher rates of psychosocial problems than those who report only allergic triggers (Block, Block, & Morrison, 1981; Mrazek & Strunk, 1984; Purcell, Turnbull, & Bernstein, 1962).

Epidemiology

Typical age of onset: The incidence of asthma fluctuates during the lifetime. Asthma is primarily diagnosed early in life – often in the newborn (Koh & Irving, 2007; Reed, 2006). Approximately half of all patients with asthma are diagnosed by 6 years of age. Those diagnosed before 3 years of age typically have a more severe course, so efforts to delay onset of the illness are important in lessening morbidity and mortality. Infants born prematurely, with low birth weight, or both, are at more risk for developing asthma. Before 6 years of age, the male-to-female ratio is about 2:1, but by puberty the rates in girls increase so that by adulthood, the ratio reverses and approximately two-thirds of patients with asthma are female (Blackwell, Collins, & Coles, 2002).

Percentage of population afflicted with this disease: Asthma is one of the most prevalent chronic conditions and causes of disability seen in children in the United States (Akinbami, 2006). In the 1980s and into the mid-1990s, there was a noticeable increase in prevalence and incidence of asthma in the United States. However, it appears that this trend is leveling off as no change has occurred in prevalence rates between 2001 and 2004 ("Trends in asthma morbidity and mortality by American Lung Association Epidemiology and Statistics Unit Research and Program Services July 2006," 2006). Currently there are roughly 6.8 million persons under the age of 18 with asthma – affecting roughly 9% (Bloom & Cohen, 2007) of all children in the United States. Certain racial or ethnic groups have shown higher prevalence rates. The highest rates are in those of Puerto Rican descent (14.5%), followed by blacks (9.2%), whites (6.9%), and those of Mexican descent (3.9%) (Beckett, Belanger, Gent, Holford, & Leaderer, 1996; Moorman et al., 2007). In 2005, approximately 3.8 million children (Akinbami, 2006) had an asthma attack, though this appears to be decreasing from recent totals of 4 million in 2003 and 3.9 million in 2004 (Akinbami, 2006). This still represents nearly 66% of all patients with asthma and roughly 5.2% of all children under the age of 18. The age group with the greatest number of attacks has been for the last several years those between the ages of 5 and 17 years of age (Akinbami, 2006).

Prognosis/Progression: Several longitudinal studies have shown that most of those diagnosed with asthma in early childhood move into remission as they grow up, with most children entering remission during adolescence (Horner & Strunk, 2007; Reed, 2006). Those who do enter remission tend to have milder cases (Horner & Strunk, 2007; Reed, 2006), thus an adolescent with active symptoms would likely have a more severe case of asthma than a younger child. Studies show that bronchial hyperresponsiveness, atopy, individual smoking, rescue medication usage, and lower lung function, have been associated with prolonged asthma symptoms (Koh & Irving, 2007). Newer evidence suggests that asthma causes remodeling of the airways, and untreated or undertreated asthma can lead to pulmonary decline over the years (Bosse, Pare, & Seow, 2008). Indeed, childhood respiratory illnesses, including asthma, are associated with a 57% greater risk of overall respiratory disease mortality in adulthood and a more than twofold increase in chronic obstructive pulmonary disease mortality (Galobardes, McCarron, Jeffreys, & Davey Smith, 2008). Given these facts, any adolescent with a history of asthma should continue to have careful monitoring of lung function even when apparently asymptomatic and not taking medications.

Symptoms of Asthma

The presentation of asthma (i.e., asthma attacks) can fluctuate greatly between two individuals and even in the same person over the time. The classic symptoms found in asthmatics include the following:

1. Coughing (which typically is worse at night)
2. Chest tightness or shortness of breath (typical complaints are "I can't catch my breath" or "I can't get enough air in or out of my lungs")

3. Wheezing – recurrent high pitched whistling sounds during exhalation
4. Faster or noisier breathing
5. Reversible airway obstruction – as shown via spirometry testing ("Expert Panel Report 3 (EPR-3): Guidelines for the Diagnosis and Management of Asthma-Summary Report 2007," 2007; "National Heart Lung and Blood Institute Asthma Signs and Symptoms of Asthma").

Frequency of symptoms: The above symptoms are normally found to be episodic in nature and can be triggered by exercise, viral infections, allergens (such as animal or human dander, house-dust mites, mold, and pollen), irritants (tobacco smoke and air pollutants), stress, menstrual cycles, and strong emotional expressions (joyful or sad in nature) ("Expert Panel Report 3 (EPR-3): Guidelines for the Diagnosis and Management of Asthma-Summary Report 2007," 2007). Individuals may have a series of days where their symptoms are worse during both day and night, or they may have sporadic symptoms only once a day.

Severity: Asthma is typically rated at four levels of severity, depending on the frequency and intensity of symptoms, as well as the types and amounts of medications necessary to maintain symptoms at that level: intermittent, mild persistent, moderate persistent, and severe persistent (Bousquet et al., 2007). However, levels of severity based on this approach change over time, and patients with any of these severity ratings may have a fatal asthma attack. Consequently, some have recommended adding past history of an asthma–related life-threatening event (Federico, Wamboldt, Carter, Mansell, & Wamboldt, 2007) to the overall assessment of severity. In general, those patients with active asthma symptoms, or poorly controlled asthma, tend to have more interference with quality of life and more likelihood of psychological symptoms (Humbert, Holgate, Boulet, & Bousquet, 2007). A teen suffering from asthma does not usually look any different than other teens, unless they are seen in an active attack, or if they are on systemic corticosteroids for therapy, in which case they will have the stigmata of steroid dependence (e.g., moon facies, obesity, and fragile skin). Asthma attacks are typically described as having "inspiratory difficulty," "chest tightness," "unsatisfied inspiration," and/or "extra work" (Lougheed, Fisher, & O'Donnell, 2006), but teens also complain of generally "feeling bad."

Lethality: While asthma has a low fatality rate, the World Health Organization (WHO) noted that in 2005 there were 300 million individuals worldwide with asthma and 255,000 deaths associated with asthma (Akinbami, 2006). The WHO estimates that asthma deaths may increase by nearly 20% over the next 10 years (Akinbami, 2006). As one may surmise, the majority of these deaths occur in less developed countries. However, asthma is far from simply a third world disease. Mortality rates rose from the early 1980s to 1998 with a noticeable decrease in 1999 owing in part to new coding of ICD-10, which more specifically captured asthma deaths (as opposed to asthma plus other respiratory illnesses) (Getahun, Demissie, & Rhoads, 2005; "Trends in asthma morbidity and mortality by American Lung Association Epidemiology and Statistics Unit Research and Program Services July 2006," 2006). It is important to note that adolescents have the highest rate of death from asthma than any other age group, including younger children (Akinbami, 2006). Risk factors for death from asthma include nonadherence, exposure to high levels of antigen, family conflict, "emotional difficulties," use of illicit drugs, delay in seeking treatment, and poor symptom recognition (Restrepo & Peters, 2008; Strunk, Mrazek, Fuhrmann, & LaBrecque, 1985).

Complications: Medical conditions associated more frequently in adolescents with asthma include the atopic illnesses – atopic dermatitis, allergic rhinitis, and food allergies. Conditions that affect asthma management include gastroesophageal reflux, chronic rhinosinusitis, and vocal cord dysfunction, and each of these conditions should be assessed for when asthma is difficult to control (Balkissoon, 2007). Hospitalization for status asthmaticus (an acute asthma attack at times necessitating intubation and ventilation) can lead to numerous complications, such as aspiration pneumonia, ventilator-associated pneumonia, pneumomediastinum, pneumothorax, and rhabdomyolysis. Intubated children are significantly more likely to experience a complication (RR 15.3; 95% CI 6.7–35) than nonintubated children (Carroll & Zucker, 2007). For chronic nonacute asthma, decrease in physical activity due to fear of exacerbation and consequent obesity is becoming a major complication (Abramson et al., 2008; Glazebrook et al., 2006), and once overweight, associated sleep apnea can add to the child's problems (Kasasbeh, Kasasbeh, & Krishnaswamy, 2007).

What is the Treatment Approach in Asthma?

Assessment: The clinical diagnosis of asthma should include a detailed assessment of current symptoms and medical history, physical exam, spirometry, along with careful consideration of other possible diagnoses ("Expert Panel Report 3 (EPR-3): Guidelines for the Diagnosis and Management of Asthma-Summary Report 2007," 2007). Spirometry is a key part in not only classifying a patient's current pulmonary functional status but also establishing the reversible nature of the patient's airflow obstruction, which is a key component of asthma. A "reversible response" is generally defined as an improvement in FEV_1 of >200 mg and >12% improvement after a short-acting β-2-agonist medication is given ("Expert Panel Report 3 (EPR-3): Guidelines for the Diagnosis and Management of Asthma-Summary Report 2007," 2007).

Treatment: A key component to asthma care is the development of an asthma action care plan. Such a plan is an outline of how to manage a particular patient's asthma and is shared with the patient. The plan helps the teen manage their asthma and medications in between doctor visits and what steps to take during an acute exacerbation. The plan is based on the patient monitoring lung function through the use of a portable peak flow meter or a portable spirometer. Based on the current lung function along with the patient's symptoms, the patient is placed in one of three zones: green (doing fine, keep on same medications), yellow (some problems – take specific additional medications), or red (dangerous symptoms – take specific medications and call physician or go to emergency room).

Currently there is no direct cure for asthma; however, most agree that asthma can be fairly well controlled with current treatment modalities. Medications used in asthma can be divided into two main groups – those used daily to decrease inflammation and prevent future exacerbations and those used for acute exacerbations on an "as-needed" basis. Long-term "controller" medications include inhaled corticosteroids, cromolyn sodium and nedocromil, and long-acting β-2 agonists (namely salmeterol and formoterol), as well as orally taken immunomodulaters (e.g., anti-IgE mAb omalizumab) and leukotriene modifiers ("Expert Panel Report 3 (EPR-3): Guidelines for the Diagnosis and Management of Asthma-Summary Report 2007," 2007). Short-term "rescue" medications include inhaled short-acting β-2 agonists, oral systemic corticosteroids used to aid recovery from acute exacerbations, and inhaled anticholinergics.

Side effects of medications: Use of short- or long-acting β-agonist medications as monotherapy (without additional anti-inflammatory or controller medications such as inhaled corticosteroids) has been associated with increased risk of asthma exacerbations and deaths (Mansfield, 2008). In general, only intermittent asthmatics should utilize β agonists as monotherapy and then only on an as needed basis. Once asthma symptoms become persistent (more than four attacks a year), the recommendation is for the patient to be on a prophylactic anti-inflammatory medication first, with β agonists only as needed. β-Agonist medications are also associated with feelings of tension or jitteriness and can be abused by teens. Steroid medications, particularly when administered systemically (i.e., orally or intravenous) or in very high inhaled doses, can cause a cascade of well-known side effects, including bone mineral loss, growth retardation, weight gain, and hypothalamic–pituitary–adrenal (HPA) axis suppression. Inhaled corticosteroids at appropriate doses minimize these side effects markedly (Barnes, 2007) but still cause patient concerns, which may lead to nonadherence or seeking alternative treatments.

Adherence issues: Managing asthma is a complex process, requiring attention to changing symptoms, avoidance of triggers, and appropriate modifications in medication as symptoms change. Adherence to each of these domains is difficult, and not necessarily correlated. For example, a teen may be proficient at taking medications but not able to avoid the family pet which triggers symptoms. Since the mainstay of persistent asthma treatment is daily anti-inflammatory medications, usually given in inhaled form daily or up to four times a day, most teens will need to have inhalers in a variety of locations, e.g., bedroom, school locker, and book bag, in order for them to have an inhaler ready when they need it. Monitoring whether those inhalers still have sufficient medication in them is tricky. Also, the prophylactic anti-inflammatory medications take days to weeks to work, so they are less "motivating" for teens to take, as opposed to the β-agonists, which provide instant relief. For this reason, teens may tend to overutilize the β-agonist inhalers, putting themselves at risk to worsen their asthma or even for asthma death, instead of complying with controller medications. Monitoring of adherence is helped with devices that range from the Doser®, which is available at many pharmacies and online for a moderate amount ($50–$75) to Medi-logs which can be up to $400. The Doser is a counter device that can be placed on metered dose inhalers which automatically records usage with each inhalation and stores information daily up to 30 days. Beeps alert the user when inhalation has been registered and when fewer than 20 inhalations remain. The Medi-logs will actually give information as to whether the inhaler was appropriately used and the date and time that each dose was inhaled. The use of these devices has documented that the range of adherence with asthma medications is great, and use of these devices may help parents and health-care providers monitor adherence and contract with adolescents to improve adherence (Rand & Wise, 1994).

A complete approach to asthma management also includes the avoidance of asthma triggers, such as tobacco smoke and allergens; the need for "pretreatments" before exercise if that is a trigger for that patient; and the prescribed exercise to avoid the frequent complication of obesity. Allergen avoidance can often be difficult for the teen and his/her family, for example, if the child is allergic to the family pet, the family may need to give the pet away or keep it outside. Other common allergens such as dust mites require mattress covers, wood floors, and attention to cleaning that can add to the family's routine duties. Interestingly, there are ethnic differences in adherence to the variety of asthma management tasks, with children from lower income families having a harder time avoiding second-hand smoke and children from higher income families having a harder time avoiding pet danders (F. S. Wamboldt et al., 2002).

Cost: It has been estimated that the total cost of asthma is around $12.7 billion per year with a projected cost of $18 billion by 2020. The cost for those under 18 years of age is around $3.2 billion dollars per year ("Center for Disease Control and Prevention, Self-reported asthma prevalence among adults – United States, 2000," 2001) *(1–4 pg 9 – Morb Mortal wkly rep 2001;50:682–686)* with 50% of the cost used to treat those with severe asthma (National Heart, 1995). Asthma may account for a staggering 30% of the spending of a family (Marion, Creer, & Reynolds, 1985). In more blunt terms, the cost of care can prevent those with lower incomes from following recommended guidelines – for example, paying for the more expensive hypoallergenic bedcovers (Denson-Lino, Willies-Jacobo, Rosas, O'Connor, & Wilson, 1993). Thus, it is not too surprising that poverty is one of the stronger predictors/risk factors for asthma outcomes (Malveaux & Fletcher-Vincent, 1995). Families with total incomes below $15,000 have significantly higher rates of asthma – 9.8% vs 5.9% ("Center for Disease Control and Prevention, Self-reported asthma prevalence among adults – United States, 2000," 2001).

Insurance coverage: While all insurances provide coverage for asthma treatment, they vary on how much they require copayments for physician visits, hospitalizations, or emergency room visits, all of which can be expensive for the family and lead them to be frugal with care. Most importantly, insurances vary widely on benefits for medications, which can be costly. We treated a teen who had numerous hospitalizations for his asthma, which led to his father needing to take on a second job in order to manage the medical bills. In working with the family, the teen admitted that he had been "rationing" the asthma medications he took, since he knew they were expensive and he was trying to save his family money. It was this poor adherence to medications that led to the frequent exacerbations necessitating hospitalization. Often teens who have not reached the cognitive level of abstract thinking can make illogical decisions like this. When we presented this case to a medical audience in the Netherlands, where health care is provided by the government, people were outraged that our medical system could put a child in such a predicament.

Frequency of necessary medical attention: The leveling off of prevalence (and decreasing mortality) in recent years does not necessarily reflect a leveling off of the burden of asthma on society. In fact, since 2000 there has been an ever-increasing rate of ambulatory care visits by children with asthma (Akinbami, 2006). In 2004, there were approximately 7 million visits secondary to asthma – (6.5 to doctors' offices and 0.5 million to hospital outpatient departments) accounting for roughly 2.5% of all ambulatory visits among children under the age of 18 (Akinbami, 2006). In 2004, there were 103 visits to the emergency room per 10,000 children, for a total of 750,000 ER visits secondary to asthma, which accounted for almost 3% of all childhood ED visits in 2004 (Akinbami, 2006). In addition, a more telling and ominous revelation is how in recent years overall hospitalization use in children has decreased (denoting a more outpatient approach to treatment) though hospitalization rates for asthma have stayed the same (i.e., an increasing percentage of childhood hospitalizations is secondary to asthma in recent years). Though this may simply reflect a more cautious approach to asthma, it more likely represents an increase in the number of severe asthma attacks in recent years (Akinbami, 2006).

Common Problems Seen with Adolescents Who Have Asthma

There have been several studies looking how asthma can impact an adolescent's life. Monhangoo et al. used the Child Health Questionnaire – Child Form to explore how wheezing may impact an adolescent's life. They administered the form to 933 teens and separated them into those that never wheezed (reference group), those reporting a history of wheezing but not within the past year (former), those wheezing within the past year but less than four episodes (mild), and those reporting four or more wheezing episodes in the past year (severe). When comparing these groups to responses on the CHQ-CF, they found that adolescents with severe wheezing (compared to those without any history of wheezing) had significantly poorer scores of bodily pain, general health, general behavior, mental health, self-esteem, and family cohesion. Of note the effect size was large ($\geq$0.8) for the bodily pain, general health, and mental health subscales with the other subscales having moderate effects sizes. Thus one can conclude, as Mohangoo et al. do, that wheezing can lead to significant pain and/or discomfort limiting one's life along with being associated with a teen having a decreased overall view of their general health and likely to worsen (Mohangoo, de Koning, Mangunkusumo, & Raat, 2007).

Forrest et al. came to similar conclusions. By using the Child Health and Illness Profile, Adolescent Edition (CHIP-AE), his group explored how acute wheezing may impact an adolescent's life. They administered the CHIP-AE to 3000 adolescents comparing three groups: those with no history of asthma, a history of asthma, and asthmatics with symptomatic wheezing in the last 28 days. They report individuals with active wheezing in the past month had significantly less satisfaction, more discomfort, were more likely to have comorbidities, less family involvement, and riskier behaviors. The effect sizes were once again greater concerning physical discomfort along with increased comorbidities (Forrest, Starfield, Riley, & Kang, 1997). This study reinforces the picture of adolescents with symptomatic asthma being in significant physical pain and having an overall bleaker outlook toward their future health, but it is not able to specify the directionality of this correlation. In other words, it may be the adolescents with less family involvement and riskier behaviors who are less likely to take the necessary steps to control their asthma, thus having active symptoms.

The physical limitations associated with asthma have been noted by others to lead to decreased ability to participate in activities such as strenuous exercise, playing music, or "hanging out with friends" (Rhee, Wenzel, & Steeves, 2007). In focus group interviews with 19 adolescents, Rhee et al. concluded asthma to have far reaching effects on a teenager's life. Common themes of missed opportunities including social activities, inability to pursue activities they would have been able to excel at (and receive social praise for), and having to work harder to obtain less emerged from their focus groups. The teens appeared to experience other people's reactions as often over protective or dismissive regarding their asthma – that is either "babying" them or "dismissing" their asthma all together. This seemed to lead to several negative emotions including embarrassment, loneliness, sadness, guilt, and anger. Though some positive coping strategies emerged, several negative ones were endorsed, namely "toughing up" where adolescents talked about ignoring symptoms or "sucking it up" to lead a more normal life and not be viewed as weak and avoid guilt they may feel for letting others down (e.g., parents, coaches, or friends) (Rhee et al., 2007).

Education: Academically, it is estimated that asthma accounts for 14 million missed school days a year (CDC, 2008) and is the leading medical cause for school absenteeism. Although studies do not necessarily show a negative effect on an asthmatic child's academic achievement (Moonie, Sterling, Figgs, & Castro, 2008; Taras & Potts-Datema, 2005), studies have shown missing school puts a child at risk of lower academic scores (Moonie et al., 2008). In 2003, there were 12.8 million days of missed school secondary to asthma.

Adolescents with asthma appear to face a difficult balancing act between acknowledging their illness and being able to modify their lives accordingly while struggling to deal with the social implications this may bring (peer pressure from friends, coaches, and families). They can be left with seeking support from others (parents, friends) – who may also be struggling to understand/accept the adolescents asthma – possibly in negative ways themselves – i.e., the overprotective parent or people who dismiss their symptoms as "attention seeking." In other words, an adolescent may not be able to get the support he/she needs from his/her support network if the network itself is struggling to accept his/her asthma diagnosis.

Is There an Increase in Psychiatric Disorders Found in Adolescents with Asthma?

As indicated in Table 1 (a detail of cited articles), increased anxiety symptoms, as well as frank anxiety disorders, have been fairly well documented in adolescents with asthma in both clinic (Bussing, Burket, & Kelleher, 1996; Kashani, Konig, Shepperd, Wilfley, & Morris, 1988; Katon et al., 2007; Silverglade, Tosi, Wise, & D'Costa, 1994; Vila, Nollet-Clemencon, de Blic, Mouren-Simeoni, & Scheinmann, 2000; Vila et al., 1999) and community samples (Blackman & Gurka, 2007; Ortega, Huertas, Canino, Ramirez, & Rubio-Stipec, 2002; Ortega et al., 2003). However, not all studies have reported increased rates of anxiety. For example, Bender Berz et al. reported no increase in internalizing symptoms for asthmatics in the Child Health Project – a 2-year longitudinal sample from five clinics. A possible reason for this different finding is that this sample included a large number of subjects with very mild asthma or nonactive asthma (i.e., no requirement that subjects need to have asthma symptoms or treatment for asthma in the last year). Another interesting finding is reported by Kashani et al. Their group did not find significantly different psychiatric symptoms (compared to normal controls) when using the DICA child version, yet did find significantly more psychiatric symptoms in the child when using parent report version of the DICA. These studies indicate that several constructs in measuring psychopathology in teens with asthma are pertinent: the severity of the asthma and who reports psychological symptoms (child, parent, or both).

Findings of rates of anxiety symptoms, such as phobias, PTSD, and panic symptoms in adolescents with asthma are mixed, with the majority indicating higher levels than non-ill controls (Craske, Poulton, Tsao, & Plotkin, 2001; Goodwin, Pine, & Hoven, 2003; Kashani et al., 1988; Kean, Kelsay, Wamboldt, & Wamboldt, 2006). Kashani found increased symptoms when asking the parent, yet no increase with patient report. Bussing et al. reported a nonsignificant difference in asthmatics vs healthy controls with regard to phobia and panic disorders. However, her sample size was small (37 asthmatics vs 31 controls) and it should be noted that although not statistically significant, there was a greater percentage of asthmatics with phobia (16.2% vs 6.5%) and panic disorder (5.4% vs 0%) which leads one to wonder if there were enough power to establish the differences. In fact, in larger studies there are statistically significant differences, e.g., Goodwin et al. reports in the MECA study

Table 1 Selected articles regarding adolescents with asthma

Author/Sample	Controls	Measures	Findings
Kashani '88			
56 subjects, 7–16 years old, referred to University Child Clinic with diagnosis of asthma	56 age, race, sex matched, presenting to acute care clinic with no history of chronic illness	DICA – child DICA – parent Child hopelessness CBCL – parent Child self concept	Trend in asthmatics to report higher psychiatric symptoms (sxs). Parents reported significantly greater overanxious sxs in asthmatic children ($p < 0.03$), and greater phobic sxs ($p<0.012$). Parents of asthmatics rated their child on CBCL as more externalizing (57 vs 53, $p=0.021$) and internalizing (54 vs 51, $p=0.38$)
Silvergrade'94			
$N=129$, private practice clinic with diagnosis of asthma, $n=41$ mild, $n=34$ moderate, $n=54$ severe	74 dental clinic patients without any chronic medical conditions	Common Beliefs Survey Multiple Affect Adjective Checklist (MAACL)	Moderate and severe asthmatics had greater anxiety sxs (on MAACL) than mild asthmatics and controls ($p<0.05$)
Bussing'96			
37 asthmatics with age range of 7–17 years old, with normal IQ, and seen in an outpatient University Clinic	31 controls with no history of chronic illness/mental illness. They were matched for age, gender, and socioeconomic status	K-SADS (p and c)	Asthmatic subjects have greater rates of anxiety disorders (43.3% vs 19.4% – $p = 0.036$)
Vila'99			
93 asthmatic outpatients from Hosp Clinic, ages 8–17, $n=51$ severe, $n=30$ moderate, $n=12$ mild persistent	93 insulin-dependent diabetics for an outpatient clinic	K-SADS-R CBCL State-Trait Anxiety Inv. for Children (STAIC) CDI Self-Esteem Inventory	Asthmatics had greater STAIC scores (33 vs 31, $p<0.05$), greater total CBCL scores (53 vs 50, $p<0.05$), greater internalization scores (57 vs 53, $p<0.01$) and greater externalization scores (51 vs 49, $p<0.05$)
Vila'00			
82 asthmatic outpatients in a hospital clinic, ages 8–15, all had moderate to severe asthma as defined by NHBLI guidelines	82 healthy controls matched for age, sex, and socioeconomic status	Anxiety/Fears Behavior Scale CDI SEI	Asthmatics had greater Anxiety/Fears mean scores (113 vs 106, $p<0.05$), though this mean was still below 124 – the cutoff for anxiety disorders, CDI, and SEI did not differ between groups
Craske'01			
$n=84$ diagnosed with panic disorder or agoraphobia (PDA), $n=225$ subjects with an anxiety diagnosis other than PDA, at 18 or 21 years of	415 controls without psychiatric diagnosis at 18 or 21 years of age	Diagnostic Interview Schedule (DIS) to diagnose panic disorder with agoraphobia, and other anxiety	Most important factor was gender, with females at greater risk than males. Females with history of respiratory problems at age 15 (from wheezing

Table 1 (continued)

Author/Sample	Controls	Measures	Findings
age, Dunedin, New Zealand Study Data: Longitudinal, Community Sample		disorders in those age 18 or 21 years of age	to severe asthma) were at a greater risk of PDA later, for females without history of asthma – having parents who had a history of asthma in adolescents greater for PDA. For males in those with history of high emotional reactivity at age 3 – having asthma by age 18 greater risk for PDA later
Ortega'02			
$n = 199$ with a history of asthma, Community sample – Data from Methods for the Epidemiology of Child/Adolescent Mental Disorders (MECA study)	Normal healthy controls	DISC 2.3 child and parent versions	Greater rate of anxiety disorders in those with asthma vs normal controls (49% vs 38%, $p<0.05$), no difference in the overall rate of psychiatric disorders in asthma vs normal controls (56% vs 49%)
Ortega'03			
Community sample of 1891 parent/child (ages of 4–17) pairs in Puerto Rico, asthma diagnosis $n = 616$, history of asthma attacks $n = 416$, history of hospitalization for asthma $n = 312$	No history of asthma $n = 1279$, no history of asthma attacks $n = 1475$, never hospitalized for asthma $n = 1570$	DISC	Asthma vs no asthma: greater percentage with any psychiatric disorder (20% vs 14%, $p = 0.01$), greater percentage with an affective disorder (3% vs 1%, $p = 0.04$), greater percentage with a disruptive disorder (15% vs 10%, $p = 0.01$). A history of an asthma attack showed greater percentage of any psychiatric disorder (22% vs 14%, $p = 0.003$), greater any anxiety disorder (11% vs 6%, $p = 0.01$), greater separation anxiety (8% vs 4%, $p = 0.04$), greater affective disorder (3% vs 1%, $p = 0.03$), greater major depressive disorder (3% vs 1%, $p = 0.04$), greater any disruptive disorder (16% vs 10%, $p = 0.003$), greater oppositional defiant disorder (9% vs 5%, $p = 0.01$). There were no significant differences between asthmatics with a history of an asthma hospitalization and those without one
Katon'07			
Adolescents aged 11–17 enrolled in HMO in Washington State, $n = 769$	$n = 582$, youth in same HMO with no history of asthma	DISC 4.0 Mood and Feelings Childhood Anxiety Sensitivity Index	Pts with asthma have greater odds ratio of *agoraphobia* (1.92, $p<0.01$),

Table 1 (continued)

Author/Sample	Controls	Measures	Findings
with history of asthma and in last year either: hospitalized, ER visit, >2 office visits and prescribed medications for asthma		(ASI) Child Health Survey Asthma Pediatric Chronic Disease Scale	greater odds ratio of any *anxiety or depressive disorder* (1.83, $p<0.001$) – results adjusted for ethnicity, education, marital status of parents, Medicaid and pediatric medical comorbidity score. Adjusted relative risk is calculated at 1.7. – i.e., asthma increases a child's risk for anxiety/depression by 1.7 times
Carpentier'07			
n = 121 College students (18–22 yo) with a history of asthma by age 12 and current prescription for asthma medications or office visits for asthma	n = 121, college students with no history of chronic illness (matched for age and gender; also compared asthma with psychiatric symptoms (sxs) to asthmatic without psychiatry sxs)	Brief Symptom Index (BSI) Mishel Uncertainty in Illness Illness Intrusiveness Scale	Asthma greater mean scores on BSI-anxiety subscale (55 vs 51, $p<0.01$), greater mean scores on BSI-GSI (58 vs 54, $p<0.01$), greater missed class (3.8 vs 2.1, $p<0.01$), greater missed work (1.86 vs 0.58, $p<0.01$) – but did NOT have greater BSI-Dep scores. Illness uncertainty predicted BSI-GSI, BSI-Anx, BSI-Depression subscale (all $p<0.001$), illness intrusiveness predicted: BSI-GSI,BSI-Anxiety (all $p<0.001$), BSI-depression ($p<0.01$), missed school days ($p<0.01$)
BenderBerz '05			
N = 48 child/parent pairs (8–12), n = 27 asthma (doctor diagnosed per parent report), Data from Childrens' Health Project – a 2-year longitudinal study involving five clinics in urban areas	n = 21 subjects without chronic illness	Behavior Assessment System for Children – Self Report of Personality (BASC) (child and parent versions) Friendship Questionnaire	Asthma was NOT linked to more internalizing problems, poor social function, but rather anxiety/depression impacted an adolescents' life (poor social network, social stress)
Goodwin'03			
MECA study data: n 1284 subjects (9–17), n = 196 with asthma – n = 75 severe asthma (history of hospitalization for asthma)	n = 1088 – those without asthma (about 85% of sample)	Child Global Assessment Scale DISC 2.3	Severe asthma OR: 2.2 of panic attacks, asthma OR: 1.5 – adjusted for gender, age, socioeconomic status, single parent, site, depressive disorders, substance abuse, anxiety disorder, cigarette smoking (note no greater OR for panic d/o)
Kean'06			
n = 49 asthma subjects with history of life-threatening asthma (LTA) , n =		UCLA PTSD Reaction Index Reynolds Depression Inventory-2	More LTA reported a traumatic event in their life compared to the other

Table 1 (continued)

Author/Sample	Controls	Measures	Findings
71 subjects with asthma without history of LTA (AC), 3 sites, clinic sample, severity based on NHBLI (also looked at the ptsd symptoms in parents)	$n = 80$ normal controls (NC) – adolescents without history of chronic medical illness	Multidimensional Anxiety Scale for Children (MASC) Functional asthma severity Impact of Events Scale BSI	groups: LTA (>90%) > AC (69%) > NC (33%). There was also greater PTSD diagnosis in LTA group vs NC (20% vs 8%, $p<0.05$). Parents of LTA pts greater PTSD (29% in LTA parents, 14% of AC parents, 2% in NC parents, $p<0.01$), PTSD sxs accounted for 9% ($p<0.001$) of the variance of asthma function, morbidity, and intrusive symptoms of PTSD appeared particularly important
Blackman'07			
$N = 101{,}778$ (2–17 yo) Community Survey (National Survey of Children's Health – NSCH 2003), $n = 5952$ minor asthma, $n = 2318$ moderate asthma, $n = 393$ severe asthma. Survey was done via telephone and questions about child health	$n = 93{,}089$ pts with no history of asthma. Normal Controls (NC) were compared to total asthma, and each of the three asthma severity groups	NSCH telephone question and answer with parents, no formal diagnostic measures given for asthma or any other illness	Total Asthma vs NC had greater ADHD/rates of depression or Anxiety, Behavior/conduct problems, Learning Disability (LD), problems with emotions/concentration/getting along with others, missing more than 10 school days for illness, repeating a grade, and parents of asthmatic kids had greater concerns about their child's achievement, self-esteem, learning difficulties, depression or anxiety (all p at least <0.01) Severe asthma had greater rates for all of the above (example: major depressive disorder/anxiety 14%, ADD/ADHD 15.5%, LD 27%, missed more than 10 days of school 50%, repeated a grade 28%) but all parents concern about substance abuse (27%) and that the child is bullied by peers (30%). All p at least <0.01

Notes: Diagnostic Interview for Children and Adolescents (DICA), Child Behavior Check List (CBCL), Kiddie Schedule for Affective Disorders and Schizophrenia for School Age Children (K-SADS), Child Depression Inventory (CDI), Diagnostic Interview Schedule for Children (DISC), $p<0.05$ significant difference.

(a large community-based study of a total $N = 1284$, using the DISC) that there were increased rates of panic attacks in asthmatics (OR: 2.2 for severe asthma, OR: 1.5 for asthma in general; all $p < 0.05$). However, their group did not find increased rates of actual panic disorder in asthmatic adolescents (Goodwin et al., 2003). One of the methodologic difficulties in such an epidemiologic study is that some panic symptoms may also be due to asthma attacks, e.g., shortness of breath, muscle tension, and chest pain. Lay interviewers (for the DISC) would not be able to sort out whether the symptom was due to panic or asthma.

Several studies have reported significantly greater depressive symptoms in adolescents with asthma (Blackman & Gurka, 2007; Ortega et al., 2003; Silverglade et al., 1994). However, there are also negative findings (Bender Berz, Murdock, & Koinis Mitchell, 2005; Carpentier, Mullins, & Van Pelt, 2007; Ortega et al., 2002; Vila et al., 2000). When comparing these studies to each other some interesting facts come to light. Carpentier et al.'s study was looking at college students with a history of asthma, thus was not directly examining adolescents and possibly missed any adolescents with severe depression that were unable to attend college. The negative depression studies as a group tended to use more simple screening measures [e.g., CDI, BASC, BSI (Bender Berz et al., 2005; Carpentier et al., 2007; Vila et al., 2000; Vila et al., 1999)] while studies reporting increased depressive symptoms used more comprehensive measures (i.e., DISC; Ortega et al., 2003). Though one cannot completely dismiss the negative reports, it is interesting to note that the large community samples have found significantly greater depressive symptoms in children and adolescents with asthma (Blackman & Gurka, 2007; Ortega et al., 2003). Studies have also reported on increased symptoms/rates of ADHD (Blackman & Gurka, 2007), agoraphobia (Katon et al., 2007), ODD (Ortega et al., 2003), and disruptive disorders (Ortega et al., 2003), although these tend to look at clinical samples where comorbidity is more likely, and not community samples.

Despite the majority of studies finding increased psychiatric symptoms, not all studies report a significantly higher rate of DSM disorder diagnoses, suggesting that while teens with asthma have higher rates of internalizing symptoms than controls, the majority still are within a normal range. For example: Vila et al. (2000) reported a higher mean on the Anxiety/Fears Behavior Scale in asthmatics (113 vs 106 in healthy controls); however, the accepted clinical cutoff for this measure is 124 (Vila et al., 2000). Another example of increased subclinical symptoms is from Carpentier's et al. study that reported increased BSI-anxiety subscale mean of 55 in asthmatics vs 51 in healthy controls, while a clinically high BSI mean is considered 63 (Carpentier et al., 2007). Furthermore, in Kashani et al. study, while they reported an increased rate of psychiatric symptoms via parent report, there was not a significantly greater number of DSM diagnoses in the asthmatic group compared to healthy controls (Kashani et al., 1988).

Are the increased rates of anxiety symptoms clinically relevant? One approach is to examine whether the increased symptoms lead to worse asthma outcomes, worse quality of life, or impairment. Another is to examine longitudinal data – do these subclinical increases in symptoms over time lead to more frank disorders? Keep in mind that several studies did find increased rates of DSM-IV anxiety disorders (Bussing et al., 1996; Katon et al., 2007; Kean et al., 2006) – in particular large community-based samples (Blackman & Gurka, 2007; Ortega et al., 2003). One may approach screening adolescents with chronic illness as looking for increased rates of particular disorders with the idea of referring these individuals to appropriate mental health services for treatment of a disorder. This is a reasonable approach; however, it fails to capture the nuances of the interplay of psychiatric symptoms and a chronic medical condition. The discussion should be more directed on identifying psychiatric symptoms that could be interfering with the adolescent's life and his medical care rather than whether a particular patient's symptom cluster meets DSM criteria. There are a number of studies that imply adolescents with asthma are more impacted by milder psychiatric symptoms (i.e., what might be considered subclinical) than healthy controls, thus warranting earlier interventions. For example, Carpentier et al.'s study on college students reported higher subclinical means on the BSI-anxiety subscale (55 vs 51; $p<0.01$) and BSI-Global Severity Score in teens with asthma

(58 vs 54; $p<0.01$), and this same group reported that there were significantly greater missed school days ($p<0.01$) which was predicted by the students' perception of illness intrusiveness (Carpentier et al., 2007).

Does "severity" of asthma matter? Several studies comment on the issue of whether more severe asthmatics are at greater risk for psychiatric symptoms. A few studies report a negative finding in this regard (Blackman & Gurka, 2007; Bussing et al., 1996; Kashani et al., 1988), while others find that severity is an important factor (Blackman & Gurka, 2007; Goodwin, Fergusson, & Horwood, 2004; Kean et al., 2006; Silverglade et al., 1994). Variance could be accounted for in the various manners in which severity was defined – from "physician rated" (Bussing et al., 1996) to "ever needing hospitalization for asthma" (Goodwin et al., 2003). However, even when severity is defined using current guidelines (Federico et al., 2007), there is a confound such that patients who are nonadherent to medications are likely to have more symptoms. Nonadherence may be associated with greater psychosocial comorbidities. For example, Katon et al. used the Health Plan Employer Data and Information Set (HEDIS) which uses four variables over the last year to define severity (medications, visits to the ER, hospitalizations, and number of ambulatory visits) (Katon et al., 2007). It is not hard to imagine that a more "severe" patient using this definition is simply a patient whose illness in not under good control. A patient with good adherence to daily medications is more likely to stay out of the hospital/ER than a patient who is not adhering to his medication regimen.

Importance of medical trauma: Kean et al. report that adolescents with asthma who reported a "life-threatening event" secondary to asthma, such as seizure or intubation, after the age of 5 years, were at more risk of developing PTSD for any reason (20%) compared to healthy controls (8%, $p<0.05$). Adolescents with persistent asthma who had not endured a life-threatening event secondary to asthma were not any more likely to develop PTSD than healthy controls (11% vs 8%; ns). This study supports the hypothesis that medically related traumas can predispose a patient to develop PTSD when exposed to future traumas. Sometimes, this PTSD reaction is a risk factor for nonadherence. For example, a child traumatized by a severe asthma attack and consequent hospitalization may get PTSD symptoms whenever exposed to an inhaler, making it more difficult to take their inhaled medications as prescribed. Assessing the teen's asthma history with an ear toward how the teen experienced their asthma events may lead to a different strategy as to how to treat the teen's nonadherence (M. Z. Wamboldt & Weintraub, 1995).

Family issues: A preponderance of studies suggests that the family climate is important in asthma management and outcome. Early studies documented that parent–child conflict and parent–staff conflict were risk factors for asthma death (Strunk et al., 1985). Further studies also implicated parental criticism of children (F. S. Wamboldt, Wamboldt, Gavin, Roesler, & Brugman, 1995) as a marker for nonadherence in the child. More recent studies (Wood et al., 2008, 2007) suggest that negative family emotional climate leads to child depressive symptoms and that child depression leads to more asthma severity directly as well as indirectly via having more emotional triggers for asthma exacerbations. Parent–child relational insecurity also directly increased asthma severity, while a secure parent–child relationship decreased asthma severity. Novel interventions in working with families with asthmatic children include trying to improve the rituals and routines in the family's life as a way to provide more security and structure for children. These approaches may work both directly, by improving a sense of secure relationships, and indirectly, by improving adherence (Fiese, Wamboldt, & Anbar, 2005).

Cultural considerations: Minority children are more likely to have limited access to outpatient care, which leads to a higher number of asthma attacks (i.e., there is a 40% higher rate of asthma attacks in black teens compared to white teens) (Akinbami, 2006). Thus it should not be surprising that black children have over 2.5 times higher ER and hospitalization rates (Akinbami, 2006). While fewer white children are dying from asthma each year, death rates in the black community have remained stable, leading to black children being five times more likely to die from asthma than their white counterparts (Akinbami, 2006). While some of this is secondary to economic matters (Willis, 2002), it has been shown that even when controlling for insurance and income, minorities have worse overall care than Caucasian individuals (Willis, 2002). One reason for the difference in care available to white children vs minority children was proposed by Hardie (Hardie, Janson, Gold, Carrieri-Kohlman, & Boushey, 2000), who showed that different ethnic groups use different words to describe the same physical symptom. This can lead to false negatives on screening tests traditionally written for Caucasian groups or miscommunication with physicians of a different ethnic group.

However, there may be additional risk factors inherent in black ethnicity that supercede issues of health-care access or neighborhood adversities. For example, Pearlman et al. (2006) found that black children living in poverty had higher rates of asthma than white or Hispanic children also living in disadvantaged neighborhoods. Indeed, there were racial differences in cord blood between children from black heritage compared to white (Willwerth et al., 2006), which indicated that a different sensitivity to allergy development may also be a risk factor for worse asthma in black children.

What is the Role of the Behavioral Health Specialist Working with Teens with Asthma?

The behavioral health specialist is a key person on the treatment team for a teen's asthma care. Given that most children with mild asthma will outgrow it by adolescence, those teens with active asthma symptoms either have more severe illness or have already had difficulties in appropriately managing the illness. Thus, one of the first goals of the behavioral specialist is to assess the teen and family's asthma management skills (McQuaid, Walders, Kopel, Fritz, & Klinnert, 2005) and target interventions for these as needed. These include ability to accurately perceive asthma symptoms, age-appropriate medication management, good working relationship with an asthma treatment team, adherence to medications, avoidance of allergens or triggers, and ability to understand and follow an asthma action plan. Most teens should be involved in taking on more of the responsibility for their asthma management, but parents need to be able to oversee this in a noninvasive manner to ensure that the teen is managing effectively.

Fights over adherence are common. Clinically, the use of pill boxes to manage oral medications, or inhalers with electronic measuring devices, e.g., Medi-logs or Dosers, is useful. A behavioral plan can be discussed with parents and the teen such that the parent agrees to not nag or question about adherence, but they can check on a nightly basis by looking at the pill box or Doser results. They may discuss only if the teen is not exhibiting good adherence. This strategy helps in shifting responsibility for care to the teen, rather than the parent.

Patients who are shown to have accurate symptom perception, e.g., by being able to tell when their lung functions are decreased and have this documented by spirometry, may be allowed to forgo daily use of peak flow meters, to which it is difficult to adhere. On the other hand, where the teen has been shown to have inaccurate symptom perception, e.g., feeling "fine" when lung functions are documented to be low, a behavioral plan to encourage daily peak flow monitoring may be crucial.

Asthma knowledge has not been shown to be necessary, or sufficient, to enhance asthma management (Ho et al., 2003). While there is a need for the teen to manage their asthma, some teens can do this without a knowledge base because they will essentially do what their physician prescribes, while others may understand a lot about asthma but choose not to use this knowledge to manage their illness. Thus, the clinician needs to individualize the necessity of asthma education.

Second, the behavioral clinician should assess family dynamics and target a decrease in family conflict and improvement in family problem-solving skills. Family conflict and nonadherence often go together, with each exacerbating the other. Multifamily group discussions, which normalize the fact that many families struggling with chronic illness do not use good problem-solving skills because they fear expressing negative emotions about the illness, are often helpful (M. Z. Wamboldt & Levin, 1995).

Third, the behavioral specialist should screen for comorbidities, most frequently anxiety and depression symptoms, although also ADHD, as teens with

ADHD will have a harder time managing their regiment, unless the ADHD is under control. If anxiety or depression is present, treatment is indicated. The use of cognitive behavior therapy for anxiety or depression symptoms is often helpful, although one also needs to assess for post-traumatic reactions to an asthma-related event, such as a frightening attack, and use targeted interventions for the PTSD symptoms so that those do not interfere with asthma management strategies (M. Z. Wamboldt & Weintraub, 1995). While SSRIs have been shown to be relatively effective and safe for treating depression in teens with asthma, the adherence to these medications is no better than adherence to older tricyclic antidepressants, in part because teens with asthma tend to report many side effects to medications (M.Z. Wamboldt, Yancey, & Roesler, 1997). The use of antidepressants needs to be monitored closely in these teens.

Finally, a good behavioral specialist should pay attention to whether the teen is getting appropriate exercise or afraid to exercise for fear of triggering asthma symptoms. Well-controlled asthma should not interfere with physical activity, and teens with asthma are at risk for being overweight. Increased body mass index is a risk factor for worse asthma outcomes (Abramson et al., 2008), as well as a risk factor for other health problems. Collaborating with a dietician, as well as a good physical therapist who can help a teen learn to pace their exercise in a manner that does not trigger asthma, is important.

Methodological considerations if conducting research with this population: Characterize asthma well with a combination of self and parent report of symptoms, pulmonary function testing, including spirometry pre- and post-bronchodilator, or the use of provocation challenge, such as methacholine or histamine challenge. Some standard asthma symptom questionnaires, such as a quality of life measure (Juniper et al., 1996) or a functional assessment (Rosier et al., 1994), are useful in comparing results across studies. If using an epidemiologic approach, in addition to self-reported symptoms, also ask if a physician diagnosis was made, and/or what medications have been used.

Research agenda: The need for more involvement of behavioral health specialists in research efforts with asthma is paramount, as despite our increased understanding of asthma physiology and treatments, the prevalence and morbidity of asthma continues to rise in developed countries. Continued research efforts to document interventions that improve adherence, self and/or family management skills, and access to care are paramount.

Understanding what in the environment of developed countries may increase the prevalence of asthma is also a critical need for research. The use of natural gene and environment interaction experiments is one methodology that provides some interesting findings. For example, the reunification of East and West Germany in 1989 was a natural experiment where two genetically similar populations which had very different cultures for 40 years were unified. Interestingly, the rates of asthma were far lower in the eastern German areas than in the west, and over the years after reunification the rates of asthma in both groups are approaching similar levels (Heinrich et al., 2002). These studies have focused on the role of indoor allergens as one potential factor implicated in the rise of asthma, but one may also wonder about different types of psychological stressors in capitalist societies than in the older communist culture.

The role of maternal stress in the perinatal period is one area that has been identified as a risk factor in the earlier development of asthma in children (Klinnert, Kaugars, Strand, & Silveira, 2008), and interventions that can target decreasing the stress load would be helpful. One area of innovative interventions may include the role of complementary and alternative medicine approaches to decreasing stress in pregnant women who carry risk factors for asthma (e.g., have asthma or atopic illness themselves). Interventions such as biofeedback, yoga, or meditation may be cost effective, and noninvasive, approaches to study in this regard. Since adolescents with asthma are a group that may soon grow into the developmental phase of parenthood, teaching these strategies to teens may allow them to develop enough skills in stress management that they can better manage their own asthma, as well as potentially decrease the risk of their children developing asthma early in life.

References

Abramson, N. W., Wamboldt, F. S., Mansell, A. L., Carter, R., Federico, M. J., & Wamboldt, M. Z. (2008). Frequency and correlates of overweight status in adolescent asthma. *Journal of Asthma, 45*(2), 135–139.

Akinbami, L. (2006). The state of childhood asthma, United States, 1980–2005. *Advance Data*, (381), 1–24.

Amelung, P. J., Scott, A. F., & Bleecker, E. R. (1996). Genetic of bronchial hyperresponsiveness. In S. B. Liggett & D. A. Meyers (Eds.). *The Genetics of Asthma* (Vol. 96, pp. 525–540). New York City: Marcel Dekker, Inc.

Arshad, S. H., & Hide, D. W. (1992). Effect of environmental factors on the development of allergic disorders in infancy. *Journal of Allergy and Clinical Immunology, 90*(2), 235–241.

Balkissoon, R. (2007). Vocal cord dysfunction, gastroesophageal reflux disease, and nonallergic rhinitis. *Clinical Allergy and Immunology, 19*, 411–426.

Barnes, N. C. (2007). The properties of inhaled corticosteroids: Similarities and differences. *Primary Care Respiratory Journal, 16*(3), 149–154.

Beckett, W. S., Belanger, K., Gent, J. F., Holford, T. R., & Leaderer, B. P. (1996). Asthma among Puerto Rican Hispanics: A multi-ethnic comparison study of risk factors. *American Journal of Respiratory and Critical Care Medicine, 154*(4 Pt 1), 894–899.

Bender Berz, J., Murdock, K. K., & Koinis Mitchell, D. (2005). Children's asthma, internalizing problems, and social functioning: An urban perspective. *Journal of Child and Adolescent Psychiatric Nursing, 18*(4), 181–197.

Blackman, J. A., & Gurka, M. J. (2007). Developmental and behavioral comorbidities of asthma in children. *Journal of Developmental and Behavioral Pediatrics, 28*(2), 92–99.

Blackwell, D. L., Collins, J. G., & Coles, R. (2002). Summary health statistics for U.S. adults: National Health Interview Survey, 1997. *Vital & Health Statistics, 10*(205), 1–109.

Block, J. H., Block, J., & Morrison, A. (1981). Parental agreement–disagreement on child-rearing orientations and gender-related personality correlates in children. *Child Development, 52*(3), 10.

Bloom, B., & Cohen, R. A. (2007). Summary health statistics for U.S. children: National Health Interview Survey, 2006. *Vital & Health Statistics, 10*(234), 1–79.

Bosse, Y., Pare, P. D., & Seow, C. Y. (2008). Airway wall remodeling in asthma: From the epithelial layer to the adventitia. *Current Allergy and Asthma Reports, 8*(4), 357–366.

Bousquet, J., Clark, T. J., Hurd, S., Khaltaev, N., Lenfant, C., O'Byrne, P., et al. (2007). GINA guidelines on asthma and beyond. *Allergy, 62*(2), 102–112.

Bussing, R., Burket, R. C., & Kelleher, E. T. (1996). Prevalence of anxiety disorders in a clinic-based sample of pediatric asthma patients. *Psychosomatics, 37*(2), 108–115.

Carpentier, M. Y., Mullins, L. L., & Van Pelt, J. C. (2007). Psychological, academic, and work functioning in college students with childhood-onset asthma. *Journal of Asthma, 44*(2), 119–124.

Carroll, C. L., & Zucker, A. R. (2007). The increased cost of complications in children with status asthmaticus. *Pediatric Pulmonology, 42*(10), 914–919.

CDC. (2008). Asthma: Children and adolescents | CDC APRHB. From http://www.cdc.gov/asthma/children.htm

Center for Disease Control and Prevention, Self-reported asthma prevalence among adults – United States, 2000. (2001). *Morbidity and Mortality Weekly Report, 50*(32), 682–686.

Craske, M. G., Poulton, R., Tsao, J. C., & Plotkin, D. (2001). Paths to panic disorder/agoraphobia: An exploratory analysis from age 3 to 21 in an unselected birth cohort. *Journal of the American Academy of Child and Adolescent Psychiatry, 40*(5), 556–563.

Denson-Lino, J. M., Willies-Jacobo, L. J., Rosas, A., O'Connor, R. D., & Wilson, N. W. (1993). Effect of economic status on the use of house dust mite avoidance measures in asthmatic children. *Annals of Allergy, 71*(2), 130–132.

Duffy, D. L., Martin, N. G., Battistutta, D., Hopper, J. L., & Mathews, J. D. (1990). Genetics of asthma and hay fever in Australian twins. *American Review of Respiratory Disease, 142*(6 Pt 1), 1351–1358.

Edfors-Lubs, M. L. (1971). Allergy in 7000 twin pairs. *Acta Allergologica, 26*(4), 249–285.

Expert Panel Report 3 (EPR-3): Guidelines for the Diagnosis and Management of Asthma-Summary Report 2007. (2007). *Journal of Allergy and Clinical Immunology, 120*(5 Suppl), S94–138.

Federico, M. J., Wamboldt, F. S., Carter, R., Mansell, A., & Wamboldt, M. Z. (2007). History of serious asthma exacerbations should be included in guidelines of asthma severity. *Journal of Allergy and Clinical Immunology, 119*(1), 50–56.

Fiese, B. H., Wamboldt, F. S., & Anbar, R. D. (2005). Family asthma management routines: Connections to medical adherence and quality of life. *Journal of Pediatrics, 146*(2), 171–176.

Forrest, C. B., Starfield, B., Riley, A. W., & Kang, M. (1997). The impact of asthma on the health status of adolescents. *Pediatrics, 99*(2), E1.

Galobardes, B., McCarron, P., Jeffreys, M., & Davey Smith, G. (2008). Association between early life history of respiratory disease and morbidity and mortality in adulthood. *Thorax, 63*(5), 423–429.

Getahun, D., Demissie, K., & Rhoads, G. G. (2005). Recent trends in asthma hospitalization and mortality in the United States. *Journal of Asthma, 42*(5), 373–378.

Glazebrook, C., McPherson, A. C., Macdonald, I. A., Swift, J. A., Ramsay, C., Newbould, R., et al. (2006). Asthma as a barrier to children's physical activity: Implications for body mass index and mental health. *Pediatrics, 118*(6), 2443–2449.

Goodwin, R. D., Fergusson, D. M., & Horwood, L. J. (2004). Asthma and depressive and anxiety disorders among young persons in the community. *Psychological Medicine, 34*(8), 1465–1474.

Goodwin, R. D., Pine, D. S., & Hoven, C. W. (2003). Asthma and panic attacks among youth in the community. *Journal of Asthma, 40*(2), 139–145.

Hardie, G. E., Janson, S., Gold, W. M., Carrieri-Kohlman, V., & Boushey, H. A. (2000). Ethnic differences: Word descriptors used by African-American and white asthma patients during induced bronchoconstriction. *Chest, 117*(4), 935–943.

Heinrich, J., Hoelscher, B., Frye, C., Meyer, I., Wjst, M., & Wichmann, H. E. (2002). Trends in prevalence of atopic diseases and allergic sensitization in children in Eastern Germany. *European Respiratory Journal, 19*(6), 1040–1046.

Ho, J., Bender, B. G., Gavin, L. A., O'Connor, S. L., Wamboldt, M. Z., & Wamboldt, F. S. (2003). Relations among asthma knowledge, treatment adherence, and outcome. *Journal of Allergy and Clinical Immunology, 111*(3), 498–502.

Horner, C. C., & Strunk, R. C. (2007). Age-related changes in the asthmatic phenotype in children. *Current Opinion in Pediatrics, 19*(3), 295–299.

Horwood, L. J., Fergusson, D. M., & Shannon, F. T. (1985). Social and familial factors in the development of early childhood asthma. *Pediatrics, 75*(5), 859–868.

Humbert, M., Holgate, S., Boulet, L. P., & Bousquet, J. (2007). Asthma control or severity: That is the question. *Allergy, 62*(2), 95–101.

Juniper, E. F., Guyatt, G. H., Feeny, D. H., Ferrie, P. J., Griffith, L. E., & Townsend, M. (1996). Measuring quality of life in children with asthma. *Quality of Life Research, 5*(1), 35–46.

Kasasbeh, A., Kasasbeh, E., & Krishnaswamy, G. (2007). Potential mechanisms connecting asthma, esophageal reflux, and obesity/sleep apnea complex – a hypothetical review. *Sleep Medicine Reviews, 11*(1), 47–58.

Kashani, J. H., Konig, P., Shepperd, J. A., Wilfley, D., & Morris, D. A. (1988). Psychopathology and self-concept in asthmatic children. *Journal of Pediatric Psychology, 13*(4), 509–520.

Katon, W., Lozano, P., Russo, J., McCauley, E., Richardson, L., & Bush, T. (2007). The prevalence of DSM-IV anxiety and depressive disorders in youth with asthma compared with controls. *Journal of Adolescent Health, 41*(5), 455–463.

Kean, E. M., Kelsay, K., Wamboldt, F., & Wamboldt, M. Z. (2006). Posttraumatic stress in adolescents with asthma and their parents. *Journal of the American Academy of Child and Adolescent Psychiatry, 45*(1), 78–86.

Klinnert, M. D., Kaugars, A. S., Strand, M., & Silveira, L. (2008). Family psychological factors in relation to children's asthma status and behavioral adjustment at age 4. *Family Process, 47*(1), 41–61.

Koh, M. S., & Irving, L. B. (2007). The natural history of asthma from childhood to adulthood. *International Journal of Clinical Practice, 61*(8), 1371–1374.

Liggett, S. B. (1996). The genetics of beta 2-andrenergic receptor polymorphisms: Relevance to receptor function and asthmatic phenotypes. In S. B. Liggett & D. A. Meyers (Eds.). *The Genetics of Asthma* (Vol. 96, pp. 455–474). New York City: Marcel Dekker, Inc.

Lougheed, M. D., Fisher, T., & O'Donnell, D. E. (2006). Dynamic hyperinflation during bronchoconstriction in asthma: Implications for symptom perception. *Chest, 130*(4), 1072–1081.

Malveaux, F. J., & Fletcher-Vincent, S. A. (1995). Environmental risk factors of childhood asthma in urban centers. *Environmental Health Perspectives, 103*(Suppl 6), 59–62.

Mansfield, L. E. (2008). The future of the long-acting beta-adrenergic bronchodilators in the treatment of asthma. *Allergy and Asthma Proceedings, 29*(2), 103–108.

Marion, R. J., Creer, T. L., & Reynolds, R. V. (1985). Direct and indirect costs associated with the management of childhood asthma. *Annals of Allergy, 54*(1), 31–34.

McQuaid, E. L., Walders, N., Kopel, S. J., Fritz, G. K., & Klinnert, M. D. (2005). Pediatric asthma management in the family context: The family asthma management system scale. *Journal of Pediatric Psychology, 30*(6), 492–502.

Mohangoo, A. D., de Koning, H. J., Mangunkusumo, R. T., & Raat, H. (2007). Health-related quality of life in adolescents with wheezing attacks. *Journal of Adolescent Health, 41*(5), 464–471.

Moonie, S., Sterling, D. A., Figgs, L. W., & Castro, M. (2008). The relationship between school absence, academic performance, and asthma status. *Journal of School Health, 78*(3), 140–148.

Moorman, J. E., Rudd, R. A., Johnson, C. A., King, M., Minor, P., Bailey, C., et al. (2007). National surveillance for asthma – United States, 1980–2004. *MMWR Surveillance Summaries, 56*(8), 1–54.

Morgan, M., & Khan, D. A. (2003). Asthma: Epidemiology, burden, and quality of life. In E. S. Brown (Ed.). *Asthma: Social and psychological factors and psychosomatic syndromes* (Vol. 24, pp. 1–15). Basel: Karger.

Mrazek, D., & Strunk, R. (1984). Psychological adjustment of severely asthmatic preschool children: Allergic considerations. *Psychosom Med, 46*.

National Heart, Lung, and Blood Institute. (1995). *NHLBI/WHO Workshop Report: Global strategy for asthma management and prevention. Global Initiative for Asthma. Bethesda, MD: Author. Publication No. 95-3659.*

National Heart Lung and Blood Institute Asthma Signs and Symptoms of Asthma. (2008) from http://www.nhlbi.nih.gov/health/dci/Diseases/Asthma/Asthma_SignsAndSymptoms.html

Ortega, A. N., Huertas, S. E., Canino, G., Ramirez, R., & Rubio-Stipec, M. (2002). Childhood asthma, chronic illness, and psychiatric disorders. *Journal of Nervous and Mental Disease, 190*(5), 275–281.

Ortega, A. N., McQuaid, E. L., Canino, G., Ramirez, R., Fritz, G. K., & Klein, R. B. (2003). Association of psychiatric disorders and different indicators of asthma in island Puerto Rican children. *Social Psychiatry and Psychiatric Epidemiology, 38*(4), 220–226.

Pearlman, D. N., Zierler, S., Meersman, S., Kim, H. K., Viner-Brown, S. I., & Caron, C. (2006). Race disparities in childhood asthma: Does where you live matter? *Journal of the National Medical Association, 98*(2), 239–247.

Purcell, K., Turnbull, J. W., & Bernstein, L. (1962). Distinctions between subgroups of asthmatic children: Psychological test and behavior rating comparisons. *Journal of Psychosomatic Research, 6*, 283–291.

Rand, C. S., & Wise, R. A. (1994). Measuring adherence to asthma medication regimens. *American Journal of Respiratory and Critical Care Medicine, 149*(2 Pt 2), S69-76; discussion S77-68.

Reed, C. E. (2006). The natural history of asthma. *Journal of Allergy and Clinical Immunology, 118*(3), 543–548; quiz 549–550.

Restrepo, R. D., & Peters, J. (2008). Near-fatal asthma: Recognition and management. *Current Opinion in Pulmonary Medicine, 14*(1), 13–23.

Rhee, H., Wenzel, J., & Steeves, R. H. (2007). Adolescents' psychosocial experiences living with asthma: A focus group study. *Journal of Pediatric Health Care, 21*(2), 99–107.

Rosier, M. J., Bishop, J., Nolan, T., Robertson, C. F., Carlin, J. B., & Phelan, P. D. (1994). Measurement of functional severity of asthma in children. *American Journal of Respiratory and Critical Care Medicine, 149*(6), 1434–1441.

Silverglade, L., Tosi, D. J., Wise, P. S., & D'Costa, A. (1994). Irrational beliefs and emotionality in adolescents with and without bronchial asthma. *Journal of General Psychology, 121*(3), 199–207.

Strunk, R. C., Mrazek, D. A., Fuhrmann, G. S., & LaBrecque, J. F. (1985). Physiologic and psychological characteristics associated with deaths due to asthma in childhood. A case-controlled study. *Journal of the American Medical Association, 254*(9), 1193–1198.

Taras, H., & Potts-Datema, W. (2005). Childhood asthma and student performance at school. *Journal of School Health, 75*(8), 296–312.

Trends in asthma morbidity and mortality by American Lung Association Epidemiology and Statistics Unit Research and Program Services July 2006. (2006). from http://www.lungusa.org/atf/cf/{7A8D42C2-FCCA-4604-8ADE-7F5D5E762256}/ASTHMA06FINAL.PDF

Vila, G., Nollet-Clemencon, C., de Blic, J., Mouren-Simeoni, M. C., & Scheinmann, P. (2000). Prevalence of DSM IV anxiety and affective disorders in a pediatric population of asthmatic children and adolescents. *Journal of Affective Disorders, 58*(3), 223–231.

Vila, G., Nollet-Clemencon, C., Vera, M., Robert, J. J., de Blic, J., Jouvent, R., et al. (1999). Prevalence of DSM-IV disorders in children and adolescents with asthma versus diabetes. *Canadian Journal of Psychiatry, 44*(6), 562–569.

Wamboldt, F. S., Ho, J., Milgrom, H., Wamboldt, M. Z., Sanders, B., Szefler, S. J., et al. (2002). Prevalence and correlates of household exposures to tobacco smoke and pets in children with asthma. *Journal of Pediatrics, 141*(1), 109–115.

Wamboldt, F. S., Wamboldt, M. Z., Gavin, L. A., Roesler, T. A., & Brugman, S. M. (1995). Parental criticism and treatment outcome in adolescents hospitalized for severe, chronic asthma. *Journal of Psychosomatic Research, 39*(8), 995–1005.

Wamboldt, M. Z., & Levin, L. (1995). Utility of multifamily psychoeducational groups for medically ill children and adolescents. *Family Systems Medicine, 13*(2), 151–161.

Wamboldt, M. Z., & Weintraub, P. (1995). Links between past parental trauma and the medical and psychological outcome of asthmatic children: A theoretical model. *Family Systems Medicine, 13*(2), 129–149.

Wamboldt, M. Z., Yancey, A. G., Jr., & Roesler, T. A. (1997). Cardiovascular effects of tricyclic antidepressants in childhood asthma: A case series and review. *Journal of Child and Adolescent Psychopharmacology, 7*(1), 45–64.

Willis, D. J. (2002). Introduction to the special issue: economic, health, and mental health disparities among ethnic minority children and families. *Journal of Pediatric Psychology, 27*(4), 309–314.

Willwerth, B. M., Schaub, B., Tantisira, K. G., Gold, D. R., Palmer, L. J., Litonjua, A. A., et al. (2006). Prenatal, perinatal, and heritable influences on cord blood immune responses. *Annals of Allergy Asthma & Immunology, 96*(3), 445–453.

Wood, B. L., Lim, J., Miller, B. D., Cheah, P. A., Simmens, S., Stern, T., et al. (2007). Family emotional climate, depression, emotional triggering of asthma, and disease severity in pediatric asthma: Examination of pathways of effect. *Journal of Pediatric Psychology, 32*(5), 542–551.

Wood, B. L., Lim, J., Miller, B. D., Cheah, P., Zwetsch, T., Ramesh, S., et al. (2008). Testing the Biobehavioral Family Model in pediatric asthma: Pathways of effect. *Family Process, 47*(1), 21–40.

Juvenile Rheumatoid Arthritis

Michael A. Rapoff and Carol B. Lindsley

Juvenile rheumatoid arthritis (JRA) is the most common type of childhood and adolescent chronic arthritis and a major cause of short- and long-term disability among the pediatric age group with chronic pediatric diseases (Cassidy & Petty, 2005) The term juvenile rheumatoid arthritis is used here because the criteria for this diagnosis (Cassidy et al., 1986) were the inclusion criteria for almost all of the studies cited (see Table 1). The newer international classification schema, Juvenile Idiopathic Arthritis (International League Against Rheumatism, ILAR), has broader inclusion criteria, including psoriatic arthritis (joint swelling or two or more of the following signs: limitation of motion, tenderness or pain on motion and increased heat), enthesitis (inflammation at the insertion site of a tendon, ligament, fascia, or bone capsule)-associated arthritis (ERA), and an undifferentiated group (Cassidy & Petty, 2005). In addition adolescents may have primarily back and hip arthritis which falls under the category of spondylitis or spondyloarthropathy (Dougadoes et al., 1991) which will also be addressed.

Table 1 Criteria for the classification of juvenile rheumatoid arthritis (Cassidy et al., 1986)

Age of onset < 16 year)
Arthritis (swelling or effusion, or presence of two or more of the following signs: limitation of range of motion, tenderness or pain on motion, and increased heat) in one or more joints
Duration of disease 6 weeks or longer
Onset type defined by disease in the first 6 months
Polyarthritis: ≥ 5 inflamed joints
Oligoarthritis (pauciarticular disease): < 5 inflamed joints
Systemic-onset: arthritis with characteristic fever
Exclusion of other forms of juvenile arthritis

Adolescents may develop any of the subtypes of JRA, but most frequently onset of either polyarticular disease (Table 1) or spondyloarthropathy (disease of the joints of the spine including hips) dominates the teenage years. Adolescents who had earlier disease onset may also have issues and perhaps complications related to any of the subtypes. This chapter reviews the medical and psychosocial aspects of JRA and spondylitis (inflammation of vertebrae) including psychosocial adjustment, chronic pain, and adherence to medical regimens. Clinical and research recommendations are also offered to address the psychosocial aspects of JRA and spondylitis.

Epidemiology

The etiology of JRA is not known, although variables thought to be important in the pathophysiology of the disease include genetic predisposition, unknown environmental triggers, and immune reactivity. The hallmark of the disease is synovitis (inflammation of the synovial membrane of a joint). There are three subtypes of JRA; the categorization is made according to the symptomatology that occurs over the first 6 months of disease (Cassidy & Petty, 2005) and includes systemic disease, polyarticular, and oligoarticular (Table 1) disease. Approximately 25% of disease onset is in adolescence.

M.A. Rapoff (✉)
Department of Pediatrics, University of Kansas Medical Center, Kansas City, KS, USA
e-mail: mrapoff@kumc.edu

W.T. O'Donohue, L.W. Tolle (eds.), *Behavioral Approaches to Chronic Disease in Adolescence*, DOI 10.1007/978-0-387-87687-0_11, © Springer Science+Business Media, LLC 2009

Symptoms

Polyarticular disease. This subtype occurs in about 40% of all JRA and is defined as involvement of more than four joints. Of the three basic subtypes, it is the most frequent in adolescents. Usually the joints involved include hands, wrists, hips, knees, ankles, and neck. If the disease has begun at an early age, there may be involvement of the mandibular growth centers that leads to facial asymmetry as an adolescent and a potential for long-term temporomandibular joint problems. About 25% of these adolescents (5–10% of JRA overall) have a positive rheumatoid factor test, which is a marker for increased risk for more severe disease. Very aggressive medical therapy is often required to control their disease symptoms and prevent disease progression. When disease begins in the adolescence, there is at least a 50% risk that it will persist into adulthood (Wallace & Levinson, 1991). The major long-term risks are continually active disease, joint destruction, osteoporosis, residual growth asymmetries, and side effects of medication.

Systemic disease. This subtype affects approximately 10% of the JRA population and is defined by the presence of a characteristic rash or high cyclic fevers, along with arthritis. Onset is unusual in adolescence. There are associated non-articular manifestations, such as lymphadenopathy (inflammation of lymph nodes), hepatosplenomegaly (enlargement of the liver and spleen), pericarditis (inflammation of the pericardium or sac enclosing the heart), serositis (inflammation of a lining membrane (e.g., the lung lining or pleura), and marked laboratory abnormalities. The systemic symptoms will generally subside over the first few months of disease as the joint symptoms persist and often progress. These children and adolescents are frequently admitted to the hospital to establish a firm diagnosis and begin therapy. The pericarditis is a potentially life-threatening manifestation. Most will respond to appropriate therapy; however, this subtype remains the most difficult group to treat, and up to 25% of those affected have a poor prognosis with continually active and poorly responsive disease. The severest involvement is generally in the hands, wrists, hips, and neck, so both mobility and dexterity are at risk.

Pauciarticular (Oligoarthritis). This subtype occurs in 40–50% of children with JRA and is defined as involvement of four or fewer joints, with the joints most frequently involved being the knees or ankles. There are two subgroups: (1) young girls who test positive for ANA (antinuclear antibody) and have a high risk for eye involvement (uveitis), and (2) older boys who have a long-term risk for developing involvement of the axial skeleton (hips and back). This type is called Enthesitis Related Arthritis in the ILAR classification.

The diagnosis of JRA is made with the demonstration of persistent arthritis in one or more joints for a minimum of 6 weeks and with the exclusion of other diagnoses. Early, accurate diagnosis is essential in order to achieve optimal outcome, which is (1) control of the arthritis and the extra-articular manifestations and (2) prevention of complications such as leg-length discrepancy, gait abnormalities, or vision impairment.

Spondyloarthropathy

Spondyloarthropathies may have onset in adolescence and include a group of diseases with arthritis focused on the back and hips (axial disease) and an association with the histocompatibility antigen, HLA-B27 (human leukocyte antigen). The disease group includes ankylosing spondylitis and psoriatic and inflammatory bowel disease-associated arthritis. There is a male predominance. The disease often presents initially with peripheral arthritis, e.g., knee or ankle, and then axial disease evolves over a period of years.

Treatment Regimens

Once the diagnosis is established, most adolescents require regular medications. The goals are to suppress inflammation and prevent complications, such as joint deformity, blindness, or growth abnormalities.... The specific therapy used depends on the maturity of the adolescent and the severity of the arthritis. Non-steroidal anti-inflammatory agents (NSAIDs) are the standard first-line therapy. Well-established drugs such as naproxen or ibuprofen are used in young children and longer acting, once-a-day drugs such as nabumetone, piroxicam or the newer COX-2 inhibitor, celecoxib, are often used in older children and adolescents. The less frequently dosed drugs make adherence easier. These drugs relieve pain, reduce inflammation, and fever (if present). The average time required for maximal response is 4–6 weeks (Lovell, Giannini, & Brewer, 1984).

Most children and adolescents with pauciarticular (Table 1) disease respond to NSAIDs, but intra-articular corticosteroids may be needed for unresponsive joints, and occasionally second-line agents such as sulfasalzaine or hydroxychloroquine are added. In polyarticular disease, NSAIDs are initial therapy, with second-line agents or disease-modifying antirheumatic drugs (DMARDs), such as hydroxychloroquine, sulfasalzaine, or methotrexate, added for poorly responsive or unresponsive disease after weeks to months. Low-dose short-term corticosteroid therapy may be used as "bridge therapy" to control symptoms during a transitional period, as when DMARDs take weeks to months to be effective.

In systemic disease, DMARDs such as hydroxychloroquine or methotrexate may be added early in the disease course, and daily corticosteroids may be required for pericarditis, macrophage activation syndrome, or severe disease. Children and adolescents with eye involvement are generally treated with corticosteroid eye drops and dilating agents. The activity of the eye disease does not usually fluctuate with that of the joint disease.

Every effort is made to avoid long-term high dose corticosteroid therapy in children or adolescents because of the serious adverse effects including growth retardation, iatrogenic Cushing's disease, osteoporosis, fractures, obesity, and hypertension. Patients with persistent, severe polyarticular or systemic disease who do not respond to combination drug therapy are candidates for biologic agents such as antitumor necrosis factor drugs (e.g., etanercept, adalimumab). However, the biologic agents are very costly and may not be an option for adolescents without insurance coverage or who are underinsured.

All adolescents with active arthritis or ongoing requirement for medication to control their disease need to be seen by their physician on a regular basis, usually every 3–6 months, depending on their specific issues and medication regimen. Adequate disease control can now be achieved in the vast majority of adolescents with use of the currently available drugs and good adherence on the part of the adolescent.

Common Problems

Psychosocial Adjustment of Children and Adolescents with JRA

Many studies have found no significant psychosocial deficits in children with JRA compared with normative or healthy control samples. Kellerman, Zeltzer, Ellenberg, Dash, and Rigler (1980) assessed 168 chronically ill adolescents (30 with rheumatic disease) and 349 healthy controls and found no significant differences between healthy and ill adolescents or between illness subgroups on measures of anxiety or self-esteem. Brace, Smith, McCauley, and Sherry (2000) compared adolescents with JRA to healthy adolescents and adolescents with chronic fatigue syndrome (CFS). The adolescents with CFS scored significantly higher on measures of internalizing problems (e.g., depression), school absences, and parental reinforcement of illness behavior than did the healthy adolescents. Adolescents with JRA scored in the intermediate range, between adolescents with CFS and healthy adolescents, on most measures, with the exception that adolescents with JRA had the lowest parental reinforcement of illness behavior.

Noll and colleagues (2000) compared 74 children and adolescents with JRA with 74 case–control classmates and found no significant differences between groups on any of the 10 measures used to assess social and emotional functioning, with both groups scoring in the normative range on all measures. Huygen, Kuis, and Sinnema (2000) conducted a study of 47 Dutch children and adolescents with JRA, 52 healthy peers, and their parents. Results indicated that self-esteem, perceived competence, body image, social competence, social support, and psychopathology were equivalent across groups despite children with JRA having less ability to participate in sports, less frequent opportunities to play with friends, and lower perceived athletic competence.

Several other studies have found significant differences between the psychosocial functioning of children and adolescents with JRA and healthy control children (McAnarney, Pless, Satterwhite, & Friedman, 1974; Mullick, Nahar, & Haq, 2005). Mullick et al. (2005) compared 40 children and adolescents with JRA to 40 age- and sex-matched and found that children with JRA were significantly more likely to have a depressive disorder (15.0%) than healthy controls (0%). In a 1-year prospective study that examined quality of life in children with JRA, children and adolescents with arthritis reported significantly lower quality of life than previously reported by healthy children in the general community (Sawyer et al., 2005). However, scores were only in the mild disability range, which the authors note is consistent with previous findings. LeBovidge, Lavigne, Donerberg, and Miller (2003) conducted a meta-analysis that reviewed 21 studies reporting on psychosocial adjustment in children and adolescents with juvenile arthritis. The authors concluded that children and adolescents with juvenile arthritis display an increased overall risk for adjustment problems and internalizing (anxious and depressive) symptoms, but no increased risk for lowered self-concept or externalizing problems. Furthermore, as indicated above, children and adolescents who report higher levels of pain report poorer overall adjustment (Sällfors, Fasth, & Hallberg, 2002) and lower quality of life (Sawyer et al., 2005, 2004) than their counterparts who experience less pain related to their JRA. Thus it appears that children and adolescents with JRA do nearly as well as their healthy peers, but that they are at increased risk for anxiety and depressive disorders.

School Attendance and Adjustment

Studies addressing school absence have found that children with JRA tend to be absent significantly more often than their healthy peers (Fowler, Johnson, & Atkinson, 1985). However, this scenario is not necessarily the case, and it seems that disease severity is related to school absence. In a study of 113 children and adolescents with JRA, Sturge, Garralda, Boissin, Dore, and Woo (1997) found the mean school attendance rate to be 92%. Children and adolescents with more severe forms of JRA were significantly more likely to miss school.

More recent studies have examined not only school attendance, but adjustment within the school setting for children with JRA. Schanberg, Anthony, Gill, and Maurin (2003) found that 56% of children and adolescents with JRA reduced their school activities at least once during a 2-month period when they experienced increased disease activity (increased pain, stiffness, and fatigue). Furthermore, increased disease activity (pain and stiffness) significantly predicted a reduction in school activities participation. Peer-support is consistently found to be important in overall adjustment. Higher classmate support predicts fewer adjustment problems and fewer depressive symptoms (von Weiss et al., 2002), while peer-rejection is associated with increased adjustment problems and increased depressive symptoms (Sandstrom & Schanberg, 2004). Fortunately, children and adolescents with JRA generally report sufficient peer-support from friends and boyfriends or girlfriends (Kyngäs, 2004).

Family Adjustment

Overall, families of children with JRA report multiple illness-related stressors, such as school difficulties, fears for the child's future, problems managing treatment regimens, and financial burdens (Degatardi, Revenson, & Ilowite, 1999). However, the majority of families appear to be fairly well-adjusted, reporting high levels of family cohesion and expressiveness and low levels of family conflict. Reid, McGrath, and Lang (2005) examined parent–child interactions among children and adolescents with juvenile fibromyalgia, JRA, and health controls during a pain-inducing exercise task. After controlling for pain, they found no significant differences across groups on parent–child interactions. Across groups, parents provided more encouraging than discouraging statements when their children voiced pain- or task-related negative statements.

Despite an overall positive picture, increased family burden and increased parental distress has been found in families of children with JRA. Henoch, Batson, and Baum (1978) compared a sample of 88 children with JRA to 2,952 control children and found that families of children with JRA were significantly more likely to have unmarried parents due to divorce, separation, or death and they experienced adoption in their families three times more frequently than the control sample. In a study of maternal functioning, Manuel (2001) assessed 92 mothers of children and adolescents with JRA. Compared with normative groups, mothers of children and adolescents with JRA reported significantly higher levels of emotional distress. Regression analyses showed that higher daily hassles and illness-related stressors were both significant predictors of greater emotional distress among mothers of children and adolescents with JRA. Higher maternal education and more positive appraisal of the child's illness (less illness-intrusiveness) on the family served to buffer against psychological distress. Although less than mothers, fathers of children with JRA also report high levels of emotional distress (McNeill, 2004) and a large number of concerns over their child's illness (Hovey, 2005). Fathers tend to report problem solving and information gathering as their primary means of coping with their emotions and concerns (Hovey, 2005; McNeill, 2004). However, fathers also tend to rely on themselves more than others for support, which may make them vulnerable to using maladaptive coping strategies, such as smoking or using alcohol (Hovey, 2005). In a sample of 45 children and adolescents with juvenile rheumatic diseases (27 with JRA), Wagner et al. (2003) found that increased parental distress and increased child reported illness-intrusiveness were both significant predictors of child depressive symptoms. When parental distress was high and children reported high levels of illness-intrusiveness (interference with daily functions), they also reported increased depressive symptoms. Helgeson, Janicki, Lerner, and Barbarin (2003) found family cohesion to be an important predictor of adjustment in children and adolescents with JRA, particularly for younger children. In a sample of 94 children and adolescents with JRA, family cohesion was related to less illness worry, and higher self-esteem, where as family conflict was related to great illness worry and lower self-esteem. Thus, parental distress, family cohesion, and cognitive appraisals of JRA are important factors in adolescent and overall family adjustment.

Daniels, Miller, Billings, and Moos (1986) compared 72 children and adolescents with a rheumatic disease (58 with JRA) and their siblings with 60 demographically matched siblings of healthy children on parent measures of psychological functioning and family functioning. Results indicated no differences between groups on any measures, with siblings of JRA children and siblings of healthy children functioning equally well. In a later study, the authors (Daniels, Moos, Billings, & Miller, 1987) compared 93 children and adolescents with rheumatic disease and 72 of their siblings with 93 demographically matched siblings of healthy controls. The authors found that across all three groups maternal depressed mood and JRA physical symptoms predicted greater adjustment problems and that high family cohesion and expressiveness were related to better functioning. Thus research indicates that JRA has little effect on siblings but likely contributes to increased stress for mothers and fathers, especially when JRA symptoms are high, daily hassles are high, illness-intrusiveness is elevated, and parental education levels are low.

Long-Term Adjustment into Adulthood

Miller, Spitz, Simpson, and Williams (1982) conducted a follow-up study of 121 individuals with JRA who had reached at least the age of 18 years and found that most of them were working, attending school full time, or a combination of the two. The authors also compared 50 patients with their siblings and found no significant differences on any demographic or psychosocial variables. However, Peterson, Mason, Nelson, O'Fallon, and Gabriel (1997) conducted a 25-year follow-up study of 44 individuals diagnosed with JRA (mean age = 33.5 years) and 102 age- and sex-matched controls. Results indicated that people with JRA had significantly lower functional status, more physical disability, higher unemployment, and less ability to exercise than controls. The major differences between these two studies are the age at assessment and the type of control group used. Miller et al. (1982) studied children with JRA around 18 years of age, whereas Peterson et al. (1997) studied patients around 33 years of age. Therefore, it is possible that children with JRA function fairly typically through the age of dependence (when they typically live with their families) but tend to have more difficulty as they progress through life. Also, the Miller et al. (1982) study compared children with JRA with their siblings, where Peterson et al. (1997) used an age- and sex-matched control group. It is possible, therefore, that using the non-sibling control group allowed other demographic features (i.e., socioeconomic status) to increase the differences between groups that were found in the Peterson et al. (1997) study.

Packham, Hall, and Pimm (2002) conducted a long-term follow-up of 246 adults who had been diagnosed with JRA (mean age = 35.4 years) and compared results to general population norms. Results indicated that adults with JRA experienced higher levels of anxiety (31.6%) than the general population (18%), but similar or lower levels of depression (5.2% current; 21.1% past) than the general population (12% current, 20% past). Approximately 38% of patients felt that their JRA had negatively impacted their emotional state. Subtype of JRA and age of onset were significant predictors of anxiety and depression levels. Those with systemic-onset JRA had higher levels of anxiety and depression; whereas those with oligoarticular JRA had lower levels of anxiety and depression. Furthermore, depression was more common when JRA onset was between 6 and 12 years of age, and anxiety was more common in the late-onset group over 12 years of age.

Chronic or Reoccurring Pain

Chronic or reoccurring pain is a primary clinical manifestation of JRA (Anthony & Schanberg, 2003; Cassidy & Petty, 2005). Children and adolescents with JRA often report mild to moderate levels of pain intensity (Gragg et al., 1996; Hagglund, Schopp, Alberts, Cassidy, & Frank, 1995; Ilowite, Walco, & Pochaczevsky, 1992; Thompson, Varni, & Hanson, 1987; Varni et al., 1996) and some (14% in one study) even report no pain (Sherry, Bohnsack, Salmonson, Wallace, & Mellins, 1990). However, about 25–30% report pain intensities in the moderate to severe range (Ross, Lavigne, Hayford, Dyer, & Pachman, 1989; Schanberg, Lefebvre, Keefe, Kredich, & Gil, 1997) and, in one study (Benestad, Vinje, Veierød, & Vandvik, 1996), 82% reported pain lasting from 30 min to 24 h a day, with a mean of 4.3 h per day. A daily dairy study over a 2-month period found that children and adolescents with JRA reported having mild to moderate pain an average of 73% of days and 31% reported pain in the severe range (Schanberg et al., 2003). Also, a long-term follow-up study from the Mayo Clinic found that the adults who were diagnosed with JRA reported significantly greater pain, fatigue, and disability relative to gender-matched healthy cases (Peterson et al., 1997). Higher levels of pain have also been linked to reductions in quality of life for children and adolescents with rheumatic diseases (Dhanani, Quenneville, Perron, Abdolell, & Feldman, 2002; Sawyer et al., 2004).

There is also some evidence that children with chronic arthritis and other rheumatic diseases come from families with a history of chronic pain. Schanberg et al. (2001) found that among 89 children and adolescents with a rheumatic disease (54 with chronic arthritis), more than 90% of their parents reported having at least one chronic pain condition. Additionally, 93% of parents reported that an extended family member experienced at least one chronic pain condition. Schanberg et al. also found that parents reporting higher levels of pain were more likely to have children reporting higher levels of pain. Thus pain is a significant problem for some children with JRA who have a family history of chronic pain and pain persists into adulthood and is associated with greater disability.

Adherence to Treatment

Children and adolescents with JRA and their parents are usually asked to adhere consistently and over a long period of time to a variety of therapeutic regimens, most notably, medications, therapeutic exercises, and splinting of joints. Many of these regimens may have delayed beneficial effects and in the short term may cause unwanted side effects, such as gastrointestinal irritation and pain. Factors associated with JRA and its treatment (i.e., the need for consistent adherence over a long period of time, delayed beneficial effects, and negative side effects) have been predictive of greater adherence problems to medical regimens for pediatric chronic diseases (Rapoff, 1999).

As can be seen in Table 2, relatively few studies have specifically addressed adherence to regimens for

Table 2 Adherence rates to treatments for JRA

Reference	Sample	Regimen	Measure	Results
April et al. (2006)	N = 50 8–18 yrs (M = 12.67 yrs)	Medications Exercise	Parent and child ratings (100-mm VAS)	Mean medication adherence = 84.9% by children and 83.1% by parents Mean exercise adherence = 61.2% by children and 57.4% by parents Adherence to medications significantly higher than adherence to exercises for both children and parents (p values <0.001)
Feldman et al. (2007)	N = 175 2–18 yrs	Medications Exercise	Caregiver rated over past 3 months	Adherence at baseline, 3, 6 , 9, and 12 months for medications was 86%, 92%, 90%, 92%, and 89%; for exercises 55%, 64%, 61%, 63%, and 54%
Giannini et al. (1990)	N = 92 1.8–15.1 yrs (M = 7.7 yrs)	Ibuprofen or aspirin	Pill count	Patients considered nonadherent if they took <60% of prescribed doses; 3% nonadherent
Hayford and Ross (1988)	N = 93 1.4–20.4 yrs (M = 8.8 yrs)	Medications Exercises	Parent and child report (five-point Likert scale but dichotomized to "always/never" = positive and "sometimes/seldom/ never" = negative)	95.1% of parents reported positive adherence to medications vs. 67.2% to exercise (p<.001); 89.2% of children reported positive adherence to medications vs. 46.9% to exercise (p<0.002)
Kvien and Reimers (1983)	N = 25 4–15 yrs	Salicylates or Naproxen	Pill count	95% adherent overall
Litt and Cuskey (1981)	N = 82 (M = 12 yrs)	Salicylates	Serum assay (<20 mg/dl defined nonadherence)	45% of patients nonadherent Mean serum level = 21.3 mg/dl
Litt , Cuskey, and Rosenberg, (1982)	N = 38 (M = 14 yrs)	Salicylates	Serum assay (<20 mg/dl defined nonadherence)	45% of patients nonadherent Mean serum level = 20.79 mg/dl
Rapoff et al. (1985)	N = 37 2–23 yrs (M = 12 yrs)	Medications Splints Exercises	Questionnaire completed by parents (rated how easy it is to get children to take medications, wear splints, or do exercises on 5-point scale, with 5 = "very easy" and 1 = "very hard")	Means: Medication adherence rating = 4.49; splints = 4.33; exercises = 3.57 43% of parents reported that their children had some negative reactions to taking medications and wearing splints; 60% reported that their children had some negative reactions to doing exercises
Rapoff et al. (2005)	N = 48 2.3–16.7 yrs	Non-steroidal anti-inflammatory drugs	Electronic monitor	Monitored over 28 consecutive days 48% nonadherent (<80% of doses taken) Median levels showed full adherence on 70% of days, partial on 14%, and no adherence on 7%

JRA. Adherence to non-steroidal anti-inflammatory medications varies depending on the measure used, with relatively higher rates by parent or child report vs. serum assays and electronic monitoring. They also vary depending on the cutpoint used to classify patients as adherent or nonadherent. Using the cutpoint convention in the literature of classifying patients as nonadherent if they took <80% of doses (Rapoff, 1999), Brewer, Giannini, Kuzmina, and Alekseev (1986) found nonadherence rates of 11–14% to active and placebo medications, while Rapoff, Belmont, Lindsley, and Olson (2005) found that 48% of newly diagnosed patients with JRA were nonadherent. Using a cutpoint of <60%, Giannini et al. (1990) found that only 3% of patients were nonadherent. There is also consistent evidence that adherence is lower to therapeutic exercise regimens than medications, at least by parent or patient report (April, Feldman, Platt, & Duffy, 2006; Feldman et al., 2007; Hayford & Ross, 1988; Rapoff, Lindsley, & Christophersen, 1985). A few studies have targeted improvements in adherence to regimens (primarily medications) for JRA.

One study tested the efficacy of a parent-managed token system program in improving adherence to medications for a 14-year-old male with polyarticular JRA (Rapoff, Purviance, & Lindsley, 1988a). Adherence was assessed by weekly pill counts obtained from the patient's mother over the phone, with independent counts by an investigator in the clinic (agreement with the mother's count was 100%). A withdrawal (reversal) single-subject design was employed to evaluate the effects of the intervention on adherence and several clinical outcome parameters (e.g., active joint counts). Medication adherence averaged 44% during baseline, increased to an average of 59% during a simplified regimen condition (in which the dosage was reduced from four to three times a day), and further increased and remained at 100% during the first token system phase. Adherence decreased during a token system withdrawal phase (mean = 77%), increased during the second token system phase (mean = 99%), and averaged 92% during the maintenance phase (in which the token system was not in effect but could be reinstated if adherence dropped below 80% for two consecutive weeks). At the 9-month follow-up (no token system in effect and no contingency for reinstatement), adherence averaged 97%. Though not as straightforward as the adherence results, improvements were shown in clinical outcomes during the token system and follow-up phases (e.g., five active joints) relative to baseline and the token system withdrawal phase (e.g., ten active joints).

Although the previously mentioned study showed that a token system could be effective in improving adherence, they are labor intensive for families and require well-trained personnel to implement and monitor. One study (Rapoff, Purviance, & Lindsley, 1988b) evaluated less complex behavioral strategies (such as self-monitoring and positive verbal feedback) combined with educational strategies (verbal and written information about medications and the importance of adherence and strategies for improving adherence). This study involved three female patients with JRA, ages 3, 10, and 13 years and adherence was again assessed by weekly pill counts obtained from parents over the phone, with independent counts by one of the investigators in the clinic (agreement was 100%). A multiple baseline across-subjects design was used to evaluate the efficacy of the intervention. Baseline medication adherence averaged 38 and 54% for two of the patients and increased during the intervention phase to an average of 97 and 92%, respectively. Adherence increased only slightly for the third patient, from an average of 44% during baseline to an average of 49% during the intervention phase. Adherence decreased for all three patients at 4-month follow-up (means ranged from 24 to 89%). Interestingly, the patient for whom the intervention was least effective was a 13-year-old who had less parental supervision of her regimen and whose mother admitted she was nonadherent to medications prescribed to treat her arthritis. Unfortunately, clinical outcomes were not reported for these patients.

The above-mentioned studies suggest that adherence can be improved by behavioral strategies alone or combined with educational strategies, a combination that has worked best for improving adherence to other chronic pediatric diseases (Rapoff, 1999). However, these studies involved small sample sizes and did not generally assess clinical outcomes, such as active joint counts. These studies also involved patients who had been diagnosed with having JRA for varying lengths of time and for whom nonadherence was implicated as interfering with the effectiveness of treatments by their pediatric rheumatologist. The success of these interventions with limited numbers of patients who were persistently nonadherent led our group to test the possible benefits of intervening with newly diagnosed patients in order to prevent the anticipated drop in adherence over time which has been reported in the pediatric adherence literature (Rapoff, 1999)

We conducted a randomized controlled trial evaluating a clinic-based, nurse-administered educational and behavioral intervention to promote adherence to non-steroidal medications among newly diagnosed patients with JRA (Rapoff et al., 2002). Thirty-four participants (mean age = 8.44 years) were matched by age and type of JRA and then randomly assigned to the experimental or (attention-placebo) control groups. Patients and parents in the experimental group were given verbal, written, and audiovisual information from a nurse about adherence improvement strategies, including prompting, monitoring, positive reinforcement, and discipline techniques (Rapoff, 1998). Control group patients and parents were given verbal, written, and audiovisual information about JRA and treatments by the same nurse, but no specific information about adherence improvement strategies. Patients and parents in both groups received their respective interventions during a 1½ h clinic visit and were then telephoned by the nurse biweekly for 2 months and then monthly for 10 months. The content of the phone calls centered on the information presented during the initial clinic visit.

Adherence was assessed using the Medication Event Monitoring System (MEMS; Aprex Corporation, Fremont, CA). This electronic medication bottle cap records the date and time of each bottle opening. It can store 1800 openings and has an 18-month battery life. MEMS data are downloaded to a portable computer and analyzed with the manufacturer's software, which provides daily and continuous data on adherence (assuming that medications are taken each time the pill cap is removed). The daily MEMS adherence score was the percent of prescribed doses taken within the recommended dosing interval, with a 2 h (plus or minus) forgiveness interval (e.g., NSAID twice daily, could be taken 10–14 h between doses). Disease activity and functional status measures were obtained during routine clinic visits where the rheumatologist recorded standard clinical indices, including number of active joints (those with pain, swelling, and limitation of motion), the number of minutes of morning stiffness, and a global disease activity rating (0 = off medication, in remission, 1 = quiescent, 2 = mild, 3 = moderate, 4 = severe). During these visits, the parents completed the Childhood Health Assessment Questionnaire (CHAQ), which is designed to assess disease-related functional limitations over the past week in eight areas: dressing and grooming, arising, eating, walking, hygiene, reach, grip, and play. The eight scores are averaged to yield the CHAQ Disability Index, ranging from 0 (no difficulty) to 3 (unable to do).

For the 52-week post-intervention follow-up, the experimental-group participants showed significantly better overall average adherence than the controls (77.7% vs. 56.9%, $p = 0.023$) and as predicted, the trend in adherence levels significantly dropped over time in the control group but not in the experimental group. There were, however, no significant post-intervention group differences on disease activity and functional status measures. The lack of significant differences in disease-related outcomes may have been due to "floor effects" (e.g., 68% of experimental participants and 67% of controls had quiescent or mild disease at baseline). This floor effect may have prevented detection of improvements that could be unambiguously attributed to the experimental adherence intervention.

A unique randomized clinical trial focused on preventing osteoporosis in children with JRA by increasing calcium (Ca) intake (Stark et al., 2005). Forty-nine children with JRA (mean age 6 years) and their parents were randomly assigned to a behavioral intervention (BI) group or an enhanced standard of care (ESC) group. Children and parents in the BI group met in separate groups for six sessions and received nutritional counseling on how to increase calcium intake and behavioral strategies (praise coupled with use of a sticker chart to track progress for reaching targeted calcium intake levels). Children and parent in the ESC group were seen individually for three visits and received nutritional counseling only. Three-day food diaries were kept by parents at baseline and posttreatment and were analyzed for calcium intake. Repeated measures analysis demonstrated a significant group by time interaction with children in the BI group achieving a greater increase in dietary Ca intake from baseline to posttreatment compared to the ESC group ($p < 0.001$). In addition, and of clinical significance, 92% of children in the BI group achieved the treatment goal of 1500 mg of Ca/day compared to 17% of children in the ESC group at posttreatment.

The above-mentioned studies suggest that behavioral strategies combined with education is the most effective way to improve adherence to regimens for JRA and to prevent deterioration in adherence over time in newly diagnosed patients. The one dietary study also suggests that behavioral strategies are a necessary adjunct to nutritional education in improving calcium intake for patients with JRA. These findings are consistent with adherence intervention studies for other chronic pediatric diseases such as asthma, cystic fibrosis, and diabetes (Rapoff, 1999). There are, however, too few adherence intervention studies and the ones which have been published involve small sample sizes, utilize less objective measures of adherence such as pill counts, and often fail to demonstrate that improvements in adherence produce improvements in disease and quality of life outcomes.

Clinical and Research Implications

Psychosocial Adjustment

The bulk of the empirical evidence suggests that children and adolescents with JRA do not appear to be at any greater risk of developing clinically significant adjustment problems. However, it is possible that this risk has been underestimated due to underreporting of psychosocial difficulties or fluctuations in psychosocial functioning concomitant with fluctuations in disease severity that may not be captured in cross-sectional studies. Children who experience more severe disease (e.g., those with increased pain and stiffness) appear to be at greater risk for adjustment problems. Alternatively, family cohesion appears to be a protective factor in both child and parent adjustment. More longitudinal studies are needed to assess psychosocial adjustment and coping among children and adolescents with JRA coupled with well-timed psychosocial interventions for those deemed to be at risk or experiencing significant distress or disruption in their daily lives.

Studies on adjustment and coping should include measures of adaptive or protective factors. Instruments to assess these types of constructs will need to be developed and validated specifically for children and adolescents with JRA. For example, Barlow and associates have reported on the development and preliminary validation of parent and child arthritis self-efficacy scales (Barlow, Shaw, & Wright, 2000, 2001). Instead of duplicating efforts to develop new instruments to measure these constructs, investigators should collaborate and pool reliability and validity data across sites. Innovative and potentially more useful approaches to assess variability in adjustment and coping might involve within-person research to examine daily fluctuations and associations between daily measures of stress, mood, and disease symptoms (as was done by Schanberg et al., 2000). Such daily measures would also provide more detailed outcome data for psychosocial intervention trials.

Pain

A biobehavioral model of pain would suggest a number of treatment options (Rapoff & Lindsley, 2000). Early and aggressive pharmacological treatment of JRA could lead to enhanced pain relief and function, both short term and long term, via a reduction in peripheral and central sensitization mechanisms. Neurochemical mechanisms also suggest the value of nonpharmacological therapies in the treatment of arthritis-related pain, such as cooling and resting inflamed joints (to control nociceptive inputs and avoid peripheral sensitization) and relaxation or other psychological treatments.

Psychological interventions that reduce negative emotional states would be expected to directly or indirectly reduce pain intensity and pain interference. Helping children to manage disease-related stressors (e.g., relaxation and problem-solving techniques) should result in concomitant reductions in negative emotions and pain. Enlisting the social support and reinforcement of family and friends should foster greater participation in social and recreational activities by patients, thereby reducing emotional distress and preoccupation with pain and suffering.

Cognitive restructuring may be helpful in countering maladaptive thinking about pain by having children identify negative thoughts (e.g., "I can't do anything to make my pain better"), challenge or question these thoughts, and substitute more helpful thoughts (e.g., "I can distract myself or do relaxation exercises to reduce my pain"). Imagery techniques (e.g., vividly imagining a relaxing place or experience) combined with relaxation exercises are often helpful in diverting attention from pain, thereby reducing pain.

Parents are important role models for their children, and they need to be made aware of how they cope with their own pain (such as headaches) and thereby influence how their children cope with pain (Rapoff & Lindsley, 2000). Parents can be taught more adaptive strategies for coping with pain so that they can model these strategies for their children (e.g., not avoiding responsibilities because of pain and using effective medical or psychological therapies to control pain). Family members and friends can be taught to respond adaptively to pain behaviors, including not being overly solicitous and attentive to pain behaviors and reinforcing alternative and adaptive coping strategies. Children with JRA can be helped to find ways (in spite of their pain) to do what they want and need to do.

There is a need for well-controlled, multisite pain intervention trials for children with JRA. Studies to date have been promising but have involved small samples and no control or alternative-treatment comparison groups (Lavigne, Ross, Berry, Hayford, & Pachman, 1992; Walco, Varni, & Ilowite, 1992). Investigators should also consider using electronic pain diaries (e-diaries), rather than paper diaries, as e-diaries are well accepted by children and adolescents with arthritis and result in fewer errors and omissions compared to paper diaries (Palermo, Valenzuela, & Stork, 2004; Stinson et al., 2006).

Adherence

Few adherence intervention studies target medical regimens for children with JRA, especially for therapeutic exercises. The studies that have been done suggest a three-tiered approach to minimizing nonadherence: primary, secondary, and tertiary prevention (Rapoff, 2000). *Primary prevention* efforts would be most relevant for those patients who have not yet exhibited clinically significant nonadherence (inconsistencies in following a particular regimen that may result in compromised health and well-being); possibly those recently diagnosed or those who are able to sustain adequate adherence over time. Interventions at this level would involve educational (e.g., stressing the importance of adherence), organizational (e.g., simplifying regimens), and relatively simple behavioral strategies (e.g., monitoring of regimen adherence by providers or parents).

Secondary prevention might be most applicable to those patients for whom clinically significant nonadherence has been identified early on in the disease course or has yet to compromise their health and well-being. Interventions at this level might include more frequent monitoring of regimen adherence by parents and patients, specific and consistent positive social reinforcement for adherence, and general discipline strategies (e.g., time-out for younger children). Pediatric psychologists could train primary health care providers, particularly nurses, to implement primary and secondary level interventions.

Tertiary prevention efforts would apply to patients with an ongoing pattern of clinically significant nonadherence. Strategies at this level might include token system programs, contingency contracting, self-management training (e.g., problem solving to anticipate and manage obstacles to adherence), and possibly psychotherapy. Because of the demanding and technical nature of these strategies, pediatric psychologists would be responsible for implementing strategies at this level.

Implementing and evaluating primary, secondary, and tertiary prevention approaches to medical nonadherence depend on a number of factors. First, prevention efforts require a valid, reliable, and clinically feasible way to detect or assess nonadherence. Although no such "ideal" measure exists, 24 h recall interviews (in clinics or by phone) may be the best option in that they have been shown to be reliable, valid, and feasible for routine and serial assessments of adherence to regimens for diabetes and cystic fibrosis and could be easily be adapted for JRA regimens (Rapoff, 1999). Second, information obtained from routine and serial assessments of adherence should also allow for the detection of clinically significant nonadherence. Previous attempts at determining the levels of adherence necessary to prevent deleterious health outcomes have been arbitrary and not biologically based (e.g., adequate adherence defined as consuming 80% of prescribed medication doses). Third, because the desired outcome of adherence interventions is that patients get better, feel better, and do better, there is a need for both traditional (e.g., clinical signs and symptoms) and quality-of-life measures of disease and health status that are valid, reliable, and clinically feasible (Rapoff, 1999). Finally, because JRA affects relatively small numbers of children and adolescents, empirical validation of primary, secondary, and tertiary prevention interventions will require multicenter collaborative research studies.

References

Anthony, K. K., & Schanberg, L. E. (2003). Pain in children with arthritis: A review of the current literature. *Arthritis Care and Research, 49*, 272–279.

April, K. T., Feldman, D. E., Platt, R. W., & Duffy, C. M. (2006). Comparison between children with juvenile idiopathic arthritis and their parents concerning perceived treatment adherence. *Arthritis Care and Research, 55*, 558–563.

Barlow, J. H., Shaw, K. L., & Wright, C. C. (2000). Development and preliminary validation of a self-efficacy measure for use among parents of children with juvenile idiopathic arthritis. *Arthritis Care and Research, 13*, 227–236.

Barlow, J. H., Shaw, K. L., & Wright, C. C. (2001). Development and preliminary validation of a children's arthritis self-efficacy scale. *Arthritis Care and Research, 45*, 159–166.

Benestad, B., Vinje, O., Veierød, M. B., & Vandvik, I. H. (1996). Quantitative and qualitative assessments of pain in children with juvenile chronic arthritis based on the Norwegian version of the Pediatric Pain Questionnaire. *Scandinavian Journal of Rheumatology, 25*, 293–299.

Brace, M. J., Smith, M. S., McCauley, E., & Sherry, D. D. (2000). Family reinforcement of illness behavior: A comparison of adolescents with chronic fatigue syndrome, juvenile arthritis, and healthy controls. *Journal of Developmental and Behavioral Pediatrics, 21*, 332–339.

Brewer, E. J., Giannini, E. H., Kuzmina, N., & Alekseev, L. (1986). Penicillamine and hydroxychloroquine in the treatment of severe juvenile rheumatoid arthritis. *The New England Journal of Medicine, 314*, 1269–1276.

Cassidy, J., Levinson, J., Bass, J., Baum, J., Brewer, E. J., Jr., Fink, C. W., et al. (1986). A study of classification criteria for a diagnosis of juvenile rheumatoid arthritis. *Arthritis & Rheumatism, 29*, 274–281.

Cassidy, J. T., & Petty, R. E. (2005). *Textbook of pediatric rheumatology* (5th ed.). Philadelphia: Saunders.

Daniels, D., Miller, J. J., Billings, A. G., & Moos, R. H. (1986). Psychosocial functioning of siblings of children with rheumatic disease. *Journal of Pediatrics, 109*, 379–383.

Daniels, D., Moos, R. H., Billings, A. G., & Miller, J. J. (1987). Psychosocial risk and resistance factors among children with chronic illness, healthy siblings, and healthy controls. *Journal of Abnormal Child Psychology, 15*, 295–308.

Degatardi, P. J., Revenson, T. A., & Ilowite, N. T. (1999). Family-level coping in juvenile rheumatoidarthritis: Assessing the utility of a quantitative family interview. *Arthritis Care and Research, 12*, 314–324.

Dougadoes, M., van der Linden, S., Juhlin, R., et al. (1991). The European Spondyloarthropathy Study Group preliminary classification criteria for the classification of spondyloarthopathy. *Arthritis & Rheumatism, 34*, 1218–1227.

Dhanani, S., Quenneville, J., Perron, M., Abdolell, M., & Feldman, B. M. (2002). Minimal difference in pain associated with change in quality of life in children with rheumatic disease. *Arthritis Care and Research, 47*, 501–505.

Feldman, D. E., De Civita, M., Dobkin, P. L., Malleson, P., Meshefedjian, G., & Duffy, C. (2007). Perceived adherence to prescribed treatment in juvenile idiopathic arthritis over a one-year period. *Arthritis Care and Research, 57*, 226–233.

Fowler, M. G., Johnson, M. P., & Atkinson, S. S. (1985). School achievement and absence in children with chronic health conditions. *Journal of Pediatrics, 106*, 683–687.

Giannini, E. H., Brewer, E. J., Miller, M. L., Gibbas, D., Passo, M. H., Hoyeraal, H. M., et al. (1990). Ibuprofen suspension in the treatment of juvenile rheumatoid arthritis. *Journal of Pediatrics, 117*, 645–652.

Gragg, R. A., Rapoff, M. A., Danovsky, M. B., Lindsley, C. B., Varni, J. W., Waldron, S. A., et al. (1996). Assessing chronic musculoskeletal pain associated with rheumatic disease: Further validation of the pediatric pain questionnaire. *Journal of Pediatric Psychology, 21*, 237–250.

Hagglund, K. J., Schopp, L. M., Alberts, K. R., Cassidy, J. T., & Frank, R. G. (1995). Predicting pain among children with juvenile rheumatoid arthritis. *Arthritis Care and Research, 8*, 36–42.

Hayford, J. R., & Ross, C. K. (1988). Medical compliance in juvenile rheumatoid arthritis: Problems and perspectives. *Arthritis Care and Research, 1*, 190–197.

Helgeson, V. S., Janicki, D., Lerner, J., & Barbarin, O. (2003). Brief report: Adjustment to juvenile rheumatoid arthritis: A family systems perspective. *Journal of Pediatric Psychology, 28*, 347–353.

Henoch, M. J., Batson, J. W., & Baum, J. (1978). Psychosocial factors in juvenile rheumatoid arthritis. *Arthritis and Rheumatism, 21*, 229–233.

Hovey, J. K. (2005). Father's parenting chronically ill children: Concerns and coping strategies. *Issues in Comprehensive Pediatric Nursing, 28* 83–95.

Huygen, A. C. J., Kuis, W., & Sinnema, G. (2000). Psychological, behavioral, and social adjustment in children and adolescents with juvenile chronic arthritis. *Annals of Rheumatic Disease, 59* 276–282.

Ilowite, N. T., Walco, G. A., & Pochaczevsky, R. (1992). Assessment of pain in patients with juvenile rheumatoid arthritis: Relation between pain intensity and degree of joint inflammation. *Annals of the Rheumatic Diseases, 51,* 343–346.

Kellerman, J., Zeltzer, L., Ellenberg, L., Dash, J., & Rigler, D. (1980). Psychological effects of illness in adolescence: I. Anxiety, self-esteem, and perception of control. *Journal of Pediatrics, 97* 126–131.

Kvien, T. K., & Reimers, S. (1983). Drug handling and patient compliance in an outpatient paediatric trial. *Journal of Clinical and Hospital Pharmacy, 8,* 251–257.

Kyngäs, H. (2004). Support network of adolescents with chronic disease: Adolescents' perspective. *Nursing and Health Sciences, 6* 287–293.

Lavigne, J. V., Ross, C. K., Berry, S. L., Hayford, J. R., & Pachman, L. M (1992). Evaluation of a psychological treatment package for treating pain in juvenile rheumatoid arthritis. *Arthritis Care and Research, 5,* 101–110.

LeBovidge, J. S., Lavigne, J. V., Donenberg, G. R., & Miller, M. L. (2003). Psychological adjustment of children and adolescents with chronic arthritis: A meta-analytic review. *Journal of Pediatric Psychology, 28* 29–39.

Litt, I. F., & Cuskey, W. R. (1981). Compliance with salicylate therapy in adolescents with juvenile rheumatoid arthritis. *American Journal of Diseases of Children, 135,* 434–436.

Litt, I. F., Cuskey, W. R., & Rosenberg, A. (1982). Role of self-esteem and autonomy in determining medication compliance among adolescents with juvenile rheumatoid arthritis. *Pediatrics, 69,* 15–17.

Lovell, D., Giannini, E., & Brewer, E. (1984). Time course of response to nonsteroidal anti-inflammatory drugs in patients with juvenile rheumatoid arthritis. *Arthritis & Rheumatism, 27,* 11433–1437.

Manuel, J. C. (2001). Risk and resistance factors in the adaptation in mothers of children with juvenile rheumatoid arthritis. *Journal of Pediatric Psychology, 26,* 237–246.

McAnarney, E. R., Pless, I. B., Satterwhite, B., & Friedman, S. B. (1974). Psychological problems of children with chronic juvenile arthritis. *Pediatrics, 53,* 523–528.

McNeill, T. (2004). Father's experience of parenting a child with juvenile rheumatoid arthritis. *Qualitative Health Research, 14,* 526–545.

Miller, J. J., Spitz, P. W., Simpson, U., & Williams, G. F. (1982). The social functioning of young adults who had arthritis in childhood. *Journal of Pediatrics, 100,* 378–382.

Mullick, M. S. I., Nahar, J. S., & Haq, S. A. (2005). Psychiatric morbidity, stressors, impact, and burden in juvenile idiopathic arthritis. *Journal of Health, Population and Nutrition, 23,* 142–149.

Noll, R. B., Kozlowski, K., Gerhardt, C., Vannatta, K., Taylor, J., & Passo, M. (2000). Social, emotional, and behavioral functioning of children with juvenile rheumatoid arthritis. *Arthritis and Rheumatism, 43,* 1387–1396.

Packham, J. C., Hall., M. A., & Pimm, T. J. (2002). Long-term follow-up of 246 adults with juvenile idiopathic arthritis: Predictive factors for mood and pain. *Rheumatology, 41,* 1444–1449.

Palermo, T. M., Valenzuela, D., & Stork, P. P. (2004). A randomized trial of electronic vs. paper pain diaries in children: impact on compliance, accuracy, and acceptability. *Pain, 107,* 213–219.

Peterson, L. S., Mason, T., Nelson, A. M., O'Fallon, W. M., & Gabriel, S. E. (1997). Psychosocial outcomes and health status of adults who have had juvenile rheumatoid arthritis. *Arthritis and Rheumatism, 40,* 2235–2240.

Rapoff, M. A. (1998). *Helping children follow their medical treatment program: Guidelines for parents of children with rheumatic diseases.* (Available from the author, University of Kansas Medical Center, Department of Pediatrics, 3901 Rainbow Boulevard, Kansas City, KS 66160–7330).

Rapoff, M. A. (1999). *Adherence to pediatric medical regimens.* New York: Kluwer/Plenum.

Rapoff, M. A. (2000). Facilitating adherence to medical regimens for pediatric rheumatic diseases: Primary, secondary, and tertiary prevention. In D. Drotar (Ed.). *Promoting adherence to medical treatment in chronic childhood illness: Concepts, methods, and interventions* (pp. 329–345). Mahwah, NJ: Erlbaum.

Rapoff, M. A., Belmont, J., Lindsley, C., Olson, N., Morris, J., & Padur, J. (2002). Prevention of nonadherence to nonsteroidal anti-inflammatory medications for newly diagnosed patients with juvenile rheumatoid arthritis. *Health Psychology, 21,* 620–623.

Rapoff, M. A., Belmont, J. M., Lindsley, C. B., & Olson, N. Y. (2005). Electronically monitored adherence to medications by newly diagnosed patients with juvenile rheumatoid arthritis. *Arthritis Care and Research, 53,* 905–910.

Rapoff, M. A., & Lindsley, C. B. (2000). The pain puzzle: A visual and conceptual metaphor for understanding and treating pain in pediatric rheumatic disease. *Journal of Rheumatology, 58*(Suppl.), 29–33.

Rapoff, M. A., Lindsley, C. B., & Christophersen, E. R. (1985). Parent perceptions of problems experienced by their children in complying with treatments for juvenile rheumatoid arthritis. *Archives of Physical Medicine and Rehabilitation, 66,* 427–430.

Rapoff, M. A., Purviance, M. R., & Lindsley, C. B. (1988a). Improving medication compliance for juvenile rheumatoid arthritis and its effect on clinical outcome: A single-subject analysis. *Arthritis Care and Research, 1,* 12–16.

Rapoff, M. A., Purviance, M. R., & Lindsley, C. B. (1988b). Educational and behavioral strategies for improving medication compliance in juvenile rheumatoid arthritis. *Archives of Physical Medicine and Rehabilitation, 69,* 439–441.

Reid, G. J., McGrath, P. J., & Lang, B. A. (2005). Parent-child interactions among children with juvenile fibromyalgia, arthritis, and healthy controls. *Pain, 113,* 201–210.

Ross, C. K., Lavigne, J. V., Hayford, J. R., Dyer, A. R., & Pachman, L. M. (1989). Validity of reported pain as a measure of clinical state in juvenile rheumatoid arthritis. *Annals of the Rheumatic Diseases, 48,* 817–819.

Sällfors, C., Fasth, A., & Hallberg, L. R.-M. (2002). Oscillating between hope and despair—a qualitative study. *Child: Care, Health & Development, 28*, 495–505.

Sandstrom, M. J., & Schanberg, L. E. (2004). Brief report: Peer rejection, social behavior, and psychological adjustment in children with juvenile rheumatic disease. *Journal of Pediatric Psychology, 29*, 29–34.

Sawyer, M. G., Carbone, J. A., Whitham, J. N., Roberton, D. M., Taplin, J. E., Varni, J. W., et al. (2005). The relationship between health-related quality of life, pain, and coping strategies in juvenile arthritis – A one year prospective study. *Quality of Life Research, 14*, 1585–1598

Sawyer, M. G., Whitham, J. N., Roberton, D. M., Taplin, J. E., Varni, J. W., & Baghurst, P. A. (2004). The relationship between health-related quality of life, pain and coping strategies in juvenile idiopathic arthritis. *Rheumatology, 43*, 325–330.

Schanberg, L. E., Anthony, K. K., Gil, K. M., Lefebvre, J. C., Kredich, D. W., & Macharoni, L. M. (2001). Family pain history predicts child health status in children with chronic rheumatic disease. *Pediatrics, 108*, e47–e53.

Schanberg, L. E., Anthony, K. K., Gil, K. M., & Maurin, E. C. (2003). Daily pain and symptoms in children with polyarticular arthritis. *Arthritis & Rheumatism, 48*,, 1390–1397.

Schanberg, L. E., Lefebvre, J. C., Keefe, F. J., Kredich, D. W., & Gil, K. M. (1997). Pain coping and the pain experience in children with juvenile chronic arthritis. *Pain, 73*, 181–189.

Schanberg, L. E., Sandstrom, M. J., Starr, K., Gil, K. M., Lefebvre, J. C., Keefe, F. J., et al. (2000). The relationship of daily mood and stressful events to symptoms in juvenile rheumatic disease. *Arthritis Care and Research, 13*, 33–41.

Sherry, D. D., Bohnsack, J., Salmonson, K., Wallace, C. A., & Mellins, E. (1990). Painless juvenile rheumatoid arthritis. *Journal of Pediatrics, 116*, 921–923.

Stark, L. J., Janicke, D. M., McGrath, A. M., Mackner, L. M., Hommel, K. A., & Lovell, D. (2005). Prevention of osteoporosis: A randomized clinical trial to increase calcium intake in children with juvenile rheumatoid arthritis. *Journal of Pediatric Psychology, 30*, 377–386.

Stinson, J. N., Petroz, G. C., Tait, G., Feldman, B. M., Streiner, D., McGrath, P. J., et al. (2006). e-Ouch: Usability testing of an electronic chronic pain diary for adolescents with arthritis. *Clinical Journal of Pain, 22*, 295–305.

Sturge, C., Garralda, M. E., Boissin, M., Dore, C. J., & Woo, P. (1997). School attendance and juvenile chronic arthritis. *British Journal of Rheumatology, 36*, 1218–1223.

Thompson, K. L., Varni, J. W., & Hanson, V. (1987). Comprehensive assessment of pain in juvenile rheumatoid arthritis: An empirical model. *Journal of Pediatric Psychology, 12*, 241–255.

Varni, J. W., Rapoff, M. A., Waldron, S. A., Gragg, R. A., Bernstein, B. H., & Lindsley, C. B. (1996). Chronic pain and emotional distress in children and adolescents. *Journal of Developmental and Behavioral Pediatrics, 17*, 154–161.

von Weiss, R. T., Rapoff, M. A., Varni, J. W., Lindsley, C. B., Olson, N. Y., Madson, K. L., et al. (2002). Daily hassles and social support as predictors of adjustment in children with pediatric rheumatic disease. *Journal of Pediatric Psychology, 27*, 155–165.

Wagner, J. L., Chaney, J. M., Hommel, K. A., Page, M. C., Mullins, L. L., White, M. M., et al. (2003). The influence of parental distress on child depressive symptoms in juvenile rheumatoid diseases: The moderating effect of illness intrusiveness. *Journal of Pediatric Psychology, 28*, 453–462.

Walco, G. A., Varni, J. W., & Ilowite, N. T. (1992). Cognitive behavioral pain management in children with juvenile rheumatoid arthritis. *Pediatrics, 89*, 1075–1079.

Wallace, C., & Levinson, J. (1991). Juvenile rheumatoid arthritis: Outcome and treatment for the 1990s. *Rheumatic Disease Clinics of North America, 17*, 891–905.

Epilepsy

Deirdre A. Caplin, Joan K. Austin, and David Dunn

Introduction

Adolescence is recognized as a developmental transition toward successful creation of an adult identity and a sense of ownership and comfort with personal beliefs and values. Adolescent emotional and cognitive resources are stretched by attempts at developing a sense of self, gaining autonomy from parents, and refining self-control. Teens with epilepsy and other chronic conditions have the additional burden of finding a way to integrate their health condition and its management into their daily lives.

Adolescents need experience, support, and a healthy mind and body to manage the challenges of rapid development. Teens with epilepsy are further challenged to find adaptive ways to cope with epilepsy, to try out independent health decisions and behaviors, and learn about how the changes in their body will affect their seizure disorder (Appleton & Neville, 1999).

Despite the unique challenges presenting in adolescence, teens with epilepsy are rarely treated as a special population (Appleton, Chadwick, & Sweeney, 1997). Although there is at least one care clinic specializing in teens with epilepsy in the United States, the vast majority of adolescents with seizure disorders do not have access to adolescent-specific care (1997). More likely, adolescents with childhood-onset seizures are treated in a pediatric clinic, whereas adolescents with new-onset seizures may be as likely to see an adult neurologist as a pediatric subspecialist (Appleton et al., 1997; Appleton & Neville, 1999). Hence, it is important for any health-care professional working with adolescents to be sensitive to their needs and challenges, especially to how those challenges affect disease management and outcomes.

Epilepsy

Although epilepsy can occur at any age, it is the most common neurologic disorder among adolescents, affecting approximately 1.5–2.0% of teens (Wheless & Kim, 2002). During adolescence the incidence of epilepsy is approximately 20–55/100,000 person-years (C. S. Camfield, Camfield, Gordon, Wirrell, & Dooley, 1996), (Kotsopoulos, van Merode, Kessels, de Krom, & Knottnerus, 2002). Higher incidence figures are found in studies that include single unprovoked seizures. Prevalence rates of epilepsy in adolescence are higher. One study from England found a prevalence of 3.9/1000 at 7 years of age, 4.9/1000 at 16 years of age, and 6.3/1000 at 23 years of age (Kurtz, Tookey, & Ross, 1998). Both the incidence and prevalence rates seem to be higher in undeveloped countries (Mbuba, Ngugi, Newton, & Carter, 2008).

A seizure is a single discrete event, whereas epilepsy is a disease category defined by two or more unprovoked seizures or, in some definitions, a single seizure with characteristic changes on the electroencephalogram (EEG) (Engel, 2006). The International League Against Epilepsy (ILAE) has defined criteria for classification of both seizures and epileptic syndromes (Engel, 2006). Seizures are defined

D.A. Caplin (✉)
Department of Pediatrics, University of Utah Health Sciences Center, Salt Lake City, UT, USA
e-mail: deirdre.caplin@hsc.utah.edu

W.T. O'Donohue, L.W. Tolle (eds.), *Behavioral Approaches to Chronic Disease in Adolescence*,
DOI 10.1007/978-0-387-87687-0_12, © Springer Science+Business Media, LLC 2009

by type, which is based on both a description of the episode and electroencephalography. Some seizure disorders can be further classified into epileptic syndromes, which are classified as localization-related, generalized, undetermined, or special syndromes. Defining epileptic syndromes requires knowledge of seizure type, presumed etiology, age of onset, EEG, and neuroimaging findings.

Seizure types. Seizures may be partial (focal or local) or generalized. Partial seizures begin in a discrete area of the brain. They are called simple partial if there is no alteration of consciousness and complex partial if there is a change in contact with the environment. With simple partial seizures, there may be motor, sensory, autonomic, or psychic symptoms (Browne & Holmes, 2001). Complex partial seizures may begin with a simple partial seizure that is followed by loss of consciousness, start with loss of consciousness, or begin with a simple partial seizure that evolves into a generalized tonic–clonic seizure (Browne & Holmes, 2001).

By contrast, generalized seizures involve both cerebral hemispheres, are characterized by loss of consciousness and, in some cases, bilateral movements (Browne & Holmes, 2001). Generalized seizures are further classified as absence, myoclonic, atonic, clonic, tonic, or tonic–clonic seizures. Absence seizures are brief staring spells, whereas myoclonic seizures consist of sudden jerks from muscle contractions and atonic seizures are drop attacks from sudden loss of muscle tone. During the tonic phase of a seizure, there is stiffness and rigidity and during the clonic phase, rhythmic contractions.

Presumed Etiology, EEG, and Neuroimaging. Syndromic epilepsies are identified in part by neuroimaging and EEG findings (Engel, 2006). From EEG findings, localization-related epilepsies begin with spikes in a single focal area of the brain, whereas in generalized epilepsies spikes appear simultaneously in both hemispheres (Browne & Holmes, 2001). The localization-related and generalized epilepsies are further divided by presumed etiology into idiopathic, symptomatic, and cryptogenic epilepsies (Engel, 2006).

Idiopathic epilepsies may have a familial, genetic, or unknown etiology (Engel, 2006). Symptomatic epilepsies are those with a defined structural etiology, and cryptogenic epilepsies are those with presumed CNS damage that is not visible on neuroimaging (Browne & Holmes, 2001). Epileptic syndromes are called undetermined when there are both focal and generalized spikes as in neonatal seizures or acquired epileptic aphasia or when it is impossible to determine the origin as in some nocturnal seizures. Many of the provoked seizures such as febrile seizures or seizures caused by toxins or infections are listed under special syndromes (Browne & Holmes, 2001).

Certain epileptic syndromes, such as childhood absence and benign rolandic epilepsy with centrotemporal spikes, tend to remit during adolescence (Browne & Holmes, 2001). By adolescence, the most common epileptic syndromes are the symptomatic and cryptogenic localization-related epilepsies, and the idiopathic generalized epilepsies (Browne & Holmes, 2001).

Localization-related seizures most commonly start in the temporal or frontal lobes. Adolescents with temporal lobe seizures usually have brief episodes lasting 1–2 minutes, with staring and motor automatisms such as lip smacking or fumbling hand movements. The seizure may be preceded by an aura, or warning, that lasts seconds. After a seizure (post-ictal) there may be a period of lethargy or confusion lasting minutes. In contrast, generalized tonic–clonic seizures start suddenly with a fall and loss of consciousness accompanied by stiffening of all extremities. This is followed by repetitive jerking of the both arms, then a post-ictal sleep and confusion. The entire episode usually lasts 1–5 min.

Juvenile absence epilepsy, juvenile myoclonic epilepsy (JME), and photosensitive epilepsy typically begin during adolescence. The juvenile absence seizures consist of a sudden onset of staring with loss of contact with the environment. There may be eye blinking or hand and arm movements, but no falls, associated with the seizures. These episodes are brief, lasting seconds, and are accompanied by 3-cycle-per-second spike and wave activity on EEG. Many of the patients with juvenile absence epilepsy will go into remission by adulthood. With JME, there are brief, repetitive jerks of the hands and arms upon awakening. In addition, most of the adolescents will have occasional generalized tonic–clonic seizures upon awakening. The EEG usually shows polyspike and wave activity seen best during the transition from sleep to wakefulness. The seizures are easily controlled but the JME persists and medication must be taken throughout life (Browne & Holmes, 2001).

Pubertal changes in seizure frequency are well documented, although the exact relationship between puberty and epilepsy is uncertain. It appears that generalized tonic–clonic seizures often increase compared to prepubertal levels, and increased seizure frequency is more common in adolescent girls than boys (Sheth, 2002).

The Cost of Epilepsy

The total annual cost of epilepsy in the United States was estimated at $12.5 billion in 1995 for all cases. These costs can be subdivided into indirect costs and direct costs associated with care, including the costs of physicians, procedures, hospital stays, and medications and indirect or costs not associated with direct care. In the United States, direct costs of epilepsy consist primarily of outpatient physician visits and medication (Begley et al., 2000). Unlike some other chronic illnesses, however, the majority of costs for epilepsy are indirect (Begley et al., 2000). The direct costs of epilepsy care tend to be small and concentrated on older adults rather than on adolescents. In contrast, indirect costs account for 86% of the burden of epilepsy in the United States.

Indirect costs are those associated with morbidity issues such as loss of productivity, loss of income, or reduced activity because of epilepsy. For adolescents, who are not yet independent physically and financially, morbidity is often measured in lost school days, lost productivity in expected activities, and to lost parent work days or lost parent productivity. This means that for adolescents with epilepsy and their families, the primary cost burden of epilepsy is likely to come from parents not meeting work hours or earning potential *and* teens not meeting expectations for their own daily responsibilities.

Prognosis

The prognosis for seizure control varies by epileptic syndrome. In general, approximately 80% of patients respond to antiepileptic drug treatment. Taking into account differences in medication choice, one very long follow-up study of seizure outcomes reported that approximately half of the patients developed a persistent remission, one-third had a relapsing-remitting course, and one-fifth never went into remission (Sillanpaa & Schmidt, 2006). The prognosis for behavior and cognition varies by etiology of seizures, presence of additional neurological deficits, and persistence of seizures. The patients with symptomatic/cryptogenic generalized epilepsy syndromes are most likely to have persistent seizures, cognitive impairment, and behavioral difficulties. The children and adolescents with benign childhood epilepsy with centrotemporal spikes (benign rolandic or benign focal epilepsy) and those with idiopathic generalized seizures have the best prognosis for seizure control without behavioral or cognitive comorbidity.

Morbidity and Mortality

Adolescents experiencing seizures are at risk for injury and, rarely, death. The most common injuries occur when there are falls during a seizure. Most injuries are mild. In one large study, the rate of accidents during a 24-month period was 27% in people with epilepsy and 17% in controls (Beghi & Cornaggia, 2002). Death is fortunately rare. In one series, the incidence of sudden unexpected death was higher in children and adolescents with epilepsy and an additional significant neurological disability. A 10-year study in Ontario found that the estimated rate of sudden unexplained death in patients with epilepsy less than 18 years of age was 2/10,000 (Donner, Smith, & Snead, 2001). Preventable causes of death in patients with epilepsy are drowning and automobile accidents.

Treating Epilepsy in Adolescents

Prior to starting treatment, most persons with seizures need an EEG and neuroimaging. The EEG is essential for classification of the epileptic syndrome and is part of the information used in choosing treatment. Neuroimaging is used to evaluate possible etiologies. Although brain tumors, arteriovenous malformations, and other progressive structural lesions are not common causes of seizures in adolescents, magnetic resonance imaging is an effective screen for these rare possibilities.

Medication. AEDs are used to prevent the recurrence of seizures. Medication may not be essential after a first isolated seizure. Adolescents with idiopathic seizures, normal development, a normal neurological examination, and normal EEG and neuroimaging may never have another seizure and are often observed without starting an AED. Medication is recommended if the seizures recur or if there are risk factors such as symptomatic seizures or an abnormal EEG.

The oldest antiepileptic medications (AEDs) currently in use are phenobarbital, ethosuximide, and phenytoin; carbamazepine and valproic acid are intermediate; and gabapentin, lamotrigine, levetiracetam, oxcarbazepine, topiramate, and zonisamide are the newest agents. AED selection should be based on epileptic syndrome or seizure type and potential medication side effects.

For adolescent patients, it is important to consider comorbid conditions, such as learning disabilities, anxiety, and depression, potential adverse effects such as lethargy, cognitive slowing, and weight gain, body image concerns, and lifestyle in decision-making about selecting and starting the appropriate AED.

Monotherapy is preferred. Evidence-based practice parameters have been developed to facilitate optimal AED use, based on data available for different seizure types and syndromes (Wilfong, 2007). For example, the treatment of localization-related epilepsies often begins with carbamazepine or oxcarbazepine. Gabapentin, lamotrigine, levetiracetam, topiramate, or valproate may also be used. Valproate is a usual first option for generalized tonic–clonic seizures. Carbamazepine, lamotrigine, and topiramate have also been used. Absence seizures are treated with ethosuximide, valproate, or lamotrigine. JME responds to valproate or lamotrigine. Phenobarbital may be effective but is often avoided because of the cognitive side effects such as inattention and hyperactivity. Phenytoin is effective but is used less often because of toxicity including rash, unsteadiness, and cosmetic side effects. Most AEDs are to be taken two or three times a day. Adherence is essential to prevent breakthrough seizures (Wilfong, 2007).

The effectiveness of AEDs is monitored by assessing seizure frequency (Wilfong, 2007). The goal is elimination of all seizures. Side effects of AEDs are monitored by the clinical history and by laboratory studies. Blood levels can be assessed for most of the AEDs currently used in clinical practice. Blood levels are used to make sure the dose of medication is adequate and not excessive and as a check on medication adherence. In addition to blood levels, routine blood counts, electrolytes, renal function, and liver function tests are often followed. The exact tests ordered depend on the side effect profile of the particular AED taken by the patient (Wilfong, 2007).

Side effects. Side effects are either dose related or idiosyncratic. Examples of dose-related side effects are sedation and ataxia. Examples of idiosyncratic side effects are allergic skin reactions, hepatotoxicity, or drop in red or white blood cell counts. The chance of side effects can be reduced by beginning with low doses of an AED and slowly increasing the dose, by using monotherapy instead of polypharmacy, and by careful monitoring of response to medication.

Approximately one-third of adolescents experience side effects from their AED, most commonly weight change and headaches (Baker et al., 2008). In adolescence, side effects can have a detrimental effect on adherence. Lethargy and cognitive dulling are associated with the more sedating AEDs and are poorly tolerated by patients. Weight gain is a common side effect of valproate and may occur with carbamazepine and gabapentin. Polycystic ovary syndrome has been seen in girls taking valproate. Acne, gingival hyperplasia, and hirsutism have been associated with phenytoin. Side effects may require modification in AED dosage or a change in AED (Baker et al., 2008).

Surgery. If the adolescent does not respond to AEDs, seizure surgery may be an option. Seizure surgery is most successful in patients with a well-defined temporal lobe focus. Seizure surgery for foci outside the temporal lobe may be an option but the rate of success in eliminating seizures is lower. Improvement in quality of life may follow surgery that results in seizure freedom and discontinuation of AEDs. However, post-surgical cognitive decline is a concern, particularly when seizures persist after surgery. Vagal nerve stimulators also have been successful in reducing seizure frequency.

Health Issues and Living with Epilepsy

Adherence to Treatment Regimens

Successful treatment of epilepsy in adolescents involves more than selecting the right AED. Appropriate adherence to medication regimen and compliance with recommendations for lifestyle are essential for optimal epilepsy treatment. Treating the whole patient improves both seizure control and quality of life but requires a long-term commitment to health promotion.

Poor adherence to medication is a major problem in adolescents with chronic illness and may be even more of a problem in adolescents with epilepsy, up to 30% in some studies (Sheth, 2002). It appears that a poor understanding of AEDs, their effects, and the adverse effects associated with not taking them is a significant factor in predicting adherence problems, especially in younger patients (Sheth, 2002).

A first step to improved adherence is education. The adolescent should learn as much as possible about the seizure condition and the proposed treatment. Assisting teens to interpret the vast amounts of information about medications, side effects, and minimizing their negative impact will do a lot to improve adherence.

Second, the choice of AED may determine adherence. Patients are more likely to adhere to medication regimes if only one medication (monotherapy) is used and if the drug can be taken once daily or at most, twice a day. Attention to specific side effects is also important when managing an adolescent patient. For example, AEDs that cause lethargy or cognitive impairment such as phenobarbital, drugs that cause weight gain such as valproate, and drugs that cause cosmetic side effects such as phenytoin are best avoided.

Healthy Behaviors and Choices

Successful epilepsy management requires adolescents have usable information, skills for how to take care of themselves, and access to the resources necessary for success (DiIorio et al., 2004). Information about medications, side effects, and the need for adherence can be integrated with recommendations for important information about making healthy choices. For example, adolescents with epilepsy should be encouraged to have regular sleep habits and to obtain adequate sleep. Information can be provided to teens about the degree to which their seizures and AEDs can disrupt sleep, because sleep deprivation can cause seizures.

Experimentation with drugs and alcohol should be expected and the adolescent with epilepsy must be given appropriate advice. Both cocaine and excess alcohol may lower the seizure threshold. Amphetamines, cocaine, hallucinogens, inhalants, and phencyclidine may cause seizures with overdose, and seizures may occur with withdrawal from alcohol and sedatives. Although neither one to two alcoholic drinks nor marijuana is likely to cause seizures, the adolescent should be warned that combining an AED with drugs or alcohol may cause a decrease in alertness.

Many teens are sensitive to their bodies and to weight gain. Weight gain is associated with certain AEDs and has been found to contribute to medication noncompliance. Exploring dietary alternatives and supplements such as a low-carbohydrate, high-protein diet or a ketogenic diet may be useful to certain adolescent patients (Sheth, 2002).

The adolescent with seizures may participate in sports but should avoid sports that might result in head injuries, skydiving, and rock climbing. Swimming must be supervised. Finally, driving is a problem for adolescents with epilepsy.

If the adolescent has uncontrolled seizures, driving is prohibited. Some studies have suggested that driving is the most difficult limitation for adolescents with epilepsy (Sheth, 2002). Once seizures are controlled, the adolescent can obtain a driver's license. The law specifying the length of time the seizures must be controlled varies by the state. Even with these restrictions, there are data to suggest that many teens are driving without a license, despite poor seizure control. All adolescents, not just those with controlled seizures and a driver's license, should be warned about factors that might increase the chance of a seizure such as sleep deprivation, febrile illness, or drugs and alcohol.

Contraception and Female Health Issues

Adolescent girls need to be aware of the reproductive health issues associated with epilepsy treatment.

Practitioners should be prepared to provide additional counseling about potential drug interactions between AEDs and oral contraceptives and about issues related to pregnancy.

Certain AEDs, such as barbiturates, phenytoin, carbamazepine and oxcarbazepine, and topiramate, may induce enzymes that increase metabolism of oral contraceptives, thus causing their failure. Oral contraceptives may cause a drop in blood levels of lamotrigine and possibly valproate. Adolescent girls should be aware of the potential teratogenic effects of AEDs. There is an increase risk of fetal malformations in women with epilepsy. The risk seems to be higher in women on polypharmacy and in those receiving valproate. Supplementation with folate should be considered for all women with epilepsy who are of childbearing age. Ideally, the woman with epilepsy should plan carefully for pregnancy. She should discuss AEDs with her physician prior to pregnancy and AED blood levels should be monitored closely during pregnancy (Kaplan, 2004).

Behavioral Issues and Living with Epilepsy

Psychosocial Issues

As young people mature they develop the knowledge, skills, and behaviors that will help them succeed as adults. Accomplishing these developmental tasks is especially challenging for adolescents with epilepsy because of the many cognitive, mental health, and social problems that are commonly associated with epilepsy.

A large number of adolescents with epilepsy have deficits in cognitive functioning such as low intelligence, slow psychomotor speed, and memory problems (Bailet & Turk, 2000). These cognitive deficits are major contributing factors to the high rates of academic underachievement that are commonly found in adolescents with epilepsy (Fastenau et al., 2004). Studies show that on average adolescents with epilepsy are about 1 year behind academically, have high rates of school failure, and have high rates of referrals for special education services. In a recent study, approximately half of children and adolescents with epilepsy had cognitive deficits that were consistent with having a learning disability (Fastenau, Jianzhao, Dunn, & Austin, 2008).

Mental health problems are also overrepresented in children and adolescents with epilepsy. Although adolescents with any chronic illness generally have high rates of mental health problems, the rate of problems in epilepsy is over twice as high as in other chronic medical health problems (Davies, Heyman, & Goodman, 2003). Common problems experienced by adolescents with epilepsy are internalizing symptoms including anxiety, depression, and social withdrawal. Depressive disorders are found in about one-fourth of adolescents with epilepsy (Ettinger et al., 1998). In a study comparing adolescents with epilepsy and healthy controls in the United Kingdom, those with epilepsy were found to have higher levels of depression, anhedonia, and social anxiety (Baker et al., 2008).

Specific behavior problems that occur more often in children and adolescents with epilepsy than in children with other chronic health conditions are attention, social, and thought problems (Rodenburg, Stams, Meijer, Aldenkamp, & Dekovic, 2005). Attention problems and social problems are more common than thought problems. ADHD occurs in about 30–40% of children and adolescents with epilepsy (Dunn, Harezlak, Ambrosius, Austin, & Hale, 2002). Both inattention and hyperactivity symptoms are common and both are probable contributors to academic underachievement. In general, children and adolescents with epilepsy are less popular and have more social problems than their peers (Hodes, Garralda, Rose, & Schwartz, 1999; Rodenburg et al., 2005). A recent study suggested that cognitive problems might contribute to social problems in adolescents with epilepsy. Psychosis is relatively uncommon in children with epilepsy. However, illogical thought processing and hallucinations have been found in approximately 10% of children with complex partial epilepsy (Caplan et al., 1998, 2005).

Adaptation Issues

Identity development is a core feature of adolescent growth. Identity formation relies on social and emotional maturation that allows an understanding of who you are relative to your peers and influential adults, and developing a sense of autonomy regarding school and future goals. The vast majority of teens are able to successfully integrate all aspects of self, including epilepsy.

The search for autonomy is often impeded by real or perceived need for supervision and restriction of activities. Overprotective parents are often to blame for stymieing their adolescent's desire for autonomy. However, many teens with epilepsy report imposing their own restrictions, including making sure they are not alone, or avoiding activities that are most likely to trigger a seizure. Concerns about living alone in the future or moving away from home are also commonly reported. In addition, the teens interviewed reported that teachers and school administrators were more likely to overreact than those who knew more about their condition (McEwan, Espie, Metcalfe, Brodie, & Wilson, 2004).

Coping with a chronic, unpredictable problem such as epilepsy can be a challenge to even a well-adjusted teen. However, the continuum of adjustment to having a seizure disorder in adolescence is likely broad. Some teens may have very few problems and manage well independently, whereas others will struggle with epilepsy in the context of much larger difficulties. Real or perceived limitations related to lifestyle, school, or activities have a significant impact on teens with epilepsy and are associated with denial, problems with compliance, and adaptation (Sheth, 2002). In addition, subthreshold psychological symptoms are often present, creating greater challenges in care and interfering with developmentally appropriate independence in epilepsy management (Wagner & Smith, 2006).

Many teens have reported difficulties with peer relationships regarding their epilepsy. Adolescents with epilepsy often report feeling different from peers, in ways that are both positive ("I am unique and this is part of me") and negative ("I have epilepsy and cannot do as much as my friends") (McEwan et al., 2004). Supportiveness of peers, seizure frequency, and concerns about personal safety are known to influence peer comparisons (McEwan et al., 2004). Worry over imagined rejection and concern about peer reactions to the diagnosis do interfere with peer relationships for some teens with epilepsy (McEwan et al., 2004). It is not uncommon for adolescents to speak to friends about epilepsy only if absolutely necessary or even refuse to talk of it at all. Others reported limiting social activities and dating because of fears about having a seizure.

Family Issues

Parenting a child with epilepsy presents unique challenges. Seizures in a child are stressful for the whole family and how they cope with the epilepsy is influenced by the severity of the epilepsy, the presence of cognitive and mental health problems, and the resources of the family. In addition to learning how to manage the seizures, parents need to provide emotional support to the child and create a family environment that helps the adolescent with epilepsy successfully accomplish developmental tasks. They need to keep the child safe without unduly restricting their activities. As adolescents are able to assume self-management of their seizure condition, the parents need to relinquish the responsibility for managing the epilepsy. The importance of a good family environment relative to the self-concept of teens with epilepsy was found in a recent study (Lee, Hamiwka, Sherman, & Wirrell, 2008). Family functioning had a stronger association with adolescent self-concept than epilepsy-related variables.

Treatment-Related Issues in Epilepsy

Patient–Practitioner Issues

Is it all right for teens to make decisions about medications? Are their opinions important? Adolescents are often trying to convey information to the people they think are going to help solve a problem. It is the job of the doctors, health specialists, and parents to acknowledge adolescents' efforts to participate, to explore their concerns, and to assist them in coming up with some reasonable alternatives to solve the problem.

Communication. Medical decision-making is most effective when decisions are a collaborative experience between patient and practitioner. Adolescents and their parents must be collaborative partners to most efficiently deal with epilepsy.

However, providing quality health care to adolescents requires an implicit understanding of adolescent development and the complex dynamics among teens, their parents, and their health-care team. Relying on parents to make decisions for their adolescent may be detrimental to patient–provider alliances, but also damaging to the relationship between parents and their teens.

Every attempt should be made to establish a collaborative relationship with adolescent patients. Small steps, such as asking their opinion, making eye contact with them, and interviewing adolescent patients independently are all steps that ensure the teen patient's position as an important member of the health-care team (Salpekar & Dunn, 2007).

In practice, many health-care professionals do a poor job of explaining epilepsy and its management to their younger patients (Choi-Kwon, Yoon, Choi, Kang, & Lee, 2001). When physicians speak to adolescents, data suggest that the information is not perceived as useful, often neglecting important issues in the daily lives of teenagers (Wilde & Haslam, 1996). As a result, adolescents without adequate information to make an informed decision may appear petulant and impulsive in their reasoning about medical matters.

Information. Knowledge is necessary to make decisions that are implementable and effective. Guiding adolescents through decision-making means providing them with the information they need, at a developmentally appropriate level that facilitates logical thinking. Numerous studies have reported that people with epilepsy want more information about their illness, their medications, and how to better manage their disease (Ridsdale, Morgan, & O'Connor, 1999). There is evidence to suggest that having sufficient knowledge about epilepsy is associated with fewer depression symptoms, higher self-esteem, and lower social anxiety (Baker et al., 2008).

Conveying information about a condition can be challenging. When a large amount of information is exchanged during a clinic visit, people often forget what they are told. Ideally, information is presented in both written and spoken formats, repeatedly over time, and with a chance for feedback to ensure understanding.

Understanding. The adolescent epilepsy patient has a perspective on illness and treatment that is unique. Adolescent desire for control and autonomy often runs counter to recommendations for treatment, especially for patients who do not have good seizure control, who experience side effects, or who are burdened by feelings of powerlessness (McEwan et al., 2004; Salpekar & Dunn, 2007).

Parents and practitioners often desire that adolescents adopt a more responsible attitude toward their health condition. Most adolescents are searching for opportunities to assert their independence. However, giving a young patient responsibility for care also means giving them the right to help make treatment decisions.

Pertinent clinical information during appointments is often directed at parents rather than at young patients (Ridsdale et al., 1999; Wilde & Haslam, 1996). Within this context, it is important that all adults working with adolescents do what they can to advocate for open discussions between all health-care professionals and their adolescent patients. Providing adolescents with opportunities to partner with their health-care team will go a long way toward improving epilepsy management long term, increasing compliance with regimens, and easing the transition from pediatric to adult care.

Psychosocial Difficulties

Despite the obvious need for evidence-based protocols for assessment and management of psychosocial problems for adolescents with epilepsy, standardized protocols for assessing the psychosocial needs of these patients are not available. There are many screening tools readily available that are adaptable to most busy practice settings. Salpekar and Dunn reviewed the ones most commonly used, including the Child Behavior Checklist, the Child Depression Inventory, The Multidimensional Anxiety Scale, and the Quality of Life in Epilepsy Inventory for Adolescents. All are available for use and have adequate psychometric value for clinical and research purposes (Salpekar & Dunn, 2007). It is recommended that until epilepsy-specific assessment tools are available, well-validated instruments such as those identified above should be used (Wagner & Smith, 2006).

Screening tools should be supplemented by a protocol-driven clinical examination and interview. Many decisions will be made based on resources available, allocation of time, and clinic structure. However, a thorough assessment will guide treatment decisions, provide a focus for clinical interventions, and provide a baseline measurement for quantifying the effects of treatment (Wagner & Smith, 2006).

Addressing Psychosocial Issues

Individual patients with epilepsy may perceive their disorder and what they need from treatment differently depending on their age, their seizure type and frequency, and other factors such as familial, educational, or cultural background. Studies have shown that physicians tend to underestimate the importance of patient stress, family adaptation, and fears on health-promoting behaviors such as following medication and management recommendations (Wagner & Smith, 2006). The concepts of self-efficacy (perceived confidence in management) and psychosocial distress are related to one another and are strongly correlated to quality of life for patients with epilepsy (Pramuka, Hendrickson, Zinski, & Van Cott, 2007). To effectively treat adolescents with epilepsy, interventions should be planned to include a psychosocial component.

Psychosocial interventions for patients with epilepsy are typically designed to target psychological adjustment, seizure management, coping skills, stress management, and seizure frequency (Wagner & Smith, 2006). Other programs provide educational experiences designed to increase knowledge, develop skills, and help adolescents with epilepsy gain independence. Psychosocial interventions typically take the form of support programs, self-management, psychoeducation, and psychological (therapeutic) interventions.

Facilitating Social Support

Support refers to providing individuals with the tools necessary to manage their epilepsy and its associated difficulties, usually through informal social relationships. For adolescents with epilepsy and their parents, a number of programs are available. Local agencies and epilepsy programs often provide age-based support groups for their young patients. In addition, there are well-organized national networks, such as the eCommunities Forum sponsored by the Epilepsy Foundation of America (EFA), which is an extensive network of easily accessed chat rooms and listserves for patients and families of all ages. Support networks offer a venue for sharing experiences, information, and resources. More importantly for teens, support groups reduce the isolation and lack of understanding they report in unaffected peer groups.

Epilepsy camps are another source of peer support for adolescents. In the United States, there are currently 38 summer camp programs for children and teens with epilepsy. Camps provide a recreational environment for teens to interact with other teens sharing a similar diagnosis. However, their efficacy is largely unknown (Wagner & Smith, 2006).

Self-Management

Self-management is defined by what individual patients do to control their disease and to integrate it into their daily lives (Dilorio & Henry, 1995). Self-management relies on three basic assumptions of health behavior change: most patients already provide for most of their own care; health-care professionals primarily provide education and support for patient efforts; changes perceived as meaningful and volitional are more likely to be sustained over time (Pramuka et al., 2007). Experts in self-management of teens with epilepsy have identified a number of factors that influence the acquisition of knowledge, skills, and strategies necessary for self-management to be successful. Behavioral health professionals need to focus on achieving a healthy balance between independence and support. Helping adolescent patients achieve independence in management *requires* facilitating parental involvement.

A recent review of self-management programs for children and adolescents with epilepsy suggests that programs that work are designed to improve patient knowledge, skills, and psychosocial adaptation in group learning formats. Results are generally positive, but outcomes for these programs are not standardized and samples are usually too small to make significant conclusions about program value (Wagner & Smith, 2006).

Epilepsy Education Programs

Most educational interventions have common elements including giving patients and families a working knowledge of seizures, treatments, and behaviors that facilitate optimal management. Some programs also provide families with supportive resources to help manage psychosocial care needs. Wagner and Smith offer a comprehensive critique of the evidence available for many of these programs (Wagner & Smith, 2006).

Available evidence suggests that small-group interventions are associated with improvements in compliance with medications, knowledge about epilepsy, self-esteem, and self-management, as well as with reductions in emergency physician visits (P. Camfield & Camfield, 2003). Empowering teens by tailoring information to individual intellectual, attentional, and interest levels is an important element of education.

Psychological Interventions

With a greater prevalence of psychosocial and psychological comorbidities, adolescents with seizure disorders are more likely than those without to require psychological intervention. However, it is not recommended that psychological intervention only be used when symptoms reach a clinically significant level. Given the increased risk posed by a diagnosis of epilepsy, routine screening for behavioral and psychosocial difficulties is recommended as a standard in epilepsy care.

The use of therapeutic interventions to target specific psychosocial factors associated with epilepsy in youth (such as perceived control, self-perception, self-efficacy, illness appraisal, compliance, and behavior problems) is commonly used. Brief psychotherapy is often used to increase acceptance of diagnosis or medical status, improve self-control and behavior management, and address concerns of teens and their families (Wagner & Smith, 2006). Cognitive-behavioral approaches to adaptation and management of psychosocial challenges are well accepted (Wagner & Smith, 2007a). Outpatient psychotherapy (individual or family) is recommended for a significant subgroup of patients whose symptoms cannot be addressed in a brief format (Wagner & Smith, 2006).

Behavior management techniques, including relaxation, habituation, and monitoring and awareness training, have all been successful interventions resulting in reduced seizure frequency for some patients. Studies of these interventions reveal that significant gains can be made and sustained long after the treatment has ended (Wagner & Smith, 2006). However, individualized treatment planning and intensive intervention schedules make it difficult to ascertain the generalizability of results to all adolescents with epilepsy.

Directions for Future Work and Research Considerations

Assessment of psychosocial difficulties is not epilepsy specific. There are few validated instruments available that evaluate psychosocial functioning specifically related to epilepsy. Assessments involving standardized protocols would be very useful in defining target symptoms for interventions and measuring the outcomes of treatment.

Identifying and addressing the barriers to adequate behavioral health care are important. Access continues to be a problem in many settings, despite the finding that appropriate epilepsy management is defined by at least 11 behavioral and psychosocial performance indicators (Caplin, Rao, Filloux, Bale, & Van Orman, 2006). When services are available they are often underutilized because of problems with stigma and reimbursement for services (Wagner & Smith, 2007b).

What data are available suggest that behavioral health is a useful resource for epilepsy management in adolescence. However, the effectiveness of specific interventions on particular outcomes is not adequately studied. Most studies of behavioral health interventions for youth with epilepsy are plagued by small sample sizes, variation and lack of control in outcome measures, and poor or no comparison groups (Wagner & Smith, 2006). Establishment of care standards for behavioral health in epilepsy management will require more collaboration with other care providers and greater integration of behavioral health issues into medical care standards.

References

Appleton, R. E., Chadwick, D., & Sweeney, A. (1997). Managing the teenager with epilepsy: paediatric to adult care. *Seizure, 6*(1), 27–30.

Appleton, R. E., & Neville, B. G. (1999). Teenagers with epilepsy. *Archives of Disease in Childhood, 81*(1), 76–79.

Bailet, L. L., & Turk, W. R. (2000). The impact of childhood epilepsy on neurocognitive and behavioral performance: A prospective longitudinal study. *Epilepsia, 41*(4), 426–431.

Baker, G. A., Hargis, E., Hsih, M. M., Mounfield, H., Arzimanoglou, A., Glauser, T., et al. (2008). Perceived impact of epilepsy in teenagers and young adults: An international survey. *Epilepsy & Behaviour, 12*(3), 395–401.

Beghi, E., & Cornaggia, C. (2002). Morbidity and accidents in patients with epilepsy: Results of a European cohort study. *Epilepsia, 43*(9), 1076–1083.

Begley, C. E., Famulari, M., Annegers, J. F., Lairson, D. R., Reynolds, T. F., Coan, S., et al. (2000). The cost of epilepsy in the United States: an estimate from population-based clinical and survey data. *Epilepsia, 41*(3), 342–351.

Browne, T. R., & Holmes, G. L. (2001). Epilepsy. *New England Journal of Medicine, 344*(15), 1145–1151.

Camfield, C. S., Camfield, P. R., Gordon, K., Wirrell, E., & Dooley, J. M. (1996). Incidence of epilepsy in childhood and adolescence: a population-based study in Nova Scotia from 1977 to 1985. *Epilepsia, 37*(1), 19–23.

Camfield, P., & Camfield, C. (2003). Childhood epilepsy: what is the evidence for what we think and what we do? *Journal of Child Neurology, 18*(4), 272–287.

Caplan, R., Arbelle, S., Magharious, W., Guthrie, D., Komo, S., Shields, W. D., et al. (1998). Psychopathology in pediatric complex partial and primary generalized epilepsy. *Developmental Medicine and Child Neurology, 40*(12), 805–811.

Caplan, R., Siddarth, P., Gurbani, S., Hanson, R., Sankar, R., & Shields, W. D. (2005). Depression and anxiety disorders in pediatric epilepsy. *Epilepsia, 46*(5), 720–730.

Caplin, D. A., Rao, J. K., Filloux, F., Bale, J. F., & Van Orman, C. (2006). Development of performance indicators for the primary care management of pediatric epilepsy: Expert consensus recommendations based on the available evidence. *Epilepsia, 47*(12), 2011–2019.

Choi-Kwon, S., Yoon, S. M., Choi, M. R., Kang, D. W., & Lee, S. K. (2001). The difference in perceptions of educational need between epilepsy patients and medical personnel. *Epilepsia, 42*(6), 785–789.

Davies, S., Heyman, I., & Goodman, R. (2003). A population survey of mental health problems in children with epilepsy. *Developmental Medicine and Child Neurology, 45*(5), 292–295.

Dilorio, C., & Henry, M. (1995). Self-management in persons with epilepsy. *The Journal of Neuroscience Nursing, 27*(6), 338–343.

Dilorio, C., Shafer, P. O., Letz, R., Henry, T. R., Schomer, D. L., & Yeager, K. (2004). Project EASE: a study to test a psychosocial model of epilepsy medication management. *Epilepsy & Behaviour, 5*(6), 926–936.

Donner, E. J., Smith, C. R., & Snead, O. C., III. (2001). Sudden unexplained death in children with epilepsy. *Neurology, 57*(3), 430–434.

Dunn, D. W., Harezlak, J., Ambrosius, W. T., Austin, J. K., & Hale, B. (2002). Teacher assessment of behaviour in children with new-onset seizures. *Seizure, 11*(3), 169–175.

Engel, J., Jr. (2006). ILAE classification of epilepsy syndromes. *Epilepsy Res, 70 Suppl 1*, S5–S10.

Ettinger, A. B., Weisbrot, D. M., Nolan, E. E., Gadow, K. D., Vitale, S. A., Andriola, M. R., et al. (1998). Symptoms of depression and anxiety in pediatric epilepsy patients. *Epilepsia, 39*(6), 595–599.

Fastenau, P. S., Jianzhao, S., Dunn, D. W., & Austin, J. K. (2008). Academic underachievement among children with epilepsy: proportion exceeding psychometric criteria for learning disability and associated risk factors. *Journal of Learning Disabilities, 41*(3), 195–207.

Fastenau, P. S., Shen, J., Dunn, D. W., Perkins, S. M., Hermann, B. P., & Austin, J. K. (2004). Neuropsychological predictors of academic underachievement in pediatric epilepsy: Moderating roles of demographic, seizure, and psychosocial variables. *Epilepsia, 45*(10), 1261–1272.

Hodes, M., Garralda, M. E., Rose, G., & Schwartz, R. (1999). Maternal expressed emotion and adjustment in children with epilepsy. *Journal of Child Psychology and Psychiatry, 40*(7), 1083–1093.

Kaplan, P. W. (2004). Reproductive health effects and teratogenicity of antiepileptic drugs. *Neurology, 63*(10 Suppl 4), S13–23.

Kotsopoulos, I. A., van Merode, T., Kessels, F. G., de Krom, M. C., & Knottnerus, J. A. (2002). Systematic review and meta-analysis of incidence studies of epilepsy and unprovoked seizures. *Epilepsia, 43*(11), 1402–1409.

Kurtz, Z., Tookey, P., & Ross, E. (1998). Epilepsy in young people: 23 year follow up of the British national child development study. *BMJ, 316*(7128), 339–342.

Lee, A., Hamiwka, L. D., Sherman, E. M., & Wirrell, E. C. (2008). Self-concept in adolescents with epilepsy: biological and social correlates. *Pediatr Neurol, 38*(5), 335–339.

Mbuba, C. K., Ngugi, A. K., Newton, C. R., & Carter, J. A. (2008). The epilepsy treatment gap in developing countries: A systematic review of the magnitude, causes, and intervention strategies. *Epilepsia, 49*(9), 1491 1503.

McEwan, M. J., Espie, C. A., Metcalfe, J., Brodie, M. J., & Wilson, M. T. (2004). Quality of life and psychosocial development in adolescents with epilepsy: A qualitative investigation using focus group methods. *Seizure, 13*(1), 15–31.

Pramuka, M., Hendrickson, R., Zinski, A., & Van Cott, A. C. (2007). A psychosocial self-management program for epilepsy: A randomized pilot study in adults. *Epilepsy & Behaviour, 11*(4), 533–545.

Ridsdale, L., Morgan, M., & O'Connor, C. (1999). Promoting self-care in epilepsy: The views of patients on the advice they had received from specialists, family doctors and an epilepsy nurse. *Patient Education and Counseling, 37*(1), 43–47.

Rodenburg, R., Stams, G. J., Meijer, A. M., Aldenkamp, A. P., & Dekovic, M. (2005). Psychopathology in children with epilepsy: A meta-analysis. *Journal of Pediatric Psychology, 30*(6), 453–468.

Salpekar, J. A., & Dunn, D. W. (2007). Psychiatric and psychosocial consequences of pediatric epilepsy. *Seminars in Pediatric Neurology, 14*(4), 181–188.

Sheth, R. D. (2002). Adolescent issues in epilepsy. *Journal of Child Neurology, 17 (Suppl 2)*, 2S23–22S27.

Sillanpaa, M., & Schmidt, D. (2006). Prognosis of seizure recurrence after stopping antiepileptic drugs in seizure-free patients: A long-term population-based study of childhood-onset epilepsy. *Epilepsy & Behaviour, 8*(4), 713–719.

Wagner, J. L., & Smith, G. (2006). Psychosocial intervention in pediatric epilepsy: A critique of the literature. *Epilepsy & Behaviour, 8*(1), 39–49.

Wagner, J. L., & Smith, G. (2007a). Pediatric epilepsy: The role of the pediatric psychologist. *Epilepsy & Behaviour, 11*(3), 253–256.

Wagner, J. L., & Smith, G. (2007b). Psychological services in a pediatric epilepsy clinic: Referral patterns and feasibility. *Epilepsy & Behaviour, 10*(1), 129–133.

Wheless, J. W., & Kim, H. L. (2002). Adolescent seizures and epilepsy syndromes. *Epilepsia, 43*(Suppl 3), 33–52.

Wilde, M., & Haslam, C. (1996). Living with epilepsy: A qualitative study investigating the experiences of young people attending outpatients clinics in Leicester. *Seizure, 5*(1), 63–72.

Wilfong, A. A. (2007). Monotherapy in children and infants. *Neurology, 69*(24 Suppl 3), S17–S22.

Migraines/Chronic Headaches

Joyce Engel

Recurrent primary (nonorganic) headaches (HAs) are one of the most common pain complaints among youths with a significant HA reported in more than 75% by the age of 15 years. Pediatric migraine occurs in up to 10.6% of youths between the ages of 5 and 15 years, further increasing to 28% of adolescents between the ages of 15 and 19 years (Hershey, 2005). The prevalence of pediatric HA has increased over the past 30 years (Sillanpaa & Antilla, 1996). Recurrent HAs significantly decrease activities and participation, thereby placing youths at risk for the development of psychopathology (Holden, Deichmann, & Levy, 1999). The World Health Organization ranked migraine as number 19 among all diseases worldwide causing disability (Headache Classification Subcommittee of the International Headache Society, 2004). Youths miss more than one million days of school per year due to HAs (National Pain Foundation, 2008). HAs often continue into adulthood (Connelly, 2003). This chapter reviews the major recurrent primary pediatric HA disorders. Headache assessment, interventions for pain control, and implications for clinical and research activities are also discussed.

Headache Classifications

The International Headache Society (2003) has identified three primary types of HA: migraine without aura (common migraine), migraine with aura (classic or complicated migraine), and tension-type (TTH). An aura is symptoms at the onset of a migraine-like disturbed vision. Migraine and TTH are differentiated primarily on the basis of vascular and muscular origins (McGrath, 1990). The type of HA disorder guides treatment. Criteria for these HA disorders are provided below in Table 1.

Prior to initiating intervention for recurrent HA, a thorough history and physical which may include diagnostic laboratory and radiological studies is prudent to rule out any life-threatening disorder (Olness & Kohen, 1996). A HA diary can be very helpful in guiding an accurate diagnosis of the HA and determining the effectiveness of intervention. The diary typically addresses HA frequency, duration, and severity, and precipitating and exacerbating pain factors as well as actions taken for relief and their effectiveness (Hämäläinen & Masek, 2003; McGrath & Larsson, 1997).

Headache Etiology

The exact mechanisms of HAs are not known. Inherited genetic factors are believed to play a role in both migraine and TTH. The risk of migraines in youths is about 45% when one parent is affected and 70% when both parents experience migraines (National Pain Foundation, 2008). HAs are probably triggered by environmental and psychosocial factors (Holden et al., 1999). Other mechanisms have also been proposed for producing and maintaining HAs.

J. Engel (✉)
Department of Rehabilitation Medicine, University of Washington School of Medicine, Seattle, WA, USA
e-mail: jmengel@u.washington.edu

W.T. O'Donohue, L.W. Tolle (eds.), *Behavioral Approaches to Chronic Disease in Adolescence*,
DOI 10.1007/978-0-387-87687-0_13, © Springer Science+Business Media, LLC 2009

Table 1 Headache classifications

	Duration	Intensity	Other characteristics
Migraine without aura	4–72 hours; 1–72 hours in children	Moderate-to-severe	Must have experienced at least five episodes. Unilateral (often bilateral up to adolescence), pulsating, exacerbated by physical activity and associated with nausea or vomiting, and/or photophobia and phonophobia
Migraine with aura	4–72 hours	Moderate-to-severe	Must have experienced at least two episodes. One or more reversible auras with visual symptoms, sensory symptoms, or dysphasic speech disorder. Aura lasts <60 minutes, pain follows aura within 60 minutes
Tension-Type (TTH)	30 minutes–7 days	Mild-to-moderate	Must have experienced at least 10 episodes <1 day/month on average. Bilateral, nonpulsatile, tightening without nausea or vomiting, photophobia, or phonophobia

Biochemical

Sustained contraction of the head and neck muscles, inflammation of cranial vascular structures, and traction (pulling) on vascular structures might result in TTH (Connelly, 2003).

There are two biomechanical theories for migraine HA. The vascular theory of migraine proposes a disorder of cerebral and extracranial blood vessel regulation, in which circulating vasoactive amines cause cerebral arteries to constrict, thereby causing some scalp vessels to dilate. Consequently, pressure in the surrounding tissue and inflammation result in a migraine. In contrast, the neurogenic model states that a migraine results from the instability of monoaminergic transmission causing individuals to be highly vulnerable to sudden internal or external states. Factors like changes in circadian rhythm are believed to impact on brain stem nuclei that project throughout the cerebral cortex. A phase of sympathetic discharge is then followed by monoamine depletion. This depletion leads to constriction of intracranial blood flow and dilation of extracranial vasculature that ultimately results in focal neurological symptoms and head pain (Connelly, 2003).

It should be noted that the above models are based on the adult population. Further research is needed to determine the evidence for these models in the pediatric population.

Stress

Physiological and psychological stressors have been hypothesized to be common etiological factors for HAs in youths (Bille, 1962; Larsson, 1999; Ross & Ross, 1988). Many HAs occur during school, at the end of the week, and after stressful events (Bille; Larsson). Neither youths nor adults with recurrent migraines differ from their peers in their level of stress but may experience a heightened response to stressors that may precipitate a HA episode (Andrasik et al., 1982; Ross & Ross). Gaffney and Gaffney (1987) stated that youths with recurrent pain have different thresholds of responsiveness to environmental stressors, which may trigger a poorly regulated nervous system. In addition, irregular eating and sleep schedules may induce a HA (Bille; Dalton & Dalton, 1979). Tyramine (e.g., contained in chocolate and cheese), nitrates, glutamate, caffeine, overexertion, fatigue, eyestrain, and hormonal changes secondary to menstruation have also been identified as migraine precipitants (Ross & Ross).

Other Considerations in Headache Disorders

Comorbidity

Fortunately, recurrent HAs are only rarely associated with underlying conditions that cause significant impairment or mortality (Connelly, 2003; Holden et al., 1999). In addition, there is little evidence of increased comorbidity with other disorders (e.g., anxiety, depression). No definitive diagnostic study involving the occurrence of migraine, depression, anxiety, or any other psychiatric disorder exists (Connelly, 2003; McGrath & Larsson, 1997).

Red flags of constant or daily HA, increased HA frequency or severity, no improvement with analgesic use, changes in mental status, altered gait, seizures, and motor weakness warrant further medical evaluation (National Pain Foundation, 2008).

Cultural Considerations

Cultural and familial influences are important factors to consider in pediatric pain assessment and treatment. Each culture has a unique system of transmitting values and attitudes to its members. As a child becomes accultured, one learns what his or her culture will expect and accept as appropriate behavior. Pain behaviors are greatly influenced by familial and cultural expectations (Weisenberg, 1977). Parents can often assist in explaining cultural and language differences and accepted practices to the health-care provider.

Interventions

Pharmacological Interventions

A treatment plan is developed based on HA activity, the degree of disability, the wishes of the adolescent, and the support of the parents (Larsson, 1999). Neinstein (1984) recommended that treatment for nonorganic HA begins with reassurance that nothing is seriously wrong and that successful treatment is possible. Symptomatic medications (e.g., simple analgesics like acetaminophen and nonsteroidal anti-inflammatory drugs such as ibuprofen) are the usual first route of treatment being used at the onset of the acute HA (Edgeworth, Bullock, Bailey et al., 1996; Holden, Levy, Deichmann, & Gladstein, 1998). Gastrointestinal bleeding, renal failure, and anaphylaxis can result from ibuprofen use (Connelly, 2003). Side effects of acetaminophen (e.g., gastrointestinal upset) are minimal. Aspirin is used with care due to the slight risk of Reye's syndrome (Larsson). Parents often give their children subtherapeutic doses of over-the-counter medications (Holden, Levy, Deichmann, & Gladstein).

Severe and recurrent migraine HAs typically warrant the use of prophylactics to prevent HA. Holden and colleagues identified the criteria for prophylaxis, which include high functional disability (e.g., school absenteeism, familial discord secondary to HA) and severe episodes. Propranolol has FDA approval for the treatment of pediatric migraine as prophylactic medication. Its side effects are minimal (e.g., fatigue, hypotension, nausea). Propranolol is contraindicated in youths with diabetes, asthma, and congestive heart failure (Connelly). In contrast, ergot preparations are often used as abortive medication at the onset of a migraine. Nausea, vomiting, and a rebound HA (intensification of pain) are typical side effects. A challenge of using abortive medication is that it is most effective at the early stage of HA when the adolescent may experience less clearly identifiable warning signals (Ross & Ross, 1988). Opiods (e.g., codeine, morphine) may be prescribed if the HA has not responded to NSAIDs (Connelly). Side effects of opiods include drowsiness, lethargy, and disphoria (Schechter, 1985). Amitriptyline and Desyrel are often prescribed for adolescents experiencing chronic TTH to alleviate possible emotional factors (Connelly; McGrath, 1990). It should be noted that few randomized controlled trials have evaluated pharmacotherapy for youths.

Behavioral Interventions

Behavioral interventions for pediatric pain control are popular for several reasons. Behavioral methods can help identify the challenges of persistent pain in youths in a precise and objective fashion, especially with regard to the role socioenvironmental factors may play in controlling pain behaviors. In addition, behavioral strategies may succeed in treating those individuals who are not likely to respond to pharmacological or medical treatments. Finally, the increasing dissatisfaction with the results of medically based treatments and the recognition of complex interactions of physiological, psychological, and pharmacological factors in the perception and elaboration of pain have prompted the continued growing interest in behavioral techniques for pain control (Engel & Rapoff, 1990).

Relaxation training. Relaxation training is believed to reduce somatic arousal. The potential benefits of relaxation rehearsal include reduction of acute anxiety, distraction from pain, alleviation of skeletal muscle tension, lessening of fatigue, and enhancement of other pain-relief measures (McCaffery, 1979). Relaxation training may involve teaching the individual to systematically contract and relax the major skeletal muscle groups (progressive muscle relaxation), the silent repetition of phrases about the physiological state of the body (autogenic training; AT), or the purposeful use of images to achieve a relaxed state (guided imagery). Consumers are instructed to use their relaxation techniques with their first awareness of the HA onset in addition to daily practice (Holden et al., 1999). There is strong evidence for the efficacy of relaxation training for reducing persistent pain in adults (National Institutes of Health, 1995) and this also appears to be true for adolescents with recurrent HA (Holden, Deichmann, & Levy). Numerous studies reported at least 50% improvement in HA rate (Engel, 1992; Engel, Rapoff, & Pressman, 1992; Larsson & Melin, 1986; McGrath et al., 1992; Wisniewski, Genshaft, Mulick, Coury, & Hammer, 1988). No relaxation technique has been found to be superior to another (Engel & Rapoff, 1990; Hämäläinen & Masek, 2003). Relaxation techniques have also been used successfully in multicomponent treatment programs (Sallade, 1980). Children as young as 7 years old can learn to master relaxation techniques (Hämäläinen & Masek, 2003). Treatment can be provided in a group format, school-based program, and minimal therapist contact format (Larsson, 1999; Larsson & Melin, 1986; McGrath et al., 1992).

Biofeedback. Biofeedback refers to instrumentation used to feedback information to an individual about his or her physiological state of which he or she may not typically be aware of (Payne, 2000). Hand warming is the physiological response to be conditioned in thermal biofeedback and is believed to correlate with reduction of cranial sympathetic activity (Blanchard & Andrasik, 1985). Children as young as age three can master thermal biofeedback (Olness, 1985). In contrast, electromyographic (EMG) biofeedback consists of teaching the individual how to relax the skeletal muscles of the face, neck, and scalp (Hämäläinen & Masek, 2003). Ultimately the goal of biofeedback training is to generalize physiological control from the clinical to the individual's natural environments. Biofeedback is typically used in conjunction with relaxation techniques.

Thermal biofeedback has been used successfully in the treatment of recurrent pediatric HA. Labbé and Williamson (1984) reported that 93% of the autogenic feedback training group improved. Similarly, Engel and Rapoff (1990) indicated that all participants ($N = 15$) achieved increased HA-free days. Numerous other studies with less rigorous experimental procedures also support the use of biofeedback for HA management (Andrasik, Blanchard, Edlund, & Rosenblum, 1982; Burke & Andrasik, 1989; Engel, 1992; Hermann, Blanchard, & Flor, 1997; Labbé & Williamson, 1983). In some cases, treatment effects were durable through at least 6-months follow-up (Burke & Andrasik; Engel et al., 1992; Labbé & Williamson, 1983, 1984; Larsson & Melin, 1986).

Hypnosis. Hypnosis consists of directing forces within the body to produce changes like analgesia (Connelly, 2003). The mechanism by which hypnosis works is not clearly understood. It has been proposed that hypnosis produces physiological changes, which mediate symptom relief. In contrast, hypnosis allows one to gain insight into how symptoms developed and ultimately how to relieve these symptoms (Turner & Chapman, 1982). Hypnosis as part of a treatment package seems promising. The combination of hypnosis and contingency management eliminated migraines in five youths aged 7–14 years (Kapelis, 1984). Likewise, Olness and MacDonald (1981) reported significant relief of HAs through the use of self-hypnosis with and without thermal biofeedback in three youths aged 9–13 years.

Contingency management. Learning factors promote and maintain the expression of pain (Labbé, 1999). When the consequences of a particular behavior are likely to be aversive, most individuals will engage in avoidance behaviors. This avoidance behavior is thereby reinforced because it successfully prevents the expected aversive consequences. All that is needed to reinforce avoidance behavior is for the aversive consequence not to occur or for its occurrence to be at a decreased frequency or intensity. In individuals who demonstrate significant learned or operant pain behavior, treatment might involve shifting positive reinforcement contingencies from "pain" to "well" (e.g., school attendance) behaviors (Fordyce, 1976). Parents therefore are instructed to eliminate the sources of reinforcement that maintain pain behaviors while promoting the child's pain-coping strategies and typical activities and participation (Hämäläinen & Masek, 2003). No adolescent HA studies were found that used only contingency management. Practitioners are cautioned that extinguishing pain behaviors cannot necessarily be equated with the absence of pain.

Cognitive behavioral techniques. These techniques target recurrent maladaptive thoughts that interfere with coping and seem to be associated with HA activity (Richardson & McGrath, 1989). The youth is first taught how to identify unhelpful (maladaptive), helpful (adaptive), and neutral thoughts related to the HA experience. After the youth identifies negative thoughts associated with pain, he or she is taught several cognitive therapy strategies that have the goal of eliminating maladaptive thoughts and increasing adaptive ones. Strategies include stopping such negative thinking, replacing maladaptive thoughts with more realistic, helpful ones, and challenging maladaptive thoughts. For example, an adolescent who responds to HAs with thoughts such as "I can't stand this" or "This is terrible" may be taught how such thoughts further exacerbate distress and pain and then how to replace such unhelpful thoughts with more realistic, helpful ones such as "I can deal with this" or "I can get through this if I practice abdominal breathing". Treatment also typically includes relaxation techniques, distraction strategies, and problem-solving methods (McGrath & Larsson, 1997). Richter et al. (1986) indicated that youths with migraines (9–18 years) responded with fewer HAs post cognitive coping groups and up to 16 weeks posttreatment. Treatment can be delivered in an individual or group format (Larsson, 1999).

Minimal therapist contact interventions. Behavioral therapists have implemented a wide range of treatment settings (e.g., school-based) and nontraditional treatment modes (e.g., minimal therapist contact, group administration) as a means to achieving advantageous cost benefit returns and interventions that are readily available (Andrasik et al., 2003; Larsson & Carlsson, 1996; McGrath et al., 1992; Richardson & McGrath, 1989). Minimal contact interventions (e.g., use of treatment manuals and relaxation CDs) aim to decrease the number of clinic visits, time spent away from school and home, demands on the family, and health-care costs. Andrasik and colleagues developed an 8-week neurologist-administered group treatment (discussion of coping strategies and progressive relaxation), which resulted in clinically meaningful improvement in HAs. Treatment gains were maintained through 1-year follow-up and without supplemental medication. More recently, Cottrell, Drew, Gibson, Holroyd, and O'Donnell (2007) determined the feasibility of providing telephone-administered behavioral treatment (TAT) to adolescents with episodic HA. All 15 participants reported large reductions in the number of HA episodes, disability equivalent hours and quality of life, as well as HA duration and severity. Participants expressed a preference for TAT over traditional in-clinic treatment. To consider a minimal contact approach, the adolescent must make the time commitment to treatment and adhere to treatment recommendations.

Psychological Counseling

Strained relationships, communication difficulties, maladaptive behaviors, situational stress, and other sources of familial distress (e.g., marital discord) can serve as predisposing, exacerbating, or maintaining pain factors (McGrath & Dade, 2004). These issues might improve with ongoing psychological counseling from someone familiar with adolescents managing chronic medical conditions like pain.

Family Counseling

The stress of living with a chronic condition is often compounded when parental and familial attitudes restrict the child's routine activities of daily living and participation. Often the child adopts a sick role. The consequent emotional distress and social isolation can exacerbate the pain and foster disability (McGrath, 1990; Walker, 1999). Families who experience significant disruption of their routines by the child's pain problems might benefit from family counseling with an emphasis on operant techniques. The family as a whole thereby is educated in how to respond to pain behaviors appropriately, alleviate suffering, and promote well behaviors.

Treatment Adherence

Very little is known about adherence in pediatric HA management. It has been estimated that about half of persons experiencing recurrent HA do not comply with prescribed pharmacological regimens that no doubt contributes to ineffective pain control. In addition, as many as two-thirds do not make optimal use of abortive medications (Connelly, 2003).

Engel (1993) reported mean adherence with progressive relaxation training as 84% (range: 36–100%). Nonadherence occurred 74% of the time when participants reported being HA-free for that day. Most of the participants had a 2–30% (mean: 15%) increase in HA-free days. Adherence with relaxation training did not result consistently in HA relief.

Conclusion

Numerous effective pharmacological and behavioral interventions exist for the treatment of recurrent HAs in adolescents. The long-standing nature of HA disorders highlights the need for early treatment. Youths would benefit from pharmacotherapy, instruction in a variety of pain-coping skills (relaxation techniques, cognitive behavioral strategies), and wellness principles (regular meal times, adequate sleep, regular exercise, and stress management). Future research that includes larger and more diverse treatment populations in randomized controlled trials will help us determine the efficacy of interventions. Component analysis of experimental groups is necessary to determine which components of treatment packages are critical and most efficacious. Strategies to enhance treatment adherence must also be explored. Modification of physical environments (e.g., reduction of bright lights) has not yet been studied. The delivery of treatment in natural settings (e.g., school) coupled with minimal therapist contact warrants further investigation. Finally, dissemination of study findings to general practitioners and neurologists, school nurses and therapists, and families of youths would allow for exploration of treatment options and matching adolescents with various characteristics to specific interventions.

References

Andrasik, F., Blanchard, E. B., Arena, J. G., Teders, S. J., Teevan, R. C., & Rodichok, L. D. (1982). Psychological functioning in headache sufferers. *Psychosomatic Medicine, 44*, 171–182.

Andrasik, F., Blanchard, E. B., Edlund, S. R., & Rosenblum, E. L. (1982). Autogenic feedback in the treatment of two children with migraine headache. *Child & Family Behavior Therapy, 4*, 13–23.

Andrasik, F., Grazzi, L., Usai, S., D'Amico, D., Leone, M., & Bussone, G. (2003). Brief neurologist-administered behavioral treatment of pediatric episodic tension-type headache. *Neurology, 60*, 1215–1216.

Bille, B. (1962). Migraine in schoolchildren. *Acta Paediatricia Scandinavia, 51* (Suppl. 136), 1–15.

Blanchard, E. B., & Andrasik, F. (1985). *Management of chronic headaches*. New York: Pergamon.

Burke, E. J., & Andrasik, F. (1989). Home- vs. clinical-based biofeedback treatment for pediatric migraine: Results of treatment through one-year follow-up. *Headache, 29*, 434–440.

Connelly, M. (2003). Recurrent pediatric headache: A comprehensive review. *Children's Health Care, 32* (3), 153–189.

Cottrell, C., Drew, J., Gibson, J., Holroyd, K., & O'Donnell, F. (2007). Feasibility assessment of telephone-administered behavioral treatment for adolescent migraine. *Headache, 47*, 1293–1302.

Dalton, K., & Dalton, M. E. (1979). Food intake before migraine attacks in children. *Journal of the Royal College of General Practitioners, 29*(208), 662–665.

Edgeworth, J., Bullock, P., Bailey, A., et al. (1996). Why are brain tumors still being missed. *Archives of Disease in Childhood, 74*, 148–151.

Engel, J. M. (1992). Relaxation training: A self-help approach for children with headaches. *The American Journal of Occupational Therapy, 46*, 591–596.

Engel, J. M. (1993). Children's compliance with progressive relaxation procedures for improving headache control. *Occupational Therapy Journal of Research, 13* (4), 219–230.

Engel, J. M., & Rapoff, M. A. (1990). A component analysis of relaxation training with vascular, muscle contraction, and mixed-headache disorders. In D. C. Tyler & E. J. Krane (Eds.), *Advances in pain research therapy* (Vol. 15, pp. 272–290). New York: Raven Press.

Engel, J. M., Rapoff, M. A., & Pressman, A. R. (1992). Long-term follow-up of relaxation training for pediatric headache disorders. *Headache: The Journal of Head and Face Pain, 32* (3), 152–156.

Fordyce, W. E. (1976). *Behavioral methods for chronic pain and illness*. St. Louis: C. V. Mosby.

Gaffney, A., & Gaffney, P. R. (1987). Recurrent abdominal pain in children and the endogenous opiates: A brief hypothesis. *Pain, 30*, 217–219.

Hämäläinen, M., & Masek, B. J. (2003). Diagnosis, classification, and medical management of headache in children and adolescents. In N. L. Schechter, C. B. Berde, & M. Yaster (Eds.), *Pain in infants, children, and adolescents* (2nd ed., pp. 707–718). Philadelphia: Lippincott Williams & Wilkins.

Headache Classification Subcommittee of the International Headache Society. (2004). The International Classification of Headache Disorders (2nd ed.). *Cephalgia, 24* (Suppl. 1), 1–160.

Hermann, C., Blanchard, E. B., & Flor, H. (1997). Biofeedback treatment for pediatric migraine: Prediction of treatment outcome. *Journal of Consulting and Clinical Psychology, 65* (4), 611–616.

Hershey, A. D. (2005). What are the impact, prevalence, disability, and quality of life of pediatric headache? *Current Pain and Headache Reports, 9* (5), 341–344.

Holden, E. W., Deichmann, M. M., & Levy, J. D. (1999). Empirically supported treatments in pediatric psychology: Recurrent pediatric headache. *Journal of Pediatric Psychology, 24* (2), 91–109.

Holden, E. W., Levy, J. D., Deichmann, M. M., & Gladstein, J. (1998). Recurrent pediatric headaches: Assessment and intervention. *Developmental and Behavioral Pediatrics, 19* (2), 109–116.

Kapelis, L. (1984). Hypnosis in a behaviour therapy framework for the treatment of migraine in children. *Australian Journal of Clinical and Experimental Hypnosis, 12*, 123–126.

Labbé, E. E. (1999). Commentary: Salient aspects of research in pediatric headache and future directions. *Journal of Pediatric Psychology, 24* (5), 113–114.

Labbé, E. E., & Williamson, D. A. (1983). Temperature biofeedback in the treatment of children with migraine headaches. *Journal of Pediatric Psychology, 8*, 317–326.

Labbé E. E., & Williamson, D. A. (1984). Treatment of childhood migraine using autogenic feedback training. *Journal of Consulting and Clinical Psychology, 52* (6), 968–976.

Larsson, B. (1999). Recurrent headaches in children and adolescents. In P. J. McGrath & G. A. Finley (Eds.), *Chronic and recurrent pain in children and adolescents* (pp. 115–140). Seattle, WA: IASP.

Larsson, B., & Carlsson, J. (1996). A school-based, nurse-administered relaxation training for children with chronic tension-type headache. *Journal of Pediatric Psychology, 21* (5), 603–614.

Larsson, B., & Melin, L. (1986). Chronic headaches in adolescents: Treatment in a school setting with relaxation training as compared with information-contact and self-registration. *Pain, 25*, 325–336.

McCaffery, M. (1979). *Nursing management of the patient with pain*. Philadelphia: Lippincott.

McGrath, P. A. (1990). *Pain in children: Nature, assessment, and treatment*. New York: Guilford Press.

McGrath, P. A., & Dade, L. A. (2004). Strategies to decrease pain and minimize disability. In D. D. Price & M. C. Bushnell (Eds.), *Psychological methods of pain control: Basic science and clinical perspectives: Vol. 29. Progress in pain research and management* (pp. 73–96). Seattle: IASP Press.

McGrath, P. J., Humphreys, P., Keene, D., Goodman, J. T., Lascelles, M. A., Cunningham, S. J., et al. (1992). The efficacy and efficiency of a self-administered treatment for adolescent migraine. *Pain, 49*, 321 324.

McGrath, P., & Larsson, B. (1997). Headache in children and adolescents. *Child and Adolescent Psychiatric Clinics of North America, 6* (4), 843–861.

National Institutes of Health. (1995, October). *Integration of behavioral and relaxation approaches into the treatment of chronic pain and insomnia*. Statement from the NIH technology assessment conference, Bethesda, MD.

National Pain Foundation. Pediatric pain: Headaches in children. http://www.medem.com/MedLB/article_detaillb.cfm?article_ID=ZZZIAZF99CC&sub_cat... Retrieved May 18, 2008.

Neinstein, L. S. (1984). *Adolescent health care: A practical guide*. Baltimore: Urban & Schwarzenberg.

Olness, K. (1985). Little swamis. *Psychology Today, 19*, 16–17.

Olness, K., & Kohen, D. P. (1996). *Hypnosis and hypnotherapy with children* (3rd ed). New York: Guilford.

Olness, K., & MacDonald, J. (1981). Self-hypnosis and biofeedback in the management of juvenile migraine. *Developmental and Behavioral Pediatrics, 2*, 168–170.

Payne, R. A. (2000). *Relaxation techniques: A practical handbook for the health care professional* (2nd ed.). New York: Churchill Livingstone.

Richardson, G. M., & McGrath, P. J. (1989). Cognitive-behavioral therapy for migraine headaches: A minimal therapist contact approach versus a clinic-based approach. *Headache, 29*, 352–357.

Richter, I. L., McGrath, P. J., Humphreys, P. J., Goodman, J. T., Firestone, P., & Keene, D. (1986). Cognitive and relaxation treatment of paediatric migraine, *Pain, 25*, 195–203.

Ross, D. M., & Ross, S. A. (1988). *Childhood pain*. Baltimore: Urban & Schwarzenberg.

Sallade, J. B. (1980). Group counseling with children who have migraine headaches. *Elementary School Guidance & Counseling, 15*, 87–89.

Schechter, N. L. (1985). Pain and pain control in children. *Current Problems in Pediatrics, 15* (5), 3 67.

Sillanpaa, M., & Antilla, P. (1996). Increasing prevalence of headache in 7-year-old schoolchildren. *Headache, 36*, 466–470.

Turner, J. A., & Chapman, C. R. (1982). Psychological interventions for chronic pain: A critical review. II. Operant conditioning, hypnosis, and cognitive-behavioral therapy. *Pain, 12*, 23–46.

Walker, L. S. (1999). The evolution of research on recurrent abdominal pain: History, assumptions, and a conceptual model. In P. J. McGrath & G. A. Finley (Eds.), *Chronic and recurrent pain in children and adolescents* (pp. 141–172). Seattle: IASP Press.

Weisenberg, M. (1977). Pain and pain control. *Psychological Bulletin, 84* (5), 1008–1044.

Wisniewski, J. J., Genshaft, J. L., Mulick, J. A., Coury, D. L., & Hammer, D. (1988). Relaxation therapy and compliance in the treatment of adolescent headache. *Headache, 28*, 612–617.

The Assessment and Management of Chronic and Recurrent Pain in Adolescents

Gary A. Walco, Helen Rozelman, and David Aaron Maroof

The International Association for the Study of Pain (IASP, 1994) defined the word *pain* as "an unpleasant sensory and emotional experience associated with actual or potential tissue damage, or described in terms of such damage." A central distinction in the assessment and often the treatment of pain has to do with its temporal characteristics. Acute pain has a fairly clear onset and importantly a reasonably clear offset, such as pain experienced post-operatively. Almost always the goal of treatment is eradication of the pain and this is typically accomplished with analgesic medications. When the offset of pain is not so distinct and the pain either frequently recurs or continues, it is referred to as recurrent or chronic. Exactly where one draws the line between acute and chronic pain is not always easy to define. In the past, arbitrary definitions were generated, such that if pain went on for 3 or 6 months, it was no longer considered to be acute, but instead chronic in nature.

A paradigm shift occurred in the latter part of the twentieth century as groundbreaking studies by Woolf and others (c.f., Woolf, Shortland, & Coggeshall, 1992; Woolf & Salter, 2000) have shown that the difference between acute pain and chronic pain is not a simple quantitative temporal issue, but that with the latter there are qualitative changes in central pain processing networks. While the details of the neurophysiology are beyond the scope of this chapter (see Zeltzer, Bursch, & Walco, 1997 for a review as related to pediatrics), suffice it to say that the assessment, impact, and often the modalities used to treat chronic pain are often distinct from approaches used to address acute pain. While the broader context of pain, including an array of genetic, developmental, environmental, and individual factors, is rarely a major focus of assessment in acute pain, these factors are essential to consider when pain is recurrent or persistent. Likewise, treatment goals may shift from pain eradication in acute pain to pain reduction, rehabilitation, and improved coping in chronic pain (American Pain Society, 1999).

In this chapter, we will discuss the epidemiology of recurrent and chronic pain in adolescents, followed by comprehensive assessment models, and then strategies for intervention, highlighting in particular the role of psychologists in this clinical arena.

The Epidemiology of Pain in Children and Adolescents

It is very difficult to ascertain specific parameters on the morbidity of various chronic pain problems in adolescence. This is due to a great deal of variability in the methodology of available epidemiological studies as well as inconsistency in definition. Just as a simple example, if we were to try to estimate the prevalence of juvenile fibromyalgia syndrome, first we would have to address the issue of definition. Do we use the widely accepted criteria published by the American College of Rheumatology in 1990 (Wolfe et al., 1990), which has principally been applied to

Gary A. Walco (✉)
Department of Pediatrics,
Hackensack University Medical Center,
30 Prospect Avenue, Hackensack, New Jersey 07601
e-mail: gwalco@humed.com

W.T. O'Donohue, L.W. Tolle (eds.), *Behavioral Approaches to Chronic Disease in Adolescence*,
DOI 10.1007/978-0-387-87687-0_14,

adults, do we use the criteria generated by Yunus and Masi (1985), which focused more specifically on juvenile fibromyalgia syndrome, or do we use a checklist of symptoms deemed to represent the condition?

Even after we define specific criteria for the syndrome, how might we ascertain if individuals fulfill those criteria? Do we conduct systematic physical examinations on all participants? Do we conduct retrospective chart reviews and seek to identify specific diagnoses? Do we use questionnaire data? And if we wish to look for biological or environmental correlates of the syndrome, how are those data gathered? How reliable and valid are the instruments? Are the analyses purely correlational or might we be able to infer some antecedent-consequence relationships, if not causality? Thus, measurement issues with specific attention to internal validity and generalizability are of great concern.

In addition to definition and measurement, the setting in which data were gathered may play a huge role. What differences in prevalence and characteristics might we observe if the study was conducted in a school setting versus a primary pediatric setting versus an adolescent medicine clinic versus a pediatric rheumatology practice versus a specialized pediatric pain program? The nature of the site would surely lead to bias in study participants. Furthermore, within those sites, what biases are introduced by those opting to participate or not? What about studies in countries with socialized medicine where huge cohorts may be followed over time (e.g., Mikkelson, Salminen, & Kautiainen, 1997)? How are those data to be compared across regions of the world or with clinically referred samples?

Finally, what about the relationship between studies on "juvenile fibromyalgia syndrome" as opposed to "idiopathic pain syndrome," "pain amplification syndrome," or "pervasive musculoskeletal pain" problems? Exactly how similar or different are these entities? Are findings from studies on one generalizable to the others and if so, with what limitations or concerns? All of these caveats are to be kept in mind as one begins to sift through data on the prevalence of pain syndromes and potential correlates or causal factors.

The prevalence of pain in children is a function of both developmental status (approximated by chronological age) and clinical condition (i.e., what type of pain is being reported). Perquin et al. (2001) demonstrated that approximately 54% of children and adolescents had experienced pain within a 3-month period, frequently leading to consultation with physicians and the use of various medications (Perquin et al., 2001). Brun Sundblad Saartok and Engstrom (2007) assessed the prevalence of self-reported pain and perceived health from a 3-month recall period, for both genders as well as at different age intervals (9, 12, and 15 years). The results indicated that within this circumscribed time frame, pain was reported as headache, abdominal, and/or musculoskeletal pain. Moreover, they revealed that girls reported headaches twice as often as boys. Abdominal pain was evinced in approximately 10% of the girls and 5% of the boys. Musculoskeletal pain was reported from 9 to 29%, depending upon the frequency of reports, and the most common form of pain was headache. Powers Gilman, and Hershey (2006) provide an excellent review of the prospective prevalence of headaches over time in children, including differences in gender as well as comorbid psychological aspects of headache pain. They make it clear that the relationship between headache and psychological dysfunction is far from direct and that a number of methodological issues limit conclusions drawn in some of the research.

Martin, McGrath, Brown, and Katz (2007) explored the impact of gender and age on the long-term results of pain management. They interviewed a clinic cohort of children who had been diagnosed with chronic pain a mean of 3 years following their last appointment at a specialized pain clinic for children. The results indicated that a high proportion of children diagnosed with chronic pain continued to experience pain for a prolonged period, with 62% of the sample reporting pain at follow-up. Over half of these individuals reported frequent pain that was adversely impacting their activities of daily living. Of note, females were more likely than males to report continuing pain, to use medication and nonpharmacologic pain control methods, and to receive treatment specifically for their pain.

Stahl et al. (2004) conducted a longitudinal study of pain-free preadolescents over a 4-year period. The results indicated that 21% at 1-year follow-up reported neck pain. However, of those that were not endorsing pain at this time, an assessment at 4 years indicated 32% experienced neck pain, half of which was experienced on a weekly basis. Additionally, half of the children with neck pain at the 1-year follow-up were pain-free at the 4-year assessment. Thus, clinically it appears that neck pain is prone to be rather fluctuating in nature. Lastly, the results indicated that neck pain was significantly more common among girls. Lower limb pain was the most common other pain in conjunction with neck pain at both follow-up assessments. As has been reiterated, lower limb pain has been found to be the most common musculoskeletal pain among children and adolescents (Mikkelson et al., 1997).

El-Metwally, Salminen, Auvinen, Kautiainen, and Mikkelson (2004) evaluated the same cohort 3 years after the 1-year follow-up to determine the extent that musculoskeletal pain recurred at adolescence. They also sought to identify baseline factors that could predict to recurrence of this pain at 4-year follow-up. The results indicated that almost two-thirds of the preadolescents complained of musculoskeletal pain at 4-year follow-up. Moreover, age, headache, hypermobility, and multiple painful musculoskeletal areas were the strongest predictive factors for pain recurrence.

Perquin et al. (2003) assessed the course of chronic "benign" pain in childhood and adolescence prospectively.[1] Chronic pain in this study was classified as a function of time (greater than 3 months of continuous or recurrent pain). These authors attempted to circumvent the possibility that chronic pain sufferers are usually seen in hospital clinics and may not be representative of sufferers in the general population. The results demonstrated that about one-third of those who had chronic benign pain at baseline still had this pain at 2-year follow-up. Girls were also twice as likely to have chronic benign pain at both time intervals. Another aim of this study was to explore pain-related consequences (e.g., quality of life) as well as to attempt to determine predictive variables for the persistence of pain. Emotional problems, mother's self-reported health in general, and the pain frequency were identified as prognostic factors.

[1] Professor John J. Bonica, an anesthesiologist who founded the International Association for the Study of Pain, said that the only pain that is benign is pain being experienced by someone else.

The extant literature is rather consistent in providing evidence that females have a much stronger tendency to experience and endorse symptoms of pain than their male counterparts. While in the past attributions were often made to socialization factors as key to this process, mounting evidence would indicate strong genetic predispositions for sex differences in pain processing that become more pronounced from adolescence into adulthood (Craig & Korol, 2008). Thus, the mechanisms underlying this phenomenon appear to have at least as great a biological basis as socioemotional, and probably far greater.

Research that focuses on multivariate models of risk and resilience for the development and maintenance of recurrent and chronic pain syndromes in children and adolescents continues to expand. In adopting a life span developmental approach (Walco & Harkins, 1999), one can begin to understand the relationship between genetics, early experiences, pain problems in childhood, and difficulties into adulthood and the elderly years. There is a substantial emerging literature that indicates that early life experiences with recurrent untreated pain sets the table for difficulties later on and a wide open area for research focuses on risk and resilience factors that may come into play. With all of that as background, a critical question becomes which of the array of genetic, temperamental, family environment, sociocultural, and broader factors provide main or interaction effects that are substantial enough to be included in clinical pain assessment?

Chronic Pain Assessment in Adolescents

As a general framework to demonstrate the range of possible approaches to assessment, consider the following perspectives. One can argue that the optimal means by which chronic pain is assessed is to "hear the patient's story." In other words, while the clinician may come armed with a great deal of knowledge about pain networks, risk and resilience factors, and specific methods of pain assessment, it is imperative to understand the role of chronic pain in the life of that specific individual. Indeed, intakes in many pediatric chronic pain programs often last close to 2 hours just so that goal may be achieved.

On the other hand, if we were to conduct research on treatment outcomes in chronic pain, such unstandardized approaches would be unacceptable. In that instance, one could turn to the recently published guidelines espoused by the Pediatric Initiative on Methods, Measurement, and Pain Assessment in Clinical Trials (PedsIMMPACT), a consensus panel of experts representing academic clinicians, the US Food and Drug Administration, the National Institutes of Health, and private industry. They reached agreement that investigators conducting pediatric clinical trials in chronic and recurrent pain should consider assessing outcomes in pain intensity; physical functioning; emotional functioning; role functioning; symptoms and adverse events; global judgment of satisfaction with treatment; sleep; and economic factors. Specific measures or measurement strategies were recommended for different age groups for each domain. Thus, depending on the purpose of the assessment, one may enter the continuum of structure as deemed optimal. That is not to say, however, that it is acceptable for the clinician–investigator to come in unarmed with appropriate models for assessment.

Chronic pain in adolescence represents a complicated interplay of "physiological" and "psychological" factors. As research progresses through modalities such as functional magnetic resonance imaging (fMRI) and positron emission tomography (PET scanning), the lines between these two general constructs become much blurrier (May, 2007). At present, however, it is generally accepted that recurrent and chronic pain in childhood and adolescence should be conceptualized dynamically, not dichotomized into either an organic or a psychogenic etiology. Models that embrace biopsychosocial and developmental factors are optimal when evaluating a child with chronic pain (Bursch, Walco, & Zeltzer, 1998).

In the process of evaluating pain, it is important to understand that children are at different stages of cognitive and emotional development. As children age, their abilities to generalize concepts and think abstractly increase. When asked to evaluate their pain, children have a tendency to provide responses that correspond to the Piagetian stages of preoperational, concrete operational, and formal operational thought processes (Gaffney & Dunn, 1986; Savedra, Gibbons, Tesler, Ward,& Wanger, 1982). A typically developing 6 year old can differentiate pain intensity and potentially may be engaged in learning to utilize cognitive strategies for dealing with pain. Between the ages of 7 and 10 years, children are able to communicate the "why" behind the pain and as they get older they begin to make value judgments relevant to their pain experience (McGrath & McAlpine, 1993).

In general, pain assessment may focus on three different channels. As one experiences pain, there are clear physiological changes that may be observed, usually representing autonomic nervous system activity. Because such responses are typically found in acute pain responses and are dampened or absent in chronic pain states, they will not be emphasized here. Second, one may observe the frequency, intensity, and duration of defined pain behaviors. Finally, there are various strategies through which one may gather self-report data from the individual experiencing pain. It is important to note that each of these strategies has its advantages and disadvantages and therefore one must focus on parameters related to the specific issues in question. Furthermore, it is clearly not the case that these parameters necessarily correlate with each other (Walco, Conte, Labay, Engel, & Zeltzer, 2005). Thus, in most clinical settings, data are gathered through a physical examination, observation of pain behaviors, and various self-report and psychometric methods. As an aside, while physical examinations have traditionally been the purview of physicians, in some institutions psychologists have been granted medical staff privileges that include limited physical examinations pertaining to the presenting pain problem.

Physical Examination

In general, the physical examination of an adolescent presenting with chronic pain focuses on the signs and symptoms of pain in the context of the child's and family's reports of the pain. Prior to seeing the patient, it is optimal to review medical records highlighting previous assessments and provisional or stated diagnoses. This helps establish what the patient and family may have been told prior to coming in. As mentioned above, it is also imperative to "hear the family's story," letting the patient and family describe in their own terms the presenting problem, previous assessments, family history of pain, and their expectations as they enter. These elements help to focus observations made as one examines the child.

As discussed by Bursch et al. (1998), the physical examination should take into consideration the child's overall physical presentation, including weight, height, posturing, and whether the child generally appears to be healthy or ill. Other general observations should include the child's mood, the degree to which the child is engaged in the evaluation, and indications of withdrawal, anxiety, distress, or general discomfort.

More specific observations would follow from the presenting problem. For example, with musculoskeletal pain, one may observe guarding, immobilization, or compensatory posturing. Range of motion or strength to resistance in limbs may be compromised as a function of pain. Joints may show indications of swelling, discoloration, mottling, or temperature change. Muscles may have specific areas of sensitivity or tension and the adolescent may demonstrate exaggerated pain responses to tender point stimulation. A comprehensive discussion of specific elements of physical assessment pertaining to the array of recurrent and chronic pain problems in adolescents is beyond the scope of this chapter and the reader is referred to Walco and Goldschneider (2008) for further details.

General Considerations in Structured Pain Assessment

When considering which pain measure to select in assisting with the evaluation of pain, issues of validity, reliability, and developmental appropriateness should be considered. Many available instruments focus on different aspects of the child's pain experience and may incorporate behavioral elements of pain as well as the individual's subjective experience. Children's and adolescents' behavior is not a passive reflection of their pain experience and interpretation of behavioral measures should be done with that in mind and considering the environmental, social and familial factors that can potentially influence one's pain experience (McGrath, 1990). von Bayer and Spagrud (2007) note that when dealing with long-term acute or chronic pain it is important to remember that over time the overt signs of pain that we are accustomed to seeing may be replaced by more covert signs and can be triggered by what the child in pain perceives as social cues. There can be increase irritability, mood fluctuations, and changes in social behaviors. All these imply that there is a need for understanding the child's baseline conditions before we can make treatment and management recommendations.

Interviews

The interview is a source of contextual data that will be critical in understanding the full picture of the child's pain. The interview should include questions reflecting the multiple aspects of pain experience, including location, sensory qualities (e.g., hot, cold, burning, pulsating, pinching, pounding, pushing), tolerability, frequency, intensity, and duration of the pain (McGrath & Gillespie, 2001). One may observe the child's engagement, interest, and level of cooperation in the interview process and how it relates to the family report of pain and behavior. Current level of the child's physical activity, levels of coping, social activity, and academic performance are important to ascertain, as well as the degree of impairment that the child may be experiencing due to the pain.

During the interview, one may also discover that families are modeling behaviors that may or may not be helping the child understand and deal with the pain experience (Dunn-Geier, McGrath, Rourke, Latter, & D'Astous, 2005). Generally, children with prolonged and severe pain do not see themselves as being able to exercise control over their pain and tend to lack adequate coping skills. It helps to have a sense of the child's ability and attitude toward problem solving, which may be ascertained by asking the child direct questions related to their pain experience. Knowing the child and family's coping strategies and styles can be incorporated into a cognitive-behavioral pain management program and a family intervention plan, should those methods prove to be appropriate. Interviews can provide a point of reference for evaluating the possibility of engaging the child in a course of rehabilitation depending on the child and family's attitudes and responses toward pain (Bursch et al., 1998).

The use of semi-structured and structured interviews and questionnaires to assess a variety of dimensions of the child's pain experience allows clinical care providers to be more consistent in collecting, sharing, and comparing information. Table 1 provides an overview of some available questionnaire and interview instruments.

Self-Report Measures and Integrated Scales

Because pain is a subjective experience, self-report measures are central to the assessment of adolescents' pain. As with any other psychometrically based endeavor, properties of reliability, validity, and clinical sensitivity of self-report measures are

Table 1 Some available questionnaire and interview instruments

Title	Age range	Population	Key elements	Reference
The Children's Comprehensive Pain Questionnaire (CCPQ)	5–19 years	Chronic pain and recurrent pain syndromes, principally headache	Semi-structured interview with areas of focus including pain history, subjective pain experience (exacerbating factors, responses, descriptors), intensity, affect, methods of calibration for young children	McGrath (1990)
The Varni–Thompson Pediatric Pain Questionnaire (PPQ) (A parent version is also available)	4–19 years	Measure chronic pain, in a developmentally appropriate way, focusing on pain intensity, emotional and sensory evaluation of pain and pain location	Questionnaire with visual analog scales, body outline, list of pain descriptors, and questions on function and environmental influences on the child's pain	Varni, Thompson, and Hanson (1987)
Functional Disability Inventory (FDI)	School age children and adolescents	Designed to assess functionality in children with recurrent abdominal pain	15 items focused on major areas of physical and psychosocial functioning and level of impairment	Walker and Greene (1991)
Pain Coping Questionnaire (PCQ)	4–17 years	Assess a wide range of pain coping strategies and behaviors	Questionnaire focuses eight types of coping (information seeking, problem solving, seeking social support, positive self-statements, behavioral distraction, cognitive distraction, externalizing, internalizing/catastrophizing) and three higher-order scales (approach, problem-focused avoidance, emotion-focused avoidance)	Reid, Gilbert, and McGrath (1998)
The Pain Experience Interview	5–16 years	Measure acute, recurrent and chronic as a preliminary screening tool and to ascertain the epidemiology of pain problems	Structured interview that includes 56 types of pain, grouped in 6 sections that correspond to pain categories, as well as intensity, affect, duration, and frequency. Relevant categories reflect recurrent pain (headache, stomachache, growing pains); chronic health conditions (sickle cell disease, arthritis, cancer, nerve damage); chronic pain	McGrath et al. (2000)

Table 1 (continued)

Title	Age range	Population	Key elements	Reference
Child Activity Limitations Interview (CALI)	8–16 years	Assessment and monitoring subjective report of functional impairment in children and adolescents with recurrent and chronic pain	Interview format, 21 items, to monitor aspects of pain experience related to sleep and rest; eating; aspects of school; ambulation; mobility; work-related tasks; physical, social, and recreational interactions	Palermo, Witherspoon, Valenzuela, and Drotar (2004)
Bath Adolescent Pain Questionnaire (BAPQ)	11–18 years	Adolescents with chronic pain	Parent rating scales that are scored on dimensions of social functioning, physical functioning, depression, general anxiety, pain-specific anxiety, family functioning, development	Eccleston et al. (2005); Eccleston, McCracken, Jordan, and Sleed (2007)

essential, as well as the important element of developmental propriety as one advances through stages of childhood into adolescence (McGrath & Gillespie, 2001; McGrath, Unruh, & Branson, 1990). Even with psychometrically sound instruments, however, there is still a possibility of bias, as adolescents may over- or under-report on certain items, depending on perceptions or anticipation of treatment goals, progress, therapeutic alliance, and desired outcomes (Williams, Davies, & Chadury, 2000).

Regardless of the pain measures chosen, it is important to keep in mind that research in the field of pain assessment is an ongoing process, scales are revised, and new measures are developed. An integrated approach to assessment and monitoring is most likely to provide the most comprehensive information regarding the dimensions that influence the child's perception of pain.

Beyond evaluating pain at a single point in time, diaries may be useful to provide important information related to the quality of life and adjustment to daily living in real time. The diary can potentially be used as an adjunct to assist with pinpointing and evaluating some of the rehabilitation goals of treatment. Newer strategies of gathering such data include electronic media, such as a personal digital assistant (PDA), that enhance the accuracy of the data as they are recorded in real time, even several times per day and at set time intervals. Such methods increase the accuracy of results as the risk of excessive prospective or retrospective recording is minimized (Palermo, Valenzuela, & Stork, 2004).

Psychometric Assessment

In some instances, additional information related to the academic functioning of an adolescent with chronic pain may be obtained through an evaluation of academic achievement, cognitive skills, and abilities. Results of neuropsychological testing can provide insight into academic and cognitive difficulties present prior to the onset of chronic pain syndromes. This can be useful information when used in combination with the interview, pain intensity measures, and physicians report to create a rehabilitation plan for the child (Bursch et al., 1998).

Logan, Simons, Stein and Chastain (2008) explored school impairment in adolescent with chronic pain. It was noted that school attendance in negatively impacted by chronic pain and that children who experienced functional abdominal pain and nonmigrainous headaches had increased school absenteeism. Chronic pain contributed to the decline in academic performance as shown by declining grades, parent report, and adolescent self-report. Although the antecedent-consequence or cause–effect relationships between learning difficulties and chronic pain are very difficult to discern, psychometric testing can be a useful tool in guiding interventions.

Finally, the specific interface between chronic pain and psychiatric comorbidity is often a thorny issue. Depression, for example, is a common presenting feature in adolescents with chronic pain, but it is impossible to define it as a cause, an effect, or as two factors with a common third etiology.

Although few studies have tested their utility in a pediatric chronic pain setting (especially in contrast to adult populations), psychometric instruments such as the MMPI-Adolescent version may be used to cast light on these issues.

Treatment Modalities

To adequately treat recurrent and chronic pain in children, one must move away from the dichotomous perspective that pain is either physiologically or psychogenically based. It is always both and, as mentioned above, as the line between the two grows increasingly faint, it is likely that in the near future these constructs will be unified. If a gastroenterologist evaluates a child with abdominal pain and gleans no clear physiological basis for the pain goes on to make a pronouncement that the child has psychological or psychiatric issues at the root of the problem, we would judge that reasoning as naïve. A psychologist who looks for specific emotional or social conflicts to be causal of abdominal pain is equally naïve and neither position is reasonable (Rosenfeld & Walco, 1997).

In order to address the range of factors involved in the assessment and treatment of chronic pain, interdisciplinary or multidisciplinary models are optimal. A pain management approach that integrates pharmacological, psychological, and physical interventions is more likely to have a higher rate of success (Weisman, 2008) in treating the majority of chronic pain problems. A critical first step is communication so that members of the treatment team, the adolescent, and the family are all "on the same page," establishing, sharing, and pursuing treatment goals (Zeltzer et al., 1997; Bursch et al., 1998).

Pharmacological Pain Management

Consideration of the most appropriate medication for the treatment of chronic pain is guided by the etiology of the pain and the neurophysiology of the pain mechanisms involved. A very general overview of the issues follows as detailed discussion of specific analgesics and matching them to clinical conditions and prescribing concerns for a pediatric or adolescent population is well beyond the scope of this chapter. The reader is referred to Walco and Goldschneider (2008) for this information.

If there is a condition in which there is a good deal of nociceptive stimulation, analgesics that minimize that stimulation or block receptor sites in the central nervous system are in order. For relatively low levels of pain, nonsteroidal anti-inflammatory medications (NSAIDs), such as acetaminophen, ibuprofen, and naproxen reduce inflammation and pain. Moderate pain typically involves the use of weaker opioids, such as oxycodone, tramadol, or codeine. Severe pain is managed with stronger opioids, such as morphine, hydromorphone, or fentanyl. Routes of administration and dosing schedules may be adjusted to best address the presenting pain problem. In addition, the advent of time-released preparations enables the clinician to get good "round the clock" coverage of pain, coupled with shorter acting preparations to treat breakthrough episodes.

If pain is deemed to have a neuropathic component, the use of antidepressants or anticonvulsants may be in order. These drugs are long acting and affect basic neural mechanisms, such as neuronal firing or neurotransmitter levels. They are not intended for short-term relief of pain. Common medications include low doses of tricyclic antidepressants (e.g. nortriptyline or amitriptyline), selective serotonin reuptake inhibitors (SSRIs), selective serotonin and norepinephrine reuptake inhibitors (SSNRIs), and anticonvulsants (e.g., gabapentin).

Finally, for specific indications, anesthesiologic agents may be introduced. This may include topical preparations of lidocaine for conditions such as complex regional pain syndrome, as well as nerve blocks at various points in the somatic or sympathetic nervous systems. The latter may be especially useful as a means to reduce or eliminate pain while aggressive physical rehabilitation is implemented, once again emphasizing the need for interdisciplinary approaches to the problem.

Psychological Strategies

Psychological strategies are generally couched within a rehabilitation model of chronic pain treatment, the goals of which are (1) to improve function and (2) to improve the patient's subjective pain experience. The former is most typically accomplished through behavioral and cognitive-behavioral programs aimed at reducing "pain behavior" and maximizing "well behavior." The latter principally involves cognitive-behavioral or self-regulatory strategies aimed at modifying the intensity, frequency, and duration of pain. Although there are few studies with large samples, random assignment, and valid control groups, available data indicate that psychological interventions show very good promise in treating multiple aspects of chronic pain in adolescents (Eccleston, Malleson, Clinch, Connell, & Sourburt, 2003; Walco, Sterling, Conte, & Engel, 1999).

Pain Behavior Regulation

The pain behavior regulation approach focuses on reducing the frequency, intensity, and duration of pain behaviors while increasing wellness behaviors (Bursch et al., 1998). Thus, the first step in this behavioral process is to clearly define these behaviors. Pain behavior includes staying home from school, resting, being excused from household activities, etc., while well behaviors include regular, full-time school attendance, socializing with peers, engaging in physical activities, etc. Structured operant approaches may then be applied to successively approximate the desired behavior.

For example, a child with pervasive musculoskeletal pain has been out of school for 2 months. The child has an erratic sleep pattern, often getting out of bed in the late morning. Physical activity is extremely limited and interactions with peers are becoming less frequent. Steps to a behavioral program may include

1. Improved sleep hygiene. The child must arise every morning (Monday through Friday) at the exact same time as would be needed to attend school. Naps are eliminated.
2. Daily routine. The child would then go into the normal morning routine, being completely dressed, having eaten, etc., so that all is in place by the usual time to leave for school.
3. Approximating the school day. At the time school starts, the child is asked to sit in a chair and do schoolwork for 45 minutes, followed by a 5 minute break and then another 45 minutes in the chair doing schoolwork. This roughly approximates first and second period in school. Over time the day is expanded until full-time re-entry into school is feasible, often time in as short as 2–3 weeks.
4. Physical activity. The child is asked to engage in aerobic exercise for 15–20 minutes every other day. Obviously this must be done in collaboration with the attending physician or rehabilitation specialist as in some conditions exercise is contraindicated. For most chronic pain problems, this is very rarely the case, however. The duration and frequency of exercise activities may then be systematically increased over time.

This entire plan is discussed with the child and parent together so that there is no disagreement about the details. Often working with school personnel is a key step so that they may cooperate with the process. In addition, school re-entry is not negotiable. Once a specific date is chosen for this to occur, the child must go daily and pain is not a reason to stay home. Because parents often have difficulty with this element, we often have the child contact us directly if they want to stay home and only with our mutual agreement may they do so. Children are not completely jokingly warned that in the past two decades, there have been extremely few instances when absenteeism was deemed appropriate.

Central to this process is helping the adolescent to problem solve. They are taught to distinguish and choose between behaviors that ultimately increase the desired outcomes and decrease the unwanted ones. Once that distinction is made, the focus turns to what elements need to be in place to move toward the goal, rather than the more typical passive and catastrophizing view of reasons "why not" or those that focus on what may happen only after the pain is better. Often these procedures need to be combined with family intervention as these behavior patterns are not only foreign to the child, but parents need to adapt as well.

Changing Pain Perceptions

Not surprisingly, if one sits down with an adolescent experiencing chronic pain and lays out the above program, a common response is "How can I do all of those things, I am in too much pain!" Thus, one must provide a detailed discussion of the relationship between pain and function, emphasizing that this is a reciprocal, not a unidirectional relationship. In other words, pain begets decreased functioning, but it is also true that diminished functioning begets more pain. Second, the adolescent may be taught self-regulatory strategies to better modulate pain. Motivation to do so is in fact elevated in the wake of discussing the above behavioral program.

The goal of cognitive-behavioral methods is to teach the child to control pain behaviors or to give the child a sense of control over the subjective pain experience. These can be accomplished through distraction, imagery, and transformation (McGrath, Dick, & Unruh, 2003; Bursch et al., 1998). Distraction is anything that takes the attention of the pain, imagery typically involves representation of scenery that the child would find pleasant, soothing, and antithetical to pain, while transformation focuses on the level of perception, attitude, and behavior related to pain, attempting to change what is typically seen as unbearable into manageable.

Progressive muscle relaxation utilizes step by step processes to induce complete body relaxation. Because one reflexively guards painful areas, often individuals with chronic pain (especially musculoskeletal) have a good deal of muscle pain. Relaxation begins to alleviate much of that pressure and it gives the child a sense of control and reduces autonomic reactivity of the body (McGrath et al., 2003).

Relaxation strategies may be enhanced with biofeedback, in which electronic equipment is used to monitor physiologic parameters (e.g. heart, rate, muscle tension) to demonstrate changes invoked by the child. Both thermal biofeedback (learning to increase skin temperature in the extremities) and EMG biofeedback (learning to reduce muscle tension, particularly in the frontalis muscles of the forehead) have been shown to be effective treatments for pediatric headache, for example (McGrath et al., 2003).

Guided imagery involves creating a scene that is pleasant, often relaxing, and that is inconsistent with pain. The image is generated with the patient, helping them to interact with the scene and invoke as many of the five senses as possible. It is used principally to distract the child away from painful and distressing sensations.

Hypnosis may be deemed more transitional in property and it has been shown to produce positive pain relief in children and adolescents. In more formal terms, there are two basic components to hypnotherapy. The preinduction stage, which requires that the clinician engage the child at an age-appropriate level to find out the child's interest, fears, and dreams. This information will be used to create an appropriate explanation of what is about to happen and to integrate the child's natural tendencies into the strategies as they are invoked. In the induction stage, the clinician uses various techniques and guides the child into a greater state of absorption and distancing from the pain experience (Kuttner & Solomon, 2003).

Rather than distracting away from pain, a goal in hypnosis is often to use metaphors to alter the perceptual experience. Standard strategies, such as the use of a "pain switch" or a "magic glove" (Kuttner, 1996), may be used to reduce pain intensity. One can also use the patient's description of the pain as a key metaphor to be used to reduce pain intensity. For example, if headache pain is described as "a tight band is wrapped around my head, squeezing it," then a reasonable image under hypnosis is to unwrap or alleviate the tension from the band. Techniques that use images to reduce pain in this manner seek to induce hypnoanalgesia; those that seek to remove sensation completely (e.g., make a limb completely numb) are called hypnoanesthesia.

Finally, one's attitude toward and perceptions of pain may be addressed with cognitive-behavioral strategies. Acceptance and Commitment Therapy (ACT) is a CBT-derived approach based on learning theory that emphasizes the acceptance of pain. The goal is to increase "psychological flexibility." The therapist guides the patient to identify and achieve value-based goals and to learn new sets of behaviors that assist in coping with pain (Wicksell, Dahl, & Olsson, 2005; McCracken, Vowles, & Eccleston, 2005). Wicksell, Melin, and Olsson (2007) conducted a pilot study with adolescents using the ACT principles and reported that given the opportunity and the training to reconceptualize their pain experience from negative events associated with avoidance into events of acceptance, adolescents were able to increase functionality and reduce pain.

Family Intervention and Social Implications of Pain

Eccleston et al. (2003) showed the treatment of chronic pain in adolescents is enhanced by a family-inclusive, broad-based, multidisciplinary approach. The family unit is an integral part of the child's environment and as such it is important to assess the family environment and involve the family as early on in the assessment and treatment process as possible.

Children learn many coping behaviors through modeling – observing and imitating those who are close to them. Parents can also influence their child's state of anxiety and cue the child's situational responses (Zeltzer et al., 1997). It is important to educate and empower the family to understand the behaviors and coping strategies used by family members that can potentially impact the pain behaviors and coping strategies of the child or adolescent. Family involvement should depend on the needs of the child or adolescent, the nature, duration and type of treatment as well as available resources (Bursch et al., 1998).

Physical Interventions

As part of a rehabilitation effort, physical and occupational therapy strategies may be exceedingly helpful. Typical regimens are designed to strengthen, increase range of motion, or increase flexibility. In addition, for complex regional pain syndrome, rehabilitation efforts also include desensitization so that allodynia and hypersensitivity may be contained and reduced.

Physical therapists may also introduce transcutaneous electrical stimulation (TENS), which is a method to stimulate nerves through electrodes applied to the skin. Although the precise mechanism of action is not clear, currents are used to "disrupt" the transmission of nociceptive impulses, typically in an extremity. TENS has no serious complications beyond allergic reactions to the application gel or the extremely rare electrical burn. TENS is most effective when pain is localized rather than diffuse, and thus has shown some good promise for complex regional pain syndrome (Sahinler, 2002).

Summary and Future Directions

Conceptual models of recurrent and chronic pain are rapidly evolving. It is clear that the dichotomy of physiological and psychological factors is passé, unhelpful, and invalid. Psychologists who seek "emotional" bases for pain symptoms are doing a huge disservice to patients as holism, emphasizing the true integration of physiological and psychological processes, is the current model of choice. Psychobiological paradigms that embrace genetic factors, temperament, developmental phenomena, the impact of life experiences, and an array of contextual factors are currently deemed most appropriate to understanding chronic and recurrent pain problems and these elements should be woven into the comprehensive assessment and treatment of recurrent and chronic pain in adolescents.

In addition being armed with conceptual and empirical models regarding chronic and recurrent pain, it is essential to understand how these symptoms fit into the broader context of one's life. This may be accomplished to some degree with standardized instruments or interviews, but it also requires a good deal of listening and observation to hear the individual's story and construct treatment strategies that are consistent with that unique constellation of elements.

Treatment approaches may include various pharmacological, psychological, physical, and complementary or alternative strategies. Although it is not expected that psychologists would have expertise in all of these areas, it is important to have sufficient understanding to function as an effective member of an interdisciplinary team. The traditional boundaries and roles of respective professionals have been challenged as the pediatric pain community is clearly quite multidisciplinary in nature and it is not clear that any constituency is more central than another.

Psychologists have a good deal to offer clinically, especially in the implementation of cognitive-behavioral strategies targeting rehabilitation and more adaptive behavioral responses. In addition, because they understand the importance of developmental processes, their expertise in research methodology is central to the field. Further, because a major focus of chronic pain treatment is assessment, both of one's perceptual experience as well as an array of contextual factors, psychologists may play a pivotal role in the development of the field. Thus, the role of psychology in clinical and research endeavors focusing on recurrent and chronic pain is extremely important and provides a major opportunity for the growth of the field.

References

American Pain Society Pediatric Chronic Pain Task Force. (1999). *Pediatric chronic pain: A position paper from the American Pain Society*. Glenview, IL: American Pain Society.

Brun Sundblad, G. M., Saartok T., & Engstrom L. M. (2007). Prevalence and co-occurrence of self-rated pain and perceived health in school-children: Age and gender differences. *European Journal of Pain, 11*, 171–180.

Bursch, B., Walco, G. A., & Zeltzer, L. (1998). Clinical assessment and management of chronic pain and pain-associated disability syndrome. *Journal of Developmental and Behavioral Pediatrics, 19*, 45–53.

Craig, K. D. & Korol, C. T. (2008). Developmental issues in understanding, assessing, and managing pediatric pain. In G. A. Walco & K. R. Goldschneider (Eds.), *Pain in children: A practical guide for primary care* (pp. 9–20). Totowa, NJ: Humana Press.

Dunn-Geier, B., McGrath, P. J., Rourke, B. P., Latter, J. D., & Astous, J. (1986). Adolescent chronic pain: The ability to cope. *Pain, 26*, 23–32.

Eccleston, C., Jordan, A., McCracken, L. M., Sleed, M., Connell, H., & Clinch J. (2005). The Bath Adolescent Pain Questionnaire (BAPQ): development and preliminary psychometric evaluation of an instrument to assess the impact of chronic pain on adolescents. *Pain, 118*, 263–270.

Eccleston, C., Malleson, P. N., Clinch, J., Connell, H., & Sourburt, C. (2003). Chronic pain in adolescents: Evaluation of a programme of interdisciplinary cognitive behavioral therapy. *Archives of Disease in Childhood, 88*, 881–885.

Eccleston, C., McCracken, L. M., Jordan, A., & Sleed, M. (2007). Development and preliminary psychometric evaluation of the parent report version of the Bath Adolescent Pain Questionnaire (BAPQ-P): A multidimensional parent report instrument to assess the impact of chronic pain on adolescents. *Pain, 131*, 48–56.

Eccleston, C., Morley, S, Williams, A., Yorke, L., & Mastroyannopoulou, A. (2003). Psychological therapies for the management of chronic and recurrent pain in children and adolescents. Cochrane Database of Systematic Reviews, (1):CD003968.

El-Metwally, A., Salminen, J. J., Auvinen, A., Kautiainen, H., & Mikkelson, M. (2004). Prognosis of non-specific musculoskeletal pain in preadolescents: A prospective 4-year follow-up still till adolescence. *Pain, 110*, 550–559.

Gaffney, A., & Dunn, E. (1986). Development components of children's definition of pain. *Pain, 26*, 105–117.

IASP Task Force on Taxonomy. (1994). *Classification of chronic pain: Descriptions of chronic pain syndromes and definitions of pain terms* (2nd ed.). Seattle, WA: IASP Press.

Kuttner, L. (1996). *A child in pain: How to help, what to do.* Point Roberts, WA: Hartly & Marks Publishers.

Kuttner, L., & Solomon, R. (2003). Hypnotherapy and imagery for managing children's pain. In N. L. Schechter, C. B. Berde, & M. Yaster (Eds.), *Pain in infants, children, and adolescents* (pp. 317–328). Philadelphia, PA: Lippincott Williams & Wilkins

Logan, D. E., Simons, L. E., Stein, M. J., & Chastain, L. (2008). School impairment in adolescents with chronic pain. *Journal of Pain, 9*, 407–416.

Martin, A. L., McGrath P. A., Brown S. C., & Katz, J. (2007). Children with chronic pain: Impact of sex and age on long term outcomes. *Pain, 128*, 13–19.

May, A. (2007). Neuroimaging: visualising the brain in pain. *Neurological Sciences, 28* (Suppl. 2), S101–107.

McCracken, L., Vowles, K., & Eccleston, C. (2005). Acceptance-based treatment for persons with complex, long standing chronic pain: a preliminary analysis of treatment outcome in comparison to a waiting phase. *Behavior Research and Therapy, 43*, 1335–1346.

McGrath, P. A. (1990). *Pain in children: Nature, assessment, and treatment*. New York, NY: Guilford Press.

McGrath, P. J., Dick, B., & Unruh, A. (2003). Psychological and behavioral treatment of pain in children and adolescents. In N. L. Schechter, C. B. Berde, & M. Yaster (Eds.), *Pain in infants, children, and adolescents* (2nd ed., pp. 303–316). Philadelphia: Lippincott Williams & Wilkins.

McGrath, P. A., & Gillespie J. (2001). Pain assessment in children and adolescents. In D. C. Turk & R. Melzack (Eds.), *Handbook of pain assessment* (2nd ed., pp. 97–118). New York, NY: Guilford Press.

McGrath, P. J., & McAlpine, L. (1993). Psychologic perspectives on pediatric pain. *Journal of Pediatrics, 122*, S2–S8.

McGrath, P. J., Unruh, A. M., & Branson, S. M. (1990). Chronic nonmalignant pain with disability. In D. C. Tyler & E. J. Krane (Eds.), *Advances in pain research and therapy: Pediatric pain* (Vol. 15, pp. 255–271). New York: Raven Press.

McGrath, P. J., Walco, G. A., Turk, D. C., Dworkin, R. H., Brown, M. T., Davidson, K., et al. (in press). Core outcome domains and measures for pediatric acute and chronic/recurrent pain clinical trials: PedIMMPACT recommendations. *Journal of Pain*.

Mikkelson, M., Salminen, J. J., & Kautiainen, H. (1997). Non-specific musculoskeletal pain in preadolescents. Prevalence and 1-year persistence. *Pain, 73*, 29–35.

Palermo, T. M., Valenzuela, D., & Stork, P. P. (2004). A randomized trial of electronic versus paper pain diaries in children: Impact on compliance, accuracy and acceptability. *Pain, 107*, 213–219.

Perquin, C. W., Hazebroek-Kampscheur, A. A. J. M., Hunfeld, J. A. M., van Suijlekom-Smit, L. W. A., Passchier, J., van der Wouden, J. C. (2001). Chronic pain among children and adolescents: physician consultation and medication use. *Clinical Journal of Pain, 16*, 229–235.

Perquin, C. W., Hunfeld, J. A., Hazebroek-Kampschreur, A. A., van Suijlekom-Smit, L. W., Passchier, J., Koes, B. W., et al. (2003). The natural course of chronic benign pain in childhood and adolescence: A two-year population-based follow-up study. *European Journal of Pain, 7*, 551–559.

Powers, S. W., Gilman, D. K., & Hershey, A. D. (2006). Headache and psychological functioning in children and adolescents. *Headache, 46*, 1404–1415.

Reid, G. J., Gilbert, C. A., & McGrath, P. J. (1998). The pain coping questionnaire: Preliminary validation. *Pain, 76*, 83–96.

Rosenfeld, W. D., & Walco, G. A. (1997). One test too many: Toward an integrated approach to psychosomatic disorders. *Adolescent Medicine State of the Art Reviews, 8*, 483–487.

Sahinler, B. A. (2002). Review of pediatric pain management in acute and chronic settings. *Pain Practice, 2*, 137–150.

Savedra, M. C., Gibbons, P. T., Tesler, M. D., Ward, J. A., & Wanger, C. (1982). How children describe pain? A tentative assessment. *Pain, 14*, 95–104.

Stahl, M., Mikkelsson, M., Kautiainen, H., Hakkinen, A., Ylinen, J., & Salminen, J. J. (2004). Neck pain in adolescence. A 4-year follow-up of pain-free preadolescents. *Pain, 110*, 427–431.

Varni, J. W., Thompson, K. L., & Hanson, V. (1987). The Varni-Thompson pediatric pain questionnaire: Chronic musculoskeletal pain in juvenile rheumatoid arthritis. *Pain, 28*, 27–38.

von Bayer, C. L., & Spagrud, L. J. (2007). Systematic review of observational (behavioral) measures of pain for children and adolescents ages 3 to 18 years. *Pain, 127*, 140–150.

Walco, G. A. (in press). Needle pain in children: Contextual factors. *Pediatrics*, Supplement 2008-1055 Optimizing the Management of Peripheral Venous Access Pain in Children: Evidence, Impact, and Implementation.

Walco, G. A., Conte, P. C., Labay, L. E., Engel, R., & Zeltzer, L. K. (2005). Procedural distress in children with cancer: Self-report, behavioral observations, and physiological parameters. *Clinical Journal of Pain, 21*, 484–490.

Walco, G. A., & Goldschneider, K. R. (Eds.) (2008). *Pain in children: A practical guide for primary care*. Totowa, NJ: Humana Press.

Walco, G. A., & Harkins, S. (1999). Life-span developmental approaches to pain. In R. J. Gatchel & D. C. Turk (Eds.), *Psychosocial factors in pain: Critical perspectives* (pp. 107–117). New York: Guilford Publications.

Walco, G. A., Sterling, C. N., Conte, P. M., & Engel, R. G. (1999). Empirically supported treatments in pediatric psychology: Disease related pain. *Journal of Pediatric Psychology, 24*, 155 167.

Walker, L. S., & Greene J. W. (1991). The functional disability inventory: Measuring a neglected dimension of child health status. *Journal of Pediatric Psychology, 16*, 39–58.

Weisman, S. J. (2008). Multidisciplinary approaches to chronic pain. In G. A. Walco & K. R. Goldschneider (Eds.), *Pain in children: A practical guide for primary care* (pp. 133–143). Totowa, NJ: Humana Press.

Wicksell, R. K., Dahl, J., & Olsson, G. L. (2005). Using acceptance and commitment therapy in a rehabilitation of an adolescent female with chronic pain: A case study. *Cognitive and Behavioral Pediatrics, 12*, 415–423.

Wicksell, R. K., Melin, L., & Olsson, G., (2007). Exposure and acceptance in the rehabilitation of adolescents with idiopathic chronic pain – A pilot study. *European Journal of Pain, 11*, 264–274.

Williams, A. C., Davies, H. T., & Chadury, Y. (2000). Simple pain rating scales hide complex idiosyncratic meanings. *Pain, 85*, 457–463.

Wolfe, F., Smythe, H. A., Yunus, M. B., Bennett, R. M., Bombardier, C., Goldenberg, D. L., et al. (1990). The American College of Rheumatology 1990 criteria for the classification of fibromyalgia: report of the multicenter criteria committee. *Arthritis and Rheumatism, 33*, 160–172.

Woolf, C. J., & Salter, M. W. (2000). Neuronal plasticity: Increasing the gain in pain. *Science, 288*, 1765–1769.

Woolf, C. J., Shortland, P., & Coggeshall, R. E. (1992). Peripheral nerve injury triggers central sprouting of myelinated afferents. *Nature, 355*, 75–78.

Yunus, M. B., & Masi, A. T. (1985). Juvenile primary fibromyalgia syndrome. A clinical study of thirty-three patients and matched normal controls. *Arthritis & Rheumatism, 28*, 138–145.

Zeltzer, L., Bursch B., & Walco G. (1997). Pain responsiveness and chronic pain: A psychobiological perspective. *Journal of Developmental and Behavioral Pediatrics, 18*, 413–422.

Adolescent Depression

Brandyn M. Street and Judy Garber

Feelings of sadness and despondency in the face of a disappointment or loss are both natural and expected. All adolescents occasionally experience distress and sadness. When such dysphoria lingers for weeks, months, or longer and limit the individual's ability to function, then the person may be suffering from major depressive disorder (MDD), which can have adverse consequences on an adolescent's academic performance, social life, and family relationships (Harrington & Dubicka, 2001; Kessler, Foster, Saunders, & Stang, 1995). MDD is also associated with several other mental health problems, suicide, and hospitalizations (Fergusson & Woodward, 2002; Lewinsohn, Rohde, & Seeley, 1998; Rohde, Kahler, Lewinsohn, Brown, 2004; Resnick et al., 1997; Weissman et al., 1999) and is the most common mental health disorder in the United States (Kessler, Berglund, Demler, Jin, & Walters, 2005).

Given the severity and chronicity of depression, it is important for health providers to learn to identify and diagnose mood disorders and to become familiar with evidence-based treatments. This chapter reviews the epidemiology, phenomenology, diagnosis, course, and treatment of depression in adolescents. We begin with a discussion of the nature, core features, and phenomenology of depression. Next, we review issues concerning the detection of MDD in community settings and provide an overview of current empirically supported psychopharmacologic and psychotherapeutic treatments. We end with suggestions for a research agenda concerning depression in adolescents.

Epidemiology

Depression is a common disorder in both community (Lewinsohn et al., 1998) and clinical populations (Birmaher, Arbelaez, & Brent, 2002). Rates of depressive disorders increase during early to middle adolescence, particularly in females (Costello, Mustillo, Erkanli, Keeler, & Angold, 2003; Hankin et al., 1998), with the peak age of onset occurring at about 13–15 years old. Whereas the rates of depression in pre-pubescent children are about equal in boys and girls (Nolen-Hoeksema & Girgus, 1994; Speier, Sherak, Hirsch, & Cantwell, 1995), by about age 14, the 2:1 female to male ratio begins to emerge (Angold, Erkanli, Silberg, Eaves, & Costello, 2002; Costello et al., 2003; Hankin et al., 1998; Lewinsohn et al., 1998).

Depressed adolescent females are more likely to experience weight or appetite disturbances, worthlessness or guilt, and suicidal ideation (Lewinsohn et al., 1998; Yorbik, Birmaher, Axelson, Williamson, & Ryan, 2004) and to have more recurrences than males (Lewinsohn & Essau, 2002). Explanations for the increased rate of depression in females starting in adolescence have included interactions among biological, psychological, and sociological factors that

Street was supported in part from an NIMH-funded training grant (T32MH18921); Garber was supported in part from an NIMH Independent Scientist Award (K02 MH66249) and grants from the National Institute of Mental Health (R01 MH57822; R01MH 064735).

B.M. Street (✉)
Vanderbilt University, Nashville, TN, USA
e-mail: brandyn.street@vanderbilt.edu

W.T. O'Donohue, L.W. Tolle (eds.), *Behavioral Approaches to Chronic Disease in Adolescence*,
DOI 10.1007/978-0-387-87687-0_15, © Springer Science+Business Media, LLC 2009

emerge over time (Cyranowski, Frank, Young, & Shear, 2000; Hankin & Abramson, 2001; Hyde, Mezulis, & Abramson, 2008; Nolen-Hoeksema & Girgus, 1994).

Lifetime prevalence rates of MDD in adolescents have been found to range from 1.9 to 18.4% (Lewinsohn & Essau, 2002; Lewinsohn, Rohde, Seeley, Klein, & Gotlib, 2000; Rao, Hammen, & Daley, 1999). In one of the most comprehensive epidemiological surveys in the United States, the National Comorbidity Study, lifetime prevalence rate of MDD in adolescents was reported to be 14%, and subsyndromal or minor depression was found in 10–20% of youth (Kessler & Walters, 2002). An even higher percentage of adolescents (20–50%) report significant levels of symptoms on questionnaires (Kessler, Avenevoli, & Merikangas, 2001). Depressive symptoms show an increasing trajectory during adolescence (Ge, Lorenz, Conger, Elder, & Simons, 1994), are associated with significant impairment (Gotlib, Lewinsohn, & Seeley, 1995), and predict the onset of subsequent clinical disorders (Angst, Sellaro, & Merikangas, 2000; Pine, Cohen, Cohen, & Brook, 1999).

Major depressive episodes (MDE) during adolescence have been found to last from 7 to 9 months in clinical samples (Birmaher et al., 2002; Rao et al., 1995), about 26 weeks in community samples (Lewinsohn, Clarke, Seeley, & Rohde, 1994), and about 24 weeks in high-risk offspring (Kaminski & Garber, 2002). Although most MDEs remit within 2 years, depression during adolescence is highly recurrent, with as many as 40% of adolescents experiencing another MDE within 2–5 years after recovery (Birmaher et al., 1996; Rao et al., 1999). Among psychotic or otherwise severely depressed adolescents, approximately 25% develop bipolar disorder within 5 years (Birmaher et al., 1996).

Evidence of continuity from adolescent to adult depression (e.g., Lewinsohn, Rohde, Klein, & Seeley, 1999; Rao et al., 1995) is stronger than for prepubertal-onset to adolescent or adult depression (Harrington, Fudge, Rutter, Pickles, & Hill, 1990). Although 75% of adults who had been diagnosed with a depressive disorder by age 26 reported having had a depressive episode during childhood or adolescence (Kim-Cohen et al., 2003), differences in the predictors and correlates of depression have been found from childhood through adulthood such as heritability (Lau & Eley, 2008; Rice, Harold, & Thapar, 2002) and family adversity (Harrington, Rutter, & Fombonnne, 1996).

Onset and Course

A common time for the first onset of depression is between 15 and 19 years old (Haarasilta, Marttunen, Kaprio, & Aro, 2001; Lewinsohn et al., 1998), with earlier age of onset associated with being female, lower parental education, the presence of psychiatric comorbidity (i.e., anxiety, conduct disorder, substance abuse), and a history of suicide attempts (Lewinsohn et al., 1998). Although adolescence often is a time of increasing self-awareness, young people with MDD and/or their parents may not recognize the possible seriousness of persistent sadness that may need evaluation and treatment. Additionally problematic is the perceived stigma many adolescents associate with the mental health care system (Jaycox et al., 2006). Jaycox et al. (2006) found that nearly half of adolescents who screened positive for depression reported that their relationships with friends would suffer more if they thought they had a recent history of depression or visited a mental health professional than if they had asthma or HIV/AIDS.

The course of MDD in adolescents is often characterized by frequent recurrence (Rao et al., 1995). Emslie et al. (1997) reported that 61% of their sample of depressed youth experienced an additional depressive episode within 2 years. Rao et al. (1999) reported that 47% of their sample experienced a recurrent MDE within 5 years, with the first year following recovery being the time of highest risk. Variables associated with recurrence include a previous depressive episode, parental psychopathology, family conflict, and negative cognitive style (Birmaher et al., 2002).

Untreated depression has been found to be a risk factor for physical health concerns, conduct problems, substance use, interpersonal conflict, educational and occupational underachievement, increasing levels of functional impairment, and recurrent episodes in adult life (Kovacs, Feinberg, Crose-Novak, Paulauskas, & Finkelstein, 1984;

Lewinsohn et al., 1998; Rohde et al., 2004; Resnick et al., 1997; Weissman et al., 1999). In addition, adolescents experiencing severe depression are at increased risk for suicidal ideation and behavior (Lewinsohn et al., 1998; Ryan et al., 1987). According to the Center for Disease Control and Prevention (2004), suicide is the third most common cause of death among adolescents and depression is the second highest predictor of completed suicide in adolescent males (Shaffer & Craft, 1999).

Studies also have shown a relation between adolescent depression and subsequent medical problems including migraine headaches, allergies, asthma, and tobacco dependence (Bardone et al., 1998; Kramer et al., 1998; Rohde, Lewinsohn, & Seeley, 1994). The link between adolescent depression and medical problems may be explained biologically, behaviorally, cognitively, and socially. For example, depression may undermine the immune system, thereby increasing susceptibility to health problems (Kiecolt-Glaser & Glaser, 2002). Symptom and behaviors that characterize depression and that can exacerbate risk for medical problems include sleep problems, lack of exercise, and poor appetite and nutrition (Cohen & Rodriguez, 1995). Further, depression is associated with maladaptive social functioning, which likely disrupts the social connectedness that can be beneficial to physical health (Cohen, 2004). Thus, untreated depression may lay the foundation for many other kinds of mental and physical disorders and impairment to develop.

Depressive symptoms among adolescents are relatively common and adolescent-onset depressive disorder tends to be recurrent (Kovacs et al., 1984). However, 70% of depressed youth go without appropriate treatment (Kataoka, Zhang, & Wells, 2002) because of multiple family, child, and healthcare system factors. Parents often do not recognize affective problems in their children (Cantwell, Lewinsohn, Rohde, & Seeley, 1997) and may mistake a child with depressive symptoms as merely quiet or irritable. In addition, youth may not communicate mental health concerns to their primary care provider, particularly when practitioners have limited time and experience with evaluating and treating depressive disorders (Jaycox et al., 2006).

Clinical Presentation

Depression in adolescents is characterized by a pervasive and persistent unhappy or irritable mood and/or loss of interest or pleasure in usual activities (i.e., anhedonia). According to the Diagnostic and Statistical Manual, fourth edition in revision (DSM-IV-TR; American Psychiatric Association, 2000), the same criteria are used to diagnose depression across development, except that in children and adolescents irritability can be one of the mood symptoms, and only 1-year duration is required for dysthymia. To qualify for a diagnosis of a major depressive disorder (MDD) five of the following symptoms are required, one of which must be either a mood disturbance or anhedonia: (1) depressed and/or irritable (in children and adolescents) mood for most of the day, (2) loss of interest or pleasure in most activities (i.e., anhedonia), (3) decreased or increased appetite and/or significant weight gain or weight loss, (4) insomnia and/or hypersomnia, (5) psychomotor agitation and/or retardation, (6) fatigue, loss of energy, (7) feelings of worthlessness and/or inappropriate or excessive guilt, (8) difficulty concentrating and/or making decisions, and (9) recurrent thoughts of death and/or suicidal ideation or behaviors. These symptoms should represent a change from previous functioning, be impairing, and persist for at least 2 weeks. The average duration of an episode of MDD in youth is reported to be between 3 and 9 months; 50–90% can be expected to recover by 12–72 months from onset (Birmaher et al., 2002). Dysthymic disorder (DD) is a chronic form of depression with fewer symptoms but lasting for at least 1 year in children and adolescents. Depression not otherwise specified (DNOS) in youth is defined by depressed mood, anhedonia, or irritability plus three depressive symptoms (i.e., problems with appetite, sleep, concentration, fatigue, low self-worth, or hopelessness). Adjustment disorders with depressed mood are the mildest mood disorder and are characterized by depressed mood that occurs within 3 months of the onset of a specific stressful situation, and lasts no longer than 6 months.

At least two important questions exist regarding the phenomenology of depression. First, some (e.g., Beach & Amir, 2003; Hankin, Fraley, Lahey, & Waldman, 2005; Ruscio & Ruscio, 2000) have argued that depression is best characterized along a severity continuum rather than as a distinct categorical entity. Using Meehl's (1995) taxometric procedures to discern whether a construct was continuous or categorical, Hankin et al. (2005) showed that the structure of depression in youth was dimensional.

A second issue is whether the experience and expression of depressive symptoms change with development. In a meta-analysis of studies comparing the occurrence of depressive symptoms across age groups, Weiss and Garber (2003) found differences in many core (e.g., agitation, retardation, fatigue, guilt, and sadness) and associated symptoms (e.g., anxiety, somatic complaints). In particular, depressed adolescents have been found to be more likely than preadolescents to experience hopelessness/helplessness, lack of energy, hypersomnia, weight loss, and suicidality (Yorbik et al., 2004), although not all of these age differences have been found in studies using longitudinal analyses (Avenevoli & Steinberg, 2001). Evidence also is mixed regarding whether the underlying structure of the depressive syndrome is similar across ages (Weiss & Garber, 2003).

Comorbidity

Depression consistently has been found to have elevated rates of comorbidity in both clinic and community samples of adolescents (Angold, Costello, & Erkanli, 1999; Essau, Conradt, & Petermann, 2000; Lewinsohn et al., 1998). Adolescents who have depression are approximately 20 times more likely to meet criteria for a diagnosis of an additional disorder (Angold & Costello, 1993). In the Oregon Adolescent Depression Project (OADP) (Lewinsohn et al., 1998), 43% of the adolescents with MDD also had a lifetime occurrence of another mental disorder.

Among clinic-referred adolescents, the most common comorbidity is anxiety disorders, particularly generalized anxiety disorders (55%), phobias (45%), and separation anxiety disorder (9%) (Birmaher et al., 1996; Simonoff, et al., 1997); indeed, anxiety disorders may serve as a risk factor for depression (Kovacs, Gatsonis, Paulauskas, & Richards, 1989). Comorbidity rates for dysthymia (30–80%), conduct problems and attention-deficit hyperactive disorder (ADHD) (10–80%), and substance use disorders (20–30%) also are quite high. Corresponding comorbidity rates for anxiety disorders, disruptive behavior disorders, substance use disorders, and ADHD (18, 8, 14, 21%, respectively) are lower in community compared to clinical samples of adolescents (Jensen, Shervette, Xenakis, & Richters, 1993; Lewinsohn, Rohde, Seeley, & Hops, 1991), although still quite high. A meta-analysis of studies of community samples of children and adolescents revealed that the odds ratios for comorbid disorders with MDD were 8.2 for anxiety disorders, 6.6 for conduct/oppositional defiant disorders, and 5.5 for attention-deficit hyperactivity disorder (Angold et al., 1999).

Compared to children, adolescent depression is more likely to co-occur with externalizing and substance use disorders (particularly in males; Lewinsohn et al., 1993; Yorbik et al., 2004) and eating disorders (particularly in females; Lewinsohn et al., 1993). For most comorbid disorders, depression typically develops after the other disorder (Lewinsohn et al., 1998), with two exceptions. MDD typically precedes the onset of substance use disorders (Birmaher et al., 1996). Second, comorbid conduct disorder often represents a complication of depression with the conduct problems persisting after the depression remits (Birmaher et al., 1996).

Impairment in cognitive and social functioning in individuals with MDD is intensified by comorbid conditions (Fergusson & Woodward, 2002; Lewinsohn et al., 1998; Rudolph & Clark, 2001). For example, Lewinsohn et al. (1998) showed that depressed adolescents with another psychiatric disorder were at increased risk for academic problems, conflict with parents, suicidal behaviors, and impaired global functioning. Depression comorbid with other disorders tends to be more severe and recurrent and is less responsive to treatment (Birmaher et al., 1996). Depressed adolescents with comorbid externalizing disorders have more interpersonal impairment (Rudolph & Clark, 2001), experience more stressful life events (Daley et al., 1997; Rudolph et al., 2000), and show lower rates of depression and higher rates of criminality/antisocial personality disorder and alcohol abuse in adulthood (Harrington, Fudge, Rutter, Pickles, & Hill, 1991) compared to those without such comorbidity.

Finally, comorbidity also complicates the treatment of depression in adolescents (Rohde, Lewinsohn, & Seeley, 1991) because it is often difficult to determine which disorder is primary, and it is not always clear which condition should be the focus of treatment first. Multiple modes of intervention likely are needed including the involvement of parents and other family members (Brent, Kolko, Birmaher, Baugher, & Bridge, 2001; Deblinger & Heflin, 1996).

Assessment

Age appropriate assessment of depressive symptoms and disorders is a key part of the treatment process. Obtaining information from multiple informants and using a variety of assessment methods including clinical interviews, questionnaires, and behavioral observation are needed to make accurate diagnoses and treatment plans. Even if information from multiple sources is available, getting report directly from the adolescent is essential (Cantwell et al., 1997). Parents often are unaware of their child's inner experience and therefore may be less accurate reporters about their child's subjective distress (Cantwell et al., 1997).

Clinical Interviews. Psychiatric interviews typically are conducted with the parent and adolescent separately and sequentially. Such detailed inquiry can help establish rapport with the adolescent and family. Observations of adolescents' nonverbal communications such as affective expressions, psychomotor restlessness or agitation, and listless speech also can be helpful in making an accurate diagnosis (Garber & Kaminski, 2000).

Several psychometrically adequate diagnostic interviews exist to assess depressive disorders in adolescents. The Schedule for Affective Disorders and Schizophrenia for School-Age Children (K-SADS; Ambrosini, 2000; Kaufman et al., 1997) is one of the most widely used and comprehensive clinician-administered interviews for diagnosing depression in youth (Hodges, 1994). Disadvantages of the K-SADS are that it can be time-consuming and resource demanding; that is, it requires extensive training and supervision (Reynolds & Kamphaus, 2003).

Other available structured clinical interviews include the Interview Schedule for Children and Adolescents (ISCA; Kovacs, 1997), the Diagnostic Interview Schedule for Children Version IV (DISC-IV; Shaffer, Fisher, Lucas, Dulcan, & Schwab-Stone, 2000), the Diagnostic Interview for Children and Adolescents-Revised (DICA-R; Reich, 1991), and the Child and Adolescent Psychiatric Assessment (CAPA; Angold & Fisher, 1999). Like the K-SADS, these structured interviews require training and are routinely used in clinical research settings.

Self-Report Questionnaires. The Center for Epidemiological Studies Depression Scale (CES-D; Radloff, 1991) is a 20-item self-report measure of depressive symptoms developed for use with adults but has been found to be reliable and valid with adolescents (Roberts, Andrews, Lewinsohn, & Hops, 1990). The CES-D assesses the degree to which the individual has experienced core symptoms of depression including negative affect, thoughts, and behaviors during the past week. Representative statements include "I felt sad" and "I did not feel like eating; my appetite was poor." Respondents rate each statement using a four-point Likert Scale from 0 (rarely or never) to 3 (most of the time). Items are summed to create a total score; total scores of 16–23 represent mild depression, 24–30 indicate moderate depression, and scores over 30 reflect more severe levels of depression (Roberts & Chen, 1995). Other self-report measures used to assess depressive symptoms in adolescents include the Beck Depression Inventory (Beck, Ward, Mendelson, Mock, & Erbaugh, 1961), the Reynolds Adolescent Depression Scale (Reynolds, 1987), the Children's Depression Inventory (Kovacs, 1985), the Mood and Feelings Questionnaire (Angold et al., 1987), the Depression Self-Rating Scale (Birleson, 1981), and the Dimensions of Depression Profile for Children and Adolescents (Harter & Nowakowski, 1987).

Depression self-report measures can be used as a quick screening test that patients can complete while in the waiting room at intake and also can be used to monitor changes in symptoms over the course of treatment (Spitzer et al., 1994). Recognition and treatment of depression are especially important in the primary care setting because for most adolescents their primary care provider may be the only health professional seen within the course of a year (Gans, McManus, & Newacheck, 1991). One study conducted in a primary care setting found that 20% of youth met criteria for a depressive disorder (Kramer & Garralda, 1998). Thus, primary care settings may be the first place that depression in an adolescent is recognized.

Treatment of Depression in Adolescents

Treatments for depression include psychopharmacologic and psychotherapeutic strategies. Although these two modalities have largely developed independently of one another, clinical practice and empirical studies (e.g., TADS, 2004) indicate that the combination of both medication and psychosocial treatments may be effective. Most studies of psychotherapy for depression in adolescents have focused on cognitive-behavioral therapy (CBT) or interpersonal psychotherapy (IPT-A). These two treatment approaches share some common components (e.g., problem solving, time-limited, attention to increasing engagement in activities), which may partially explain why both approaches have been found to be effective in improving outcomes for depressed youth (Blagys & Hilsenroth, 2002).

Cognitive-Behavioral Therapy. Beck (1967, 1976) suggested that individuals with depression hold beliefs and use information processing styles that are maladaptive, such that they interpret the self, the world, and the future in a negative manner. CBT teaches individuals how to recognize and challenge their automatic negative thoughts and the beliefs underlying them (Kaslow, McClure, & Connell, 2002). CBT for depression in adolescents also aims to improve coping, emotion regulation, problem solving, and social skills. Typically, treatment begins with a few sessions of psychoeducation about depression and the cognitive model underlying the CBT approach. Adolescents are taught to monitor their moods, thoughts, behaviors, and events. Such monitoring helps to identify the links among them, particularly the relations between thoughts and feelings. Additionally, patients are taught to monitor "mastery" and "pleasurable" activities that also may alter their mood. If there is a dearth of pleasurable events, then they are encouraged to increase them. Such pleasurable activities can provide a wider range of potential reinforcers, which then may serve to improve their depressed mood.

In CBT, depressed adolescents also learn to identify, monitor, and challenge their negative thoughts, which lead to more realistic and adaptive ways of thinking. This process is facilitated through Socratic-like dialogue between the adolescent and the therapist. Role-plays provide in-session practice of cognitive restructuring skills and "safe" exposure to situations the adolescent may have avoided in the past. Structured out-of-session practice assignments also are used throughout treatment so that adolescents gain experience applying the cognitive restructuring strategies and problem-solving skills in their natural environment.

In clinical trials with depressed adolescents, positive findings for CBT generally have been reported in comparison to no treatment (Butler, Miezitis, Friedman, & Cole, 1980; Stark, Reynolds, & Kaslow, 1987). When CBT has been compared to other treatments (e.g., relaxation training), results indicate that CBT is better or equally as effective at reducing depressive symptoms (Brent et al., 1997; Kahn, Kehle, Jenson, & Clark, 1990; Reynolds & Coats, 1986; Vostanis, Feehan, Grattan, & Bickerton, 1996; Wood, Harrington, & Moore, 1996). For example, Reynolds and Coats (1986) reported that both CBT and relaxation training reduced depressive symptoms and produced higher academic self-concept in depressed adolescents, and both approaches were superior to a wait-list control. Wood et al. (1996) tested a six-session individual therapy format of CBT versus relaxation training and found that adolescents in CBT reported greater change in depressive symptoms, greater self-esteem, higher global functioning, and greater satisfaction with the treatment compared to adolescents who received relaxation training. Kahn et al. (1990) compared CBT to relaxation and to self-modeling in a sample of depressed middle school students and found significant decreases in depressive symptoms for adolescents in all treatment groups, and CBT and relaxation were superior to a wait-list control.

In one of the most carefully conducted randomized controlled trials with depressed adolescents treated in an outpatient clinic, Brent et al. (1997) found that CBT was superior to systematic behavioral family therapy and nondirective supportive therapy with regard to the rates of improvement and remission. No differences in depression were found among conditions, however, at a 2-year follow-up (Birmaher et al., 2000). In a study comparing CBT to supportive therapy, Vostanis et al. (1996) found a significant decrease in depressive symptoms among adolescents in both conditions at post-treatment and at the 9-month follow-up.

To date, the largest randomized controlled trial of clinically depressed youth (n = 439) is the Treatment for Adolescents with Depression Study (TADS, 2007), which was conducted in 13 academic and community sites in the United States. To be eligible for this study, adolescents (ages 12–17) had to meet diagnostic criteria for moderate to severe MDD. Adolescents were randomly assigned to one of four conditions: fluoxetine hydrochloride alone, CBT alone, the combination of fluoxetine and CBT, and placebo medication. Administration of placebo and fluoxetine was double-blind through 12 weeks, after which treatments were unblinded. Patients assigned to placebo were treated openly after week 12, and not included in further analyses. Cognitive-behavioral and combination therapies were not masked.

CBT (in both the CBT alone and combined conditions) encompassed adolescent and family modules. The CBT intervention consisted of six required skill-building sessions and six subsequent optional modules. The initial skill-building sessions focused on psychoeducation about depression, goal setting, mood monitoring, behavioral activation, problem solving, and cognitive restructuring. The optional modules addressed adolescent-identified social skills concerns such as communication, assertiveness, and negotiation. In addition, parents could receive psychoeducation about depression and conjoint sessions in which the adolescent and parent collaboratively selected issues to discuss.

The primary dependent measures were the Children's Depression Rating Scale-Revised (CDRS-R) total score and the response rate defined as a Clinical Global Impressions-Improvement score of "much" or "very much" improved. Intent-to-treat analyses on the CDRS-R identified a significant time by treatment interaction. Rates of response at weeks 12, 18, and 36 are shown in Table 1. Suicidal ideation decreased with treatment, but less so with fluoxetine therapy than with combination therapy or CBT alone. The conclusion from this study is that for adolescents with moderate to severe depression, treatment with fluoxetine alone or in combination with CBT accelerates response; CBT alone is as effective but takes a little longer. CBT alone or in combination with medication may be safer than medication alone.

Thus, the overall evidence is promising regarding the efficacy of CBT for depressed adolescents. Several important unresolved questions remain. To what extent does CBT prevent relapse and recurrence? What are the essential mechanisms of change in CBT? Are the effects of combined fluoxetine and CBT additive or do some patients respond better to one than the other producing a greater percent of responders overall. How much training is necessary for CBT to be disseminated effectively in the field?

Interpersonal Psychotherapy for Adolescents (IPT-A). Although IPT-A and CBT include some similar components, IPT-A differs from CBT in its particular focus on interpersonal problems and conflicts rather than on cognitive restructuring per se (Stark, Laurent, Livingston, Boswell, & Swearer, 1999). Issues addressed in IPT-A include separating from parents, negotiating relationships, and interpersonal deficits (Moreau, Mufson, Weissman, & Klerman, 1991). Once the adolescent and therapist identify an issue, they collaboratively examine the problem and how it impacts the adolescent's depression.

Several studies have examined the effectiveness of IPT-A for depressed adolescents (Mufson & Fairbanks, 1996; Mufson et al., 1994; Mufson, Moreau, Weissman, & Garfinkel, 1999; Rosello & Bernal, 1999; Santor & Kusumakar, 2001). In the first open clinical trial of IPT-A, Mufson et al. (1994) evaluated its effectiveness with 14 clinically

Table 1 Response rates at weeks 12, 18, and 36, and suicide events in the Treatment for Adolescents with Depression Study (TADS, 2007) as a function of treatment condition

	12 weeks (%)	18 weeks (%)	36 weeks (%)	Suicide events (%)
Fluoxetine hydrochloride	62	69	81	14.7
Cognitive-Behavioral Therapy (CBT)	48	65	81	6.3
Combined fluoxetine + CBT	73	85	86	8.4

depressed adolescents. At the end of the 12 individual IPT-A sessions, adolescents reported significantly fewer depressive symptoms, decreased physical distress, and improved global functioning; none met criteria for a diagnosis of depressive disorder. At a 1-year follow-up, participants continued to maintain treatment gains.

In a randomized controlled clinical trial comparing 12 sessions of IPT-A to clinical monitoring in a sample of 48 clinically referred, depressed adolescents, Mufson et al. (1999) found that adolescents who received IPT-A were more likely to meet recovery criteria, reported significantly fewer depressive symptoms and had better global and interpersonal functioning than those in the control condition. In an attempt to examine whether these promising findings could be replicated in a different sample and by a different investigator, Rosello and Bernal (1999) compared IPT-A, CBT, and a wait-list control in a sample of depressed Puerto Rican youth. Results indicated that both IPT-A and CBT produced greater improvement in depressive symptoms compared to the control condition. IPT-A also was more effective than the wait-list control at increasing self-esteem and social adaptation.

Mufson et al. (2004) conducted another randomized, controlled trial of 63 adolescents with diagnoses of MDD, DD, adjustment disorder with depressed mood, or DNOS. IPT-A delivered in an urban school-based health clinic over 12 weeks was compared to mental health treatment as usually provided in this clinic. Participants who received IPT-A reported significantly fewer depressive symptoms and were more likely to meet recovery criteria than were youth who received treatment as usual. At a 1-month follow-up, IPT-A participants continued to be doing significantly better.

Thus, studies of both CBT and IPT-A have yielded promising short-term findings for the treatment of depressed adolescents. More research is needed to determine the long-term maintenance of treatment gains. Moreover, a better understanding of the moderators and mediators of change will facilitate the further refinement of these treatment approaches. More research also is needed to explore the effects of comorbidity and the efficacy of these interventions with adolescents from diverse cultural groups.

Pharmacotherapy. Research investigating the effectiveness of specific pharmacological agents in treating depressive disorders in adolescents is still relatively limited. This chapter emphasizes medications that have received the most attention and have been subjected to the most rigorous empirical trials (double-blind, placebo controlled). These medication types include tricyclic antidepressants (TCAs), selective serotonin reuptake inhibitors (SSRIs), and nontricyclic antidepressants.

Tricyclic Antidepressants (TCAs) were among the first type of medications to be used and evaluated in the treatment of depression in children and adolescents. Unfortunately, little evidence exists to support the efficacy of TCAs in youth. Two studies were stopped prematurely due to poor treatment response (Geller et al., 1992; Puig-Antich & Gittleman, 1982). Reviews of this literature (Hazell, O'Connell, Heathcote, & Henry, 2004; Sommers-Flanagan & Sommers-Flanagan, 1996) have reported that double-blind placebo-controlled studies have not shown significant effects of TCAs compared to placebo in youth. In their meta-analysis, the Cochrane Group (Hazell et al., 2003) concluded that TCAs failed to alleviate depression in youth. Thus, because there is little evidence of the effectiveness of TCAs in youth, and because of their adverse side-effect profile, including cardiac conduction delays (Gutgesell et al., 1999), their use in treating depression in adolescents has declined.

Selective Serotonin Reuptake Inhibitors (SSRIs) are better tolerated and more easily managed than TCAs. Concerns emerged in the 1990s, however, regarding the association between SSRIs and increased suicidality in adolescents. In 2003, the British Medicines and Healthcare products Regulatory Agency responded by issuing a statement that SSRIs, with the exception of fluoxetine (Prozac), should not be prescribed to children and adolescents (Coffey, 2006). Fluoxetine was excluded from the warning due to its demonstrated efficacy in controlled studies. The U.S. Food and Drug Administration, in turn, advised that paroxetine (Paxil) not be used to treat depression in individuals under age 18, and that other SSRIs and nontricyclic antidepressants should be used cautiously among youth.

Fluoxetine is the most studied SSRI in youth. Open trials consistently have demonstrated the efficacy of fluoxetine for the treatment of depression in adolescents (Butcher, Kutcher, Gardner, & Young,

1992; Colle, Belair, DiFeo, Weiss, & LaRoche, 1994; Riggs, Mikulich, Coffman, & Crowley, 1997; Waslick et al., 1999). Response rates have ranged from 52 to 88% of depressed youth. In contrast, double-blind, placebo-controlled studies have produced more mixed results. For example, Simeon, Dinicola, Ferguson, and Copping (1990) found in a sample of adolescents diagnosed with MDD that fluoxetine failed to show a benefit over placebo at post-treatment and at the 24-month follow-up. In a larger sample, however, Emslie et al. (1997) reported that after 8 weeks, fluoxetine was superior to placebo in the reduction of depression in adolescents. Similarly, in TADS March et al. (2004) showed that fluoxetine alone and in combination with CBT was more effective at reducing depression than placebo.

Studies of paroxetine also have produced mixed results. The efficacy and safety of paroxetine in treating MDD in adolescents has been demonstrated in several open trials (Masi, Marchesi, & Pfanner, 1997; Nobile, Bellotti, Marino, Molteni, & Battaglia, 2000; Rey-Sanchez & Gutierrez-Casares, 1997). In a placebo-controlled study of adolescents with MDD, however, clinician ratings, but not self- or parent-report, of adolescents' depressive symptoms revealed greater improvement for youth randomly assigned to paroxetine than to placebo after 8 weeks (Keller et al., 2001).

Open-label trials also have found that sertraline is effective at reducing symptoms of depression in adolescents (Ambrosini et al., 1999; McConville et al., 1996). In a placebo-controlled trial, Wagner and Ambrosini (2003) randomly assigned adolescents to 10 weeks of sertraline or placebo, and found that youth treated with sertraline had significantly greater improvement in depressive symptoms compared to those in the placebo group.

Citalopram has been evaluated in one open trial of depressed adolescents and yielded positive results (Bostic, Prince, Brown, & Place, 2001). Additionally, in a placebo-controlled study of depressed adolescents, Wagner et al. (2004) randomly assigned participants to citalopram or placebo and found after 8 weeks a greater reduction in clinicians' ratings of depressive symptoms for youth in the citalopram treatment group compared to those in the placebo group. A different placebo-controlled trial examining escitalopram in depressed children and adolescents (Wagner, Jonas, Findling, Ventura, & Saikali, 2006) found that among adolescent completers, treatment with escitalopram reduced depressive symptoms to a significantly greater extent than placebo.

In a study of fluvoxamine in combination with psychosocial treatment for inpatient adolescents with MDD and comorbid diagnoses, all participants reported reductions in depressive symptoms (Apter et al., 1994). An open trial of fluvoxamine with dysthymic adolescent outpatients found that 44% of the participants achieved symptom reduction after 26 weeks (Rabe-Joblanska, 2000); one-third, however, failed to maintain their gains.

The efficacy of alternative antidepressants also is beginning to be investigated in the treatment of depression in youth. Studies of Serotonergic Noradrenergic Reuptake Inhibitors (SNRIs) for treating depression in children and adolescents are still in the early stages. One 6-week, randomized, placebo-controlled trial comparing venlafaxine in combination with psychotherapy to placebo plus psychotherapy in children and adolescents with MDD found no between-group differences (Madoki, Tapia, Tapia, & Sumner, 1997). More recently, Emslie, Findling, Yeung, Kinz, and Li (2007) reported that venlafaxine produced greater improvements in depression compared to placebo among adolescents with MDD.

Mirtazapine is classified as a noradrenergic and specific serotonergic antidepressant (NaSSA). Two placebo-controlled studies examining mirtazapine for youth with depression have found no significant group differences between mirtazapine and placebo (US Food and Drug Administration).

Although limited, some clinical evidence indicates that adolescents with MDD treated with bupropion show improvement in depressive symptoms. In an 8-week open trial, Glod, Lynch, Flynn, Berkowitz, and Baldessarini (2003) used bupropion extended release form (bupropion SR) to treat adolescents with MDD. Depressive symptoms, as assessed with both self-report and clinician ratings, were found to decrease. In a study of substance abusing adolescents with comorbid ADHD and depression, 93% of participants treated with bupropion showed a significant reduction in depressive symptoms (Solhkhah et al., 2005).

Finally, Nefazodone, although not considered an SSRI, acts similarly to them. A series of case reports demonstrated that nefazodone was effective in treating younger patients with MDD (Wilens, Spencer, Biederman, & Schleifer, 1997). A trial testing nefazodone for the treatment of depression in children and adolescents found significant improvement in depressive symptoms (Findling et al., 2000). Nefazodone, however, has been found to be associated with liver abnormalities, which has led to a black box warning.

Overall, fluoxetine has the most evidence of efficacy in the treatment of depression in adolescents and is FDA approved for use. Although other SSRIs and alternative agents are being studied, further randomized, placebo-controlled trials with sufficiently large samples of adolescents are needed before they can be approved for widespread use in clinical practice. Studies also are needed that examine the efficacy of combined medication and psychotherapy.

Prevention of Depression in Adolescents

Historically, prevention was categorized as primary, secondary, or tertiary (Caplan, 1964). Reducing the incidence of new cases of disorder in individuals who have not had the disorder is *primary prevention*; reducing the duration and severity of symptoms is *secondary prevention* (i.e., treatment), and reducing the recurrence of the disorder and its associated impairment in those who have already had it is *tertiary prevention* (maintenance). The Institute of Medicine (IOM) found this distinction to be too broad, and instead introduced the classification of prevention based on the population groups to whom the interventions are directed (Mrazek & Haggerty, 1994). *Universal preventive intervention* is administered to all members of a population and does not select participants based on risk. *Selective prevention* is given to subgroups of a population whose risk is deemed to be above average (e.g., offspring of depressed parents). *Indicated prevention* is provided to individuals who have detectable, sub-threshold levels of signs or symptoms of the disorder, but who do not currently meet criteria for the diagnosis.

Qualitative (e.g., Garber, 2009; Gillham, Shatté, Freres, 2000; Merry & Spence, 2007; Sutton, 2007) and quantitative (e.g., Horowitz & Garber, 2006; Merry, McDowell, Hetrick, Bir, & Muller, 2004) reviews of studies testing interventions to prevent depression in children and adolescents have concluded that (a) some targeted (i.e., selective, indicated) depression prevention programs are efficacious; (b) targeted preventions have effect sizes greater than those found for universal programs; (c) the effect sizes for targeted prevention programs generally have been small to moderate; and (d) the effects tend not to endure. Most studies have measured change in depressive symptoms. Far fewer studies have prevented the subsequent occurrence of depressive disorders, and none has yet been shown to prevent the first onset of a mood disorder.

The most extensively tested preventive intervention with youth is the *Penn Prevention Program* (PPP) (Gillham, Reivich, Jaycox, & Seligman, 1995; Jaycox, Reivich, Gillham, & Seligman, 1994), which has been administered to universal, selective, and indicated samples. PPP has shown both short- and long-term significant effects and has been replicated several times and by independent researchers (e.g., Cardemil, Reivich, Beevers, Seligman, & James, 2007; Quayle et al., 2001; Yu & Seligman, 2002). Most studies of PPP have assessed depressive symptoms, although a few have evaluated depressive disorders (Gillham et al., 2006). Samples sizes have been generally adequate, and evidence of satisfactory fidelity has been demonstrated.

The second most replicated depression prevention program in youth is based on the *Coping with Depression course* developed by Clarke, Lewinsohn, and Hops (1990). Short-term efficacy was found when a modified version of the program was tested in a universal sample (Horowitz, Garber, Ciesla, Young, & Mufson, 2007), and both short- and long-term efficacy have been found in selective and indicated samples (Clarke et al., 1995; 2001). Significant effects have been replicated by independent researchers (Garber et al., 2008); depressive diagnoses have been assessed; sample sizes have been generally adequate, and adherence to the program protocol has been demonstrated.

Two depression prevention programs have been developed and evaluated in Australia and New Zealand. The *Resourceful Adolescent Program* (RAP) (Merry, McDowell, Wild, Bir, & Cunliffe, 2004; Shochet et al., 2001) has been tested in large universal samples, was found to be efficacious both at post-intervention and follow-up, was replicated by independent researchers, and was found to have satisfactory adherence. The *Problem Solving for Life program* (PSFL) (Spence, Sheffield, & Donovan, 2003) is administered by teachers and has been tested in large universal school samples. PSFL was found to have significant short-term effects in one study (Spence et al., 2003), although this was not replicated (Sheffield et al., 2006), and it has not shown significant long-term effects (Spence, Sheffield, & Donovan, 2005).

Recently, evidence of short-term efficacy of the *Interpersonal Psychotherapy-Adolescent Skills Training program* (IPT-AST) in both a large universal (Horowitz et al., 2007) and a small indicated (Young, Mufson, & Davies, 2006) sample has been found. Young et al. also showed that the significant effects endured through the 6-month follow-up. They found a marginally significant trend for adolescents in the IPT-AST group to have fewer depressive diagnoses during the 6-month follow-up compared to controls.

Overall, results of prevention studies with adolescents suggest the benefit of CBT-based interventions, such as the Penn Resiliency program, and interpersonal-based approaches like IPT-AST (Young et al., 2006). Further study of the inclusion of parent and/or family components in preventative interventions with adolescents is warranted (Compas, Keller, & Forehand, in press; Gillham et al., 2006). Modification and evaluation of depression prevention programs with youth from diverse ethnic and racial backgrounds also is needed.

Treatment of Adolescent Depression in Primary Care

Traditional models of treatment consist of a child being seen individually by a therapist for a limited number of sessions to address an identified problem. These models, however, ignore another available option; that is, providing mental health treatment within the primary care setting (Asarnow et al., 2005; DeBar, Clarke, O'Connor, & Nichols, 2001; Shatin & Drinkard, 2002; Wells, Kataoka, & Asarnow, 2001). Given that about 70% of youth typically visit a primary care provider within the course of a year, primary care settings may be an ideal site for identification of and intervention with adolescents who have mood disorders (Monheit & Cunningham, 1992).

An interdisciplinary task force of experts developed Guidelines for Adolescent Depression in Primary Care (GLAD-PC; Cheung et al., 2007) to assist primary care clinicians in managing depression in youth 10–21 years of age. They recommended that primary care providers should consider a period (about 6–8 weeks) of active support and monitoring before implementing or referring for further treatment. For appropriate treatment to occur, adequate assessment of depression and suicidality is needed. Although 90% of pediatricians believe that it is their responsibility to identify depression, 46% lack confidence that they can recognize the disorder and 56% report that appointment times are too short to gather information about psychiatric history and current status (Olson, Kelleher, Kemper, Zuckerman, Hammond, & Dietrich, 2001).

In an effort to address these assessment concerns, Zuckerbrot et al. (2007) evaluated the feasibility and acceptability of a 2-stage adolescent depression identification method at three sites of a pediatric primary care practice. The first stage involved adolescents completing the Columbia Depression Scale (CDS) while in the waiting room. During the second stage, providers reviewed the screens and could request that the patient take the youth-informant Columbia voice DISC-IV, a computer assisted self-interview version of the present state version of the Columbia Diagnostic Interview Schedule for Children, which generates a diagnostic report for providers. Patients expressed satisfaction with the procedure, and providers expressed a willingness and desire to continue using the CDS (Zuckerbrot et al., 2007).

In a review of studies that examined the efficacy of psychosocial interventions delivered to adolescents by primary care physicians or their staff in a "real-world" primary care setting, Stein, Zitner, and Jensen (2006) concluded that relatively simple primary care-based interventions can improve outcomes of adolescents with subclinical depression. For example, in a study of eight general practices in which 1,516 teens completed a variety of questionnaires including the CES-D, Walker et al. (2002) offered youth an opportunity to receive general practice consultations to discuss health behavior concerns. Interested adolescents were randomly assigned to either a 20-minute consultation with a nurse aimed at improving self-efficacy for behavior change or to "standard care." Walker et al. found that among teens with subclinical levels of depressive symptoms, those who received the consultation from the medical practice nurse had significantly lower CES-D scores at the 3-month and 1-year follow-ups compared to youth not receiving the consultation.

An important issue for primary care is the implementation of quality improvement programs (QIP), which are interventions aimed at increasing access to evidence-based treatments by providing training and education to patients and providers (Wells et al., 2001). In the Youth Partners-in-Care study, Asarnow et al. (2005) conducted one of the most carefully executed, quality improvement investigations for youth depression to date in five health care organizations with 418 adolescent primary care patients. Youth with current depressive symptoms were randomly assigned to either "usual care" or a quality improvement program (QIP). In usual care, primary care clinicians were provided with training and educational materials about depression evaluation and treatment. The QIP included teams of experts as well as care managers who supported primary care clinicians with patient evaluation, education, evidence-based psychosocial treatment, medication when needed, and links to mental health services. At the 6-month follow-up, adolescents in QIP had significantly lower CES-D scores, a lower rate of severe depression, higher mental health-related quality of life, and greater satisfaction with mental health care compared to youth receiving usual care. This study was the first to demonstrate that depression in adolescents can be improved in primary care settings.

In a study testing the effectiveness of a depression prevention program, the Penn Resiliency Program (PRP), when delivered by therapists in a primary care setting, Gillham, Hamilton, Freres, Patton, and Gallop (2006) randomized 271 children (11–12 years old) with elevated depressive symptoms on the CDI to either PRP or usual care. Over the 2-year follow-up, PRP significantly prevented depression, anxiety, and adjustment disorders (when combined) among high-symptom children. Stronger effects were found when the intervention was delivered with high compared to low fidelity, and girls benefited more from PRP than boys.

One concern about providing intervention in managed care settings is the issue of safety. When teens are at risk of harming themselves or others, the option for hospitalization needs to be available to provide treatment and ensure safety. Many communities, however, lack inpatient hospital beds for the crisis care of youth (Thomas, 1999). Addressing this need should be a priority for the mental health service system. Unfortunately, due to features of managed care, the time-limited nature of pediatric visits, and the low rates of specialty referral from primary care settings, the detection and outcomes for adolescents with mental health needs in primary care settings have not been as good as they could be (Burns, 1996; Chang, Warner, & Weissman, 1988; Lavigne et al., 1993; Wells et al., 1989).

Is it possible to address this unmet need by extending coverage to the uninsured and establishing parity laws that mandate equivalent coverage for mental health and physical health conditions among the insured (Wells et al., 2001)? Many low income youth have decreased access to mental health services because they are uninsured, and for those who are insured, costs for mental health services commonly exceed coverage limits (Sturm, 1997).

Primary care settings hold considerable promise for addressing unmet needs for identification and treatment of depression in adolescents. There is still a serious dearth of information about how to implement and maintain depression screening as part of routine clinical practice. Additional research on the financial implications and clinical benefits of such screening is imperative (Zuckerbrot et al., 2007). In addition, longitudinal research within primary care settings is needed to develop effective intervention strategies for youth with depression and to address issues of sustainability and dissemination (Wells et al., 2001).

Summary and Directions for Future Research

Depression among adolescents is common, recurrent, highly comorbid with other disorders, and associated with significant impairment. Approximately 70% of depressed youth do not receive any or appropriate treatment (Kataoka et al., 2002). Optimal assessment of depression can be achieved with clinical interviews, behavioral observation, and questionnaires completed by adolescents, parents, and teachers.

Treatments for depression include psychopharmacology and/or psychotherapy. Central to treatment of depression is the recognition that dysfunctional thinking and interpersonal relationships are core features of depression that need to be addressed in treatment. CBT focuses on cognitive restructuring, behavioral activation, and problem solving, and IPT-A emphasizes building and strengthening interpersonal relationships. Both approaches have been found to be efficacious in the treatment of depression in adolescents. The long-term maintenance of treatment gains, the impact of comorbidity on outcome, and the transportability of these interventions still need to be established.

Several medications including TCAs, SSRIs, and other nontricyclic antidepressants also have been used to treat depression in adolescents. Fluoxetine is FDA approved for the treatment of depression in youth and has the most empirical evidence of its efficacy. The efficacy and safety of other psychopharmacological interventions need to be investigated further. In addition, studies need to evaluate whether and which medications should be combined with psychotherapy, and how medication regimens can be administered safely.

Prevention of depression in youth represents another important area of inquiry. Evidence of short-term effects of some preventive interventions has been found, particularly cognitive and/or interpersonal approaches with high-risk populations (Horowitz & Garber, 2006; Merry et al., 2004). Nevertheless, research is needed to develop and test depression prevention programs that have more enduring effects.

Recent research on the provision of mental health treatments within the primary care setting has shown promise (Asarnow et al., 2005; Gillham et al., 2006; Jaycox et al., 2006; Wells et al., 2001; Zuckerbrot et al., 2007). Several barriers to appropriate treatment in primary care exist, however, including short duration of pediatric visits, limited insurance coverage, and absence of therapists on site (Wells et al., 2001). Nevertheless, given that most youth visit primary care providers at least once a year (Monheit & Cunningham, 1992), the setting represents a logical area for intervention, and an opportunity to reduce the burden of depression on young people.

References

Ambrosini, P. J. (2000). Historical development and present status of the Schedule for Affective Disorders and Schizophrenia for School-Age Children (K-SADS). *Journal of the American Academy of Child and Adolescent Psychiatry, 39*, 49–58.

Ambrosini, P. J., Wagner, K. D., Biederman, J., Glick, I., Tan, C., & Elia, J. (1999). Multicenter open-label sertraline study in adolescent outpatients with major depression. *Journal of the American Academy of Child and Adolescent Psychiatry, 38*, 566–572.

American Psychiatric Association. (2000). *Diagnostic and statistical manual of mental disorders* (4th ed.). Washington, DC: American Psychiatric Publishing.

Angold, A., & Costello, E. J. (1993). Depressive comorbidity in children and adolescents: Empirical, theoretical, and methodological issues. *American Journal of Psychiatry, 150*, 1779–1791.

Angold, A., Costello, E. J., & Erkanli, A. (1999). Comorbidity. *Journal of Child Psychology and Psychiatry, 40*, 57–87.

Angold, A., Erkanli, A., Silberg, J., Eaves, L., & Costello, E. J. (2002). Depression scale scores in 8–17-year-olds: Effects of age and gender. *Journal of Child Psychology and Psychiatry, 43*, 1052–1063.

Angold, A., & Fisher, P. W. (1999). Interviewer-based interviews. In D. Shaffer, C. Lucas, & J. Richters (Eds.), Diagnostic assessment in child and adolescent psychopathology (pp. 34–64). New York: Guilford Press.

Angold, A., Weissman, M. M., John, K., Merikangas, K. R., Prusoff, B. A., & Wickramaratne et al. (1987). Parent and child reports of depressive symptoms in children at low and high risk of depression. *Journal of Child Psychology and Psychiatry and Allied Disciplines, 28*, 901–915.

Angst, J., Sellaro, R., & Merikangas, K. R. (2000). Depressive spectrum diagnoses. *Comprehensive Psychiatry, 41*, 39–47.

Apter, A., Ratzoni, G., King, R. A., Weizman, A., Iancu, I., Binder, M. et al. (1994). Fluvoxamine open-label treatment of adolescent inpatients with obsessive-compulsive disorder or depression. *Journal of the American Academy of child and Adolescent Psychiatry, 33*, 342–348.

Asarnow, J. R., Jaycox, L. H., Duan, N., LaBorde, A. P., Rea, M. M., Murray, P., et al. (2005). Effectiveness of a quality improvement intervention for adolescent depression in primary care clinics. *Journal of the American Medical Association, 293*, 311–319.

Avenevoli, S., & Steinberg, L. (2001). The continuity of depression across the adolescent transition. In H. W. Reese & R. Kail (Eds.). *Advances in Child* Development (pp. 139–173). San Diego: Academic Press.

Bardone, A. M., Moffit, T. E., Caspi, A., Dickson, N., Stanton, W. R., & Silva, P. A. (1998). Adult physical health outcomes of adolescent girls with conduct disorder, depression, and anxiety. *Journal of the American Academy of Child and Adolescent Psychiatry, 37*, 594–601.

Beach, S. R. H., & Amir, N. (2003). Is depression taxonic, dimensional, or both? *Journal of Abnormal Psychology, 112*, 228–236.

Beck, A. T. (1967). *Depression: Causes and treatment*. New York: Harper and Row.

Beck, A. T. (1976). *Cognitive Therapy and the emotional disorders*. Oxford: International Universities Press.

Beck, A. T., Ward, C. H., Mendelson, M., Mock. J., & Erbaugh, J. (1961). An inventory for measuring depression. *Archives of General Psychiatry, 4*, 561–571.

Birleson, P. (1981). The validity of depressive disorder in childhood and the development of a self-rating scale: A research report. *Journal of Child Psychology and Psychiatry, 22*, 73–88.

Birmaher, B., Arbelaez, C., & Brent, D. (2002). Course and outcome of child and adolescent major depressive disorder. *Child and Adolescent Psychiatric Clinics of North America, 11*, 619–638.

Birmaher, B., Brent, D. A., Kolko, D., Baugher, M., Bridge, J. Holder, D., et al. (2000). Clinical outcome after short-term psychotherapy for adolescents with major depressive disorder. *Archives of General Psychiatry, 57*, 29–36.

Birmaher, B., Ryan, N. D., Williamson, D. E., Brent, D. A., Kaufman, J., Dahl, R. E., et al. (1996). Childhood and adolescent depression: A review of the past 10 years. Part I. *Journal of the American Academy of Child and Adolescent Psychiatry, 35*, 1427–1439.

Blagys, M. D. & Hilsenroth, M. J. (2002). Distinctive activities of cognitive-behavioral therapy: A review of the comparative psychotherapy process literature. *Clinical Psychology Review, 22*, 671–706.

Bostic, J. Q., Prince, J., Brown, K., & Place, S. (2001). A retrospective study of citalopram in adolescents with depression. *Journal of Child and Adolescent Psychopharmacology, 11*, 159–166.

Brent, D. A., Holder, D., Kolko, D., Birmaher, B., Baugher, M. Roth, C., et al. (1997). A clinical psychotherapy trial for adolescent depression comparing cognitive, family, and supportive therapy. *Archives of General Psychiatry, 54*, 877–885.

Brent, D. A., Kolko, D. J., Birmaher, B., Baugher, M., & Bridge J. (2001). A clinical trial for adolescent depression: Predictors of additional treatment in the acute and follow-up phases of the trial, *Journal of the American Academy of Child and Adolescent Psychiatry, 38*, 263–271.

Burns, B. (1996). What drives outcomes for emotional and behavioral disorders in children and adolescents? *New directions for Mental Health Services, 71*, 89–102.

Butcher, D., Kutcher, S., Gardner, D., & Young, E. (1992). An open naturalistic trial of fluoxetine in adolescents and young adults with treatment-resistant major depression. *Journal of child and Adolescent Psychopharmacology, 2*, 103–111.

Butler, L., Miezitis, S., Friedman, R., & Cole. E. (1980). The effect of two school-based intervention programs on depressive symptoms in preadolescents. *American Educational Research Journal, 17*, 111–119.

Cantwell, D. P., Lewinsohn, P. M., Rohde, P., & Seeley, J. R. (1997). Correspondence between adolescent report and parent report of psychiatric diagnostic data. *Journal of the American Academy of Child and Adolescent Psychiatry, 36*, 610–619.

Caplan G. (1964). *Principles of preventive psychiatry*. New York: Basic Books.

Cardemil, E. V., Reivich, K. J., Beevers, C. G., Seligman, M. E. P., & James, J. (2007). The prevention of depressive symptoms in low-income, minority children: Two-year follow-up. *Behaviour Research and Therapy, 45*, 313–327.

Centers for Disease Control and Prevention. (2004). Suicide in the United States fact sheet. Atlanta, GA.

Chang, G., Warner, V., & Weissman, M. M. (1988). Physicians' recognition of psychiatric disorders in children and adolescents. *American Journal of Diseases of Children, 142*, 736–739.

Cheung, A., Zuckerbrot, R. A., Jensen, P. S., et al. (2007). Guidelines for Adolescent Depression in Primary Care (GLAD-PC): Part II – treatment and ongoing management. *Pediatrics, 120*(5). DOI: 10.1542/peds.2006–1395. http://www.pediatrics.org/cgi/content/full/120/5/e1313

Clarke, G. N., Hawkings, W., Murphy, M., Sheeber, L., Lewinsohn, P. M., & Seeley, J. R. (1995). Targeted prevention of unipolar depressive disorder in an at-risk sample of high school adolescents: a randomized trial of a group cognitive intervention. *Journal of the American Academy of Child and Adolescent Psychiatry, 34*, 312–321.

Clarke, G. N., Hornbrook, M., Lynch, F., Polen, M., Gale, J., Beardslee, W., et al. (2001). A randomized trial of a group cognitive intervention for preventing depression in adolescent offspring of depressed parents. *Archives of General Psychiatry, 58*, 1127–1134.

Clarke, G. N., Lewinsohn, P. M., & Hops, H. (1990). *Instructor's manual for the Adolescent Coping with Depression Course* . Eugene, OR: Castalia Press.

Cohen, S. (2004). Social relationships and health. *American Psychologist, 59*, 676–684.

Cohen, S., & Rodriguez, M. S. (1995). Pathways linking affective disturbances and physical disorders. *Health Psychology, 7*, 269–297.

Colle, L. M., Belair, J. F., DiFeo, M., Weiss, J., & LaRoche, C. (1994). Extended open-label fluoxetine treatment of adolescents with major depression. *Journal of Child and Adolescent Psychopharmacology, 4*, 225–232.

Coffey, C. E. (2006). *Pediatric neuropsychiatry*. Philadelphia: Lippincott, Williams & Wilkins.

Costello, E. J., Mustillo, S., Erkanli, Keeler, G., & Angold, A. (2003). The prevalence and development of psychiatric disorders in childhood and adolescence. *Archives of General Psychiatry, 60*, 837–844.

Cyranowski, J. M., Frank, E., Young, E., & Shear, K. (2000). Adolescent onset of the gender difference in lifetime rates of depression. *Archives of General Psychiatry, 57*, 21–27.

Daley, S. E., Hammen, C., Burge, D., Davilla, J., Paley, B., Lindberg, N., & Herzberg, D. S. (1997). Predictors of the generation of episodic stress: A longitudinal study of late adolescent women. *Journal of Abnormal Psychology, 106*, 251–259.

Debar, L. L., Clarke, G. N., O'Connor, E., & Nichols, G. A. (2001). Treated prevalence, incidence, and pharmacotherapy of child and adolescent mood disorders in an HMO. *Mental Health Services Research, 3*, 73 89.

Deblinger, E., & Heflin, A. H. (1996). *Treating sexually abused children and their nonoffending parents: A cognitive behavioral approach*. Thousand Oaks, CA: Sage Publications.

Emslie, G. J., Findling, R. L., Yeung, P. P., Kinz, N. R., & Li, R. (2007). Venlafaxine ER for the treatment of pediatric subjects with depression: Results of two placebo-controlled trials. *Child and Adolescent Psychiatry, 46*, 479–488.

Emslie, G. J., Rush, J., Weinberg, W. A., Kowatch, R. A., Hughes, C. W., Carmody, T., et al. (1997). A double-blind, randomized, placebo-controlled trial of fluoxetine in children and adolescents with depression. *Archives of General Psychiatry, 54*, 1031–1037.

Essau, C. A., Conradt, J., & Petermann, F. (2000). Frequency, comorbidity, and psychosocial impairment of depressive disorders in adolescents. *Journal of Adolescent Research, 15*, 470–481.

Fergusson, D. M., & Woodward, L. J. (2002). Mental health, educational, and social role outcomes of adolescents with depression. *Archives of General Psychiatry, 59*, 225–231.

Findling, R. L., Preskorn, S. H., Marcus, R. N., Magnus, R. D., D'Amico, F., Marathe, P., & Reed, M. D. (2000). Nefazodone pharmokinetics in depressed children and adolescents. *Journal of the American Academy of Child & Adolescent Psychiatry, 39*, 1008–1016.

Gans J. E., McManus M. A., & Newacheck P. W. (1991). *Adolescent health care: Use, costs, and problems of access*. Chicago: American Medical Association.

Garber, J., (2009). Prevention of depression and early intervention with subclinical depression. In J. M. Rey & B. Birmaher (Eds.). *Treating childhood depression*. (pp. 274–292). Philadelphia: Lippincott Williams & Wilkins.

Garber, J., Gladstone, T.R.G., Weersing, V.R., Clarke, G., Brent, D.A., Beardslee, W.R., Hollon, S.D., Debar, L., & D'Angelo, E. (2008, May). *The prevention of depression in at-risk adolescents: Rationale, design, & preliminary results*. Presented at the annual meeting of the Society for Prevention Research, San Francisco.

Garber, J., & Kaminski, K. M. (2000). Laboratory and performance-based measures of depression in children and adolescents. *Journal of Clinical Child Psychology, 29*, 509–525.

Ge, X., Lorenz, F. O., Conger, R. D., Elder, G. H., & Simons, R. L. (1994). Trajectories of stressful life events and depressive symptoms during adolescence. *Developmental Psychology, 30*, 467–483.

Geller, B., Cooper, T. B., Graham, D. L., Fetner, H. H., Marsteller, F. A., & Wells, J. M. (1992). Pharmacokinetically designed double-blind placebo-controlled study of nortriptyline in 6- to 12-year-olds with major depressive disorder. *Journal of the American Academy of child and Adolescent Psychiatry, 31*, 34–44.

Gillham, J. E., Hamilton, J., Freres, D. R., Patton, K., & Gallop, R. (2006). Preventing depression among early adolescents in the primary care setting: A randomized controlled study of the Penn Resiliency Program. *Journal of Abnormal Child Psychology, 34*, 203–219.

Gillham, J. E., Reivich, K. J., Freres, D. R., Lascher, M., Litzinger, S., Shatté, A.J. et al. (2006). School-based prevention of depression and anxiety symptoms in early adolescence: A pilot of a parent intervention component. *School Psychology Quarterly, 21*, 323–348.

Gillham, J. E., Reivich, K. J., Jaycox, L. H., & Seligman, M. E. P. (1995). Prevention of depressive symptoms in schoolchildren: Two-year follow-up. *Psychological Science, 6*, 343–351.

Gillham, J. E., Shatté, A. J., & Freres, D. R. (2000). Preventing depression: A review of cognitive-behavioral and family interventions. *Applied and Preventive Psychology, 9*, 63–88.

Glod, C. A., Lynch, A., Flynn, E., Berkowitz, C., & Baldessarini, R. J. (2003). Open trial of bupropion sr in adolescent major depression. *Journal of Child and Adolescent Psychiatric Nursing, 16*, 123–130.

Gotlib, I. H., Lewinsoh, P. M., & Seeley, J. R. (1995). Symptoms versus a diagnosis of depression: Differences in psychosocial functioning. *Journal of Consulting and Clinical Psychology, 63*, 90–100.

Gutgesell, H., Atkins, D., Barst, R. Buck, M., Franklin, W., Humes, R., et al. (1999). AHA scientific statement: Cardiovascular monitoring of children and adolescents receiving psychotropic drugs. *Journal of the American Academy of Child and Adolescent Psychiatry, 28*, 1047–1050.

Haarasilta, L., Marttunen, M., Kaprio, J., & Aro, H. (2001). The 12-month prevalence and characteristics of major depressive episode in a representative sample of adolescents and young adults. *Psychological Medicine, 31*, 1169–1179.

Hankin, B. L., & Abramson, L. Y. (2001). Development of gender difference in depression: An elaborated cognitive vulnerability-transactional stress theory. *Psychological Bulletin, 127*, 773–796.

Hankin, B. L., Abramson, L. Y., Moffit, T. E., Silva, P. A., McGee, R., & Angell, K. E. (1998). Development of depression from preadolescence to young adulthood: Emerging gender differences in a 10-year longitudinal study. *Journal of Abnormal Psychology, 107*, 128–140.

Hankin, B. L., Fraley, R. C., Lahey, B. B., & Waldman, I. D. (2005). Is youth depressive disorder best viewed as a continuum or discrete category? A taxometric analysis of childhood and adolescent depression in a population-based sample. *Journal of Abnormal Psychology, 114*, 96–110.

Harrington, R., & Dubicka, B. (2001). Natural history of mood disorders in children and adolescents. In I. M. Goodyer (Ed.), *The depressed child and adolescent* (2nd ed., pp. 353–381). New York, NY: Cambridge University Press.

Harrington, R., Fudge, H., Rutter, M., Pickles, A., & Hill, J. (1990). Adult outcomes of childhood and adolescent depression: I. Psychiatric status. *Archives of General Psychiatry, 47*, 465–473.

Harrington, R., Fudge, H., Rutter, M., Pickles, A., & Hill, J. (1991). Adult outcomes of childhood and adolescent depression: II. Links with antisocial disorders. *Journal of the American Academy of Child & Adolescent Psychiatry, 30*, 434–439.

Harrington, R. Rutter, M., & Fombonne, E. (1996). Developmental pathways in depression: Multiple meanings, antecedents, and endpoints. *Development and Psychopathology, 8*, 601–616.

Harter, S., & Nowakowski, M., (1987). Manual for the dimensions of depression profile for children and adolescents. University of Denver.

Hazell, P., O'Donnell, D., Heathcote, D., & Henry, D. (2004). Tricyclic drugs for depression in children and adolescents. *Cochrane Database of Systematic Reviews*. The Cochrane Library, 3.

Hodges, K. (1994). Evaluation of depression in children and adolescents using diagnostic clinical interviews. In H. F. Johnston & W. M. Reynolds (Eds.), *Handbook of depression in children and adolescents* (pp. 209–234). New York: Plenum Press.

Horowitz, J. L., & Garber, J. (2006). The prevention of depressive symptoms in children and adolescents: A meta-analytic review. *Journal of Consulting and Clinical Psychology, 74*, 401–415.

Horowitz, J. L., Garber, J., Ciesla, J. A., Young, J. F., & Mufson, L. (2007). Prevention of depressive symptoms in adolescents: A randomized trial of cognitive-behavioral and interpersonal prevention programs. *Journal of Consulting and Clinical Psychology, 75*, 693–706.

Hyde, J. S., Mezulis, A. H., & Abramson, L. Y. (2008). The A-B-Cs of depression: Integrating affective, biological, and cognitive models to explain the emergence of the gender difference in depression. *Psychological Review, 115*, 291–313.

Jaycox, L. H., Asarnow, J. R, Sherbourne, C. D., Rea, M. M., LaBorde, A. P., & Wells, K. B. (2006). Adolescent primary care patients' preferences for depression treatment. *Administration and Policy in Mental Health and Mental Health Services Research, 33*, 198–207.

Jaycox, L. H., Reivich, K. J., Gillham, J., & Seligman, M. E. P. (1994). Prevention of depressive symptoms in school children. *Behavior Research and Therapy, 32*, 801–816.

Jensen, P. A., Shervette, R. E., Xenakis, S. N., & Richters, J. (1993). Anxiety and depressive disorders in attention deficit disorder with hyperactivity: New findings. *American Journal of Psychiatry, 150*, 1203–1209.

Kahn, J. S., Kehle, T. J., Jenson, W. R., & Clark, E. (1990). Comparison of cognitive-behavioral, relaxation, and self-modeling interventions for depression among middle-school students. *School Psychology Review, 19*, 196–211.

Kaminski, K. M., & Garber, J. (2002). Depressive spectrum disorders in high-risk adolescents; Episode duration and predictors of time to recovery. *Journal of the American Academy of Child & Adolescent Psychiatry, 41*, 410–418.

Kaslow, N. J., McClure, E. B., & Connell, A. M. (2002). Treatment of depression in children and adolescents. In C. L. Hammen & I. H. Gotlib (Eds.). *Handbook of depression* (pp. 441–464). New York: Guilford Press.

Kataoka, S. H., Zhang, L., & Wells, K. B. (2002). Unmet need for mental health care among U. S. children: Variation by ethnicity and insurance status. *American Journal of Psychiatry, 159*, 1548–1555.

Kaufman, J., Birmaher B., Brent, D., Rao, U., Flynn, C. Moreci, P. et al. (1997). Schedule for affective disorders and schizophrenia for school-age children-present and lifetime version (K-SADS-PL): Initial reliability and validity data. *Journal of the American Academy of Child and Adolescent Psychiatry, 36*, 980–988.

Keller, M. B., Ryan, N. D., Strober, M., Klein, R. G., Kutcher, S. P., Birmaher, B., et al. (2001). *Journal of the American Academy of Child and Adolescent Psychiatry, 40*, 762–772.

Kessler, R. C., Avenevoli, Sh., & Merikangas, K. R. (2001). Mood disorders in children and adolescents: An epidemiologic perspective. *Biological Psychiatry, 49*, 1002–1014.

Kessler, R. C., Berglund, P., Demler, O., Jin, R., & Walters, E. E. (2005). Lifetime prevalence and age-of-onset distributions of DSM-IV disorders in the national comorbidity survey replication. *Archives of General Psychiatry, 62*, 593–602.

Kessler, R. C., Foster, C. L., Saunders, W. B., & Stang, P. E. (1995). Social consequences of psychiatric disorders I: Educational attainment. *American Journal of Psychiatry, 152*, 1026–1032.

Kessler R. C., & Walters E. E. (2002). The National Comorbidity Survey. In: M. T. Tsaung & M. Tohen M (Eds.). *Textbook in Psychiatric Epidemiology. 2nd ed.* (pp. 343–362). New York: John Wiley & Sons Inc.

Kiecolt-Glaser, J. K., & Glaser, R. (2002). Depression and immune function: Central pathways to morbidity and mortality. *Journal of Psychosomatic Research, 53*, 873–876.

Kim-Cohen, J., Caspi, A., Moffitt, T. E., Harrington, H., Milne, B. J., & Poulton, R. (2003). Prior juvenile diagnoses in adults with mental disorder: Developmental follow-back of a prospective-longitudinal cohort. *Archives of General Psychiatry, 60*, 709–717.

Kovacs, M. (1985). The children's depression inventory. *Psychopharmacology Bulletin, 21*, 995–998.

Kovacs, M. (1997). The Interview Schedule for Children and Adolescents (ISCA): Current and Lifetime (ISCA-C & L) and Current and Interim (ISCA-C & I) Versions. Pittsburgh: Western Psychiatric Institute and Clinic

Kovacs, M., Feinberg, L., Crouse-Novak, M. A., Paulauskas, S. L., & Finkelstein, R. (1984). Depressive disorders in childhood. I. A longitudinal prospective study of characteristics and recovery. *Archives of General Psychiatry, 41*, 229–237.

Kovacs, M., Gatsonis, C., Paulauskas, S. L., & Richards, C. (1989). Depressive disorders in childhood: IV. A longitudinal study of comorbidity with and risk for anxiety disorders. *Archives of General Psychiatry, 46*, 776–782.

Kramer, T., & Garralda, M. E. (1998). Psychiatric disorders in adolescents in primary care. *British Journal of Psychiatry, 173*, 508–513.

Kramer, R. A., Warner, V., Olfson, M., Ebanks, C. E., Chaput, F., & Weissman, M. M. (1998). General medical problems among the offspring of depressed parents: A 10-year follow-up. *Journal of the American Academy of Child and Adolescent Psychiatry, 37*, 602–612.

Lau, J. Y. F., & Eley, T. C. (2008). Disentangling gene–environment correlations and interactions in adolescent depression. *Journal of Child Psychology and Psychiatry, 49*, 142–150.

Lavigne, J. V., Binns, H. J., Christoffel, K. K., Rosenbaum, D., Arend, R., Smith, K., et al. (1993). Behavior and emotional problems among preschool children in pediatric primary care: Prevalence and pediatric recognition. *Pediatrics, 91*, 649–655.

Lewinsohn, P.M., Clarke, G.N., Seeley, J.R., & Rohde, P. (1994), Major depression in community adolescents: age at onset, episode duration, and time to recurrence. *Journal of the American Academy of Child and Adolescent Psychiatry, 33*, 809–818.

Lewinsohn, P. M., & Essau, C. A. (2002). Depression in adolescents. In I. H. Gotlib & C. L. Hammen (Eds.), *Handbook of depression* (pp. 541–559). New York, NY: Guilford.

Lewinsohn, P. M., Hops, H., Roberts, R. E., Seeley, J. R., & Andrews, J. A. (1993). Adolescent psychopathology: I. Prevalence and incidence of depression and other DSM-III-R disorders in high school students. *Journal of Abnormal Psychology, 102*, 133–144.

Lewinsohn, P. M., Rohde, P., Klein, D. N., & Seeley, J. R. (1999). Natural course of adolescent major depressive disorder: I. Continuity into young adulthood. *Journal of the American Academy of Child and Adolescent Psychiatry, 38*, 56–63.

Lewinsohn, P. M., Rohde, P., & Seeley, J. R. (1998). Major depressive disorder in older adolescents: Prevalence, risk factors, and clinical implications. *Clinical Psychology Review, 18*, 765–794.

Lewinsohn, P. M., Rohde, P., Seeley, J. R., & Hops, H. (1991). Comorbidity of unipolar depression: I. Major depression with dysthymia. *Journal of Abnormal Psychology, 100*, 205–213.

Lewinsohn, P. M., Rohde, P., Seeley, J. R., Klein, D. N., & Gotlib, I. H. (2000). Natural course of adolescent major depressive disorder in a community sample: Predictors of recurrence in young adults. *American Journal of Psychiatry, 157*, 1584–1591.

Madoki, M. W., Tapia, M. R., Tapia, M. A., & Sumner, G. S. (1997). Venlafaxine in the treatment of children and adolescents with major depression. *Psychopharmacology Bulletin, 33*, 149–154.

Masi, G., Marchesi, M., & Pfanner, P. (1997). Paroxetine in depressed adolescents with intellectual disability: An open label study. *Journal of Intellectual Disability Research, 41*, 268–272.

McConville, B. J., Minnery, K. L., Sorter, M. T., West, S. A., Friedman, L. M., & Christian, K. (1996). An open study of the effects of sertraline on adolescent major depression. *Journal of Child and Adolescent Psychopharmacology, 6*, 41–51.

Meehl, P. E. (1995). Bootstraps taxometrics: Solving the classification problem in psychopathology. *American Psychologist, 50*, 266 –275.

Merry, S., McDowell, H., Hetrick, S., Bir, J., & Muller, N. (2004). Psychological and/or educational interventions for the prevention of depression in children and adolescents. *Cochrane Database of Systematic Reviews*, Issue 2., 1–103, Art. No.: CD003380. DOI: 10.1002/14651858. CD003380.pub2.

Merry, S. N., McDowell, H., Wild, C. J., Bir, J., & Cunliffe, R. (2004). A randomized placebo controlled trial of a school-based depression prevention program. *Journal of the American Academy of Child and Adolescent Psychiatry, 43*, 538–547.

Merry, S. N., & Spence, S. H. (2007). Attempting to prevent depression in youth: A systematic review of the evidence. *Early Intervention in Psychiatry, 1*, 128–137.

Monheit, A. C., & Cunningham, P. J. (1992): Children without health insurance. *Future Child, 3*, 154–170.

Moreau, D., Mufson, L., Weissman, M. M., & Klerman, G. L. (1991). Interpersonal psychotherapy for adolescent depression: Description of modification and preliminary application. *Journal of the American Academy of Child and Adolescent Psychiatry, 30*, 642–651.

Mrazek, P. J., & Haggerty, R. J. (1994). *Reducing risks for mental disorders: Frontiers for preventive intervention research*. Washington, DC: National Academy Press.

Mufson, L., & Fairbanks, J. (1996). Interpersonal psychotherapy for depressed adolescents: A one-year naturalistic follow-up study. *Journal of the American Academy of Child and Adolescent Psychiatry, 35*, 1145–1155.

Mufson, L., Moreau, D., Weissman, M. M., & Garfinkel, R. (1999). Efficacy of interpersonal psychotherapy for depressed adolescents. *Archives of General Psychiatry, 56*, 573–579.

Mufson, L., Moreau, D., Weissman, M. M., Wickramartne, P., Martin, J., & Samoilov, A. (1994). Modification of interpersonal psychotherapy with depressed adolescents (IPT-A): Phase I and II studies. *Journal of the American Academy of Child and Adolescent Psychiatry, 33*, 695–705.

Mufson, L., Pollack-Dorta, K., Wickramaratne, P., Nomura, W., Olfson, M., & Weissman, M. (2004). A randomized effectiveness trial of interpersonal psychotherapy for depressed adolescents. *Archives of General Psychiatry, 61*, 577–584.

Nobile, M., Bellotti, B., Marino, C., Molteni, M., & Battaglia, M. (2000). An open trial of paroxetine in the treatment of children and adolescents diagnosed with dysthymia. *Journal of Child and Adolescent Psychopharmacology., 10*, 103–109.

Nolen-Hoeksema, S., & Girgus, J. S. (1994). The emergence of gender differences in depression during adolescence. *Psychological Bulletin, 115*, 424–443.

Olson, A. L., Kelleher, K. J., Kemper, K. J., Zuckerman, B. S., Hammond. C.S., & Dietrich, S. J. (2001). Primary care pediatricians roles and perceived responsibilities in the identification and management of depression in children and adolescents. *Ambulatory Pediatrics, 1*, 91–98.

Pine, D. S., Cohen, E., Cohen, P., & Brook, J. (1999). Adolescent depressive symptoms as predictors of adult depression: Moodiness or mood disorder? *American Journal of Psychiatry, 156*, 133–135.

Puig-Antich, J., & Gittleman, R. (1982). Depression in childhood and adolescence. In E. Paykel (Ed.), *Handbook of affective disorders* (pp. 379–392). New York: Guilford Press.

Quayle, D., Dzuirawiec, S., Roberts, C., Kane, R., & Ebsworthy, G. (2001). The effect of an optimism and life skills program on depressive symptoms in preadolescence. *Behaviour Change, 18*, 194–203.

Rabe-Joblanska, J. (2000). Therapeutic effects and tolerability of fluvoxamine treatment in adolescents with

dysthymia. *Journal of Child and Adolescent Psychopharmacology, 10*, 9–18.
Radloff, L. S. (1991). The use of the Center for Epidemiologic Studies Depression Scale in adolescents and young adults. *Journal of Youth and Adolescence, 20*, 149–166.
Rao, U., Hammen, C., & Daley, S. (1999). Continuity of depression during the transition to adulthood: A 5-year longitudinal study of young women. *Journal of the American Academy of Child and Adolescent Psychiatry, 38*, 908–915.
Rao, U., Ryan, N. D., Birmaher, B., Dahl, R. E., Williamson, D. E., Kaufman, J., et al. (1995). Unipolar depression in adolescents: Clinical outcomes in adulthood. *Journal of the American Academy of Child and Adolescent Psychiatry, 34*, 566–578.
Reich, W. (1991). *The diagnostic interview for children and adolescents – revised.* St. Louis, MO: Washington University.
Resnick, M. D., Bearman, P. S., Blum, W., Bauman, K. E., Harris, K. M., Jones, J. et al. (1997). Protecting adolescents from harm: Findings from the National Longitudinal Study on Adolescent Health. *Journal of the American Medical Association, 278*, 823–832.
Rey-Sanchez, F., & Gutierrez-Casares, J. R. (1997). Paroxetine in children with major depressive disorder: An open trial. *Journal of the American Academy of Child and Adolescent Psychiatry, 36*, 1443–1447.
Reynolds, W. M. (1987). *Reynolds adolescent depression scale: Professional manual.* Odessa, FL: Psychological Assessment Resources.
Reynolds, W. M., & Coats, K. I. (1986). A comparison of cognitive-behavioral therapy and relaxation training for the treatment of depression in adolescents. *Journal of Consulting and Clinical Psychology, 54*, 653–660.
Reynolds, C. R., & Kamphaus, R. W. (2003). *Handbook of psychological and educational assessment of children: Personality, behavior, and context* (2nd ed.). New York: Guilford Press.
Rice, F., Harold, G. T., & Thapar, A. (2002). Assessing the effects of age, sex and shared environment on the genetic aetiology of depression in childhood and adolescence. *Journal of Child Psychology and Psychiatry and Allied Disciplines, 43*, 1039–1051.
Riggs, P. D., Mikulich, S. K., Coffman, L. M., & Crowley, T. J. (1997). Fluoxetine in drug-dependent delinquents with major depression: An open trial. *Journal of Child and Adolescent Psychopharmacology, 7*, 87–95.
Roberts, R. E., Andrews, J. A., Lewinsohn, P. M., & Hops, H. (1990). Assessment of depression in adolescents using the Center for Epidemiologic Studies Depression Scale. *Psychological Assessment, 2*, 122–128.
Roberts, R. E., & Chen, Y. W. (1995). Depressive symptoms and suicidal ideation among Mexican-origin and Anglo adolescents. *Journal of the American Academy of Child and Adolescent Psychiatry, 34*, 81–90.
Rohde, P., Kahler, C. W., Lewinsohn, P. M., & Brown, R. A. (2004). Psychiatric disorders, familial factors, and cigarette smoking: III. Associations with cessation by young adulthood among daily smokers. *Nicotine and Tobacco Research, 5*, 509–522.
Rohde, P., Lewinsohn, P. M., & Seeley, J. R. (1991). Comorbidity of unipolar depression: II. Comorbidity with other mental disorders in adolescents and adults. *Journal of Abnormal Psychology, 100*, 214–222.
Rohde, P., Lewinsohn, P. M., & Seeley, J. R. (1994). Are adolescents changed by an episode of depression? *Journal of the American Academy of Child and Adolescent Psychiatry, 33*, 1289–1298.
Rosello, J., & Bernal, G. (1999). The efficacy of cognitive-behavioral and interpersonal treatments for depression in Puerto Rican adolescents. *Journal of Consulting and Clinical Psychology, 67*, 734–745.
Rudolph, K. D., & Clark, A. G. (2001). Conceptions of relationships in children with depressive and aggressive symptoms: Social-cognitive distortion or reality? *Journal of Abnormal Child Psychology, 29*, 41–56.
Rudolph, K. D., Hammen, C., Burge, D., Lindberg, N., Herzberg, D., & Daley, S. E. (2000). Toward an interpersonal life-stress model of depression: The developmental context of stress generation. *Development and Psychopathology, 12*, 215–234.
Ruscio, J., & Ruscio, A. M. (2000). Informing the continuity controversy: A taxometric analysis of depression. *Journal of Abnormal Psychology, 109*, 473–487.
Ryan, N. D., Puig-Antich, J., Ambrosini, P., Rabinovich, H., Robinson, D., Nelson, B., et al. (1987). The clinical picture of major depression in children and adolescents. *Archives of General Psychiatry, 44*, 854–861.
Santor, D. A., & Kusumakar, V. (2001). Open trial of interpersonal therapy in adolescents with moderate to severe major depression: Effectiveness of novice IPT therapists. *Journal of the American Academy of Child and Adolescent Psychiatry, 40*, 236–240.
Shaffer, D., & Craft, L. (1999). Methods of adolescent suicide prevention. *Journal of Clinical Psychiatry, 60*, 70–74.
Shaffer, D., Fisher, P., Lucas, C., Dulcan, M., & Schwab-Stone, M. (2000). NIMH Diagnostic Interview Schedule for Children Version IV (NIMH DISC-IV): Description, differences from previous versions and reliability of some common diagnoses. *Journal of the American Academy of Child and Adolescent Psychiatry, 39*, 28–38.
Shatin, D., & Drinkard, C. R. (2002). Ambulatory use of psychotropics by employer-insured children and adolescents in a national managed care organization. *Ambulatory Pediatrics, 2*, 111–119.
Sheffield, J. K., Spence, S. H., Rapee, R. M., Kowalenko, N., Wignall, A., Davis, A. et al. (2006). Evaluation of universal, indicated, and combined cognitive-behavioral approaches to the prevention of depression among adolescents. *Journal of Consulting and Clinical Psychology, 74*, 66–79.
Shochet, I., Dadds, M., Holland, D., Whitefield, K., Harnett, P., & Osgarby, S. (2001). The efficacy of a universal school-based program to prevent adolescent depression. *Journal of Clinical Child Psychology, 30*, 303–315.
Simeon, J. G., Dinicola, V. F., Ferguson, H. B., & Copping W. (1990). Adolescent depression: A placebo-controlled fluoxetine treatment study and follow-up. *Progress in Neuro Psychopharmacology and Biological Psychiatry, 14*, 791–795.
Simonoff, E., Pickles, A., Meyer, J. M., Silberg, J. L., Maes, H. H., Loeber, R., et al. (1997). The Virginia twin study of adolescent behavioral development Influences of age, sex,

and impairment on rates of disorder. *Archives of General Psychiatry, 54*, 801–808.

Solhkhah, R., Wilens, T. E., Daly, J., Prince, J. B., Van Patten, S. L., & Biederman, J. (2005). Bupropion SR for the treatment of substance-abusing outpatient adolescents with attention-deficit/hyperactivity disorder and mood disorders. *Journal of Child and Adolescent Psychopharmacology, 15*, 777–786.

Somers-Flanagan, J., & Sommers-Flanagan, R. (1996). Efficacy of antidepressant medication with depressed youth: What psychologists should know. *Professional Psychology: Research and Practice, 27*, 145–153.

Speier, P. L., Sherak, D. L., Hirsch, S., & Cantwell, D. P. (1995). Depression in children and adolescents. In W. R. Leber & E. E. Beckham (Eds.), *Handbook of depression* (2nd ed.,. pp. 467–493). New York: Guilford Press.

Spence, S. H., Sheffield, J. K., & Donovan, C. L. (2003). Preventing adolescent depression: An evaluation of the Problem Solving for Life Program. *Journal of Consulting and Clinical Psychology, 71*, 3–13.

Spence, S. H., & Sheffield, J. K., & Donovan, C. L. (2005). Long-term outcome of a school-based, universal approach to prevention of depression in adolescents. *Journal of Consulting and Clinical Psychology, 73*, 160–167.

Spitzer, R. L., Williams, B., Kroenke, K., Linzer, M., deGruy, F. V., Hahn, S. R., et al. (1994). Utility of a new procedure for diagnosing mental disorders in primary care. The PRIME-MD 1000 study. *The Journal of the American Medical Association, 272*, 1749–1756.

Stark, K. D., Laurent, J. Livingston, R., Boswell, J., & Swearer. S. (1999). Implications of research for the treatment of depressive disorders during childhood. *Applied and Preventive Psychology, 8*, 79–102.

Stark, K. C., Reynolds. W. M., & Kaslow, N. J. (1987). A comparison of the relative efficacy of self-control therapy and a behavioral problem-solving therapy for depression in children. *Journal of Abnormal of Child Psychology, 15*, 91–113.

Stein, R. E. K., Zitner, L. E., & Jensen, P. S. (2006). Interventions for adolescent depression in primary care. *Pediatrics, 118*, 669–682.

Sturm, R. (1997). How expensive is unlimited mental health care coverage under managed care? *Journal of the American Medical Association, 278*, 1533–1537.

Sutton, J. M. (2007). Prevention of depression in youth: A qualitative review and future suggestions. *Clinical Psychology Review, 27*, 552–571.

Thomas, C. R. (1999). National distribution of child and adolescent psychiatrists. *Journal of the American Academy of Child and Adolescent Psychiatry, 38*, 9–15.

Treatment for Adolescents with Depression Study (TADS) Team. (2004). Fluoxetine, cognitive-behavioral therapy, and their combination for adolescents with depression: Treatment for Adolescents with Depression Study (TADS) randomized controlled trial. *Journal of the American Medical Association, 292*, 807–820.

US Food and Drug Administration. Executive Summary. Available at: http://www.fda.gov/cder/. Accessed November 8, 2007.

Vostanis, P., Feehan, C., Grattan, E., & Bickerton, W. L. (1996). A randomised controlled out-patient trial of cognitive-behavioural treatment for children and adolescents with depression: 9-month follow-up. *Journal of Affective Disorders, 40*, 105–116.

Wagner, K. D., & Ambrosini, P. J. (2003). Efficacy of sertraline in the treatment of children and adolescents with major depressive disorder: Two randomized controlled trials. *Journal of the American Medical Association, 290*, 2033–1041.

Wagner, K. D., Jonas, J., Findling, R. L., Ventura, D., & Saikali, K. (2006). A double-blind, randomized, placebo-controlled trial of escitalopram in the treatment of pediatric depression. *Journal of the American Academy of Child and Adolescent Psychiatry, 45*, 280–288.

Wagner, K. D., Robb, A. S., Findling, R. L., Jin, J. Guierrez, M. M., & Heydorn, W.E. (2004). A randomized, placebo-controlled trial of citalopram for the treatment of major depression in children and adolescents. *American Journal of Psychiatry, 161*, 1079–1083.

Walker, Z., Townsend, J., Oakley, L., et al. (2002). Health promotion for adolescents in primary care: randomized controlled trial. *British Medical Journal, 325*, 524–529.

Waslick, B. D., Walsh, B. T., Greenhill, L. L., Ellenberg, M., Capasso L., & Lieber, D. (1999). Open trial of fluoxetine in children and adolescents with dysthymic disorder or double depression. *Journal of Affective Disorders, 56*, 227–236.

Weiss, B., & Garber, J. (2003). Developmental differences in the phenomenology of depression. *Development and Psychopathology, 15*, 403–430.

Weissman, M. M., Wolk, S., Goldstein, R. B., Moreau, D., Adams, P., Greenwald, S., et al. (1999). Depressed adolescents grown up. *Journal of the American Medical Association, 281*, 1707–1713.

Wells, K. B., Kataoka, S. H., & Asarnow, J. R. (2001). Affective disorders in children and adolescents: Addressing unmet need in primary care settings. *Biological Psychiatry, 49*, 1111–1120.

Wells, K. B., Stuart, A., Hays, R. D., Burnam, M. A., Rogers, W., Daniels, M. et al. (1989). The functioning and well-being of depressed patients: Results from the medical outcomes study. *Journal of the American Medical Association, 262*, 914–919.

Wilens, T. E., Spencer, T. J., Biederman, J., & Schleifer, D. (1997). Case study: Nefazodone for juvenile mood disorders. *Journal of the American Academy of Child and Adolescent Psychiatry, 36*, 481–485.

Wood, A., Harrington, R., & Moore, A. (1996). Controlled trial of a brief cognitive-behavioural intervention in adolescent patients with depressive disorders. *Journal of Child Psychology and Psychiatry, 37*, 737–746.

Yorbik, O., Birmaher B., Axelson D., Williamson, D. E., & Ryan, N. D. (2004). Clinical characteristics of depressive symptoms in children and adolescents with major depressive disorder. *Journal of Clinical Psychiatry, 65*, 1654–1659.

Young, J. F., Mufson, L., & Davies, M. (2006). Efficacy of interpersonal psychotherapy-adolescent skills training: An indicated preventive intervention for depression. *Journal of Child Psychology and Psychiatry, 47*, 1254–1262.

Yu, D. L., & Seligman, M. E. P. (2002). Preventing depression in Chinese students. *Prevention & Treatment, 5*, Article 9.

Zuckerbrot, R. A., Maxon, L., Pagar, D., Davies, M., Fisher, P. W., & Shaffer, D. (2007). Adolescent depression screening in primary care: Feasibility and acceptability, *Pediatrics, 119*, 101–108.

Cancer

Lisa A. Schwartz, Anne E. Kazak, and Ifigenia Mougianis

Childhood cancer is a potentially traumatic experience for youth and their families. The impact of cancer on adolescents is especially significant given the critical developmental stage of adolescence and its expanding ecology encompassing school, friends, work, and romantic partners. Comprehensive care that includes physicians (pediatric oncologists and other medical subspecialists), nurses, social workers, child life specialists, nutritionists, teachers and tutors, psychologists, and other mental health professionals is critical for optimal treatment of adolescent cancer patients. In addition to curative treatment, the objectives of such care include behavioral interventions to improve quality of life, improve adherence, facilitate "normal" adolescent development, provide support to the patient and their families, and manage distress, pain, and other symptoms. The present chapter describes the characteristics of and medical issues related to adoles cent cancer, the impact on adolescents and their families, related interventions, future research implications, and methodological considerations. The focus of this chapter is on those with cancer while they are in their teens and early twenties, or long-term survivors in the same age range.

Epidemiology and Related Issues

Cancer has many forms and types and is always potentially life threatening. It represents a broad spectrum of malignancies that vary by histology and site of disease and is the leading cause of disease-related deaths in adolescents [U.S. Department of Health and Human Services (USDHHS), National Institutes of Health, National Cancer Institute, Livestrong, 2006]. Cancer may be related to genetic, constitutional, behavioral, and environmental causes. However, cancer risk and etiology are not well understood for children and adolescents who have less exposure to the behavioral (e.g., smoking, diet) and environmental risks (e.g., sun, chemical exposures) relative to adults.

The incidence of cancer in 15- to 30-year-old adolescents is almost three times more than incidence in the first 15 years of life with 1 out of every 168 adolescents and young adults developing cancer (Bleyer, 2007). The most common cancer diagnoses in 15- to 19-year-olds (representing 90% of the cases) include acute leukemias, lymphomas, central nervous system tumors, bone and soft tissue sarcomas, germ cell and other gonadal tumors, thyroid carcinoma, and malignant melanoma (Stiller, 2002). Of these, leukemias and lymphomas are most common, occurring in over 30% of adolescents, although the incidence declines across adolescence. However, survival from acute lymphoblastic leukemia (ALL) is worse in teens (range of 53.5–79% 5-year event-free survival) than in younger children (80% 5-year event-free survival) (Ramanujachar, Richards, Hann, & Webb, 2008). Osteosarcoma (bone cancer) peaks in incidence in 15- to 19-year-olds – a cancer which often results is long-term physical impairments. Cancer incidence for males and females during adolescence is similar although the incidence is 50% higher for White, Non-Hispanics than African-Americans.

The 5-year relative survival rates for 15- to 19-year-olds is excellent, over 75%, and higher than that for

L.A. Schwartz (✉)
The Children's Hospital of Philadelphia, University of Pennsylvania, Philadelphia, PA, USA
e-mail: schwartzl@email.cnop.edu

W.T. O'Donohue, L.W. Tolle (eds.), *Behavioral Approaches to Chronic Disease in Adolescence*, DOI 10.1007/978-0-387-87687-0_16, © Springer Science+Business Media, LLC 2009 younger children. Among 15- to 29-year-olds, survival is highest for non-Hispanic whites, whereas African-Americans have the lowest survival rate, with a 20% difference apparent by 5 years (USDHHS et al., 2006). Although overall survival rate is high, improvements in survival rates for this group have lagged behind that in younger patients for many reasons (Bleyer, 2002). For one, there is a lack of attention to the differences in the biology of cancers in adolescence (Bleyer et al., 2008). Another significant concern is the delay in diagnosis for many adolescents (Albritton & Eden, 2008). The number of days between symptom onset and diagnosis increases with age in pediatric and adolescent patients. Reasons for this delay include embarrassment by symptoms and/or lack of communication about symptoms to parents or providers, lack of a primary-care provider, lack of insurance – especially for those who are no longer dependents, and misattribution of symptoms to stress, normal injuries, or insignificant illnesses. Physicians, too, often misdiagnose symptoms and may not consider a potential diagnosis of cancer (USDHHS et al., 2006; Bleyer, 2002).

Furthermore, there are unique issues of adolescents that affect outcomes once they are diagnosed. Unlike younger children, of whom most are enrolled in clinical trials, only 20% of 15–19 year olds are seen at institutions with NCI clinical trials and 10% are enrolled in clinical trials (USDHHS et al., 2006; Bleyer, 2002). A similar problem is the lack of standardization of where to treat adolescents. Many are treated in adult institutions, despite research demonstrating improved survival rates for those treated at pediatric institutions, where there is more access to clinical trials and more available supportive services (Albritton & Eden, 2008). Lastly, as discussed later, a significant issue for adolescents is adherence to treatment, especially oral chemotherapy and antibiotic regimens. Nonadherence to medication regimens is most common in adolescents (Rapoff, McGrath, & Smith, 2006) and is life threatening (Kennard et al., 2004).

Treatment

Improved success in curing children and adolescents with cancer is related to the intensive treatments that they must receive. The course of the cancer treatment is variable depending on the type of malignancy. Treatments may last up to 3 years or longer and may include combinations of chemotherapy, radiation, and surgery. Because of the potentially long treatment duration and long-term medical sequelae from treatment, cancer is often considered a chronic health condition. There are, however, potential acute periods within the disease's courses, depending on the diagnosis. As an example, treatment for ALL typically involves three phases of chemotherapy: approximately 4 weeks of induction, 6 months of consolidation, and 2–3 years of maintenance. Patients often receive an intravenous line to facilitate chemotherapy. Such lines require close attention including dressing changes and flushing to prevent infection. Furthermore, treatment often requires hospital admissions and may include blood count checks multiple times a week. In addition to frequent blood draws, patients may undergo periodic lumbar punctures and bone marrow aspirations, which can be anxiety producing and potentially painful. Bone marrow/stem cell transplants may also be part of treatment regimen, especially for those diagnosed with acute myelogenous leukemia (AML) or for those who have relapsed. Because many of the treatments leave adolescents immunocomprimised, they are often required to limit contact with others including friends and pets. Overall, the treatment regimen for pediatric cancer is intense, intrusive in one's life given the many appointments and in-patient stays, and can last years. Furthermore, it is recommended that long-term survivors of childhood cancer attend, at minimum, annual follow-up visits with an oncologist or provider familiar with long-term issues of childhood cancer survivors (Children's Oncology Group, http://www.survivorshipguidelines.org).

Symptoms and Long-Term Medical Problems

Symptoms of cancer and its treatment are generally similar to those of children and adults. Unlike many other diseases, the treatment for cancer may produce more debilitating symptoms than the cancer itself. Fortunately, teens are better able to describe symptoms than younger children (Bleyer, 2002). The most common symptoms experienced include pain, nausea and vomiting, nutritional concerns, mucositis, and fatigue (Hockenberry, 2004). More than half of pediatric patients with cancer report moderate-to-severe cancer-related pain (Hellsten, 2000) with the majority experiencing pain at some point related to procedures such as blood draws and bone marrow aspirations. Furthermore, chemotherapy treatments can cause changes in appearance such as weight gain or hair loss. Such changes can exacerbate distress experienced by adolescents with cancer given inherent insecurities about appearance in adolescence.

Those who have completed treatment may suffer from medical problems that result from the cancer or cancer treatment and are known as physical late effects. Even if late effects are not present, survivors may be at increased risk for long-term medical morbidities, many of which are life threatening and can include a second cancer diagnosis. Late effects can impact any organ or system of the body. Examples are cardiac or pulmonary disease, short stature, infertility, dermatologic problems, and problems with senses of hearing and vision. Such problems may not emerge until years after treatment and can increase in severity over time (Oeffinger et al., 2006). Problems such as pain and fatigue also persist into survivorship. Furthermore, permanent disfigurement or altered appearance is an issue for many survivors and heighten self-consciousness due to problems such as scars from surgery, orthopedic difficulties or amputations, visible dermatological late effects related to skin or hair, dental irregula rities, physical asymmetry, and growth problems (Bottomley & Kassner, 2003). Because of such physical late effects, survivors have also reported more functional limitations compared to siblings (Ness et al., 2005). These include lower ability to attend work or school, engage in self-care activities, and routine activities.

Psychosocial and Behavioral Challenges of Adolescents with Cancer

For the most part, adolescents on treatment and long-term adolescent survivors are resilient and report positive overall adjustment. Nonetheless, patients that are diagnosed during adolescence may experience their illness and treatment quite differently than younger children. Reasons for this include the following (1) they are more likely to have direct conversations with their parents and medical team members about their disease, treatment, side effects, and prognosis, (2) they may participate directly in decision making about treatment, (3) their cognitive ability and life experience may enable them to better understand the cancer diagnosis and its implications, and 4) their ability to cope with the challenges of treatment may be greater than for younger children given their larger repertoire of coping strategies (Decker, 2006). The potential impact on development and potential psychosocial sequelae and challenges that are experienced by some adolescents and their families, are described next.

General Developmental Challenges

Adolescence is a period of development characterized by the emergence of autonomy in setting and striving for personal goals. Such goal striving is critical for identity development, planning to transition to adulthood, and overall well-being (Nurmi, 1993). Cancer-related disruptions (e.g., long hospitalizations, frequent medical appointments, invasive procedures, surgeries, nausea, fatigue, and pain) of these critical developmental processes are likely to affect identity development and cause psychological distress that may have lasting effects into adulthood (Rowland, Pfefferbaum, Adams-Greenly, & Redd, 1989; Zeltzer, 1993). For example, research has demonstrated that (1) cancer impacts identity development (Gavaghan & Roach, 1987; Madan-Swain et al., 2000), (2) adolescents with cancer often report worse quality of life than healthy peers or long-term survivors (Wu et al., 2007), and (3) young adult survivors are more likely to experience psychosocial problems in early adulthood when their cancer occurred during adolescence (Felder-Puig et al., 1998; Kupst et al., 1995; Wu et al., 2007). Furthermore, preliminary data shows that, compared to healthy controls, adolescents with cancer report more health-related hindrance of pursuit of personal goals (Schwartz & Wolf, 2008).

Indeed, research suggests that AYA survivors identify "maintaining normalcy" as an important priority in order to continue on their planned adolescent developmental trajectory (Ward-Smith, Hamlin, Bartholomew, & Stegenga, 2007; Zebrack, Bleyer, Albritton, Medearis, & Tang, 2006). This is consistent with the general message provided to patients and their families at diagnosis – maintain, as much as possible, a "normal" life during treatment and minimize disruptions to usual routines to the extent possible. This is a challenging message when life changes abruptly and in significant ways at a critical developmental period. For teens with cancer, this means ongoing attention to processes of self-acceptance and cognitive maturation, emotional and physical changes, individuation from family, focus on school and academic achievement, and peer and social relationships. Any or all of these areas of development may be impacted by cancer and its treatment. For example, increased parental monitoring of medication and vigilance about health may collide with taking more responsibility for one's health and well-being. Normal processes of conflict and negotiation within the family may also become amplified when "life and death" considerations intrude, and changes in physical appearance may be particularly upsetting at a time of heightened self-consciousness about physical attractiveness and comparison to peers. While some of these disruptions in normal development may be transient, some adolescents and their families face significant challenges through treatment and survival.

Psychological Problems

Although research has found low levels of anxiety and depression among adolescents with cancer, concerns about their psychological well-being are common (Allen, Newman, & Souhami, 1997; Noll, LeRoy, Bukowski, Rogosch, Kulkarni, 1991). In the majority of cases, expressions of fear and sadness are expected responses to diagnosis, initiation of treatment, and the related side effects and limitations imposed on adolescents. One recent study demonstrated that increased risk for depression among female adolescents at least 2 years from diagnosis and that a past-negative time perspective (focusing negatively on the past) mediated the relationship between gender and depression (Bitsko, Stern, Dillon, Russell, & Laver, 2008). Female gender has also been shown to be a risk factor for worse quality of life in adolescents on active treatment (Ward-Smith et al., 2007). In addition, illness uncertainty contributes to distress in adolescents (Neville, 1998). Newly diagnosed adolescents have been found to have higher uncertainty about future pain, course of illness, staff responsibilities, and when they would be able to care for themselves (Decker, Haase, & Bell, 2007). Long-term adolescent survivors in the study also had many unanswered questions and felt uncertain about the impact of illness on their daily lives, success of treatment, and the course of their illness, despite being cured and far out from treatment (Decker et al., 2007). Such illness uncertainty has been found to relate to posttraumatic stress symptoms (PTSS) and to mediate the relationship between posttraumatic stress and health behaviors (Santacroce & Lee, 2006).

PTSS are a helpful way to understand the psychosocial responses of children with cancer and their families. Although adolescents with cancer do not demonstrate consistent elevations in PTSS, rates of PTSS and posttraumatic stress disorder (PTSD) for mothers and fathers suggest that intrusive thoughts, avoidance, and physiological arousal can be persistent for many family members (see Kazak, Schneider, & Kassam-Adams, in press, for a recent review). Nearly half of mothers and fathers of children newly diagnosed with cancer meet criteria for a diagnosis of Acute Stress Disorder (ASD; Patiño-Fernández et al., 2008) and two-thirds of mothers and 40% of fathers in an independent sample of families during treatment experienced moderate to severe PTSS (Kazak, Boeving, Alderfer, Hwang, & Reilly, 2005).

In long-term adolescent survivors and their families, elevated levels of PTSS are usually reported among survivors, mothers, fathers, and siblings (Alderfer, Labay & Kazak, 2003; Brown, Madan-Swain, & Lambert, 2003; Kazak et al., 1997; Kazak, Alderfer, Rourke et al., 2004). Furthermore, parents of survivors often meet criteria for PTSD. In one study of adolescent survivors, almost 30% of mothers met diagnostic criteria since their child's diagnosis, with 14% currently experiencing PTSD (Kazak, Alderfer, Rourke et al., 2004). Nearly 20% of families had at least one parent with current PTSD. While adolescent survivors are unlikely to meet criteria for PTSD, research shows that up to 20% of young adult survivors meet criteria for PTSD (Hobbie et al., 2000; Rourke, Hobbie, Schwartz, & Kazak, 2007; Schwartz & Drotar, 2006a). PTSD has also been found to relate to depressive symptoms, quality of life, mood, and impact of cancer on goals in a sample of 18- to 28-year-old survivors (Schwartz & Drotar, 2006a). When entering adulthood, risk for PTSD may increase as survivors gain the cognitive ability and perspective to process and comprehend the implications of the cancer experience in terms of physical and psychosocial vulnerabilities. In addition to findings of PTSS/PTSD, data from the Childhood Cancer Survivor Study (CCSS – a national epidemiological study) revealed that adolescent survivors were 1.5 times more likely than siblings to have symptoms of depression and anxiety and 1.7 more times likely to have antisocial behaviors and higher attention problems (Schultz et al., 2007). Those with brain tumors and ALL (who were likely to be treated with intrathacal methotrexate or cranial radiation) were most at-risk.

Of course, not all pediatric oncology patients will survive and end of life care in pediatric oncology has only recently been the focus of research. Although not widely studied, adolescent emotional and cognitive maturity, relative to younger patients, allows more reflection about dying and the related processes. In a retrospective study of bereaved parents, psychological symptoms they reported in their children undergoing palliative care included sadness, difficulties talking about feelings regarding illness and death with parents, fear to be alone, loss of perspective, and loss of independence (Theunissen et al., 2007). Forty-three percent of the symptoms were addressed by health professionals and 34% partially or completely resolved after intervention. Children over 12 years old suffered more psychological problems than young children under age of 7. Symptoms reported more frequently for adolescents than other age groups were loss of perspective, fear of physical symptoms, fear of death, and feelings of guilt. The most frequent symptoms of parents were fear of death of child, fear of physical problems, sadness, somberness, and anger. Fifty-six percent of the symptoms were addressed by health professionals and 25% partially or completely resolved after intervention. Another retrospective study found that when parents did not agree on the primary goal of lessening suffering during end of life care, both parents were more likely to report that the child suffered significantly from cancer-directed treatment (Edwards et al., 2008). Furthermore, research has found that a delay exists from the time physicians recognize that children have no realistic chance for cure to the time parents realize this, which delays collaborative goal setting between parents and providers to lessen suffering at end of life (Wolfe et al., 2000). Thus, the collective findings indicate the significant child and family stress experienced at end of life care and emphasize the importance of family centered care.

Social and Family Functioning

Social support from family and friends and optimal family functioning is critical for the positive adjustment of adolescents and their parents. Qualitative research findings have highlighted that adolescents perceive support as more than just "being there"; it is a psychosocial–emotional presence that includes emotional and instrumental support (Woodgate, 2006). Mothers have been found to be the most significant source of social support by doing things such listening, being with them at appointments and in the hospital, and helping to manage their life (Ritchie, 2001). Indeed, conflict with mothers, but not other supports (friends, fathers, siblings), was found to relate to distress in adolescent patients, which highlights the enhanced importance of mothers in adolescent adjustment (Manne & Miller, 1998). Adolescents have also reported feelings of guilt about someone always "being there" (Woodgate, 2006). Woodgate (2006) also notes that this closeness with parents and related guilt may actually represent independence from family. They have a mature appreciation for their family for "being there," and they, in turn, wanted to "be there," for them. In terms of parent outcomes, social support and positive family functioning (e.g., flexibility, low conflict, communication) have been shown to be resilience factors for PTSS (Brown, Fuemmeler, & Forti, 2003) and general distress (Speechley & Noh, 1992).

Peers are also an important source of social support. Qualitative findings revealed that peers are needed as confidants and to help facilitate continued participation in school and social activities as much as possible (Ritchie, 2001). Another qualitative study reported that adolescents needed their friends as a "peer-shield" – to help them feel accepted and integrated and to shield them from negativity of others (Larouche & Chin-Peuckert, 2006). There is some evidence that the social networks of teens with cancer is smaller than networks of healthy peers, and teens with cancer are less satisfied with cancer-related support from friends (Nichols, 1995; Noll et al., 1991). Clearly, their limited ability to participate in school, sports, and leisure during treatment may inhibit their interactions with peers (Novakovic et al., 1996). Moreover, side effects such as hair loss and weight changes may affect confidence and impact body image. Impaired body image has been found in many studies of adolescents with cancer and adolescent long-term survivors (Puukko, Sammallahti, Siimes, & Aalberg, 1997; Wallace, Harcourt, Rumsey, & Foot, 2007) and has been found to relate to reductions in peer activities and increase the risk for depression and social anxiety (Larouche & Chin-Peuckert, 2006; Novakovic et al., 1996; Varni, Katz, Colegrove, & Dolgin, 1995)

There is mixed evidence about the impact of cancer on social functioning for adolescent long-term survivors. Research has shown that childhood and adolescent survivors' social skills are similar to their peers when excluding brain tumor patients (Noll, Bukowski, Davies, Koontz, & Kulkarni, 1993). However, reduced social activities or confidence to engage with others in adolescence may have long-term impact on adolescents with cancer as they enter adulthood. Unique challenges that impact relationships into adulthood include how and when to disclose information related to their health and fertility, a past history of relationship disruptions or less opportunity to develop relationships, and potential changes in appearance that may become more salient to a survivor with age. Examples of long-term deleterious social outcomes include reduced social activities, living longer with their parents and being less independent from their parents than peers, difficulty forming relationships with same-sex peers and romantic partners, and being less satisfied with both types of relationships (Boman & Bodegard, 2004; Mackie, Hill, Kondryn, & McNally, 2000; Pendley, Dahlquist, & Dreyer, 1997; Stam, Grootenhuis, & Last, 2005).

Treatment Adherence and Health Promotion

Research to date suggests that many children and adolescents with cancer do not take their oral mediations in accord with their prescribed regime. Adherence in adolescents with cancer may be especially difficult given the likelihood for medications to cause intense side effects. Also, the maintenance phase of ALL is especially challenging as it lasts 2–3 years and requires multiple pills taken throughout the day. Adolescents, despite risk of relapse, may become relaxed in taking their medication when their disease is in remission and they have no symptoms. In one study, clinical and lab measures of 6-MP (a maintenance chemotherapy taken orally) revealed that 33.3% were nonadherent, and the rate was highest in adolescents (de Oliveira, Viana, Zani, & Romanha, 2004). Nonadherence to prednisone (a steroid and chemotherapy agent which often causes distressing symptoms such as increase in weight and mood/behavior difficulties) has been found to range from 19 to 52% (see Rapoff et al., 2006, for a review). One study assessed adherence in adolescents and found that 52% were nonadherent to prednisone using serum assay and 48% were nonadherent to penicillin using urine samples (Festa, Tamaroff, Chasalow, & Lanzkowsky, 1992). Using serum assay, another study found that 27% of adolescents tested for the chemotherapy agents trimethoprim or sulfamethoxazome had no detectable drug in their system (Kennard et al., 2004). Those with no trace of the drug had higher levels of depression, lower self-esteem, and higher levels of parent-child incongruence. Six years later, survival rates were lower for those who were nonadherent.

Increasing communication about treatment and disease with adolescents usually elicits increase in cooperation and adherence (Windebank & Spinetta, 2008). In fact, study findings have revealed that adolescents desire more information related to their disease and treatment (Dunsmore & Quine, 1995; Stegenga & Ward-Smith, 2008). Nonadherence may result from a lack of information about the treatment, in addition to not wanting to suffer side effects, feeling depressed, and wanting to be normal. For a select few, nonadherence may be a form of rebellion or assertion of autonomy (Windebank & Spinetta, 2008). A focus group study with adolescents found the following barriers to adherence: wanting to be normal, egocentric thinking, concrete thinking that prevented them from understanding long-term implications of missing pills, and lack of parental involvement (Malbasa, Kodish, & Santacroce, 2007).

For survivors, health-promoting behaviors and long-term medical follow-up are critical given the risk for second cancers and later chronic health conditions such as cardiac and pulmonary disease, diabetes, and osteoporosis. For example, smoking and other tobacco use may exacerbate risk of cardiac and pulmonary disease, including lung cancer; alcohol may exacerbate liver and cardiac damage resulting from various therapies; and ultraviolet exposure may increase risk of skin cancer heightened by radiation (Clarke & Eiser, 2007). Thus, for all teens, and especially those with a history of cancer, medical counseling should implement a preventative approach that increases proactive, health-promoting behavior, and promotes the avoidance of unhealthy behaviors. Health-promoting practices to emphasize include eating a balanced diet, exercising regularly, avoidance of tobacco, minimizing alcohol intake, sunscreen use, and safe sex practices to avoid sexually transmitted diseases. Fortunately, many studies have demonstrated that survivors engage in health-risk behaviors at equal or lower rates as same age peers (see Clarke & Eiser, 2007 for a review). However, survivors still engaged in smoking, drinking, and marijuana use at a rate that should be concerning based on their increased risk for new cancer diagnoses and other diseases. Exercise, diet, and health-screening practices are also not at optimal levels for most survivors (Florin et al., 2007; Finnegan et al., 2007; Yeazel et al., 2004). Moreover, despite recommendations to receive follow-up care at lease once a year (Children's Oncology Group, http://www.survivorship-guidelines.org), the CCSS found that only 71% of survivors reported having a general physical exam and less than half reported a cancer-related medical visit in the previous 2 years (Oeffinger et al., 2004).

Cognitive/Academic Challenges

In addition to the potential negative social outcomes associated with school absences during treatment, adolescents with cancer may have difficulty with educational achievement and school re-entry following intensive treatment (Katz, & Madan-Swain, 2006; Prevatt, Heffer, & Lowe, 2000). Repeating a grade and feeling left out from their cohort of peers is not uncommon for such teens (Gerhardt et al., 2007). Long-term adolescent cancer survivors may also suffer cognitive late effects as a result of the cancer, related treatments involving the central nervous system, and the cumulative impact of cancer on school attendance and achievement. Lower IQ and impairments in attention and concentration, processing speed (e.g., more time required to complete work, slower to understand), visual perceptual skills (e.g., difficulty with writing, interpretation of visual information such as maps or puzzles), executive functioning (e.g., problems with planning, insight, organization), memory, and cognitive fatigue (difficulty with concentrating for long periods of time and being more tired than expected after a day at work or school) may be present (Katz & Madan-Swain, 2006; Nathan et al., 2007). Risk is highest for central nervous system malignancies, and those treated with cranial radiation therapy, intrathecal therapy, or a bone marrow/stem cell transplant (Nathan et al., 2007).

A study from the CCSS showed that 23% of survivors utilized special education services, and those who survived leukemia, non-Hodgkin lymphoma, brain tumors, and neuroblastoma were less likely than their siblings to graduate high school if they did not utilize special education services (Mitby et al., 2003). Unfortunately, many families have difficulty securing appropriate support services for their children given the lack of awareness by schools and some parents of the potential cognitive late effects. Even with best efforts, teenagers may resist services in favor of being "normal". Some evidence suggests that survivors catch-up academically with their peers with regards to high-school graduation rates (Boman & Bodegard, 2004; Gerhardt et al., 2007) and parent-reported academic competence (Gerhardt et al., 2007). Others have found that young adult survivors are less likely than controls to have educational goals beyond high school (Boman & Bodegard, 2004), are less likely to attend college than when compared to the general population or siblings (Boman & Bodegard, 2004; Zeltzer et al., 1997), and less often hold an advanced degree (Langeveld et al., 2003). In addition to educational support services, adolescents should pursue evaluation of their neuropsychological status and psychoeducational strengths and weaknesses to help inform college and career choices. Those with significant impairments will need vocational planning.

Sociocultural Considerations

While theoretically important to disease management and adaptation, little empirical work has studied sociocultural influences in youth with cancer and their families. Proposed sociocultural influences on family management include personal/individual, health-care provider/health system, economics, and cultural practices/beliefs (Thibodeaux & Deatrick, 2007). These elements, which may translate to factors such as various personal values, financial resources, and complicated health systems, can potentially impact adjustment and medical outcomes. Specifically, sociocultural factors may influence communication style, how diagnosis/prognosis is discussed, coping styles, support, and how treatment and family goals are prioritized (Schwartz & Drotar, 2006b; Thibodeaux & Deatrick, 2007). Language barriers, especially if medical translators are not consistently available, may also pose a barrier to optimal care (Crom, 1995). Stigma, too, may impact treatment and adaptation. For example, Taiwanese parents reported stigma associated with death and valued religion as a treatment option (Yeh, 2001). Another study found that Chinese-American parents experienced much self-blame about the diagnosis and were subsequently less likely to tell the grandparents (Martinson et al., 1999).

As reported earlier, minority patients are less likely to be diagnosed with cancer, but have worse survival rates. While the reasons for lower survival rates are not completely understood, delayed diagnoses and lower access to optimal care for treatment may contribute to lower survival rates of minorities (Brown et al., 2003; USDHHS et al., 2006). However, the CCSS study found that minority survivors, for the most part, were as likely or more likely to engage in health-promoting behaviors (Castellino et al., 2005). African-American survivors reported less risky behaviors (smoking and drinking) and better preventative practices. Hispanic survivors were also less likely to smoke. However, female Hispanic survivors were also less likely to have a recent pap smear.

Psychosocial Care for Adolescents with Cancer and Their Families

The importance of psychosocial care for all youth with cancer and their families has been long recognized and endorsed by major professional organizations, including the American Academy of Pediatrics (American Academy of Pediatrics, 2004), the Children's Oncology Group (COG; Noll & Kazak, 2004) and, most recently, the Institute of Medicine (IOM, 2007). These recommendations, while generally developmentally oriented and comprehensive, have not been widely implemented. Psychosocial care across and even within pediatric oncology treatment programs is variable and often relatively infrequent. For example, in a recent survey, only 11% of COG institutions used evidence-based psychosocial care (Selove, 2007). There are many understandable obstacles to a comprehensive behavioral treatment approach for adolescents. These include the need to provide care to patients across a wide spectrum of age groups, limited availability of evidence-based approaches, and the fiscal and administrative challenges of providing psychosocial care. Psychosocial treatments provided to adolescents are often delivered by social workers, child life specialists, pediatric psychologists, and sometimes psychiatrists or medical providers. Our group has developed a model for the delivery of psychosocial care in pediatric oncology that is based on two dimensions – the phase of treatment (diagnosis and early treatment initiation, ongoing treatment, after treatment ends) and the Preventative Pediatric Psychosocial Health Model (PPPHM) which describes three levels of psychosocial risk (based on a public health framework of universal, targeted, and clinical needs; Kazak et al., 2007). The PPPHM has also been applied to end of

Fig. 1 Pediatric psychosocial preventative health model

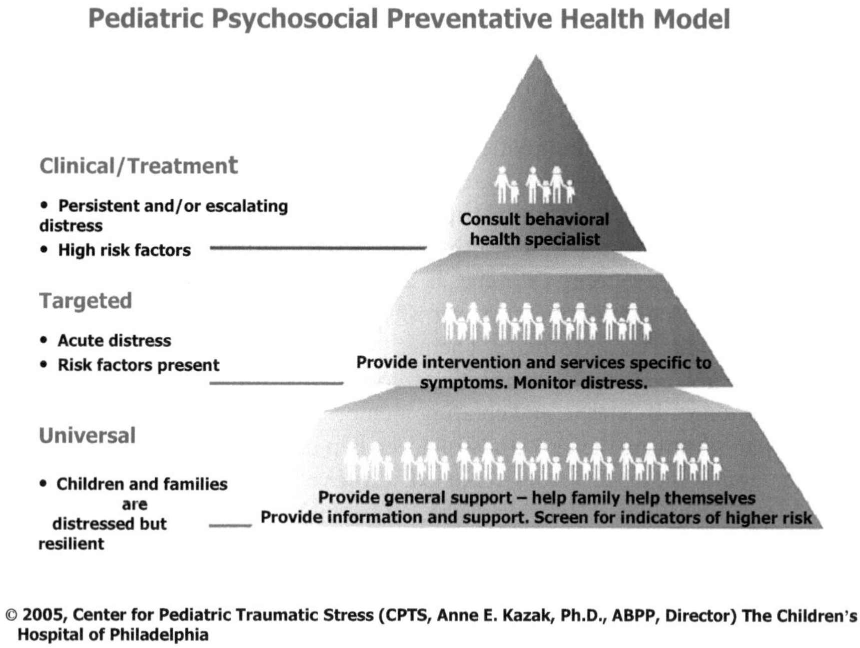

life and bereavement in pediatric cancer (Kazak & Noll, 2004). Universal, targeted, and clinical interventions with adolescents with cancer are described next (Fig. 1).

Universal Care

Universal psychosocial care for adolescents and their families may enhance the treatment experience for all families, regardless of psychosocial risk status. This generally includes assessment by social workers, nurses, or other care providers that helps to identify general psychosocial concerns (e.g., coping and adjustment, emotional and financial resources, family concerns) of the adolescent and family. The Psychosocial Assessment Tool (PAT) is one example of a universal tool to assess potential risk factors at the outset of treatment (Pai et al., 2008). Universal care also includes educational materials and access to resources in the hospital such as child life specialists, teachers, and chaplains, along with programs consistent with family-centered care. Ongoing collaboration among schools, families, and health-care settings and helping adolescents with cancer remain connected with their teachers and classmates is also universally important (Katz & Madan-Swain, 2006; Power, DuPaul, Shapiro, & Kazak, 2003). A review of school reintegration programs for children with cancer emphasized the importance of providing education to the school personnel and peers about the cancer experience, yet few of the programs have tested empirical outcomes (Prevatt et al., 2000).

Given the evidence for traumatic stress responses among patients and family members, resources that advance trauma-informed care offer other approaches to enhancing universal care. For example, the Medical Traumatic Stress Toolkit provides evidence-based materials that are intended for use by health-care providers (physicians, nurses, other providers) to deliver medical care in a way that promotes adaptive psychological outcomes by reducing the likelihood of ongoing traumatic stress responses (Stuber, Schneider, Kassam-Adams, Kazak, & Saxe, 2006). This includes providing brief psychoeducation to providers about traumatic stress in parents and patients, tips for providers, and handouts that can be given to patients and families. As described next, a few health promotion and coping interventions have also demonstrated initial efficacy.

Novel interventions with adolescents to enhance quality of life and "normalcy" have begun to emerge. As an example, The Teen Outreach Program helps to facilitate social connections among teens with lymphoma/leukemia and with affected teens and their healthy peer network (Shama & Lucchetta, 2007). Teenagers report benefits from the program and reinforce the need for programming to do normal teenage activities. Another novel and creative approach is adventure therapy. One study described an outward bound trip to the Arctic with 11 adolescents to enhance health-related quality of life and self-esteem (Stevens et al., 2004). Documentary footage of the trip was shot in an unstructured interview format. Themes yielded from the data were forming connections, togetherness, rebuilding self-esteem, and creating memories. In a similar adventure therapy study of a jeep trip in Greece, young adult survivors reported improvements in self confidence, independence, and social contracts (Elad, Yagil, Cohen, & Meller, 2003). While relatively qualitative in nature, such evidence points to the fact that young cancer patients and survivors interacting with one another in collaborative activities may provide a therapeutic forum to discuss and process similar thoughts, beliefs, and experiences with cancer.

Computer-based interventions are also promising. One intervention tested the efficacy of a video game called Re-Mission which was developed to enhance disease and treatment knowledge of adolescents and young adults with cancer (Beale, Kato, Marin-Bowling, Guthrie, & Cole, 2007). Treatment participants were asked to play Re-Mission for 1 hour each week for 3 months while controls played a regular video game for the same amount of time. At 1- and 3-month follow-up assessments, those playing Re-Mission scored higher on cancer-related knowledge than the control group. Another study evaluated 21 personal web pages of adolescents with cancer (Suzuki & Beale, 2006). Common themes identified from material on the pages were discussion of positive benefits of the cancer experience, sharing advice, and networking with others. Thus, computers provide an important mode of intervention that is accessible and comfortable for most teenagers and may help to educate them and keep them engaged with others.

Many brief interventions to enhance health promotion, medical follow-up, and disease knowledge have also been implemented. These have included written materials (e.g., brochures and treatment summaries), risk counseling, and health-behavior training (Absalom, Eiser, Greco, & Davies, 2004; Cox, McLaughlin, Rai, Steen, & Hudson, 2005; Donze & Tercyak, 2006; Eiser, Hill, & Blacklay, 2000; Hudson et al., 2002; Tyc et al., 2003). Two randomized control trials to improve health-promoting behaviors (Hudson et al., 2002) and to reduce the intention to smoke (Tyc et al., 2003) found success in using a brief but multi-component approach that included goal setting and goal modifying related to personal health. They also included follow-up telephone counseling to reinforce goals. These findings highlight the importance of enhancing adolescent motivation to change health behaviors and attitudes and facilitating the internalization of related goals (Cox, McLaughlin, Steen, & Hudson, 2006). Another pilot study tested an intervention to enhance psychosexual development and related knowledge in adolescents and young adults with cancer (Canada, Schover, & Li, 2007). The intervention consisted of two sessions and included discussion and support around sexual development and functioning, body image, fertility, and prevention of sexually transmitted infections and unwanted pregnancies. Compared to a wait-list control, benefits gained by the treatment group included increased knowledge related to cancer-specific sexual issues, improved body image, reduction in anxiety related to romantic relationships, and reduction in general distress.

Targeted Care

Generally, about a quarter of families of newly diagnosed children require more intensive psychosocial interventions at diagnosis and/or during treatment. Key issues and interventions include treatment for distress and adjustment difficulties, cognitive and academic-related interventions, pain and procedural distress, and adherence. Survivors may also benefit from selected interventions to reduce health-risk behaviors such as smoking. The most evidence-based treatments to date include interventions for traumatic stress, cognitive remediation, and procedural distress. Treatment of anxious and depressive symptoms, social skills training, and psychosocial interventions at end of life care are less well established in adolescents.

There are few reports of interventions specific to adolescents with cancer with regard to anxious and depressive symptoms. Worry and sadness are normal responses to cancer and treatment, thus careful assessment is necessary to determine symptom severity and frequency. In general, cognitive-behavioral (Kendall, 2005) and family therapy (Diamond & Josephson, 2005) approaches used more generally for adolescents can be adapted for use in cancer. Given the presence of illness uncertainty and the potential impact of cancer on adolescent development, it is important to explore beliefs (modifiable targets of intervention) associated with developmentally relevant issues such as body image and appearance, school and peer issues, worries about mortality, and the impact of cancer on normal developmental processes in families.

With respect to traumatic stress, elevated rates suggest the importance of intervening with parents in ways that are consistent with treating acutely distressed individuals (e.g., care in presenting information in a calm and clear manner, repeating information as needed, offering services that may help parents tolerate strong anxiety symptoms). There is evidence that more severe traumatic stress reactions at diagnosis are predictive of ongoing distress (Kazak et al., in press). Surviving Cancer Competently Intervention Program (SCCIP) is an intervention that combines cognitive-behavioral and family therapy treatment approaches to reduce ongoing traumatic stress symptoms in adolescent cancer survivors and their families. SCCIP was tested in a randomized controlled trial (RCT) of 150 families. Participation in the SCCIP trial was associated with reductions in traumatic stress symptoms across members of the family (Kazak, Alderfer, & Streisand et al., 2004). A pilot study of an adaptation of SCCIP for parents/caregivers of patients newly diagnosed with pediatric cancer was promising (Kazak et al., 2005), although more recent data from a larger RCT highlights the difficulties inherent in conducting intervention research close to the time of cancer diagnosis (Lutz Stehl et al., 2008).

Interventions to improve impairments related to neurocognitive deficits in childhood cancer survivors are an important area of work. Based on the adult literature on cognitive remediation approaches for brain injury, a Cognitive Remediation Program (CRP) for 6- to 17-year-old cancer survivors with attention deficits was tested in a multisite randomized clinical trial (Butler et al., 2008). The CRP treatment uses hierarchically graded mass practice activities, strategy acquisition, and cognitive-behavioral approaches in order to potentially impact academic achievement, attention, working memory, memory recall, and vigilance. The 20 session treatment approach was shown to be most effective in improving academic achievement and less impactful on neuropsychological outcomes (Butler et al., 2008). Despite the equivocal findings from this RCT, sufficient evidence exists for the tailoring of interventions to address specific learning and attentional difficulties in adolescents with or at risk for neurocognitive difficulties (based on disease or treatment) and to explore expanded treatment models that may include other pharmacological, behavioral, and family treatment approaches (Butler et al., 2008). There is, for example, emerging evidence for the use of methylphenidate in pediatric cancer survivors for memory and attentional concerns (Butter & Copeland, 2005).

Physical symptoms and procedural distress have also been targeted in interventions. Cognitive–behavioral interventions such as relaxation, guided imagery, and distraction are key for reducing chemotherapy side effects, anticipatory nausaea, and reducing anxiety and pain during procedures (see the following reviews: McQuaid & Nassau, 1999; Powers, 1999, Spirito & Kazak, 2006). An example of a novel approach to distraction is virtual reality – a medium of human–computer interaction. A randomized controlled trial testing a virtual reality distraction intervention for youth getting their venous port accessed showed lower physiological and reported levels of anxiety compared to the no distraction control group (Gershon, Zimand, Pickering, Rothbaum, & Hodges, 2004). Collaboration with child life specialists and also with parents to help support patients who experience such difficulties is also important. Fatigue, another side effect of cancer and treatment, was also the target of a successful pilot study of inpatients using a stationary bicycle-style exerciser (Hinds et al., 2007). This represents a promising downward extension of interventions in adult cancer using yoga and exercise to improve fatigue and quality of life (Mock, 2004).

There is increasing appreciation for nonadherence to treatment among adolescents, which is not surprising given that many of the treatments cause significant symptoms that impair quality of life. However, there are no known published reports of interventions for adherence specific to pediatric cancer. Indeed, adherence issues for cancer have much in common with other pediatric illnesses and emphasize the importance of determining reliable and valid means of assessing adherence to treatment, including laboratory assays, observation, microelectronic monitors, pill counting, staff report and self and parent report (Rapoff et al., 2006). Effective interventions are likely to entail application of a cognitive–behavioral approach involving education, goal setting and monitoring, strategies for remembering and organizing treatments, positive reinforcement, and partnerships among patients, families, and staff to promote adherence when difficulties emerge (Spirito & Kazak, 2006). Other familial barriers to adherence such as family dysfunction, lack of financial resources, and lack of comprehension of treatment plan should also be assessed with the family. Additionally, providers may inadvertently reinforce nonadherence in some instances. In a focus group study on adherence to ALL maintenance therapy, teens acknowledged that positive blood counts may occur and be reinforced by their providers, despite teen nonadherence (Malbasa et al., 2007). Thus, providers should carefully assess teen and parent routine around taking medication and barriers to adherence in addition to monitoring biological markers. Furthermore, the teens in the study acknowledged that parent involvement was critical for positive adherence, thus emphasizing the important role of parents in adolescents' health management (Malbasa et al., 2007).

Clinical Care

In general, less than 10% of the pediatric cancer population will require more intensive clinical intervention. However, some psychosocial risks are more likely to be seen in adolescent patients than in younger age groups. For example, while suicidality is rare in pediatric cancer in general, psychosocial care should include attention to potential suicidal risk both during treatment and in survivors (Pao & Kazak, in press; Recklitis, Lockwood, Rothwell, & Diller, 2006). Similarly concerns about substance use, other high risk activities, and more serious psychopathology that increase during adolescents in general, irregardless of health status, are important considerations when evaluating and treating adolescents with cancer and adolescent cancer survivors. Not only are addressing these problems important for adolescent well-being, but they may also be critical for medical management and outcomes. For example, disordered eating or substance abuse may affect chemotherapy and increase the risk for poor outcomes, risky sexual behaviors may enhance an immunocompromised teen's risk for acquiring a sexually transmitted disease, significant parent–child conflict may hinder optimal disease management, and significant PTSD may increase adolescent and parent avoidance of follow-up care.

In many instances, patients with the highest level of psychological distress are the patients that are referred for consultation and potential treatment by behavioral health providers. Our group has developed a systems-oriented consultation model that can be applied across problem areas and across diseases (Kazak, Simms & Rourke, 2002). Using a social ecological approach to understanding adolescents with childhood cancer, the treatment framework guides the consultant to view presenting problems (e.g. depression, conflict, nonadherence) in the context of the patient, family, and health-care provider team triad. The consultant joins with the system (patient, parents, providers) to promote positive adaptation by framing the presenting problem interpersonally and identifying a collaborative solution that promotes changes in behavior (Kazak et al., 2002). This model may work in tandem with general evidence-based treatments that are problem focused and target issues such as anxiety, depression, oppositional defiant disorder, and eating disorders. Pharmacotherapy may also be used as there is some evidence from small trials for the safety of antidepressants in pediatric oncology (DeJong & Fombonne, 2007; Gothelf et al., 2005). However, accurate recognition of emotional problems in children with cancer by health-care providers, even at the end of life, lags behind identification of other health concerns (Hedström, Kreuger, Ljungman, Nygren, & von Essen, 2006; Hilden et al., 2001). There is also evidence that pediatric oncologists prescribe antidepressants at rates in excess of the likely incidence of depression in childhood cancer (Kersun & Kazak, 2006). While intending treatment to alleviate suffering from depression, these data suggest the importance of conducting a complete assessment and determining the presence of clinical symptoms, with appropriate and multimodal treatments offered as indicated (Pao & Kazak, in press).

On some occasions, it is more evident that, although an adolescent may be upset or symptomatic, the problem is broader and a family intervention is necessary. Some families are seen by staff as "difficult," particularly when parents are verbally or physically threatening or aggressive, or when the behavior of family members is seen as obstructing the safe delivery of medical care. In these cases, mechanisms to address concerns can be protocalized and implemented by staff (Rourke et al., 2006). These include regularly scheduled contact times with families, goal setting with families and staff, developing a consistent team to work with families, and having clear lines of communication among nurses, physicians, psychologists, and other staff members. It is also important for parents who experience psychopathology to receive mental health treatment outside the pediatric setting as their mental health problems may compromise the care of the adolescent on treatment. In these instances, it is essential that a member of the adolescent care team (a behavioral health professional if possible) communicates with the parent's therapist or physician in order to assure the safety of the child, convey the situation related to cancer treatment and relevant parent responsibilities to the practitioner, and to support the parent's treatment.

Methodological Considerations

Sampling, Recruitment, and Retention

There are significant challenges to recruitment and retention of adolescents and their families, especially in cancer research. Adolescents with cancer may be resistant to participate in research, given their desire to be "normal" and limit reminders of the cancer experience, their need to attend to other areas such as school and friends, and lack of interest in health promotion (Tercyak, Donze, Prahlad, Mosher, & Shad, 2006). For parents, participation in intervention research raises worries about whether this may take away time from their care of the sick child and infringe on other family responsibilities (Lutz Stehl et al., 2008; Schwartz & Drotar, 2004). Parents may not want to leave their child in the hospital room alone or do not want to (or cannot) come back to the hospital for research participation. For survivors and their families, PTSS may impact their willingness to participate in clinical intervention research. Again, this could serve as a traumatic reminder of the cancer experience and limit the ability to recruit and retain families most in need of clinical intervention (Lutz Stehl et al., 2008).

A related issue is the source of the sample. For adolescents on treatment, recruitment can take place in the hospital setting as patients are frequently visiting for clinic appointments or inpatients stays. However, it is often more difficult to attain a representative sample of adolescent long-term survivors. Many adolescents may not be receiving follow-up care, especially if they live far from the medical center where they were treated or have symptoms of avoidance (e.g., PTSS). Furthermore, those with frequent oncology appointments may have more late effects or a significant medical problem compared to those who have been "lost to follow-up." In these instances, recruitment in the hospital setting may not always yield a representative sample of survivors.

Another sampling issue is heterogeneity of diseases represented and homogeneity in ethnic/racial representation. Because pediatric cancer is relatively rare, most samples include participants with many different kinds of malignancies and treatments. This may obscure differences and needs specific to one diagnosis or form of treatment. For example, the experience and needs of adolescents with osteosarcoma who had an amputation may be quite different than an adolescent with ALL. Furthermore, because the majority of pediatric cancer patients are Caucasian, and subsequently reflected in study samples, it is difficult to yield a large minority sample in order to test culturally relevant and sensitive interventions.

Taken together, it is important at the outset of the study to define the desired sample and address any potential barriers to its recruitment. For example, if a representative sample of adolescent survivors is desired, then it will be important to recruit them in various communities rather than solely relying on recruitment of those coming to clinic. Or, if a sample of at least 50% minorities is desired to test the efficacy of an intervention among various ethnic groups, then plans to oversample minorities will be required. To address potential recruitment and retention issues, including needs for larger samples that oversample a particular group, planful strategies are necessary. Such strategies may include locating and reaching previous patients lost to follow-up, joining with community groups to identify participants and promote the interventions, advertising efforts, home-based or computer-based assessment and intervention, and multisite studies encompassing a diverse geographic area. Flexibility in scheduling of interventions may also be necessary to recruit and retain participants. The physical or psychological status of adolescents on treatment may limit their ability or their parents' ability to participate in an intervention at regularly scheduled times. For families who do not want another appointment scheduled, interventions may need to take place during days of other visits to the hospital for medical appointments or stays. Home-based intervention may be necessary when more regular intervention intervals are required for research design.

Outcomes and Related Analyses

Outcomes of interventions are also an important consideration. Because of the resiliency and lack of psychopathology of most adolescents and families affected by pediatric cancer, outcomes sensitive to specific and important issues and behaviors of adolescents are indicated. Qualitative research has identified the subtle, yet important, effects of cancer on adolescents that are not easily captured in available standardized assessments. However, relevant measurement development has lagged behind and, consequently, valid and reliable measures of psychosocial outcomes in pediatric oncology are sparse (see exceptions: Kazak et al., 2001, Kazak, McClure, Alderfer et al., 2004, Pai et al., 2008, Wu et al., 2007). In turn, intervention researchers often use generic outcome measures or newly developed measures with limited psychometric properties, thus limiting findings and the conclusions that can be drawn from them. In order to advance intervention research in pediatric oncology, measurement development research needs to advance in terms of validating existing measures and creating new psychometrically sound measures specific to targets of interventions. Furthermore, it is imperative for descriptive research to employ control groups in order to identify the developmental and psychosocial outcomes that are unique, and possibly impaired, in adolescents affected by cancer compared to peers.

Data analytic plans should also be carefully composed from the outset in terms of specific outcome variables to assess and subgroups to analyze. Outcomes may differ by demographic variables (e.g., gender, age, socioeconomic status), disease-related variables, or psychological status. Thus, to attain sufficient statistical power, subgroup analyses should be planned ahead of time in order to accrue an adequate and representative sample. Furthermore, clinically meaningful outcomes for intervention analysis should be carefully defined and considered. This may include subscale or single-item analysis, which may be warranted if the outcomes are particularly relevant and meaningful for the adolescents or families. As an example, a health promotion intervention reported no significant outcomes of the study based on a composite score of health behaviors (Hudson et al., 2002). However, re-analysis of the data revealed significant improvements in specific and important behaviors for the population such as self-exams (Cox et al., 2005). Again, such analyses are best planned from the outset of the study given the multiple comparisons involved with many analyzed outcomes and the need for statistical corrections to reduce likelihood of Type 1 error.

Clinical Research Agenda

The research agenda for adolescents with cancer and their families reflects areas in need of clinical attention that are understudied in adolescents. Targets of intervention are described below.

Communication

Communication broadly refers to that among adolescents, families, and providers about treatment, symptoms, and late effects. Studying and enhancing communication is critical for many reasons. From a provider perspective, treating adolescents may be challenging given the intense involvement of parents, which may conflict with the importance of respecting the autonomy and perspective of the adolescent. Enhancing communication with adolescents is critical to best understand their symptoms, concerns, and maladaptive behaviors (e.g., nonadherence, smoking, sex, end-of-life plans, treatment preferences). Providers also must convey sensitive information to adolescents and families such as prognosis and plans for end-of-life care, and fertility challenges and other late effects. Given the presence of illness uncertainty and PTSS for many adolescents, long-term survivors, and their families, knowing how best to and when to communicate these issues to adolescents and families is critical (Decker et al., 2007). Moreover, families face significant challenges to optimal communication when dealing with a teenager, in general, which may be magnified when the teen has cancer. Lack of congruence among family members (adolescent, mother, father, other caregivers) and the medical team about treatment plans and goals can impact the delivery and outcomes of care (Edwards et al., 2008). Thus interventions to study and enhance communication among the adolescent, parents, and providers are essential for improving medical and psychological outcomes.

Developmental Competencies and Tasks

The "normalcy" that adolescents with cancer strive for relates to achievement of developmental tasks of adolescence such as social competence, academic achievement, autonomy from parents, and pursuing romantic/sexual relationships. While studies have described the needs of adolescents and provided some program information and initial findings (as described in this chapter), few interventions to enhance developmental competencies are evidence based and adolescent focused. Randomized control trials are needed to test interventions to improve social skills (for an example with children, see Barakat et al., 2003), school re-integration, vocational/college planning, peer networking, family functioning after cancer, and body image and sexuality. These targets of intervention are also critical for improving optimal transition to adulthood as independence and competence is promoted.

Health Promotion

In addition to typical health-promoting behaviors prescribed to all teens (no drug use, no unprotected sex, healthy diet, etc.), adolescents with cancer or long-term survivors must adhere to treatment regimens and/or comply with long-term medical follow-up needs. While work in this area has increased with adult survivors of childhood cancer, long-term positive behavior changes are difficult to maintain (as with other health behavior change interventions). Approaches typically used with healthy individuals may not be effective with cancer survivors (Tyc, Hudson, & Hinds, 1999) and an increase in novel approaches such as peer-counseling (Emmons et al., 2005) or computer-based programming (Beale et al., 2007) is needed. Furthermore, there is increasing evidence that survivors' worries and concerns about their cancer and late effects is an important target of interventions to improve health behaviors (Cox et al., 2006). Unfortunately, little work has focused on adolescents despite the advantage of targeting this age range prior to adulthood when maladaptive health behaviors may be more easily modified. Intervention work investigating approaches to keep survivors engaged and committed to long-term follow-up care is also needed. Given the need for lifelong follow-up care, attention to readiness for transition to adult care is particularly important and remains a significant challenge for reasons including lack of awarenesss of survivorship issues on the part of adult providers, limited insurance, and patient attachment to pediatric providers (Freyer & Brugieres, 2008). Finally, as discussed earlier, adherence among adolescents is often poor, despite its importance for managing and curing cancer. Thus, interventions to promote adherence among adolescents are paramount.

End-of-Life Care

Research comparing a cohort of patients from 1990–1997 to 1997–2004 demonstrated that children dying of cancer are currently receiving care that is more consistent with comprehensive palliative care and are experiencing less suffering per parent report (Wolfe et al., 2008). However, end of life care for adolescents presents unique challenges. It may be unclear what role the adolescents want in treatment decisions and how to determine advance directives for older adolescents (Bearison, 2006). Also, because adolescents are better able to understand death and the implications of their situation, they may experience more psychological distress during this time (Theunissen et al., 2007). These issues, combined with normal complex adolescent/parent relationships, may exacerbate the decision-making process of treatment and the psychological symptoms of the affected adolescent and family. Unfortunately, little is known about patient concerns or symptoms given the paucity of research on patient reported outcomes in pediatric oncology palliative care (Hinds et al., 2007). Research is necessary to better understand the issues for adolescents and their families in end-of-life care and to provide clinically sensitive and timely interventions to improve the process and related distress.

Summary

In summary, adolescents with cancer, long-term adolescent survivors, and their families are generally doing well. However, many experience ongoing physical and psychological distress that warrants intervention. Unfortunately, few intervention studies have focused on adolescents, in particular. More adolescent-focused research is needed to better understand and address the impact of cancer on adolescent and early adult developmental outcomes, disease management, and distress.

References

Absalom, K., Eiser, C., Greco, V., & Davies, H. (2004) Health promotion for survivors of childhood cancer: a minimal intervention. *Patient Education and Counseling, 55*, 379–384.

Albritton, K. H., & Eden, T. (2008). Access to care. *Pediatric Blood and Cancer, 50*, 1094–1098.

Alderfer, M. A., Labay, L. E., & Kazak, A. E. (2003). Brief report: does posttraumatic stress apply to siblings of childhood cancer survivors? *Journal of Pediatric Psychology, 28*, 281–286.

Allen, R., Newman, S. P., & Souhami, R. L. (1997). Anxiety and depression in adolescent cancer: findings in patients and parents at the time of diagnosis. *European Journal of Cancer, 33*, 1250–1255.

American Academy of Pediatrics. (2004). Guideline for pediatric cancer centers. *Pediatrics, 113*, 1833–1835.

Barakat, L. P., Hetzke, J. D., Foley, B., Carey, M. E., Gyato, K., & Phillips, P. C. (2003). Evaluation of a social-skills training group intervention with children treated for brain tumors: A pilot study. *Journal of Pediatric Psychology, 28*, 299–307.

Beale, I. L., Kato, P. M., Marin-Bowling, V. M., Guthrie, N., & Cole, S. W. (2007). Improvement in cancer-related knowledge following use of a psychoeducational video game for adolescents and young adults with cancer. *Journal of Adolescent Health, 41*, 263–270.

Bearison, D. J. (2006). Palliative care at the end of life. In R. Brown (Ed.). *Comprehensive handbook of childhood cancer and sickle cell disease*. (pp. 341–357). New York, NY: Oxford University Press.

Bitsko, M. J., Stern, M., Dillon, R., Russell, E. C., & Laver, J. (2008). Happiness and time perspective as potential mediators of quality of life and depression in adolescent cancer. *Pediatric Blood and Cancer, 50*, 613–619.

Bleyer, W. A. (2002). Cancer in older adolescents and young adults: Epidemiology, diagnosis, treatment, survival, and importance of clinical trials. *Medical and Pediatric Oncology, 38*, 1–10.

Bleyer, A. (2007). Young adult oncology: The patients and their survival challenges. *Cancer, 57*, 242–255.

Bleyer, A., Barr, R., Hayes-Lattin, B., Thomas, D., Ellis, C., & Anderson, B. (2008). The distinctive biology of cancer in adolescents and young adults. *Nature Reviews Cancer, 8*, 288–298.

Boman, K. K., & Bodegard, G. (2004). Life after cancer in childhood: Social adjustment and educational and vocational status of young-adult survivors. *Journal of Pediatric Hematology and Oncology, 26*, 354–362.

Bottomley, S. J., & Kassner, E. (2003). Late effects of childhood cancer therapy. *Journal of Pediatric Nursing, 18*, 126–133.

Brown, R. T., Fuemmeler, B., & Forti, E. (2003). Racial and ethnic disparity and access to health care. In M. C. Roberts (Ed.), *Handbook of pediatric psychology* (3rd ed., pp. 683–685). New York, NY: Guilford Press.

Brown, R. T., Madan-Swain, A., & Lambert, R. (2003). Posttraumatic stress symptoms in adolescent survivors of childhood cancer and their mothers. *Journal of Traumatic Stress, 16*, 309–318.

Butler, R., & Copeland, D. (2005). Neurocognitive interventions for children and adolescents surviving cancer. *Journal of Pediatric Psychology, 30*, 65–78.

Butler, R. W., Copeland, D. R., Fairclough, D. L., Mulhern, R. K., Katz, E. R., Kazak, A. E., et al. (2008). A multicenter, randomized clinical trial of a cognitive remediation program for childhood survivors of a pediatric malignancy. *Journal of Consulting and Clinical Psychology, 76*, 367–378.

Canada, A. L., Schover, L. R., & Li, Y. (2007). A pilot intervention to enhance psychosexual development in adolescents and young adults with cancer. *Pediatric Blood and Cancer, 49*, 824–828.

Castellino, S. M., Casillas, J., Hudson, M. M., Mertens, A. C., Whitton, J., Brooks, S. L., et al. (2005). Minority adult survivors of childhood cancer: a comparison of long-term outcomes, health care utilization, and health-related behaviors from the childhood cancer survivor study. *Journal of Clinical Oncology, 23*, 6549–6507.

Children's Oncology Group. Long-Term Follow-Up Guidelines for Survivors of Childhood, Adolescent, and Young Adult Cancers, Version 2.0. Children's Oncology Group; 2006. http://www.survivorshipguidelines.org. Accessed July 15, 2006.

Clarke, S. A., & Eiser, C. (2007). Health behaviours in childhood cancer survivors: A systematic review. *European Journal of Cancer, 43*, 1373–1384.

Cox, C. L., McLaughlin, R. A., Rai, S. N., Steen, B. D., & Hudson, M. M. (2005) Adolescent survivors: A secondary analysis of a clinical trial targeting behavior change. *Pediatric Blood and Cancer, 45*, 144–154.

Cox, C. L., McLaughlin, R. A., Steen, B. D., & Hudson, M. M. (2006) Predicting and modifying substance use in childhood cancer survivors: Application of a conceptual model. *Oncology Nursing Forum, 33*, 51–60.

Crom, D. (1995). The experience of South American mothers who have a child being treated for malignancy in the United States. *Journal of Pediatric Oncology Nursing, 12*, 104–112.

de Oliveira, B., Viana, M., Zani, C., & Romanha, A. (2004). Clinical and laboratory evaluation of compliance in acute lymphoblastic leukaemia. *Archives of Disease in Childhood, 89*, 785–788.

Decker, C. L. (2006). Coping in adolescents with cancer: A review of the literature. *Journal of Psychosocial Oncology, 24*, 123–140.

Decker, C. L., Haase, J. E., & Bell, C. J. (2007). Uncertainty in adolescents and young adults with cancer. *Oncology Nursing Forum, 34*, 681–688.

DeJong, M., & Fombonne, E. (2007). Citalopram to treat depression in pediatric oncology. *Journal of Child & Adolescent Psychopharmacology, 17*, 371–377.

Diamond, G., & Josephson, A. (2005). Family-based treatment research: A 10-year update. *Journal of American Academy of Child & Adolescent Psychiatry, 44*, 872–887.

Donze, J. R., & Tercyak, K. P. (2006). The survivor health and resilience education (SHARE) program: Development and evaluation of a health behavior intervention for adolescent survivors of childhood cancer. *Journal of Clinical Psychology in Medical Settings, 13*, 169–176.

Dunsmore, J., & Quine, S. (1997). Information, support, and decision making needs and preferences of adolescents with cancer: Implications for health professionals. *Journal of Psychosocial Oncology, 13*, 39–56.

Edwards, K. E., Neville, B. A., Cook, E. F., Aldridge, S. H., Dussel, V., & Wolfe, J. (2008). Understanding of prognosis and goals of care among couples whose child died of cancer. Journal of *Clinical Oncology, 26*, 1310–1315.

Eiser, C., Hill, J. J., & Blacklay, A. (2000) Surviving cancer; what does it mean for you? An evaluation of a clinic based intervention for survivors of childhood cancer. *Psycho-Oncology, 9*, 214–220.

Elad. P., Yagil, Y., Cohen., L., & Meller, I. (2003). A jeep trip with young adult cancer survivors: lessons to be learned. *Support Care Cancer, 11*, 201–206.

Emmons, K. M., Puleo, E., Park, E., Gritz, E. R., Butterfield, R. M., Weeks, J. C., et al. (2005) Peer-delivered smoking counseling for childhood cancer survivors increases rate of cessation: The partnership for health study. *Journal of Clinical Oncology, 23*, 6516–6523.

Felder-Puig, R., Formann, A. K., Mildner, A., Bretschneider, W., Bucher, B., Windhager, R., et al. (1998). *Quality of life and psychosocial adjustment of young patients after treatment of bone cancer. Cancer, 83*, 69–75.

Festa, R. S., Tamaroff, M. H., Chasalow, F., & Lanzkowsky, P. (1992). Therapeutic adherence to oral medication regimens by adolescents with cancer. I. Laboratory assessment. *Journal of Pediatrics, 120*, 807–811.

Finnegan, L., Wilkie, D. J., Wilbur, J., Campbell, R. T., Zong, S., & Katula, S. (2007). Correlates of physical activity in young adult survivors of childhood cancers. *Oncology Nursing Forum, 34*, 60–69

Florin, T. A., Fryer, G. E., Miyoshi, T., Weitzman, M., Mertens, A. C., Hudson, M. M., et al. (2007). Physical inactivity in adult survivors of childhood acute lymphoblastic leukemia: a report from the childhood cancer survivor study. *Cancer Epidemiology Biomarkers and Prevention, 16*, 1356–1363.

Freyer, D. R., & Brugieres, L. (2008). Adolescent and young adult oncology: Transition of care. *Pediatric Blood and Cancer, 50*, 1116–1119.

Gavaghan, M. P., & Roach, J. E. (1987). Ego identify development of adolescents with cancer. *Journal of Pediatric Psychology, 12*, 203–213.

Gerhardt, C. A., Dixon, M., Miller, K., Vannatta, K., Valerius, K. S., Correll, J., et al. (2007). Educational and occupational outcomes among survivors of childhood cancer during the transition to emerging adulthood. *Journal of Developmental and Behavioral Pediatrics, 28*, 448–455.

Gershon, J., Zimand, E., Pickering, M., Rothbaum, B. O., & Hodges, L. (2004). A pilot and feasibility study of virtual reality as a distraction for children with cancer. *Journal of the American Academy of Child & Adolescent Psychiatry, 43*, 1243–1249.

Gothelf, D., Rubinstein, M., Shemesh, E., Miller, O., Farbstein, I., Klein, A., et al. (2005). Pilot study: fluvoxamine treatment for depression and anxiety disorders in children and adolescents with cancer. *Journal of the American Academy of Child and& Adolescent Psychiatry, 44*,1258–1262.

Hedström, M., Kreuger, A., Ljungman, G., Nygren, P., & von Essen, L. (2006). Accuracy of assessment of distress, anxiety, and depression by physicians and nurses in adolescents recently diagnosed with cancer. *Pediatric Blood and Cancer, 46*, 773–779.

Hellsten, M. B. (2000). All the king's horses and the king's men: Pain management from hospital to home. *Journal of Pediatric Oncology Nursing, 17*, 149–159.

Hilden, J. M., Emanuel, E. J., Fairclough, D. L., Link, M. P., Foley, K. M., Clarridge, B. C., et al. (2001). Attitudes and practices among pediatric oncologists regarding end-of-life care: results of the 1998 American Society of Clinical Oncology survey. *Journal of Clinical Oncology, 19*, 205–212.

Hinds, P. S., Brandon, J., Allen, C., Hijiya, N., Newsome, R., & Kane, J. R. (2007). Patient-reported outcomes in end-of-life research in pediatric oncology. *Journal of Pediatric Psychology, 32*, 1079–1088.

Hobbie, W. L., Stuber, M., Meeske, K., Wissler, K., Rourke, M. T., Ruccione, K., et al. (2000). Symptoms of posttraumatic stress in young adult survivors of childhood cancer. *Journal of Clinical Oncology, 18*, 4060–4066.

Hockenberry, M. (2004). Symptom management research in children with cancer. *Journal of Pediatric Oncology Nursing, 21*, 132–136.

Hudson, M. M., Tyc, V. L., Srivastava, D. K., Gattuso, J., Quargnenti, A., Crom, D. B., et al. (2002) Multi-component behavioral intervention to promote health protective behaviors in childhood cancer survivors: The protect study. *Medical and Pediatric Oncology*, 39, 2–11.

Institute of Medicine. (2007). *Cancer care for the whole patient: Meeting psychosocial health needs*. Washington, DC: The National Academies Press.

Katz, E. R., & Madan-Swain, A. (2006). Maximizing school, academic, and social outcomes in children and adolescents with cancer. In R. Brown (Ed.). *Comprehensive handbook of childhood cancer and sickle cell disease*. (pp. 313–338). New York, NY: Oxford University Press.

Kazak, A. E., Alderfer, M., Rourke, M. T., Simms, S., Streisand, R., & Grossman, J. R. (2004). Posttraumatic stress disorder (PTSD) and posttraumatic stress symptoms (PTSS) in families of adolescent childhood cancer survivors. *Journal of Pediatric Psychology, 29*, 211–219.

Kazak, A., Alderfer, M., Streisand, R., Simms, S., Rourke, M., Barakat, L., et al. (2004). Treatment of posttraumatic stress symptoms in adolescent survivors of childhood cancer and their families: A randomized clinical trial. *Journal of Family Psychology, 18*, 493–504.

Kazak, A., Barakat, L, Alderer, M., Rourke, M., Meeske, K., Gallagher, P., et al. (2001). Posttraumatic stress in survivors of childhood cancer and their mothers: Development and validation of the Impact of Traumatic Stressors Interview Schedule (ITSIS). *Journal of Clinical Psychology in Medical Settings, 8*, 307–323.

Kazak, A. E., Barakat, L. P., Meeske, K., Christakis, D., Meadows, A. T., Casey, R., et al. (1997). Posttraumatic stress, family functioning, and social support in survivors of childhood leukemia and their mothers and fathers. *Journal of Consulting and Clinical Psychology, 65*, 120–129.

Kazak, A., Boeving, A., Alderfer, M., Hwang, W. T., & Reilly, A. (2005). Posttraumatic stress symptoms in parents of pediatric oncology patients during treatment. *Journal of Clinical Oncology, 23*, 7405–7410.

Kazak, A., McClure, K., Alderfer, M., Hwang, W. T., Crump, T., Le, L., et al. (2004). Cancer-related parental beliefs: The Family Illness Beliefs Inventory. *Journal of Pediatric Psychology, 29*, 531–542.

Kazak, A., & Noll, R. (2004). Child death from pediatric illness: Conceptualizing intervention approaches from a family/systems and public health perspective. *Professional Psychology, 35*, 219–226.

Kazak, A. E., Rourke, M. T., Alderfer, M. A., Pai, A., Reilly, A. F., & Meadows, A. T. (2007) Evidence-based assessment, intervention and psychosocial care in pediatric oncology: A blueprint for comprehensive services across treatment. *Journal of Pediatric Psychology 32*, 1099–1110.

Kazak, A., Schneider S., & Kassam-Adams N. (in press). Pediatric medical traumatic stress. In M. Roberts & R. Steele (Eds.) *Handbook of pediatric psychology* (4th ed.). New York: Guilford.

Kazak, A., Simms, S., & Rourke, M. (2002). Family systems practice in pediatric psychology. *Journal of Pediatric Psychology, 27*, 132–143.

Kendall, P. C. (2005). *Child and adolescent therapy: Cognitive-behavioral procedures*. New York: Guilford.

Kennard, B. D., Stewart, S. M., Olvera, R., Bawdon, R. E., Ohailin, A., Lewis, C. P., et al. (2004). Nonadherence in adolescent oncology patients: Preliminary data on psychological risk factors and relationships too outcome. *Journal of Clinical Psychology in Medical Settings, 11*, 30–39.

Kersun, L. S., & Kazak, A. E. (2006). Prescribing practices of selective serotonin reuptake inhibitors (SSRIs) among pediatric oncologists: a single institution experience. *Pediatric Blood & Cancer 47*, 339–342.

Kupst, M. J., Natta, M. B., Richardson, C., Schulman, J. L., Lavigne, J. V., & Das, L. (1995). Family coping with pediatric leukemia: Ten years after treatment. *Journal of Pediatric Psychology, 20*, 601–617.

Langeveld, N. E., Ubbink, M. C., Last, B. F., Grootenhuis, M. A., Voute, P. A., & De Haan, R. J. (2003). Educational achievement, employment and living situation in long-term young adult survivors of childhood cancer in the Netherlands. *Psycho-Oncology, 12*, 213–225.

Larouche, S. S., & Chin-Peuckert, L. (2006). Changes in body image experienced by adolescents with cancer. *Journal of Pediatric Oncology Nursing, 23*, 200–209.

Lutz Stehl, M., Kazak, A. E., Alderfer, M. A., Rodriguez, A., Hwang, W. T., Pai, A. L. H., et al. (2008). The feasibility of conducting a randomized clinical trial of an intervention for parents/caregivers of children newly diagnosed with cancer. *Journal of Pediatric Psychology*. Advance online publication. Retrieved March 2, 2009. doi:10.1093/ipepsy/jsn130.

Mackie, E., Hill, J., Kondryn, H., & McNally, R. (2000). Adult psychosocial outcomes in long-term survivors of acute lymphoblastic leukaemia and Wilms' tumour: a controlled study. *Lancet, 355*, 1310–1314.

Madan-Swain, A., Brown, R. T., Foster, M. A., Vega, R., Byars, K., Rodenberger, W., et al. (2000). Identity in adolescent survivors of childhood cancer. *Journal of Pediatric Psychology, 25*, 105–115.

Malbasa, T., Kodish, E., & Santacroce S. J., (2007). Adolescent adherence to oral therapy for leukemia: A focus group study. *Journal of Pediatric Oncology Nursing, 24*, 139–151.

Manne, A., & Miller, D. (1998). Social support, social conflict, and adjustment among adolescents with cancer. *Journal of Pediatric Psychology, 23*, 121–130.

Martinson, I. M., Leavitt, M., Liu, C., Armstrong, V., Hornberger, L., Zhang, I., et al. (1999). Comparison of Chinese and Caucasian families caregiving to children with cancer at home: Part I. *Journal of Pediatric Nursing, 14*, 99–109.

McQuaid, E. L., & Nassau, J. H. (1999). Empirically supported treatments of disease-related symptoms in pediatric psychology: Asthma, diabetes, and cancer. *Journal of Pediatric Psychology, 24*, 305–328.

Mitby, P. A., Robison, L. L., Whitton, J. A., Zevon, M. A., Gibbs, I. C., Tersak, J. M., et al. (2003). Utilization of special education services and educational attainment among long-term survivors of childhood cancer: A report from the Childhood Cancer Survivor Study. *Cancer, 97*, 1115–1126.

Mock, V. (2004). Evidence-based treatment for cancer-related fatigue. *Journal of the National Cancer Institute Monographs, 32*, 112–118.

Nathan, P. C., Patel, S. K., Dilley, K., Goldsby, R., Harvey, J., Jacobsen, C., et al. (2007). Guidelines for identification of, advocacy for, and intervention in neurocognitive problems in survivors of childhood cancer: A report from the Children's Oncology Group. *Archives of Pediatrics and Adolescent Medicine, 161*, 798–806.

Ness, K. K., Mertens, A. C., Hudson, M. M., Wall, M. M., Leisenring, W. M., Oeffinger, K. C., et al. (2005) Limitations on physical performance and daily activities among long-term survivors of childhood cancer. *Annals of Internal Medicine, 143*(9), 639–647.

Neville, K. (1998). The relationships among uncertainty, social support, and psychological distress in adolescents recently diagnosed with cancer. *Journal of Pediatric Oncology Nursing, 15*, 37–46.

Nichols, M. L. (1995). Social support and coping in young adolescents with cancer. *Pediatric Nursing, 21*, 235–240.

Noll, R. B., Bukowski, W. M., Davies, W. H., Koontz, K., & Kulkarni, R. (1993). Adjustment in the peer system of adolescents with cancer: a two-year study. *Journal of Pediatric Psychology, 18*, 351–364.

Noll, R., & Kazak, A. (2004). Psychosocial Care. In A. Altman (Ed.). *Supportive care of children with cancer: Current therapy and guidelines from the children's oncology group* (pp. 337–353). Baltimore, MD: The Johns Hopkins University Press.

Noll, R. B., LeRoy, S., Bukowski, W. M., Rogosch, F. A., & Kulkarni, R. (1991). Peer relationships and adjustment in children with cancer. *Journal of Pediatric Psychology, 16*, 307–326.

Novakovic, B., Fears, T. R., Wexler, L. H., McClure, L. L., Wilson, D. L., McCalls, J. L., et al. (1996). Experiences of cancer in children and adolescents. *Cancer Nursing*, 19(1), 54–59.

Nurmi, J. (1993). Adolescent development in an age-graded context: The role of personal beliefs, goals and strategies in the tackling of developmental tasks and standards. *International Journal of Behavioral Development, 16*, 169–189.

Oeffinger, K. C., Mertens, A. C., Hudson, M. M., Gurney, J. G., Casillas, J., Chen, H. et al. (2004). Health care of young adult survivors of childhood cancer: A report from the childhood cancer survivor study. *Annals of Family Medicine, 2*, 61–70.

Oeffinger, K. C., Mertens, A. C., Sklar, C. A., Kawashima, T., Hudson, M. M., Meadows, A. T., et al. (2006). Chronic health conditions in adult survivors of childhood cancer. *New England Journal Medicine, 355*(15), 1572–1582.

Pai, A. L., Patiño-Fernández, A. M., McSherry, M., Beele, D., Alderfer, M. A., Reilly, A. T., et al. (2008). The psychosocial assessment tool (PAT2.0): psychometric properties of a screener for psychosocial distress in families of children newly diagnosed with cancer. *Journal of Pediatric Psychology, 33*, 50–62.

Pao, M., & Kazak, A. (2009). Anxiety and Depression. In L. Wiener, M. Pao, A. Kazak, M. J. Kupst, & A. F. Patenaude (Eds.), *Quick reference for pediatric oncology clinicians: The psychiatric and psychological dimensions of pediatric cancer symptom management.* Charlottesville, VA: IPOS Press.

Patiño-Fernández, A. M., Pai, A. L., Alderfer, M., Hwang, W. T., Reilly, A., & Kazak, A. E. (2008). Acute stress in parents of children newly diagnosed with cancer. *Pediatric Blood and Cancer, 50*, 289–292.

Pendley, J. S., Dahlquist, L. M., & Dreyer, Z. (1997). Body image and psychosocial adjustment in adolescent cancer survivors. *Journal of Pediatric Psychology, 22*, 29–43.

Power, T. J., DuPaul, G. J., Shapiro, E. S., & Kazak, A. E. (2003). *Promoting children's health: Integrating school, family, and community.* New York, NY: The Guilford Press.

Powers, S. W. (1999). Empirically supported treatments in pediatric psychology: Procedure related pain. *Journal of Pediatric Psychology, 24*, 131–145.

Prevatt, F. F., Heffer, R. W., & Lowe, P. A. (2000). A review of school reintegration programs for children with cancer. *Journal of School Psychology, 38*, 447–467.

Puukko, L., Sammallahti, P. R., Siimes, M. A., & Aalberg, V. A. (1997). Childhood Leukemia and body image: Interview reveals impairment not found with a questionnaire. *Journal of Clinical Psychology, 53*, 133–137.

Ramanujachar, R., Richards, S., Hann, I., & Webb, D. (2008). Review: Adolescents with acute lymphoblastic leukaemia: Emerging from the shadow of paediatric and adult treatment protocols. *Pediatric Blood and Cancer, 47*, 478–756.

Rapoff, M., McGrath, A., & Smith, S. (2006). Adherence to treatment demands. In R. Brown (Ed.). *Comprehensive handbook of childhood cancer and sickle cell disease* (pp. 138–169). New York, NY: Oxford University Press.

Recklitis, C. J., Lockwood, R. A., Rothwell, M. A., & Diller, L. (2006). Suicidal ideation and attempts in adult survivors of childhood cancer. *Journal of Clinical Oncology 24*, 3852–3857.

Ritchie, M. A. (2001). Sources of emotional support for adolescents with cancer. *Journal of Pediatric Oncology Nursing, 18*, 105–110.

Rourke, M. T., Hobbie, W. L., Schwartz, L., & Kazak, A. E. (2007). Posttraumatic stress disorder (PTSD) in young adult survivors of childhood cancer. *Pediatric Blood and Cancer, 49*,177–182.

Rourke, M. T., Reilly, A., Kersun, L. S., McSherry, M., Ingram, M., & Tracy, E. (2006). *Understanding and managing challenging families in pediatric oncology.* Poster presented at the American Psychosocial Oncology Society (APOS) 3rd Annual Conference, Amelia Island, FL.

Rowland, J. H., Pfefferbaum, B., Adams-Greenly, M., & Redd, W. H. (1989). Childhood cancer: Psychological issues and their management. In J. C. Holland & J. H.

Rowland (Eds.), *Handbook of psycho-oncology: Psychological care of the patient with cancer* (pp. 517–581). NY: Oxford University Press.

Santacroce, S. J., & Lee, Y. (2006). Uncertainty, posttraumatic stress, and health behavior in young adult childhood cancer survivors. *Nursing Research, 55*, 259–266.

Schultz, K. A., Ness, K. K., Whitton, J., Recklitis, C., Zebrack, B., Robison, L. L., et al. (2007). Behavioral and social outcomes in adolescent survivors of childhood cancer: A report from the childhood cancer survivor study. *Journal of Clinical Oncology, 25*(24), 3649–3656.

Schwartz, L., & Drotar, D. (2004). The effects of written emotional disclosure on caregivers of children and adolescents with chronic illness. *Journal of Pediatric Psychology, 29*, 105–118.

Schwartz, L., & Drotar, D. (2006a). Posttraumatic stress and related impairment in survivors of childhood cancer in early adulthood compared to healthy peers. *Journal of Pediatric Psychology, 31*, 356–366.

Schwartz, L., & Drotar, D. (2006b). Defining the nature and impact of goals in children and adolescents with a chromic health condition: a review of research and a theoretical framework. *Journal of Clinical Psychology in Medical Settings, 13*(4), 390–402.

Schwartz, L. A., & Wolf, J. (2008, April). *Health-related hindrance of personal goals of adolescents with cancer.* Poster presented at the National Conference on Child Health Psychology Conference, Miami, FL.

Selove, R. (2007, October). *Psychosocial services in the first 30 days.* Presentation at the Children's Oncology Group Meeting, Denver, CO.

Shama, W., & Lucchetta, S. (2007). Psychosocial issues of the adolescent cancer patient and the development of the teenage outreach program (TOP). *Journal of Psychosocial Oncology, 25*, 99–112.

Speechley, K. N., & Noh, S. (1992). Surviving Childhood Cancer, Social Support, and Parents' Psychological Adjustment. *Journal of Pediatric Psychology*, 17, 15–31.

Spirito, A., & Kazak, A. (2006). *Effective and emerging treatments in pediatric psychology.* New York: Oxford University Press.

Stam, H., Grootenhuis, M. A., & Last, B. F. (2005). The course of life of survivors of childhood cancer. *Psycho-Oncology, 14*, 227–238.

Stegenga, K., & Ward-Smith, P. (2008). The adolescent perspective on participation in treatment decision making: a pilot study. *Journal of Pediatric Oncology Nursing*, 25, 112–117.

Stevens, B., Kagan, S., Yamada, J., Epstein, I., Beamer, M., Bilodeau, M., et al. (2004). Adventure therapy for adolescents with cancer. *Pediatric Blood & Cancer, 43*, 278–284.

Stiller, C. (2002). Epidemiology of cancer in adolescents. *Medical and Pediatric Oncology, 39*(3), 149–155.

Stuber, M. L., Schneider, S., Kassam-Adams, N., Kazak, A. E., & Saxe, G. (2006). The medical traumatic stress toolkit. *CNS Spectrums, 11*, 137–142.

Suzuki, L. K., & Beale, I. L. (2006). Personal web home pages of adolescents with cancer: Self-presentation, information dissemination, and interpersonal connection. *Journal of Pediatric Oncology Nursing, 23*, 152–161.

Tercyak, K. P., Donze, J. R., Prahlad, S., Mosher, R. B., & Shad, A. T. (2006). Identifying, recruiting, and enrolling adolescent survivors of childhood cancer into a randomized controlled trial of health promotion: Preliminary experiences in the survivor health and resilience education (SHARE) program. *Journal of Pediatric Psychology, 31*, 252–261.

Theunissen, J. M., Hoogerbrugge, P. M., van Achterberg, T., Prins, J. B., Vernooij-Dassen, M. J., & van den Ende, C. H. (2007). Symptoms in the palliative phase of children with cancer. *Pediatric Blood and Cancer, 49*, 160–165.

Thibodeaux, A. G., & Deatrick, J. A. (2007). Cultural influence on family management of children with cancer. *Journal of Pediatric Oncology Nursing, 24*, 227–233.

Tyc, V. L., Hudson, M. M., & Hinds, P. (1999) Health promotion interventions for adolescent cancer survivors. *Cognitive and Behavioral Practice, 6*, 128–136.

Tyc, V. L., Rai, S. N., Lensing, S., Klosky, J. L., Stewart, D. B., & Gattuso, J. (2003). Intervention to reduce intentions to use tobacco among pediatric cancer survivors. *Journal of Clinical Oncology, 21*, 366–1372.

U.S. Department of Health and Human Services, National Institutes of Health, National Cancer Institute, & Livestrong. (2006). Closing the gap: Research and care imperative for adolescnts and young adults with cancer, report of the adolescent and young adult oncology progress review group. NIH Publication No. 06-6067.

Varni, J. W., Katz, E. R., Colegrove, R. Jr., & Dolgin, M. (1995). Perceived physical appearance and adjustment of children with newly diagnosed cancer: A path analytic model. *Journal of Behavioral Medicine, 18*, 261–278.

Wallace, M. L., Harcourt, D., Rumsey, N., & Foot, A. (2007). Managing appearance chances resulting from cancer treatment: resilience in adolescent females. *Psycho-Oncology, 16*, 1019–1027.

Ward-Smith, P., Hamlin, J., Bartholomew, J., & Stegenga, K. (2007). Quality of life among adolescents with cancer. *Journal of Pediatric Oncology Nursing, 24*, 166–171.

Windebank, K. P., & Spinetta, J. J. (2008). Do as I say or die: Compliance in adolescents with cancer. *Pediatric Blood and Cancer, 50*, 1099–1100.

Wolfe, J, Grier, H. E., Klar, N., Levin, S. B., Ellenbogen, J. M., Salem-Schatz, S., et al. (2000). Symptoms and suffering at the end of life in children with cancer. *The New England Journal of Medicine, 342*, 326–333.

Wolfe, J., Hammel, J. F., Edwards, K. E., Duncan, J., Comeau, M., Breyer, J., et al. (2008). Easing of suffering in children with cancer at the end of life: Is care changing? *Journal of Clinical Oncology, 26*, 1717–1723.

Woodgate, R. L. (2006). The importance of being there: Perspectives of social support by adolescents with cancer. *Journal of Pediatric Oncology Nursing, 23*, 122–134.

Wu, E., Robison, L. L., Jenney, M. E., Rockwood, T. H., Feusner, J., Friedman, D., et al. (2007). Assessment of health-related quality of life of adolescent cancer patients using the Minneapolis-Manchester Quality of Life Adolescent Questionnaire. *Pediatric Blood and Cancer, 48*, 678–686.

Yeazel, M. W., Oeffinger, K. C., Gurney, J. G., Mertens, A. C., Hudson, M. M., Emmons, K. M., et al. (2004). The cancer screening practices of adult survivors of childhood cancer: A report from the Childhood Cancer Survivor Study. *Cancer, 100*, 631–640.

Yeh, C. H. (2001). Development and testing of the Parental Coping Strategy Inventory (PCSI) with children with cancer in Taiwan. *Journal of Advanced Nursing, 36*, 78–88.

Zebrack, B., Bleyer, A., Albritton, K., Medearis, S., Tang, J. (2006). Assessing the health care needs of adolescent and young adult cancer patients and survivors. *Cancer, 107*, 2915–2923.

Zeltzer, L. K. (1993). Cancer in adolescents and young adults psychosocial aspects. Long-term survivors. *Cancer, 15*, 3463–3468.

Zeltzer, L. K., Chen, E., Weiss, R., Guo, M. D., Robison, L. L., Meadows, A. T., et al. (1997). Comparison of psychological outcome in adult survivors of childhood acute lymphoblastic leukemia versus sibling controls: A cooperative Children's Cancer Group and National Institutes of Health study. *Journal of Clinical Oncology, 15*, 547–556.

Cystic Fibrosis in Adolescents

Anthony A. Hains, W. Hobart Davies, Diana Quintero, and Julie A. Biller

Folklore from central Europe recounts that infants who taste salty with their mother's kiss will not survive infancy. This is felt to be the first description of cystic fibrosis. Centuries later in 1938, the first description of CF in the medical literature noted pancreatic abnormalities, malnourishment, and associated pneumonia in infants who died usually in the first year of life (Andersen, 2008). The disease was noticed to be more prevalent among Caucasians, with affected individuals dying in early childhood. For years, families were told of grim outcomes until the late 1980 s when the affected gene was discovered, along with new therapies. Since then, life expectancy has dramatically improved with a current median survival age of 36.5 years as reported by the Cystic Fibrosis Foundation in 2005 (http://www.cff.org).

Genetic Factors

Cystic fibrosis is the most common genetic disease among Caucasians, affecting 1 in 2500 individuals. In contrast, CF affects 1:9000 Hispanics, 1:12,000 Blacks, and 1:90,000 Asians (Andersen, 1949; Collins, 1992). Nearly 30,000 individuals in the United States and 70,000 around the world have been diagnosed with this disease (FitzSimmons, 1993).

A.A. Hains (✉)
Department of Educational Psychology, University of Wisconsin-Milwaukee, Milwaukee, WI, USA
e-mail: aahains@uwm.edu

CF is an autosomal recessive condition where two carriers with the defective gene will pass it on to their offspring. With each pregnancy there is a 25% chance of having a child with CF. The gene is located on the long arm of chromosome 7 (Kerem et al., 1989), and it encodes for a large protein called cystic fibrosis transmembrane regulator (CFTR). This protein forms the major chloride channel across the cell membranes of the sweat glands, sinuses, lungs, pancreas, gastrointestinal tract, and reproductive organs. The main function of CFTR is to pump excess intracellular chloride ions out of the cell. When the CFTR is not working appropriately, the chloride negative charges forces sodium and water to move into the cell (Quinton, 1990). CFTR has another important function of inhibiting sodium reabsorption across the cell membrane. This inhibition is lost with dysfunctional CFTR in CF. This abnormal shift of ions and water results in thick secretions that plug the lumen or tube-like portions of different organs resulting in the clinical findings described below. CFTR may be affected in various ways depending on the location of the mutation in the gene with more than 1500 mutations described so far. The mutations are classified into five types depending on which part of the process of CFTR formation is affected, starting in the nucleus and ending on the surface of the cell (Welsh & Smith, 1995). The most common mutation is the delta F508, which affects 70% of all individuals with CF. The severity of the disease depends on the inherited mutations; however, there may be variations among individuals with the same genotype. It is difficult to predict the severity of the disease even when knowing an individual's genotype.

W.T. O'Donohue, L.W. Tolle (eds.), *Behavioral Approaches to Chronic Disease in Adolescence*,
DOI 10.1007/978-0-387-87687-0_17,

Clinical Manifestations

Clinical findings will depend on the underlying gene mutation and age of the patient. The most severe forms – classical CF – will present with multiple organ manifestations, whereas nonclassical or atypical CF will have either milder symptoms or some organs not affected at all.

Early Childhood

Individuals with classical CF will experience symptoms very early in life. Approximately 10–15% may have meconium ileus at birth. This happens when the flow through the gastrointestinal track becomes so thick that it causes a mechanical obstruction. This abnormality may be detected prenatally by ultrasound, with hyperechoic images suggesting meconium ileus. Once born, the neonate will experience abdominal distension and feeding intolerance with vomiting and no passage of meconium or gas (Littlewood, 1992).

Respiratory symptoms are uncommon at this age, but chest films suggest evidence of air trapping. In addition, asymptomatic small airway disease has been documented in autopsies of newborns with CF who died of meconium ileus at birth (Zuelzer & Newton, 1949). Moist cough or respiratory symptoms may appear at any time, however, and a thorough evaluation for infection is warranted.

Pancreatic insufficiency is evident at birth but can be difficult to distinguish from normal frequent stooling in a newborn. It occurs because of obstruction of pancreatic ducts that do not allow the enzymes produced in the pancreas to reach the small intestine. As enzymes cannot be released, pancreatitis can ensue and autodestruction of pancreatic tissue can occur (Kopelman, Durie, Gaskin, Weizman, & Forstner, 1985). Since lipase and amylase are enzymes that are vital for the absorption of food and fat-soluble vitamins (vitamin A, D, E, and K), newborns will have frequent, bulky, greasy stools with pancreatic insufficiency. They experience poor weight gain despite appropriate caloric intake. Failure to thrive is usually the most common manifestation at this point, leading to the diagnosis of pancreatic insufficiency. Manifestations of vitamin deficiency will include skin rash, bleeding, and rickets among others (Feranchak et al., 1999).

Childhood and Adolescence

As the child with CF grows, symptoms typically worsen and other clinical findings of CF will become more evident and progress through adulthood. One common feature of this disease is loss of salt through sweat glands especially during summer months. Parents will mention their child tastes "salty". If sweating is profuse, it will lead to dehydration and electrolyte imbalance. Prompt correction by providing electrolyte-rich fluid helps stabilize this abnormality (Ballestero et al., 2006).

Sinus disease is found in 100% of affected patients and is a consequence of their inability to clear thick mucus from the sinuses, leading to infection and inflammation. However, despite significant involvement of sinuses, individuals with CF rarely complain of symptom unless there is mucus impaction. This may lead to headache, sinus pressure, and throat clearing. Treatment includes daily nasal irrigation, antibiotics, or surgery if symptoms are persistent or if they affect lung function (Wang et al., 2000).

Nasal polyps may also be found in individuals with CF. They are caused by chronic inflammation of the nasal mucosa, which leads to tissue overgrowth. They appear as gray, shiny, well-circumscribed tissue. The size may vary and can become clinically evident with protrusion out of the sinus into the upper portion of the nose. Surgery is indicated especially if obstruction of the airway occurs (Wang et al., 2000).

As the child grows, respiratory symptoms may become recurrent and finally persistent. Thick mucus accumulates in the airway, leading to increased daily productive cough and increased production of thick, green phlegm. These secretions are rich in carbohydrates that facilitate bacterial growth. Many organisms, but more commonly *Staphylococcus aureus* and *Pseudomonas aeruginosa*, reproduce easily in this environment (Abman et al., 1991). If untreated, they colonize the airway and chronic inflammation occurs. This leads to recurrent episodes of bronchopneumonia, airway destruction, and bronchiectasis (abnormal dilatation and weakening of the airways). Bronchiectasis furthers the recurrent airway obstruction and retention of the thickened secretions so that a vicious cycle of obstruction, inflammation, and infection develops in the lungs (Konstan & Berger, 1992). Eventually, casual colonization with *P. aeruginosa* becomes chronic, which begins the exorable decline in lung function. Other respiratory complications include hemoptysis (coughing up blood) and asthma. Lung disease is progressive and is the main cause of death among patients with CF (Ramsey, 1996). Available treatments to try to prevent lung deterioration will be discussed later.

Multiple organs in the gastrointestinal tract are also affected (Welsh, Tsui, Boat, & Beaudet, 1995). Despite supplemental enzymes, pancreatic insufficiency may become an ongoing problem through life. Common symptoms include malabsorption of food manifested by frequent bulky, greasy, foul-smelling stools. Failure to thrive is the most common consequence of malabsorption as the body does not absorb the necessary amount of nutrients that are vital for growth and development. Malnourishment can affect the immune system impairing the ability to fight infection. There is a clear correlation between good nutrition and optimal lung function. Monitoring of appropriate weight gain by using body mass index (weight/height^2) is done during each visit to the CF clinic. Children and adolescents should maintain their body mass index (BMI) above the 50th percentile for their age. Adults are felt to have optimal nutritional status when a BMI greater than 22 for women and 23 for men is achieved. In 20% of individuals with CF, the endocrine function of the pancreas is impaired by chronic scarring, leading to diabetes requiring chronic insulin therapy (Lanng, Hansen, Thorsteinsson, Nerup, & Koch, 1995). This adds a significant treatment burden to those affected.

Other gastrointestinal manifestations include involvement of the large intestine by impaired lubrication during passage of stools, which leads to abdominal pain and constipation. Episodes of the so-called distal intestine obstruction syndrome (DIOS) happen when the constipation is so severe that it causes obstruction with bowel distension and pain (Dik, Nicolai, Schipper, Heijerman, & Bakker, 1995; Littlewood, 1992). This requires clean-out of the intestine that may take hours to days to clear up. Rarely, it may require surgery to relieve the obstruction.

Cirrhosis may occur due to chronic obstruction of liver bile ducts, which leads to stasis of abnormally thick bile and subsequent inflammation (Corbett et al., 2004). Careful annual evaluations are necessary to diagnose this complication as it usually does not have any presenting symptoms that will help make an early diagnosis.

Rectal prolapse happens in 10% of patients with CF and usually manifests early in life, especially during toilet-training years. It presents as a protrusion of the rectum through the anus and needs immediate reduction. The use of enzymes may help resolve the events; however, surgery maybe indicated if symptoms persist (Littlewood, 1992).

Reproductive organs are also affected in this disease. In affected males, 98% have congenital bilateral absence of van deferens (CBAVD), which leads to infertility (Taussig, Lobeck, di Sant'Agnese, Ackerman, & Kattwinkel, 1972). Females may also have problems with conception due to increased thickness of the cervical mucus or reproductive hormone abnormality (Kotloff, FitzSimmons, & Fiel, 1992).

Adults

All of the clinical problems discussed above continue and worsen as individuals age with CF. Some complications such as diabetes and DIOS increase in frequency in adulthood. Pulmonary functions tend to decline in most adults. Eventually many become so ill that they may not be able to continue to work. When lung involvement becomes so severe, lung transplantation may be an option to prolong life in suitable candidates.

Diagnosis

A diagnosis of CF is made when the following conditions occur (Rosenstein & Cutting, 1998):

1) Clinical findings
2) History of CF in the family

3) Abnormal sweat test done twice
4) Confirmation of the above by a DNA genetic testing showing two abnormal genes
5) Abnormal newborn screen test with confirmed DNA and/or sweat test.

Treatment

Early and significant complications of cystic fibrosis maybe avoided or delayed by very close follow-up. There are 120 CF centers in the United States which are closely monitored by the CF Foundation (CFF). This nonprofit organization has developed the guidelines and standards of care that each center should follow. These recommendations include quarterly visits to an accredited CF center, where a team of experienced multidisciplinary providers evaluates patients to assure optimal health and intervene with appropriate therapies as needed. During these visits, patient's weight, height, and development are routinely assessed. A thorough interview addressing possible complications is also done. Routine testing including pulmonary function tests and sputum cultures are done to detect any lung deterioration or new organisms that may indicate the need for antibiotics. Other tests to monitor liver disease, renal function, and diabetes are done yearly.

Medications prescribed to delay lung disease are started early in life (Flume et al., 2007). The main purpose is to facilitate expectoration of thick secretions by reducing the viscosity of respiratory mucus and improving ciliary function of airway-lining cells to facilitate clearance of respiratory secretions. They are commonly prescribed twice a day. However, during CF exacerbations – which consist of increased productive cough, worsening dyspnea, or a drop in lung function tests – it is recommended that these medications and clearance techniques be used up to four times a day. The most common medications to maintain lung function include the following (Ramsey, 1996):

1) *Albuterol*: A bronchodilator that helps facilitate expectoration of mucus. It may be given through a nebulizer machine, which takes about 10 minutes, or by a metered dose inhaler (MDI), a quicker method. It needs to be taken at least twice a day before other respiratory treatments. Its most common side effects are tremors and palpitations.
2) *Hypertonic saline*: A concentrated salt water solution that rehydrates mucus by allowing water to shift from the epithelial or lining cells to the lumen of the airway where the mucus resides. Once this happens, secretions are thinner and easier to expectorate. This solution is given at least twice a day through a nebulizer machine and usually takes 15 minutes for the entire dose to be delivered. Patients may experience persistent cough that is somewhat relieved by predosing with albuterol.
3) *Pulmozyme*: This nebulized medication is used to help reduce the viscosity of the abnormally thick mucus and facilitates expectoration. It is used once a day and takes 10–15 minutes to be delivered. The main side effects include hoarseness and transient increase of cough. However, this medication is usually very well tolerated.

In addition to medications, airway clearance is also recommended (Main, Prasad, & Schans, 2005). The classic and most common technique used is clapping and vibration of all areas of the chest. Other modes include devices where patients may blow against resistance (PEP and acapella are the most common) or a high-frequency chest wall oscillation device. The latter is a vest that covers the patient's entire chest wall and is connected to a compressor through two hoses. The compressor inflates the vest and vibrates making the entire chest move. This helps the mucus become dislodged from the airway walls and facilitates expectoration.

These modes of airway clearance are done for at least 20 minutes twice a day when patients are healthy; they are used longer or more frequently when they are ill with an exacerbation. Nebulized medications may be given at the same time to help reduce the time-consuming nature of the treatments.

Antibiotics are frequently prescribed during CF exacerbations in an attempt to decrease the bacterial density in the airways, given the instrumental role bacterial load plays in causing exacerbations (Ramsey, 1996). Oral antibiotics are one of the options and are usually prescribed for at least 10 days, depending on the organism and the overall clinical findings. Frequent follow-up is necessary to make sure that symptoms are resolved and lung function is back to baseline.

If patients are significantly ill, or their lung function drops by at least 15% of their baseline, consideration for an admission to the hospital for a course of IV antibiotics is undertaken. The average length of stay during such hospitalizations is 10–14 days and during this stay, the frequency of inhaled medications and airway clearance is increased. Careful monitoring of lung function test is done until the patient get close to their baseline. Frequency of admission to the hospital depends of how sick the individual is. As more lung disease develops, the likelihood of frequent clinic visits and prolonged hospitalizations increases. These individuals may also need to undergo placement of a long-term intravenous catheter to facilitate the delivery of medications and blood draws. It also facilitates home treatments with antibiotics.

Pancreatic insufficiency is treated with enzymes. They should be started as soon as a diagnosis of classical CF is confirmed to prevent further weight loss and are a lifelong treatment. Enzymes come in capsules and are dosed based on the patient's weight. As the child or the adolescent grows, dosing is adjusted accordingly. Quantity of how many capsules they take may vary. Prescribed doses should be taken before eating meals and snacks, especially those with high fat content. If poor nutritional status becomes a persistent problem despite an appropriate dose of enzymes, oral supplements, i.e., Pediasure®, Boost®, or Ensure®, may be indicated (Poustie, Russell, Watling, Ashby, & Smyth, 2006).

Some patients do not gain weight despite these measures or they have chronic poor appetite with inadequate caloric intake. In such cases, it may be necessary to place a gastrostomy feeding tube. This tube is placed under anesthesia and is inserted through the abdominal skin directly into the stomach. With this tube in place, supplemental feeding to achieve higher caloric intake becomes easier and may be given as a night drip. The main concern especially among adolescent girls is aesthetic. Other complications that may occur are local pain, skin infections around the tube, and uncommonly, intestinal perforation.

Other treatments include symptom management for CF-related complications such as insulin for diabetes or stool softeners for constipation.

Cost

As expected, the cost of frequent clinic visits, laboratory tests, radiology studies, admissions to the hospital, and medications is quite high. Coverage for services and medications is variable depending on the type of insurance. Government-based health-care insurance like Medicaid and Medicare usually provides adequate coverage for these high costs. However, many patients are underinsured with poor coverage, causing financial and emotional hardship, furthering the strain of this chronic illness on the entire family.

Medical Summary

Great strides have been made in the life expectancy of individuals with CF with survival improving from 20 years of age to nearly 40 years in just the last two decades. This has been due to an ever-increasing number of treatments available to help those with CF. Individuals with CF are encouraged to plan on reaching adulthood, with a strong emphasis on vocational planning to assure a satisfying work life with health-care benefits to cover the costs of their expensive care. Marriage and having families occurs with increasing frequency as the CF population ages. This is all tempered by the time-consuming and demanding daily treatment regimen required by those with CF to remain healthy. This dichotomy, the desire to have a full life like those without chronic health problems, can cause conflict with family and health-care providers. It is the unintended consequence of the advances of health care in CF and one we hope can be improved in the years to come.

Developmental Aspects and the CF Medical Care Team

Historically, the very limited life span of individuals with CF meant that treatment of CF was almost exclusively the province of pediatric pulmonology and pediatric gastroenterology, along with affiliated pediatric professionals. As life expectancies began to increase, most patients continued to be treated by a pediatric team. Gradually, the field began to realize that the pediatric environment was not ideal for these patients in terms of promoting independent adult functioning and self-image. Nor was the increased expense of multidisciplinary pediatric care always needed. We began to see the development of adult CF centers, and this has become the standard of care. Most patients today are with an adult treatment team longer than they are with the pediatric team.

This has been a very positive development for centers treating CF, but it begs the question: When and how do you make the transition to adult care? This is a question that most centers have addressed carefully and on a case-by-case basis, ideally with decision-making involving discussion between the pediatric and the adult medicine providers. The transition to the adult center may be gradual or abrupt and can begin before the patient has even entered adolescence, if that seems best for an individual patient (to facilitate a good match with a particular provider during adolescence, for example). Decisions about the transition to adult care become one of the numerous decisions that have to be made in keeping with the goal of achieving independent and adaptive functioning by young adulthood. Given the long-term and intensive nature of the relationship with the pediatric treatment team, the transition to adult care can be a significant stressor.

The Range of Intervention Targets in CF

Behavioral health clinicians working with adolescents with CF and their families are faced with a complex range of potential foci for intervention. Youths with CF obviously face the same range of issues with psychopathology and development that physically healthy youths face (anxiety, depression, substance abuse and dependence, and identity development) and that may lead to a referral for psychotherapy. However, these "normative issues" must be looked at from within the lens of CF. For example, identity development and choices about education and career are certainly influenced by knowledge of one's relatively limited, yet constantly increasing, life expectancy. Choices made in pursuing intimate relationships will be affected by life expectancy, sensitivity about one's appearance, and knowledge of an increased risk of infertility.

Other problems are encountered in families of adolescents battling CF that arise much more directly from the demands of the very complicated and multidimensional treatment regimen(s) described above (Quittner et al., 1996). Referrals may come about because of adolescents who resist taking medications or avoid doing chest physical therapy, who are not eating adequate calories to maintain their growth and health, who refuse to do self-care activities when around their peers, or who begin smoking. There are also frequent problems identified in the gradual transition from pediatric caregivers to adult medicine caregivers, and in the shift from parent-directed adherence of the medical regimen to patient-directed adherence and self-management.

Figure 1 outlines these key intervention themes of considering (1) the range of presenting problems from age-normative to CF-specific, with most problems involving an interaction of both; (2) the

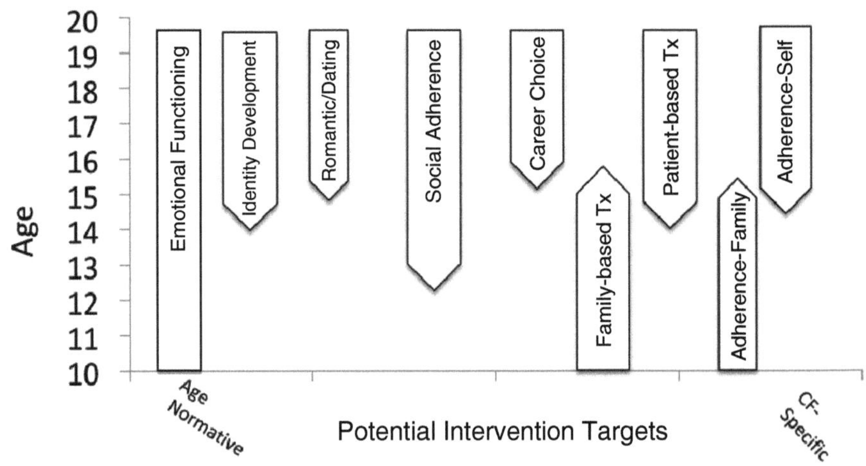

Fig. 1 Developmental model of intervention targets for adolescents with cystic fibrosis

chronological age of the adolescent; and (3) related to that, the move from family-based interventions and parent-directed adherence to a focus on promoting optimal individual functioning and self-management. This reflects an enormously wide range of possible presenting problems and interventions for a condition with a relatively small population. Consideration of the specifics of CF treatment implies that we must proceed with caution in assuming that interventions developed for physically healthy youths and families, or even interventions developed for youths with other chronic illnesses, can simply be inserted into treatment plans for youths with CF (Quittner et al., 2000). An additional complication is the inadequacy of the current DSM-IV-TR diagnoses in reflecting the context specificity of working with this population.

Behavioral Health Interventions for Adolescents with CF

The role of a behavioral health clinician working with adolescents who have CF is comparable to working with other chronic illness populations. Issues like disease knowledge and awareness, coping with health concerns, emotional distress, and regimen adherence are seen as potential intervention targets. Unfortunately, very little intervention research has been conducted with the CF population as a whole, and this is especially true for adolescents with CF (Glasscoe & Quittner, 2003; Quittner et al., 2000). Until relatively recently, the life expectancy of children with CF was rather short. While there have been steady increases in life expectancy over the past two decades, investigation of psychosocial factors and treatments has not kept pace. More attention and grant resources have naturally been focused on developing treatments to prolong life, as opposed to emotional or behavioral issues. Therefore, the science of psychosocial intervention for adolescents with CF remains in its infancy, and empirically supported treatments which could serve as examples of best practice for mental health providers are lacking.

The empirically evaluated interventions conducted with adolescents have targeted CF-related knowledge, support, coping, exercise, adherence, and relieving emotional distress. Each of these areas has an overarching agenda of helping adolescents develop coping and self-management skills to facilitate improved quality of life, adjustment, and/or physical health.

Intervention Research: Knowledge, Support, and Coping

Johnson, Ravert, and Everton (2001) developed a web-based electronic support group to facilitate interactions among adolescents with CF, change youths' perceptions of peer support and their disease, and improve communication between adolescents and the medical team. Eighteen participants with a mean age of 13 years had access to the site, and on average, they logged in four times per month. At the completion of the study, the youths thought that their access to peers with CF had improved. In addition, they felt that bonding opportunities became available and that there was an increase in their ability to talk about teen issues. The sections of the site that permitted socialization opportunities were the most active, and frequent e-mails were common among participants. There was, however, no change in CF-related knowledge in the participants.

Davis, Quittner, Stack, and Yang (2004) evaluated the effectiveness of a STARBRIGHT CD-ROM program entitled *Fitting CF into Your Everyday Life*. This educational CD-ROM was designed to teach children and adolescents about CF and to increase the generation of CF-related coping strategies related to such issues as adherence to a treatment regimen, peer relationships, and dealing with hospitalizations. The CD-ROM takes 30 minutes to complete and contains three modules focusing on Eating (e.g., the importance of taking enzymes), Breathing (e.g., the importance of adhering to breathing exercises), and Questions and Answers (e.g., involving the presentation of hypothetical dilemmas involving CF and suggestions for dealing with them). The 47 participants ranging in age from 7 to 17 years (mean age 13 years) were randomly assigned to a treatment group and a waiting-list control group. The adolescents in the treatment group showed increases in knowledge of CF and the generation of competent coping strategies after viewing the CD-ROM. Similar improvements were found in the waiting-list group after they viewed the program.

A comprehensive psychoeducational program directed at both parents and patients to improve CF self-management was developed by Bartholomew et al. (1997). They examined the efficacy of the *Cystic Fibrosis Education Program* across early childhood, middle childhood, and adolescence on a variety of knowledge, self-efficacy, self-management, health, and quality of life measures. The program was family centered and self-paced and emphasized interventions based on social cognitive theory such as modeling, skill training, goal setting, self-monitoring, and reinforcement. The instructional modules included topics on respiratory care, nutrition and malabsorption, communication, and coping. In comparison to a control group, those families participating in the program showed increased knowledge in CF care among parents and patients at all three age levels. Also, there were slight decreases in parent-rated problem behavior, and both adolescents and parents showed improvement on a self-reported, self-management questionnaire. There was little intervention impact, however, on the various health, quality of life, problem solving, and social cognitive measures.

Intervention Research: Adherence

Problems with adherence in adolescents with CF are a consistent source of concern and frustration for parents and members of the medical team (Drotar, 2006). This issue is hardly surprising, as adherence difficulties in adolescents are common across a variety of chronic illness groups (La Greca & Bearman, 2003), such as diabetes (Thomas, Peterson, & Goldstein, 1997). The regimen process for CF is complex, including daily chest physiotherapy (CPT), taking enzymes, frequent aerobic exercise, improving nutrition through diet, and administering oral and aerosol antibiotic treatments (Stark, Mackner, Patton, & Acton, 2003). Rates of adherence vary depending on the type of behavior involved, with greater compliance for taking oral medications and lesser compliance for CPT and diet needs (DiGirolamo, Quittner, Ackerman, & Stevens, 1997; Foster et al., 2001; Gudas, Koocher, & Wypij, 1991; Quittner et al., 2000; Passero, Remor, & Solomon, 1981).

Despite the critical nature of maintaining the adherence regimen, very little research has been conducted on interventions to improve this self-care behavior in adolescents. While some research has examined behavioral interventions for increasing caloric intake and facilitating weight gain in younger children (Stark et al., 2003), the few studies with adolescents have targeted exercise programs.

Selvadurai et al. (2002) examined the effectiveness of two different exercise training programs in children and adolescents aged 8–16 years (mean of 13 years) who were hospitalized for infectious pulmonary exacerbation. A total of 66 youths were randomly assigned to three groups: aerobic training (AT), resistance training (RT), and a control group. The AT group participated in aerobic activities for five 30-minute sessions. The RT group exercised their arms and legs against a graded resistance machine completing five sets of 10 repetitions. The control group did not receive any training other than the standard chest physiotherapy. Participants in the AT group showed greater improvement than the youths in both the RT and control groups on measures of peak aerobic activity, quality of life, and activity level. Those in the RT group showed greater improvement than the AT and control groups on measures of lung functioning, weight gain, and leg strength. The improvements noted at the end of training were maintained for 1 month after leaving the hospital. The findings of this study indicated that various forms of exercise have differing impacts on youths with CF. Consequently, to obtain desired results, adolescents should be trained and encouraged to adhere to an exercise schedule that offers a variety of physical activities, therefore facilitating enjoyment and motivation.

Two other studies examined the impact of home exercise training using cycling programs. Gulmans et al. (1999) worked with 14 adolescents, ranging in age from 10 to 16 years. The training period ran 6 months, preceded by a baseline of 6 months. Weekly supervision was provided by a physiotherapist. Compared to baseline, the youths showed improvements on muscle strength in their knees and ankles along and in oxygen consumption. In fact, the positive change in oxygen consumption during the training reversed a slight decrease during the baseline period. In addition, there were improvements in feelings about personal appearance and overall self-worth. Unfortunately, the participants reported that they did not find the cycling program an acceptable form of exercise. This finding may partially account for adherence problems by adolescents on the exercise aspect of their self-care. That is, adolescents may simply become frustrated or bored with the repetitive nature of some exercise plans.

In the second home exercise study, de Jong et al. (1994) examined the impact of a 3-month training program with 10 participants described as adolescents (but who were over the age of 15 years with a mean age of 20 years). Compared to baseline, these participants showed an improvement in exercise tolerance and a self-reported decrease of limitations in activities of daily living. A 4-week follow-up showed that eight of the participants maintained their treatment gains, and seven reported that they continued to exercise at home.

The results of the exercise training studies indicate a variety of positive consequences in terms of physical health. In addition, the seven young adults who continued to exercise after the completion of the de Jong et al. (1994) study may provide an interesting contrast to the adolescents in the Gulmans et al. (1999) study who did not find their program acceptable. While these findings are not directly comparable, one could assume that the young adults who maintained their exercise regimen found it acceptable, purposeful, or important. In order to maintain adolescents' adherence to exercise, it appears that multiple forms and varying options of exercise be encouraged. Clinicians may need to explore alternative ways of exercising and reinforce participation in activities that youths find fun or interesting. These activities are likely different across youths and are likely to change within individual youths during the teenage years.

Intervention Research: Emotional Adjustment

The research examining psychosocial and emotional adjustment of adolescents with CF has produced mixed results. Some research has shown that roughly 50–60% of CF patients can be diagnosed as having adjustment or psychiatric problems, with these primarily being anxiety-based internalizing problems (Thompson, Gustafson, George, & Spock, 1994; Thompson, Gustafson, Hamlett, & Spock, 1992). Others have found that adolescents with CF were not any more distressed than healthy peers (Blair, Cull, & Freeman, 1994; Carew, 2001). Adolescents report feelings of stress related to coping with adherence and declining health, especially while trying to navigate the developmental transition and markers of the teenage years (D'Auria, Christian, Henderson, & Haynes, 2000; DiGirolamo et al., 1997; Mullins, et al., 1994). These concerns include school absences and related consequences (e.g., falling behind in school work), conflicts with parents over adherence, peer and dating challenges, transitions from middle to high school and high school to college, and clinic or hospital visits. However, these stressors do not necessarily result in emotional distress or adjustment problems (Drotar, 2006).

Even though there is not a clear picture indicating significant emotional distress in adolescents, they are still seen as at-risk for adjustment problems and CF-related stressors and are therefore potential targets for interventions (Thompson et al. 1994, 1992; Mullins et. al, 1994). Cognitive behavioral approaches to intervention have the potential for significant potential impact on youths with CF. In the cognitive behavioral model, an individual responds to appraisals or interpretations of events instead of the events themselves. Identification and modification of negative cognitions, attributions, and other cognitive activities are central to the intervention process (Kendall et al., 1992). Treatment typically involves restructuring distorted cognitions, developing more adaptive problem solving, and increasing more functional coping (Kendall et al., 1997). Cognitive behavioral interventions have been shown to be effective in reducing anxiety, depression, and anger-control problems in children and adolescents (Feindler, Ecton, Kingsley, & Dubey, 1986; Kendall, 1994; Kendall et al., 1997; Lewinsohn, Clarke, Hops, & Andrews, 1990). In addition, cognitive behavioral interventions for stress, anxiety, and family conflict in other chronic illness groups such as type 1 diabetes have been reported (Hains, Davies, Parton, & Silverman, 2001; Wysocki et al., 2008).

Cognitive processes may play a major contributing role in the internalizing disorders of adolescents with CF (Thompson et al., 1992). Therefore, the acquisition of cognitive behavioral strategies may be beneficial to adolescents' efforts to manage stress related to CF (e.g., conflicts with parents, body image problems, feeling left out by peers, and maintaining adherence to a complex regimen) or anxiety and depression over their (potentially worsening) health.

Hains, Davies, Behrens, and Biller (1997) examined the effectiveness of a cognitive behavioral intervention to help adolescents with CF cope with anxiety, daily stressors, and health issues. The nine-session intervention involved training cognitive restructuring and problem-solving skills and was implemented across five youths, aged 13–15 years, at staggered intervals in a multiple baseline design. Treatment impact was assessed on measures of trait anxiety and coping and behavioral functioning in the form of functional disability. Four out of the five participants showed decreases in anxiety with treatment, all of them reported an increase in the use of positive coping techniques and a decrease in negative coping techniques on problems related to cystic fibrosis, and all of them showed a decrease in perceived functional disability. The improvements seen on trait anxiety were maintained at follow-up, and three youths maintained improvements on perceived functional disability at follow-up. The training gains on coping with CF-related problems generally were not maintained. Another study examining the effectiveness of the same cognitive behavioral program with four young adults in their early to mid twenties obtained mixed results (Hains, Davies, Behrens, Freeman, & Biller, 2001). One young adult showed improvement on measures of emotional distress, and two others showed slight improvement on functional disability.

Future Research

Overall, the amount of research investigating intervention programs for adolescents with CF has been sparse. This is consistent with the limited psychosocial research examining any CF-related issues with adolescents. As a result, conclusions are difficult to draw, but some suggestions can be made.

Specific focus of intervention studies. First, with the general lack of research showing marked psychopathology in this population, further research searching for ties with general maladjustment really is not warranted. Rather, efforts should extend toward identifying how to target youths with situation or contextually specific problems related to their CF (Quittner et al., 1996, 2000). For instance, some youths may have anxiety about peer relationships, others may have fears about deteriorating health, and others may have questions about disclosing disease status to potential romantic partners. Finding out how to recognize these issues in adolescents and developing individualized interventions will have a greater impact (Modi & Quittner, 2006).

An example from our intervention research highlights this individualized or context-specific approach. In our intervention studies, we noted that many of the issues discussed by the adolescents in the cognitive behavioral treatment programs involved worry or frustration over maintaining adherence in various situations (Hains et al., 1997). Our experience has been that adolescent fears about performing self-care in public are not restricted to teenagers with CF. We found similar patterns in youths with type 1 diabetes (Hains, Davies, Parton et al., 2001). Specifically, it seemed that many of the adherence issues occurred within social contexts, especially around friends and other peers. The adolescents often reported that they anticipated their friends would act negatively (e.g., shun them, abandon them) or think negatively about them (e.g., consider them weak, not fun, or somehow unworthy) if they engaged in public self-care behavior. As a result, some would engage in rather ill-advised impression management strategies (e.g., not adhere to the required behavior) in order to avoid peer sanctions.

As an illustration, consider the behavior of Jake, a 14-year-old boy participating in one of our intervention studies. Jake's most recent FEV1 was 79%, suggesting mild pulmonary disease. He came from an intact, close-knit family with supportive and encouraging parents. He generally maintained his regimen well at home, displaying mature self-management skills for his age. In addition, Jake was a rather sociable teen with a cohort of close friends. While his friendship network was a prosocial one and played an important role in his positive adjustment, Jake was very apprehensive about performing self-care when he was around his friends. For instance, Jake would often play basketball with friends after school. He knew that he should take a preventive dose of albuterol before playing, but did not want to be seen using his inhaler. Many of his friends knew that he had a "lung disease," but they thought it was asthma and Jake did not correct this mistaken impression. Jake thought that his friends would think he was somehow abnormal or sickly if they knew he needed this medication and would not hang out with him anymore. Ultimately, he feared that he would lose all of his friends. Ironically, Jake would often become winded which interfered with his playing (and drew attention to himself), but weighed against the possibility of losing his friends, this was a risk he was willing to take.

The cognitive behavioral intervention with Jake made use of cognitive restructuring and problem solving to address this issue. The cognitive restructuring process involved training Jake to identify and monitor negative cognitions related to his feelings and behavior choices. These included worries about friends not liking him anymore if they knew he had a serious chronic illness and that the other kids would think he was weird, strange, or a weakling (not the words he used) or the catastrophic belief that he would end up friendless if he used his inhaler. Once Jake recognized the role that these thoughts had in his anxiety and poor adherence in public, the therapist helped Jake with a series of cognitive change strategies to challenge these beliefs. For instance, Jake was taught to look for evidence supporting or disconfirming his thoughts, trained to look for alternative interpretations of the situation, or assess the likelihood of the catastrophic outcomes. With practice, Jake began to realize and believe that his friends were actually very supportive (some friends would even prompt him to use his inhaler when he was playing), valued him more for his friendship than his sickness – in fact, they often overlooked his disease, and much preferred a "well" Jake who would play basketball than a "wheezing" Jake who would often prematurely end the basketball game.

The cognitive restructuring description above makes the process sound rather straightforward. The course of the therapy was actually more complex. Jake's appraisals of his friends' reactions were very resistant to change. It took a few sessions for Jake to collect the evidence to allow him to entertain the idea that his thinking might be negative and then successfully challenge these thoughts. In the meantime, in order to improve his adherence and maintain his health, a problem-solving strategy was implemented to help Jake consider alternative ways to use his inhaler before playing but to not do so in public. Oddly enough, Jake never considered other ways of maintaining his inhaler use; instead, he was just avoiding it altogether. Through problem-solving practice, the therapist and Jake considered alternative solutions and devised a series of plans to use his inhaler out of view of his friends (e.g., detouring to the bathroom before the start of the game, act like he is digging something out of his backpack). This exercise quickly improved his adherence in these situations until Jake was able to restructure his cognitions and decrease his anxiety about being more open with his inhaler use.

Based on our anecdotal experiences in our intervention research, we wanted to systematically examine the relationship between negative appraisals of friend reactions and adherence behavior (Hains, Berlin, Davies, Parton, & Alemzadeh, 2006; Hains et al., 2007). While this research was conducted on adolescents with diabetes, we suspect that similar relationships may exist in youths with other chronic conditions, including CF. In a series of studies, we found that adolescents with diabetes who make negative attributions about expected friend reactions to their diabetes-care efforts are more likely to anticipate adherence difficulties (Hains et al., 2006, 2007). A similar pattern of results is found when youths considered self-care behavior around peers other than friends in school settings (Hains et al., 2007). Furthermore, negative attributions of friend and other peer reactions and anticipated adherence difficulties have significant indirect effects on metabolic control through associations with stress (Hains et al., 2007). Friend support does not seem to have a large impact on the relationship between expected friend and peer sanctions for public self-care behavior and anticipated adherence difficulties (Hains et al., 2007). Thus, youths' problems with adherence may be related in part to their own inaccurate thoughts and beliefs.

The findings of this research indicate the importance of examining individual patient characteristics or situational contexts that might contribute to emotional distress and adherence problems. In the case of some adolescents, negative cognitive appraisals of situations in the form of anxiety over peer reactions may result in poor adherence. Cognitive behavioral interventions geared toward identifying, monitoring, and restructuring potentially distorted attributions (such as misattributions of others' reactions) may prove a valuable resource in working with adolescents with CF.

Interventions to improve adherence. Second, more focus should be directed toward developing and assessing adherence interventions. While the research showing the positive impact of exercise training illustrated the benefits of increasing this important self-care behavior, additional efforts at improving adherence to other behaviors is needed. As stated numerous times in this review, very few studies have been conducted to examine the effectiveness of adherence interventions (Quittner et al., 2000). Recently a large-scale randomized, controlled trial was undertaken by Quittner et al. (2000) to compare the effectiveness of the *Family Learning Program*, adapted from the *Cystic Fibrosis Education Program* (Bartholomew et al., 1997) described earlier, and *Behavioral Family Systems Therapy* (BFST; Robin & Foster, 1989) developed to address parent–adolescent conflict. BFST involves training all family members in the use of problem-solving and communication skills, employing cognitive restructuring to target parent-and/or youth-distorted cognitions about one another, and using functional and structural family therapy interventions to address dysfunctional family system interactions. Previously, BFST has been adapted for use with families who have an adolescent with diabetes (Wysocki et al., 2008) with promising outcomes. Families receiving the intervention were found to improve family communication and problem solving, and these improvements were associated with improvements in metabolic control (Wysocki et al., 2008).

At this point, the results of the Quittner et al (2000) randomized, controlled trial for CF families have not been published. In an earlier review, however, Drotar (2006) indicated preliminary results suggesting that families in the BFST group reported fewer CF-related problems, improved communication, and decreased family conflict. Recently, research has indicated that relationship quality among family members and not family problem-solving skills per se was predictive of adherence behavior (DeLambo, Ievers-Landis, Drotar, & Quittner, 2004). Consequently, interventions involving problem-solving training as a target skill to improve adherence should emphasize the quality of family relationships. Thus, positive family communication skills and more functional interpretations by individual family members regarding sources of family conflict (as opposed to individuals expressing distorted and negative attributions) should be given strong emphasis in therapy.

Summary

There is a pressing need for research on effective psychosocial interventions for adolescents with CF. As outlined above, there are a wide variety of presenting problems that affect teens with CF, and these challenges differ from those facing younger children with CF and their families. Taken together, the evidence suggests that the interventions that have been investigated have been shown to be effective. Yet the controlled interventions reviewed here reflect the participation of less than 100 adolescents with CF. With concerted effort of pediatric psychologists, CF center staffs, and federal and private funders, this could be the area where we comment on the most progress over the next 20 years.

References

Abman, S. H., Ogle, J. W., Harbeck, R. J., Butler-Simon, N., Hammond, K. B., Accurso, F. J. (1991). Early bacteriologic, immunologic, and clinical courses of young infants with cystic fibrosis identified by neonatal screening. *Journal of Pediatrics, 119*, 211–217.

Andersen, D. H. (1949). The present diagnosis and therapy of cystic fibrosis of the pancreas. *Proceedings of the Royal Society of Medicine, 42*, 25–32.

Andersen, D. H. (2008). Cystic fibrosis of the pancreas and its relation to celiac disease. *American Journal of Diseases of Children, 56*, 344.

Ballestero, Y., Hernandez, M. I., Rojo, P., Manzanares, J., Nebreda, V., Carbajosa, H., et al. (2006). Hyponatremic dehydration as a presentation of cystic fibrosis. *Pediatric Emergency Care, 22*, 725–727.

Bartholomew, L. K., Czyzewski, D. I., Parcel, G. S., Swank, P. R., Sockrider, M. M., & Mariiotto, M. J. (1997). Self-management of cystic fibrosis: Short-term outcomes of the Cystic Fibrosis Family Education Program. *Health Education & Behavior, 24*, 652–666.

Blair, C., Cull, A., & Freeman, C. P. (1994). Psychosocial functioning of young adults with cystic fibrosis and their families. *Thorax, 49*, 798–802.

Carew, L. D. (2001). The adolescent with cystic fibrosis: A psychosocial perspective. *South African Journal of Child and Adolescent Mental Health, 13*, 23–29.

Collins, F. S. (1992). Cystic fibrosis: molecular biology and therapeutic implications. *Science, 256*, 774–779.

Corbett, K., Kelleher, S., Rowland, M., Daly, L., Drumm, B., Canny, G., et al. (2004). Cystic fibrosis-associated liver disease: a population-based study. *Journal of Pediatrics, 145*, 327–332.

D'Auria, J. P., Christian, B. J., Henderson, Z. G., & Haynes, B. (2000). The company they keep: The influence of peer relationships on adjustment to cystic fibrosis during adolescence. *Journal of Pediatric Nursing, 15*, 175–182.

Davis, M. A., Quittner, A. L., Stack, C. M., Yang, M. C. (2004). Controlled evaluation of the STARBRIGHT CD-ROM program for children and adolescents with cystic fibrosis. *Journal of Pediatric Psychology, 29*, 259–267.

de Jong, W., Grevink, R. G., Roorda, R. J., Kaptein, A. A., & van der Schans, C. P. (1994). Effect of a home exercise training program in patients with cystic fibrosis. *Chest, 105*, 463–468.

DeLambo, K. E., Ievers-Landis, C. E., Drotar, D., & Quittner, A. L. (2004). Association of observed family relationship quality and problem-solving skills with treatment adherence in older children and adolescents with cystic fibrosis. *Journal of Pediatric Psychology, 29*, 343–353

DiGirolamo, A. M., Quittner, A. L., Ackerman, V., & Stevens, J. (1997). Identification and assessment of ongoing stressors in adolescents with a chronic illness: An application of the behavior-analytic model. *Journal of Clinical Child Psychology, 26*, 53–66.

Dik, H., Nicolai, J. J., Schipper, J., Heijerman, H.G., & Bakker, W. (1995). Erroneous diagnosis of distal intestinal obstruction syndrome in cystic fibrosis: Clinical impact of abdominal ultrasonography. *European Journal of Gastroenterology & Hepatology, 7*, 279–281.

Drotar, D. (2006). *Psychological interventions in childhood chronic illness*. Washington DC: American Psychological Association.

Feindler, E. L., Ecton, R. B., Kingsley, D., & Dubey, D. (1986). Group anger control training for institutionalized psychiatric male adolescents. *Behavior Therapy, 17*, 109–123.

Feranchak, A. P., Sontag, M. K., Wagener, J. S., Hammond, K. B., Accurso, F. J., & Sokol, R. J. (1999). Prospective, long-term study of fat-soluble vitamin status in children with cystic fibrosis identified by newborn screen. *Journal of Pediatrics, 135*, 601–610.

FitzSimmons, S. C. (1993). The changing epidemiology of cystic fibrosis. *Journal of Pediatrics, 122*, 1–9

Flume, P. A., O'Sullivan, B. P., Robinson, K. A., Goss, C. H., Mogayzel, P. J., Willey-Courand, D. B., et al. (2007). Cystic fibrosis pulmonary guidelines: chronic medications for maintenance of lung health. *American Journal of Respiratory & Critical Care Medicine, 176*, 957–969.

Foster, C., Eiser, C., Oades, P., Sheldon, C., Tripp, J., Goldman, P., et al. (2001). Treatment demands and differential treatment of patients with cystic fibrosis and their siblings: Patient, parent and sibling accounts. *Child: Care Health & Development, 27*, 349–364.

Glasscoe, C. A., & Quittner, A. L. (2003). Psychological interventions for cystic fibrosis. Cochrane Database of Systematic Reviews. Retrieved April 4, 2008, from http://web.ebscohost.com.

Gudas, L. J., Koocher, G. P., & Wypij, D. (1991). Perceptions of medical compliance in children and adolescents with cystic fibrosis. *Journal of Developmental & Behavioral Pediatrics, 12*, 236–242.

Gulmans, V.A. M., de Meer, K., Brackel, H. J. L., Faber, J. A. J., Berger, R., & Helders, P. J. M. (1999). Outpatient exercise training in children with cystic fibrosis: Physiological effects, perceived competence, and acceptability. *Pediatric Pulmonology, 28*, 39–46.

Hains, A. A., Berlin, K. S., Davies, W. H., Parton, E. A., & Alemzadeh, R. (2006). Attributions of adolescents with Type 1 diabetes in social situations: Relationship with expected adherence, diabetes stress, and metabolic control. *Diabetes Care, 29*, 818–822.

Hains, A. A., Berlin, K. S., Davies, W. H., Smothers, M. K., Sato, A. F., & Alemzadeh, R. (2007). Attributions of adolescents with Type 1 diabetes related to performing self-care around friends and peers: The moderating role of friend support. *Journal of Pediatric Psychology, 32*, 561–570.

Hains, A. A., Davies, W. H., Behrens, D., & Biller, J. A. (1997). Cognitive behavioral interventions for adolescents with cystic fibrosis. *Journal of Pediatric Psychology, 22*, 669–687.

Hains, A. A., Davies, W. H., Behrens, D., Freeman, M. E., & Biller, J. A. (2001). Effectiveness of a cognitive behavioral intervention for young adults with cystic fibrosis. *Journal of Clinical Psychology in Medical Settings, 8*, 325–336.

Hains, A. A., Davies, W. H., Parton, E., & Silverman, A. H. (2001). A cognitive behavioral intervention for distressed adolescents with Type 1 diabetes. *Journal of Pediatric Psychology, 26*, 61–66.

Johnson, K. B., Ravert, R. D., & Everton, A. (2001). Hopkins teen central: Assessment of an internet-based support system for children with cystic fibrosis. *Pediatrics, 107*, e24.

Kendall, P. C. (1994). Treating anxiety disorders in children: Results of a randomized clinical trial. *Journal of Consulting and Clinical Psychology, 62*, 100–110.

Kendall, P. C., Chansky, T. E., Kane, M. T., Kim, R. S., Kortlander, E., Ronan, K. R. et al. (1992). *Anxiety disorders in youth: Cognitive-behavioral interventions*. New York: Allyn & Bacon.

Kendall, P. C., Flannery-Schroeder, E., Panichelli-Mindel, S. M., Southam-Gerow, M., Henin, A., Warman, M. (1997). Therapy for youths with anxiety disorders: A second randomized clinical trial. *Journal of Consulting & Clinical Psychology, 65*, 366–380.

Kerem, B., Rommens, J. M., Buchanan, J. A., Markiewicz, D., Cox, T. K., Chakravarti, A., et al. (1989).

Identification of the cystic fibrosis gene: Genetic analysis. *Science, 245*, 1073–1080.

Konstan, M. W., & M. Berger. (1992). Infection and Inflammation of the lung in cystic fibrosis. In P. Davis (Ed.), *Cystic fibrosis: Lung biology in health and disease* (pp. 219–276). New York: Marcel Dekker.

Kopelman, H., Durie, P., Gaskin, K., Weizman, Z., & Forstner G. (1985). Pancreatic fluid secretion and protein hyperconcentration in cystic fibrosis. *New England Journal of Medicine, 312*, 329–334.

Kotloff, R. M., FitzSimmons, S. C., & Fiel, S. B. (1992). Fertility and pregnancy in patients with cystic fibrosis. *Clinics in Chest Medicine, 13*, 623–635.

La Greca, A. M., & Bearman, K. J. (2003). Adherence to pediatric treatment regimens. In M. C. Roberts (Ed.), *Handbook of pediatric psychology* (3rd ed., pp. 119–140). New York: Guilford Press.

Lanng, S., Hansen, A., Thorsteinsson, B., Nerup, J., & Koch, C. (1995). Glucose tolerance in patients with cystic fibrosis: Five year prospective study. *British Medical Journal, 311*, 655–659.

Lewinsohn, P. M., Clarke, G. N., Hops, H., & Andrews, J. (1990). Cognitive-behavioral treatment for depressed adolescents. *Behavior Therapy, 21*, 385–401.

Littlewood, J.M. (1992). Gastrointestinal complications in cystic fibrosis. *Journal of the Royal Society of Medicine, 85*(Suppl. 19), 13–19.

Main, E., Prasad, A., & Schans, C. (2005). Conventional chest physiotherapy compared to other airway clearance techniques for cystic fibrosis. *Cochrane Database of Systematic Reviews*, (1):CD002011

Modi, A. C., & Quittner, A. L. (2006). Barriers to treatment adherence for children with cystic fibrosis and asthma: What gets in the way? *Journal of Pediatric Psychology, 31*, 846–858.

Mullins, L. L., Pace, T. M., & Keller, J. (1994). Cystic fibrosis: Psychological issues. In R. A. Olson, L. L. Mullins, J. B. Gillman, & J. M. Chaney (Eds.), *The sourcebook of pediatric psychology* (pp. 204–217). Boston: Allyn & Bacon.

Passero, M. A., Remor, B., & Solomon, J. (1981). Patient reported compliance with cystic fibrosis therapy. *Clinical Pediatrics, 20*, 264–268.

Poustie, V. J., Russell, J. E., Watling, R. M., Ashby, D., & Smyth, R. L. (2006) Oral protein energy supplements for children with cystic fibrosis: CALICO multicentre randomised controlled trial. *British Medical Journal, 332*, 632–636.

Quinton, P. M. (1990). Cystic fibrosis: A disease in electrolyte transport. *The FASEB Journal, 4*, 2709–2717.

Quittner, A. L., Drotar, D., Ievers-Lands, C., Slocum, N., Seidner, D., & Jacobsen, J. (2000). Adherence to medical treatments in adolescents with cystic fibrosis: The development and evaluation of family based interventions. In D. Drotar (Ed.), *Promoting adherence to medical treatment in childhood chronic illness* (pp. 383–407). Mahwah, NJ: Lawrence Erlbaum Assoc.

Quittner, A. L., Tolbert, V., Regoli, M. J., Orenstein, D., Hollingsworth, J. L., & Eigen, H. (1996). Development of the Role-Play Inventory of Situations and Coping Strategies (RISCS) for parents of children with cystic fibrosis. *Journal of Pediatric Psychology, 21*, 209–235.

Ramsey, B. W. (1996). Management of pulmonary disease in patients with cystic fibrosis. *New England Journal of Medicine, 335*, 179–188.

Robin, A. L., & Foster, S. L. (1989). *Negotiating parent-adolescent conflict: A behavioral family systems approach.* New York: Guilford Press.

Rosenstein, B. J., & Cutting, G. R. (1998). The diagnosis of cystic fibrosis: A consensus statement. *Journal of Pediatrics, 132*, 589–595.

Selvadurai, H. C., Blimkie, C. J., Meyers, N., Mellis, C. M., Cooper, P. J., & Van Asperen, P. P. (2002). Randomized controlled study of in-hospital exercise training programs in children with cystic fibrosis. *Pediatric Pulmonology, 33*, 194–200.

Stark, L. J., Mackner, L. M., Patton, S. R., & Acton, J. D. (2003). Cystic fibrosis. In M. C. Roberts (Ed.), *Handbook of pediatric psychology* (3rd ed., pp. 286–303). New York: Guilford Press.

Stark, L. J., Opipari, L. C., Spieth, L. E., Jelalian, E., Quittner, A. Q., Higgins, L., et al. (2003). Contribution of behavior therapy to dietary treatment in cystic fibrosis: A randomized controlled study with a 2-year follow-up. *Behavior Therapy, 34*, 237–258.

Taussig, L. M., Lobeck, C. C., di Sant'Agnese, P. A., Ackerman, D. R., & Kattwinkel, J. (1972). Fertility in males with cystic fibrosis. *New England Journal of Medicine, 287*, 586–589.

Thomas, A. M., Peterson, L., & Goldstein, D. (1997). Problem solving and diabetes regimen adherence by children and adolescents with IDDM in social pressure situations: A reflection of normal development. *Journal of Pediatric Psychology, 22*, 541–561.

Thompson, R. J., Gustafson, K. E., George, L. K., & Spock, A. (1994). Change over a 12-month period in the psychological adjustment of children and adolescents with cystic fibrosis. *Journal of Pediatric Psychology, 19*, 189–203.

Thompson, R. J., Gustafson, K. E., Hamlett, K. W., & Spock, A. (1992). Psychological adjustment of children with cystic fibrosis: The role of child cognitive processes and maternal adjustment. *Journal of Pediatric Psychology*, 17, 741–755.

Wang, X., Moylan, B., Leopold, D. A., Kim, J., Rubenstein, R. C., Togias, A., et al. (2000). Mutation in the gene responsible for cystic fibrosis and predisposition to chronic rhinosinusitis in the general population. *Journal of the American Medical Association, 284*, 1814–1819.

Welsh, M. J., & Smith, A. E. (1995). Cystic fibrosis. *Scientific American, 273*, 52–59.

Welsh, M. J., Tsui, L. C., Boat, T. F., & Beaudet, A. L. (1995). Cystic fibrosis. In C. R. Scriver, A. L. Beaudet, W. S. Sly, & D. Valle (Eds.), *The metabolic and molecular basis of inherited disease* (7th ed., pp 3799–3876). New York: McGraw-Hill.

Wysocki, T., Harris, M. A., Buckloh, L. M., Mertlich, D., Lochrie, A. S., Taylor, A., et al. (2008). Randomized, controlled trial of behavioral family systems therapy for diabetes: Maintenance and generalization of effects on parent-adolescent communication. *Behavior Therapy, 39*, 33–46.

Zuelzer, W. W., & Newton, W. A. (1949). The pathogenesis of fibrocystic disease of the pancreas: A study of 36 cases with special reference to the pulmonary lesions. *Pediatrics, 4*, 53–69.

Chronic and End-Stage Renal Disease

Michelle A. Meade, Sarah Tornichio, and John D. Mahan

The kidneys perform four major functions: (1) elimination of waste products and toxins from the blood; (2) control of chemical and fluid balances within the body; (3) regulation of blood pressure; and (4) regulation of red blood cell production (Clearinghouse, 2008). Chronic damage to or reduced functioning of these organs, then, can affect every aspect of a child's life – growth and development, learning, appetite, energy, exercise capacity, muscle strength, psychological adaptability, and health. Unlike adults, who have completed their physiologic and cognitive development, children are in formative stages of development and therefore are particularly vulnerable to the adverse effects of Chronic Kidney Disease (CKD). With chronic kidney dysfunction, every cell in the body is ultimately affected – altered by the deranged internal milieu, toxin accumulation, and imbalances in fluid and blood pressure.

In the past, the term *chronic renal insufficiency* was used to describe patients with an impaired ability to filter toxins from the body, as measured by glomerular filtration rate (GFR). More recently, clinical practice guidelines developed by the National Kidney Foundation (NKF) Kidney Disease Outcomes Quality Initiative (K/DOQI) introduced the term *chronic kidney disease* (CKD) and a classification system to promote early disease detection, delay disease progression, and prevent related complications (National Kidney Foundation, 2002). This classification identifies five stages of CKD based on the presence of permanent kidney damage and the degree of functional impairment observed, irrespective of the underlying etiology (Table 1). In CKD stage 3, functional impairment results in a reduction of GFR by at least 50% and clinical complications become more prevalent. At CKD stage 5, kidney failure or *end-stage renal disease* (ESRD) is present and renal replacement therapy (dialysis or transplantation) is needed.

Table 1 NKF KDOQI classification of the stages of chronic kidney disease

Stage	GFR (mL/min/ 1.73 m^2)[a]	Description
1	≥90	Kidney damage and comorbid conditions
2	60–89	Kidney damage with mild reduction of GFR
3	30–59	Moderate reduction of GFR
4	15–29	Severe reduction of GFR
5	<15 (or dialysis)	Kidney failure

[a]GFR ranges apply to children aged 2 years and older.

Epidemiology

It is estimated that 26 million people in the United States have CKD and another 20 million are at increased risk of developing CKD in the future (The National Kidney Foundation of Ohio, 2008). The overall incidence of CKD is clearly increasing in the United States and children less than 20 years of age account for about 2% of the population of over 200,000 individuals with ESRD in the United States. The prevalence, or at least diagnosis, of children with

M.A. Meade (✉)
Rehabilitation Psychology and Neuropsychology, Department of Physical Medicine and Rehabilitation, University of Michigan, Ann Arbor, MI, USA
e-mail: mameade@unich.edu

W.T. O'Donohue, L.W. Tolle (eds.), *Behavioral Approaches to Chronic Disease in Adolescence*,
DOI 10.1007/978-0-387-87687-0_18,

CKD 5 appears to be increasing, as there was a 22% higher incidence in 2004 than in 1992 (USRDS, 2008).

The underlying causes for CKD are quite different in children compared to adults (NAPRTCS, 2008). Diabetic nephropathy and hypertension, which are the most common causes of CKD in adults, are uncommon in children. The leading causes of CKD in children are congenital and urologic anomalies, especially in the youngest age groups (Ardissino et al., 2004; NAPRTCS, 2008). As age increases, the proportion of children with congenital urologic abnormalities decreases and those with glomerular diseases increases (NAPRTCS, 2008). Of the 6,794 children of all ages registered in the North American Pediatric Renal Transplant Cooperative Study (NAPRTCS), males are affected more than females, accounting for 64% of the total population. Adolescents accounted for 31.9% of this total population and the racial distribution for adolescents included 58.8% Caucasians, 23.2% African-Americans, and 12.0% Hispanics.

The incidence and prevalence of CKD and particularly ESRD in children is affected by economic status, social factors, geography, and family and ethnic/racial background. Improved survival of low birth weight infants and older children with acute renal failure insults has increased the numbers of children with CKD in pediatric nephrology centers in developed countries. Since children may spend many years in CKD, and many children are not detected early in the course of CKD, the incidence and prevalence of CKD undoubtedly exceeds published figures. The best incidence data for CKD in children are derived from the report from northern Virginia that reported 20 new cases per million children per year (Chan, Mendez-Picon, & Landehr, 1981). In Central and Southeastern Ohio, where there is only one pediatric nephrology center for an estimated population of 500,000 children, the incidence of new patients detected with CKD averaged 36 per million children per year from 2001 to 2005 (Mahan & Smith, 2008).

In children with congenital disorders, CKD is often present early in life and profoundly affects growth and development throughout childhood and adolescence. These children tend to display more protean effects from CKD compared to children with glomerular causes of CKD, who often present with CKD later in childhood after many years of normal growth. Relative ages of onset of CKD in the NAPRTCS registry are 0–1 year of age – 20.1%; 2–5 years of age – 15.9%; 6–12 years of age – 32.1%; 13–17 years of age – 28.2%; over 17 years of age – 3.7% (NAPRTCS, 2008).

Prognosis

For many children and adolescents, CKD inevitably progresses to more severe renal impairment, particularly when complicating features like hypertension and recurrent infections occur. The value of interventions to control such complicating features is less well established in children than in adults. There is some evidence that sharp decline in renal functioning in children with CKD is associated with puberty and that approximately two-thirds of children with CKD require renal replacement therapy by the age of 20 years (Ardissino et al., 2004; Gonzalez Celedon, Bitsori, & Tullus, 2007). However, some children maintain relative stability in renal functioning even during puberty. The presence of proteinuria (abnormal levels of protein in the urine), hypertension, urinary tract infections, and lower GFR at onset were associated with deteriorating renal function over the 10 years of follow-up for affected children (Ardissino et al., 2004).

Complicating the specter of CKD for adolescents and their families is the altered chances for survival to adulthood. The mortality associated with ESRD in children who receive dialysis is estimated to be at least 30 times higher than that in the general pediatric population (USRDS, 2008). The mortality rate in adolescents with CKD pre-dialysis or transplantation was 2.4% over the 20 years of follow-up in the NAPRTCS registry which compares to the overall death rate of 3.8% for all ages (NAPRTCS, 2008).

Clinical Manifestations and Treatment Options

The variability of signs and symptoms of renal disease in children with CKD is primarily related to the etiology of the renal disorder, age and severity of involvement, and complications of appropriate therapies. Different children tolerate uremia (toxin buildup) and fluid excess differently and the complications tend to be more prominent with more severe GFR impairment over a longer duration. Other modifying factors include frequency (does the sign or symptom occur all day/every day?); severity (are daily activities altered? is the problem visible or associated with pain?); duration (is it likely to resolve? will it go away?); lethality (is it or can it be life threatening? if so, how and when?); and complications (number, significance, permanence). Table 2 provides a list of the most common clinical manifestations.

The type of treatment depends on the options to delay progression and the severity of disease manifestations. For individuals with mild to moderate kidney disease, management typically involves medication, dietary/nutritional management, and attention to physical activity. Children with CKD 5 need to have renal function replaced through either dialysis or transplantation, with transplantation being the most frequent treatment of choice (Furth, Gerson, Neu, & Fivush, 2001). Table 3 provides an overview of the treatment issues relevant to each stage of CKD.

Table 2 Clinical manifestations of CKD in children

Symptoms	Signs
Polyuria/polydipsia	Hypertension
Fatigue/muscle weakness	Poor growth
Delayed development	Delayed puberty
Poor psychosocial development	Seizures
Impaired learning	Metabolic acidosis
Bone pain/fractures	Renal osteodystrophy
Poor exercise ability	Anemia
Poor caloric intake	Delayed gastric emptying/gastritis
Decreased appetite	Edema
Decreased taste	Left ventricular hypertrophy/heart failure
	Arrhythmias
	Hyperlipidemia
	Increased infections
	Bruising/increased bleeding

Table 3 Overview of treatment modalities for adolescents with CKD

Disease severity	Type of treatment	Adherence required to	Frequency of medical attention	Cost/insurance coverage	Positives	Negatives
CKD 1 (minimal)	Typically none	Follow-up visits/monitoring	Every year	Parents' policy/Medicaid	Minimal needs	Specter of more renal disease in future
CKD 2 (mild)	Typically none, may need antihypertensive Rx	Follow-up visits/monitoring; medications	Two to three times a year	Parents' policy/Medicaid	Minimal needs	Some medications; specter of more renal disease in future
CKD 3 (moderate)	Medications; may need diet modifications	Follow-up visits/monitoring; medications; diet	Three to four times a year	Parents' policy/Medicaid	More visits and monitoring provide opportunities for education	More involved medications, disease concerns
CKD 4 (severe)	Medications; diet modifications; may need fluid restrictions	Follow-up visits/monitoring; medications; diet; fluids	Three to four times a year	Parents' policy/Medicaid	More visits and monitoring provide opportunities for education	More involved medications, disease concerns; concern about imminent dialysis
CKD 5 (ESRD)	Hemodialysis	Fluid restrictions; medications; diet restrictions	*Home dialysis* – 6–7 nights/week *In-center dialysis* – 3 times/week, each time lasting 3–4 hours	Parents' policy/Medicaid/Medicare coverage	Many visits and more intensive monitoring provide opportunities for education	Many medications, frequent disease concerns; concern about transplant options
CKD 5 (ESRD)	Peritoneal dialysis	Dietary restrictions; medications	Home peritoneal dialysis – 6–7 nights/week; ambulatory peritoneal dialysis – 4 exchanges/day	Parents' policy/Medicaid/Medicare coverage	Many visits and more intensive monitoring provide opportunities for education	Many medications, frequent disease concerns; concern about transplant options
	Renal transplant	Medications; monitoring BP/signs of infections/rejection	Regular lab work	Parents' policy/Medicaid/Medicare coverage; Medicare drops off after 3 years	Many visits and more intensive monitoring provide opportunities for education	Many medications, rejection concerns; medication complications

Nutritional Management: Evaluation and management of nutritional issues is an essential component of care for children with CKD. Dietary assessment will help direct dietary recommendations to achieve optimal calorie, protein, mineral, and vitamin intake. There is no evidence that extra calories are required for growth in CKD but adequate caloric intake may be difficult for children with CKD 3–5. For patients with polyuria or salt wasting, supplemental fluids and/or sodium is needed to achieve normal growth. Oliguric children (children with an abnormally small production of urine) often require fluid restrictions and moderation of salt intake to avoid fluid overload and hypertension. Although protein restriction has been shown to help delay progression of renal insufficiency in adults (Kasiske, Lakatua, Ma, & Louis, 1998), there is no evidence that protein restriction is of benefit in children with CKD (Wingen, Fabian-Back, Schaefer, & Mehls, 1997). For some children with CKD 4, poor nutrition may be adequately addressed only by initiation of dialysis with fluid removal to allow provision of more calories.

Medications: Medications may be useful to delay or prevent progression to renal insufficiency (ACE inhibitors or ARBs) or may be needed to control the manifestations of CKD (phosphate binders, vitamin D analogs, erythropoietin). Medication prescriptions are tailored to the adolescent's underlying needs – related to CKD stage but also very much related to particular disease characteristics (extra bicarbonate in tubular disorders with alkali wasting; more erythropoietin in tubular disorders). For some teens, the burden of many required medications may detract from the ability to eat and ingest adequate nutrition. The frustrations and impact of multiple medications taken at multiple times each day clearly play a part in the psychological stress of CKD. Table 4 presents the medications most frequently used by adolescents with CKD and their side effects.

Table 4 Medications most frequently used by children and adolescents with CKD

Categories of medications	Medication	Effects	Side effects
Stool softener	Docusate (Colace)	Prevents constipation	Loose, watery stools, extra gas, cramping
Loop diuretics	Furosemide (Lasix) Bumetanide (Bumex)	Rids body of excess fluids	Lowered potassium levels, dry mouth, weakness, excessive thirst
Antibiotics	Varying types	Destroys or inhibits growth of infectious organisms, such as bacteria	Vary
Nystatin	Nystatin (Mycostatin)	Prevents or treats yeast infections (thrush) in mouth	Nausea or vomiting, stomach ache, diarrhea
Antacids	Varying types	Decreases the amount of acid secreted by the stomach and relieves symptoms of pain or burning in stomach	Diarrhea
Alkali	Sodium bicarbonate	Buffers excess acid	Abdominal distension, bloating
Phosphate binders	Calcium carbonate Calcium acetate (PhosLo) Sevelamer carbonate (Renagel)	Buffers phosphate and promotes good bone health	Poor taste, abdominal distension
Vitamin D analogs	Calcitriol (Rocaltrol) Zemplar (paracalcitol)	Promotes good bone health	Hypertension, extraosseous calcifications, pruritis
Erythropoietin	Erythropoietin (Epogen) Darbepoietin (Darbo)	Corrects anemia of kidney disease	Hypertension
Calcium channel blockers	Isradipine (Dynacirc) Amlodipine (Norvasc) Nifedipine XL (Procardia XL)	Antihypertensive; improves BP by dilating blood vessels	Postural hypotension, swelling, headache, lightheadedness, fatigue, or lethargy
ACE inhibitors	Enalapril (Vasotec) Lisinopril (Prinivil) Benazepril (Lotensin)	Antihypertensive: improves BP by preventing blood vessels from narrowing	Angioedema, recurrent cough, fatigue or lethargy, hyperkalemia
ARB (angiotensin receptor blocker)	Valsartan (Diovan) Losartan (Cozaar)	Antihypertensives: improves BP by preventing blood vessels from narrowing	Fatigue or lethargy, hyperkalemia

Activity/Restrictions: Normal activities can often be maintained through the stages of CKD for many children. Exercise and physical activity should be encouraged and emphasized in the care of these adolescents. There is no evidence that physical exercise is deleterious to kidney function or outcome (Johansen, 2005). In terms of maintaining good muscle strength, normal body weight, and psychological health, regular physical activity should be stressed. With advanced CKD restrictions based on limited exercise endurance may need to be promoted – but it is important that affected teens continue to exercise up to their ability. For adolescents with dialysis catheters, specific restrictions in terms of contact sports or activities may be warranted.

Promoting Growth: Growth failure is a common and significant clinical problem in children and adolescents with CKD. Short teens with CKD exhibit a range of potentially serious medical and psychological complications as well as increased mortality (Furth et al., 2002; Postlethwaite, Eminson, Reynolds, Wood, & Hollis, 1998). The etiology of growth failure in this population is multifactorial, reflecting both abnormalities in the growth hormone (GH)–insulin-like growth factor (IGF)-I axis and a variety of nutritional and metabolic problems, each requiring specific management to improve growth potential. Recombinant human GH therapy is safe and effective in promoting growth in teens with CKD (Mahan, Warady, & The Consensus Committee, 2006). It is important that all modifiable factors to improve growth are addressed before GH therapy is initiated; in teens where growth potential may last for only a few more years, the timing and urgency to address these concerns is high. Final adult height is improved by GH treatment in teens and this fact should be understood by affected teens and families (Haffner et al., 2000).

ESRD/CKD 5 Therapies: Unlike the medical treatment available for failure of other solid organs, renal failure offers several treatment alternatives: (a) dialysis (peritoneal and hemodialysis) or (b) transplantation (either from a deceased or a living related donor). Many factors influence the choice of one therapy over another, including differential psychosocial and economic burdens for patients, their families, and society (Binik & Devins, 1986; Christensen & Ehlers, 2002; Goldstein et al., 2008). *Dialysis* is the process through which blood is artificially cleaned. Hemodialysis is the more common modality for adults, while peritoneal dialysis is the modality most commonly chosen for pediatric patients. Both types require continued medications, like regular doses of phosphate-binding medications and diets that limit phosphorus-rich food (National Kidney Foundation, 2005).

Hemodialysis involves circulating the blood through a machine (dialyzer) outside of the body where the blood is filtered and returned to the circulatory system. This process requires vascular access via a subcutaneous catheter or a created arteriovenous fistula or synthetic graft. For teens, hemodialysis typically requires three treatments a week, with each treatment lasting between 3–4 hours. Because of the time period between treatments, diet and fluid intake must be carefully monitored. In particular, prolonged fluid overload is associated with congestive heart failure, pulmonary edema, and shortened survival (Brunner et al., 1988; Parekh et al., 2002). Different levels of care are available to patients receiving hemodialysis. Full dialysis care is provided at hospitals or outpatient clinics for teens who require medical supervision or who are limited in their ability to care for themselves. Home hemodialysis is available for adolescents who have the support and resources to perform dialysis at home. These children and their caregivers (e.g., parents) must participate in an intensive training program. Self-care dialysis allows adolescents more flexibility with regard to the treatment schedule in a familiar atmosphere.

Peritoneal dialysis is the process by which blood is cleaned within the abdominal cavity or peritoneum of the child's own body rather than through an outside machine. In this process, dialysis fluid is introduced into the abdominal cavity by a peritoneal catheter and the peritoneum serves as a filter for the blood. Metabolic byproducts are filtered into the dialysate (through diffusion) and excess fluids are removed. In continuous ambulatory peritoneal dialysis (CAPD) the dialysate is exchanged every 4–6 hours in a process that takes up to 40 minutes (10–20 minutes to introduce and 10–20 minutes to drain the dialysate). The tube through which the dialysate is exchanged can be easily covered by clothing, and the exchange can be performed in private. While this option allows greater mobility for the adolescent and typically requires few dietary restrictions, infection from improper or unsanitary handling of the equipment is relatively common. Continuous cycling peritoneal dialysis (CCPD) is typically performed for 8–10 hours with four to six exchanges that occur while the child sleeps. It is similar to CAPD, except that exchanges are facilitated by an automatic cycling machine. This alternative reduces the likelihood of infection that occurs from improper handling of equipment (Will & Johnson, 1994) and requires less work for the child and parent, facilitating more normal activity during the day (Fine & Ho, 2002).

Renal transplantation is the second major treatment alternative for ESRD and the treatment of choice for most child and adolescent patients (NAPRTCS, 2008). Renal transplants are usually considered, however, only when the adolescent is medically stable. The renal allograft is taken from either a living donor (LD), usually a relative (LRD), or a deceased donor (DD) and typically placed beneath the lower abdominal muscles. Receiving a kidney from a relative is the best option, as it is usually a better match, results in longer graft survival, and may reduce the amount of immunosuppressive medication that is needed to prevent rejection of the organ for the rest of the recipient's life, or the life of the graft (Collaborative Transplant Study, 2006; Seikaly et al., 2001). The medications required to prevent rejection, however, may lead to secondary disorders such as diabetes and hypertension and other concerns (NAPRTCS, 2008). Renal transplantation is the treatment option that is thought to provide the best quality of life and the least interference with life functioning for individuals with kidney failure (Goldstein, Gerson, Goldman, & Furth, 2006). Compared with dialysis, management of and by the adolescent after the renal transplant involves less time and fewer intrusive procedures after the initial operations. This is not to imply that transplantation is a cure for ESRD; rather it is an ongoing treatment process.

Morbidity and mortality associated with renal transplants: Survival of renal allografts and survival of children and adolescents who undergo renal transplantation continue to improve. Data from North America for the last decade point to the high expectations that many patients and families should have for this treatment. The 1-year survival rates for renal allografts is 95.1% for living related donors (LD) and 93.4% for deceased donors; at 5 years, these numbers reduce to 85.2 and 76.9%, respectively. Patient survival was 98.3, 97.5, 95.7 and 93.6% for LD at 1, 2, 5, and 7 years post-transplant, respectively; for DD, the rates were 97.2, 96.2, 92.7, and 90.5%, respectively (NAPRTCS, 2008). Patient survival has improved over time but is still influenced by age at renal transplantation, with 3-year survival rates being lowest for individuals who receive their transplants before the age of 1 year. The reasons for patient death include infection (28.6% of deaths), cancer/malignancy (10.6%), cardiopulmonary (15.4%), and dialysis-related complications (3.0%), with 46.5% of children having died with a functioning graft (NAPRTCS, 2008).

The leading cause for improved transplant survival has been the development of new immunosuppressive medications. The introduction of cyclosporine (CSA) and tacrolimus (calcineurin inhibitors), in particular, has resulted in dramatic increases in allograft survival (Ettenger, Rosenthal, Marik, Grimm et al., 1991; Ettenger, Rosenthal,

Table 5 Most frequently used post-transplant immunosuppressive medications

Medication	Side effects
Prednisone (Deltasone)	Aseptic necrosis at hips and knees, GI bleeding, hyperlipidemia, diabetes mellitus, acne, stomach pain; vomiting; nausea; increased appetite, increased sweating, muscle weakness; joint pain, increased sensitivity to sun, slowed growth and sexual maturation, cataracts, pancreatic, hyperphagia/obesity, cushingoid faces, emotional lability
Cyclosporine (Neoral); **Tacrolimus** (Prograf)	Hypertrichosis, nephrotoxicity, hair growth on face and body, numbness or tingling of hands or feet, gingival hypertrophy, fever, chills, or sore throat, oily skin or acne, excess gum growth
Azathioprine (Imuran)	Decreased white blood cell count, fever, chills, sore throat, or infection, loss of appetite; nausea; vomiting, diarrhea, skin rash
Mycophenolate (Cellcept, Myfortic)	Abdominal pain, nausea, decreased appetite, bone marrow suppression
Rapamycin (Rapammune)	Bone marrow suppression, hyperlipidemia, skin rash

Marik, Malekzadeh et al., 1991; Knechtle et al., 1994; Tan, 1992). After receiving renal transplants, most patients receive triple immunosuppressive therapy; prednisone, tacrolimus and mycophenolate were used in 53% of children transplanted in 2003–2006 and induction therapy with cell-specific agents were used in 69.4% of the children. Increasingly, the trend is to use medications, such as tacrolimus, with lower disfiguring side effects (NAPRTCS, 2008); in particular, there is increasing attention to the use of steroid-sparing regimens. The side effects for the immunosuppressive medications are included in Table 5.

Common Issues Seen with Adolescents with Chronic Kidney Disease

Developmental and Cognitive Issues: Chronic kidney disease (CKD) can negatively impact academic achievement and school performance as well as intellectual and cognitive development (Fennell, Rasbury, Fennell, & Morris, 1984; Fox, McDowall, Neale, Morrison, & Hatfield, 1993; Gelb, Shapiro, Hill, & Thornton, 2008; Gerson et al., 2006; Gipson et al., 2006; Madero, Gul, & Sarnak, 2008; Rasbury, Fennell, & Morris, 1983; Slickers, Duquette, Hooper, & Gipson, 2007). The number of students with CKD receiving special education services, though, is approximately 10–15%, similar to national average. Declines in verbal IQ have been noted and language problems have been seen to result from poor renal functioning, as well as sensorineural hearing loss and medication toxicity (Warady, 2002), though increases in the rates of mental retardation have not been shown (Gerson et al., 2006). In general, adolescents with CKD show an IQ distribution that is shifted downward compared to that seen in normal adolescents (Lawry, Brouhard, & Cunningham, 1994). The cognitive delays appear to relate to the extent of renal dysfunction and the developmental stage in which it occurs (Bawden et al., 2004). Severe acute impairment of renal function can result in delirium, as can high-dose steroid toxicity. In addition, frequent school absences for medical appointments and hospitalizations may lower academic achievements (Gerson et al., 2006).

However, research comparing individuals with CKD with age-matched controls does suggest that there are specific areas that are affected by renal insufficiency, including attention, visual–spatial processing, memory, and initiation (Gerson et al., 2006; Gipson et al., 2006; Slickers et al., 2007). Attention problems can interfere with both the acquisition of new skills and the demonstration of previously acquired skills (Gerson et al., 2006). Visual–spatial problems can manifest as mild to moderate deficits in visual perception and visual–motor abilities (Gerson et al., 2006). Problems with both immediate and delayed memory can limit retention of information. These difficulties can lead to impaired academic performance and effect adherence to medical regimen. Renal transplantation, through the improvement in the filtration rate of the kidneys and thus better control of uremia, is thought to improve cognitive functions, such as attention and executive functions (Gerson et al., 2006).

Emotional Distress: Emotional distress can be thought of on a continuum from no concerns to mild adjustment difficulties to severe depression, anxiety, or behavioral problems. Many adolescents with CKD have good emotional health and normal peer relationships (Fadrowski et al., 2006; Gerson et al., 2004, 2005; Madden, Ledermann, Guerrero-Blanco, Bruce, & Trompeter, 2003). Adjustment problems, when they occur, appear related to age at transplant (with problems less likely to occur if transplant occurred before the age of 8 years), degree of functional impairment caused by illness, and general family functioning. Few reports document increased problems with behavior or substance abuse for this population, though depression and anxiety are significant concerns (Soliday, Kool, & Lande, 2000, 2001).

Major depression affects 5–50% of adults with ESRD (Binik, 1983; Devins et al., 1982; Tossani, Cassano, & Fava, 2005); adolescents appear to be equally affected although specific findings are less available. Adult ESRD patients have suicide rates up to 15 times higher than the general population (Welch, 1994; Will & Johnson, 1994); these figures include individuals who withdraw from dialysis (Neu & Kjellstrand, 1986). In adolescents with CKD, depression is most manifested as depressed affect, withdrawal from usual activities, social isolation, and negative cognitions. As fatigue associated with CKD can also result in withdrawal and nonparticipation in activities, it is important to explore the thoughts and reasons that underlie such phenomena as depressed affect and withdrawal from activities in a child with CKD (Tossani et al., 2005).

Fear of rejection of the transplant can also be a significant worry. Transplant recipients live with the knowledge that their graft may not be a permanent solution, i.e., that they may have to begin or return to dialysis (Will & Johnson, 1994). This may cause anxiety and worry on the part of patients and their parents (Schweitzer & Hobbs, 1995). Rejection or the threat of rejection can cause emotional stress and feelings of loss, including loss of desired form of treatment, loss of an object of attachment, and loss of a sense of control (Viswanathan, 1991). These losses, as well as uncertainty, may lead to profound sense of helplessness and depression.

Additional emotions that may be problematic involve feelings toward the transplanted organ (Schweitzer & Hobbs, 1995). Some adolescents have questions about how having another person's kidney in their body will affect them. They may wonder if they will begin to take on the characteristics of the donor, especially if the donor is of the opposite sex. If the patient has received the kidney from a cadaver, feelings of guilt may arise. If the kidney was from a living related donor, issues of worthiness for the sacrifice and responsibility toward that person may occur. These issues are further complicated if acute or chronic rejection of the graft occurs.

Of course, CKD does not just affect individuals but entire families. Research has shown that parents of children and adolescents with ESRD are at increased risk for emotional distress and depression. In particular, parents in lower SES households, those with large families, limited support, or young children are particularly likely to show poor adjustment (Fielding & Brownbridge, 1999). A systematic review of qualitative studies conducted with parents of children with CKD found that parental concerns could be grouped into three areas: intrapersonal issues, interpersonal issues, and external issues (Tong, Lowe, Sainsbury, & Craig, 2008). Intrapersonal concerns of parents included living with constant stress and uncertainty. Interpersonal concerns involved how relationships with their child, with the medical staff, and with peers were affected by the demands of disease management. Finally, external issues were generally associated with managing the practical details of medical regimen management as well as domestic responsibilities.

Adherence: When focusing on CKD, adherence to medical regimens is probably the psychosocial and behavioral issue that is most often discussed in the literature. In part, this reflects the significant potential for preventing disease advancement and minimizing symptoms when guidelines are well followed; at the same time, there is high morbidity and mortality when recommendations are not followed. For individuals on hemodialysis, the focus of adherence is primarily fluid and diet compliance. As seen in studies conducted with adults, few adolescent patients are totally noncompliant and do not show up for dialysis sessions. In particular, the stress and strain of adherence to multiple medications, many of which do not appear to the adolescent to have any obvious effects, and the burden of repeated medical visits and treatments are part of the issue with non-adherence to therapy.

For adolescents with a renal transplant, the focus is usually on adherence to immunosuppressive medications. Non-immunological risk factors account for more than one-third of graft losses in children, with non-adherence being especially significant for rejection in adolescent recipients (Gagnadoux, Niaudet, & Broyer, 1993) and ranging from 5 to 78% (Morgenstern et al., 1994). In fact, until proven otherwise, it is assumed that a late rejection episode is due to non-adherence (Ettenger, Rosenthal, Marik, Grimm et al., 1991; Ettenger, Rosenthal, Marik, Malekzadeh et al., 1991). The consequences of non-adherence include financial costs for rejection episodes, loss of the graft/transplanted organ, difficulties in acquisition of another transplant kidney, the costs and stress related to return to dialysis therapy, and possible death (Dunn et al., 1990; Gagnadoux et al., 1993; Rovelli et al., 1989).

Age, race/ethnicity, and gender have all been found to be related to non-adherence in transplant recipients. Younger recipients, especially adolescents, are generally found to be less compliant (Didlake, Dreyfus, Kerman, Van Buren, & Kahan, 1988). While some studies show no racial differences in adherence rates (Dunn et al., 1990),

African-Americans have been found less adherent with the therapeutic regimens in others (Didlake et al., 1988; Kiley, Lam, & Pollak, 1993), though investigators have been unable to separate the impact of socioeconomic status from that of race. The influence of gender on compliance is also unclear. Some studies report that males are more likely to be noncompliant (Dunn et al., 1990), while other investigations found higher noncompliance rates in females (Korsch, Fine, & Negrete, 1978).

Contrary to expectations, it has been found that neither a patient's knowledge about their disease (Masur, 1981) nor their educational level (Gagnadoux et al., 1993) is related to whether or not they will adhere to treatment (Korsch et al., 1978). However, specific factors of the medical condition and therapeutic regimen are associated with higher rates of noncompliance. Complexity of regimen appears to be a primary cause of non-adherence (Kiley et al., 1993), although it is unclear whether this results from confusion, misinformation, or other reasons. The medical factor most commonly associated with noncompliance is severity of side effects, particularly those that alter appearance (Schweitzer & Hobbs, 1995). No differences in compliance rates have been found between recipients of cadaver kidneys and those who received the organ from living donors (Schweizer et al., 1990). Frequency of transplant, or at least a history of significant non-adherence, however, may be a factor, with patients who have lost one kidney due to non-adherence being more likely to lose a second one (Fine, 1987; Fine, Salusky, & Ettenger, 1987). Non-adherence with dialysis and pre-transplant therapies also tends to predict poor compliance with medication regimen after the transplant (Schweitzer & Hobbs, 1995).

Finally, various psychosocial factors have been linked to higher rates of non-adherence. Adolescents experiencing significant anger or depressive symptoms are both thought to be more noncompliant with treatment regimen (Kiley et al., 1993). In addition, low self-esteem, cognitive impairment, poor social adjustment and social support, poor pre-morbid family equilibrium and communication, and locus of control attributed to powerful others have all been associated with increased non-adherence (Christensen & Ehlers, 2002; Fine et al., 2004; Kiley et al., 1993; Korsch et al., 1978).

Other Psychosocial Factors: Other psychosocial effects of CKD vary according to current age, age at onset, severity of condition, and effects and demands of the medical regimen. If the adolescent was first diagnosed and treated for CKD as a child, he or she may have carryover effects from disruptions in various developmental stages caused by frequent medical appointments, long-term hospitalizations, or reduced physical stamina. These children may not have had the opportunity to explore or gain mastery over their environment or acquire age-appropriate skills. They may also have limited social interactions and skills and have developed social systems composed of family and health care professionals rather than peers (Schweitzer & Hobbs, 1995). On the other hand, diagnosis of CKD in adolescence generally occurs when there is increased severity and disease progression that cause signs and symptoms that cannot be overlooked or ignored. In these cases, social development may be more normal, though academic achievement may have deteriorated for some time, potentially related to the cognitive dysfunction caused by undiagnosed chronic uremia.

Adolescents with CKD have been found, in some studies, to have smaller social networks than their age-matched peers and appear to have significantly fewer friends or acquaintances of the opposite sex. Instead, their support networks consist of family members and health care personnel. This lack of peer support may result in difficulty with parent–child individuation, the developmental stage appropriate for this time of life (Manificat et al., 2003). This stage/milestone may be delayed because of the dependence on family support and lack of interaction with and support from peers. Parents are likely to be concerned about their children's health and become overprotective, allowing little room for independence (Siegel, Mahan, & Johnson, 1994). Issues of privacy also become important to the adolescent who resents both the well-meaning parental supervision and the intrusiveness of medical professionals. Orders from physicians and parents become evidence of the lack of control that adolescents exert over his or her own life (Schweitzer & Hobbs, 1995).

While quality of life is generally improved after transplantation, the teenager inevitably must still deal with the residual physical and psychosocial effects of ESRD (Goldstein, Gerson et al., 2006).

In addition, the transplant and subsequent medical regimen introduces additional burdens. For example, while the retardation of growth caused by ESRD may lessen for some patients, growth may continue to be impeded by the effects of corticosteroid medications (Siegel et al., 1994).

Body Image: Dissatisfaction with physical appearance and issues of body image can also be an issue for adolescents with CKD, though possibly less of one now than in decades past (Melzer, Leadbeater, Reisman, Jaffe et al., 1989). Older immunosuppressive medications, particularly prednisone, can produce cosmetic disfigurements such as cushingoid features (particularly in adolescent females), obesity, and increased growth of hair on the face and body. These changes affect both psychological adjustment (Korsch et al., 1978) and compliance with medications (Schweitzer & Hobbs, 1995). Satisfaction with growth and height remains an issue, despite increased treatment with growth hormone (Rosenkranz et al., 2005). Poor body image may lead to or reflect low self-esteem, self-consciousness, and a sense of distinctiveness, anxiety, and unhappiness (Korsch et al., 1978; Rosenkranz et al., 2005). Distorted body image may cause difficulties in negotiating issues of sexuality and sexual relationships (Siegel et al., 1994).

Dating and Sex: Teenagers with chronic illnesses such as CKD, like most adolescents, are likely to have questions about sexuality and sexual functioning (Waite & Laraque, 2006) and be interested in dating and eventually marriage and having children. These concerns can sometimes be overlooked as teens with CKD may be developmentally more immature than their age-matched peers or have delayed growth or short stature that may cause them to look younger than their actual age.

What the research tells us is that individuals with CKD can have good sex lives. That is, while sexual desire and activity may be affected by fatigue and depression, both can increase to normal levels once these side effects or symptoms are addressed. Specifically, sexual desire and activity generally improve after transplantation for younger patients (Kinnaert, Vereerstaeten, & Toussaint, 1985). However, since it has been found that adolescents with transplants date less and are less likely to report having sexual relations (Melzer, Leadbeater, Reisman, & Jaffe, 1989; Schweitzer & Hobbs, 1995), specific attention to social skill development and promotion of peer interaction may be beneficial. In any discussion, however, it is important to emphasize safe sex practices (Hergenroeder & Brewer, 2001). Conception is feasible in adolescent females with CKD, with fertility returning as soon as 3 weeks post-transplant. Method of birth control should be discussed, as intrauterine devices are more likely to fail in patients taking immunosuppressive medications. Condoms should be used (when individuals with CKD who are not in a monogamous, committed relationship and know the health status of their partners engaging in sexual activity), as adolescents with CKD can have compromised immune systems which may make them more vulnerable to the effects of sexually transmitted diseases (Waite & Laraque, 2006).

Getting married and having children are also reasonable expectations that the adolescent with CKD can consider, especially those with renal transplantations and individuals who are able to maintain good management of their health. While marriage rates for adults who were diagnosed as having CKD as children may be lower than the general population, they have still been recorded at 50% in some studies though they have been as low as 15% in others (Kaplan-DeNour, 1994). Ideally, conception should be postponed for at least 1 year post-transplant, or longer if the allograft function is not stable or if rejection episodes have occurred in the past year. Pregnancies are often complicated by hypertension, preterm delivery, and low birth weight infants (Waite & Laraque, 2006).

Motivation, Planning for the Future, and Vocational Preparation/Employment: Developing goals and plans for the future must be addressed with adolescents with CKD. A significant percentage of teens – particularly those on dialysis or with poorly managed renal transplants – have difficulty seeing beyond the present and making plans for future jobs, careers, or other goals (Soliday et al., 2000). Despite this, vocational rehabilitation for ESRD patients ranges from fair to good, especially following renal transplantation (Broyer et al., 2004; Kinnaert et al., 1985; Rosenkranz et al., 2005). Reasons for unemployment included perception of disability (patients perceived themselves as "invalids"), classified as unable to work by Social Security, and the reluctance of employers to hire individuals requiring medical supervision.

Transition to Adult Renal Care: Individuals who get diagnosed with CKD and ESRD as children and adolescents and survive to grow into adulthood eventually have to transition to adult health care services. While this is a process and milestone that many adolescents with chronic health conditions traverse, the skills needed to be successful in an adult medical environment are especially critical for the adolescent with renal disease to master (Watson, 2005). Adolescents in the adult medical environment must be able to schedule appointments and arrive at them on time, take and refill medications, and find and work within an insurance system. While social workers are sometimes available within adult clinics, the level of psychosocial support and assistance provided by the adult nephrology team is greatly reduced (McDonagh & Viner, 2006; Viner, 2003, 2008). Transition can be a period of increased infections and graft loss as adolescents and young adults struggle to master the skills required for more self-care. It is clear that the timing of transfer to adult care needs to be individualized (Watson, 2005) and a process developed to ensure success in meeting the concerns and needs of the patient. In particular, some suggest that the transition wait until all objectives related to growth and development are achieved (McDonagh & Viner, 2006; Viner, 1999, 2000, 2001, 2008; Watson, 1996, 2005).

Cultural Issues: Relatively little is known about how race and ethnicity influence reactions to or outcomes of chronic kidney disease in adolescents. Some studies suggest that African-American adolescents are likely to be seen as less adherent by physicians and therefore less likely to be placed on transplantation lists (Furth et al., 2000; Furth, Hwang, Neu, Fivush, & Powe, 2003). For adults, additional research exists about the willingness to ask or likelihood of receiving kidneys for transplantation from living related donors Another study found ethnic and racial differences in the relationship between depression and coping strategies; that is, while avoidant coping style (which includes denial and behavioral and mental disengagement) was related to depression across adult kidney transplantation candidates, active and social support coping strategies were negatively related to depression only for non-Hispanic white candidates. Racial and ethnic differences in rates of depression, measured by cognitive symptoms, were not significant once the influence of education was controlled for, though physical symptoms of depression were higher among non-Hispanic black candidates. These results suggest ethnic/ racial variations in both coping strategies and depression in adults with ESRD, including possible variations in expression of depressive symptoms (Greco, Brickman, & Routh, 1996).

In any event, the realities of working with multiethnic populations are that the health care providers must attempt to tailor treatment and communication styles to those of the adolescent and their family (Washington, 1999). Family structure, expectations, and functioning may differ based on ethnicity, education, and religion. Within different family structures, individuals may be given different roles such that one individual within the family may act as spokesperson in interacting with health care providers while another acts as family medic, dispensing medications and insuring adherence (Washington, 1999). Health care providers should explore cultural identity, health beliefs, and treatment expectations at varying points during the medical relationship.

Role of the Behavioral Health Specialist

Behavioral health specialists are critically important to the management of ESRD and should play a prominent role for individuals with mild to moderate forms of CKD. Once a child, adolescent, and/or family begins to work with a pediatric nephrology team, they usually have more access to services to assist with addressing psychosocial and behavioral issues. In fact, Medicare regulations mandate that psychosocial issues are addressed and that all individuals with ESRD see a social worker (Furr, 1998). Social workers and pediatric specialty nurses are regular members of a pediatric nephrology team and the ones most frequently called upon to address psychosocial and behavioral issues. Social workers assist the patient and family with managing both financial and psychosocial issues by using solution-focused approaches to identify problems and then locate or rally internal or environmental resources to address the specific issues or concerns. Pediatric nurses have regular interactions with both the patient and the family and may assist with educating the child and family about treatment regimens and monitoring techniques.

Child development and educational specialists, psychologists, psychiatrists, and pediatric neuropsychologists are less frequent team members, but regular meetings and established consultation and liaison services with these specialists can benefit both patients and staff (North & Eminson, 1998). Neuropsychologists can identify learning disorders and cognitive difficulties. Child development and educational specialists can assist with education, facilitate academic advancement, and work with school systems to address concerns and facilitate scholastic achievement and vocational planning. Pediatric and child psychologists and psychiatrists can provide more formal assessment and therapy for adolescents with psychiatric diagnoses (i.e., depression, eating disorder, conduct disorder) and adjustment disorders as well as family therapy to address systemic issues. Their expertise has also been found useful in program development, guiding the management of specific situations and providing an objective and informed perspective on difficult cases, especially those in which significant adherence issues exist.

Best practices for assessment: There have not been any definitive texts or guidelines developed to suggest specific assessment measures or techniques for adolescents with CKD. Published research has used any number of measures to assess similar constructs. Recently, attempts are being made to standardize the approach to assessment of children and adolescents with CKD – primarily not only to allow for increased comparison within the research literature but also to provide norms and standards relevant to this population (Furth et al., 2006; Gerson et al., 2006). Table 6 provides an outline of the measures that are currently being advocated for, as well as those most prevalent in the literature. In addition, social workers on the pediatric nephrology team gather information about family structure, personal and financial resources, school performance, perception of illness by both the adolescent and the parent(s), and coping mechanisms used by both the

Table 6 Psychosocial and cognitive assessments

Measure	Age range	Domains/Functions
*Behavioral Assessment System for Children – 2nd edition (BASC-2) – parental rating scales	**2–18**	Behavior, conduct, development
*BASC-2 – Self-report of personality	**8–18**	Personality, coping
*Child depression inventory	**7–18**	Overall depression and related symptoms
State Trait Anxiety Inventory for Children (STAIC)		Anxiety
*Pediatric quality of life – parent	**2–18**	Assesses five domains of health – physical, emotional, psychosocial, social, and school functioning
*Pediatric quality of life – child	**8–18**	Overall QOL
2005 Youth risk behavior survey	**12–18**	Physical activity, smoking, alcohol and drug use
Kidney Disease Quality of Life (KDQOL) scale		Quality of life
*Adaptive Behavior Assessment System – 2nd edition (ABAS-II) – Parent Form	**1–18**	Overall adaptive behavior and functioning in specific areas such as communication and community use
*Wechsler abbreviated scales of intelligence	**6–18**	Verbal, nonverbal, overall IQ
*Behavioral Rating Inventory for Executive Functions (BRIEF) – parent	**6–18**	Parent report of executive functions such as inhibition, shift of set, emotional control, initiation, working memory, planning, organization, and monitoring
*Connors continuous performance Test-II	**6–18**	Selective attention, sustained attention, impulsivity, and reaction time
*Wechsler individual achievement Test-II abbreviated	**6–18**	Reading recognition, spelling, and arithmetic skills

* Measure is included in the CKiD battery (Furth et al., 2006; Gerson et al., 2006).

adolescent and the parent(s). In cases where medical neglect is suspected, social workers may be called upon to contact Child Protective Services.

Best practices for treatment: Just as there are few established guidelines for assessment of adolescents with CKD, so little evidence is available for behavioral and psychosocial interventions with this population. The research literature is devoid of large-scale interventions and the few studies that do exist with adolescents use descriptive and quasi-experimental designs to document interventions that address adherence among dialysis patients and renal transplant recipients. In general, these interventions use a combination of education, skill building, behavioral cues, and either peer modeling or social support to produce improvements related to knowledge, adherence, and emotional distress (Beck et al., 1980; Fennell, Foulkes, & Boggs, 1994; Meade, 1999; Meade, Creer, & Mahan, 2003). The evidence-based practices described below, then, rely heavily on existing clinical practice and the translation of approaches found beneficial in working with adolescents with other types of chronic disease.

Best practices for treatment of the adolescent with CKD involve the behavioral health specialist working as part of an inter-disciplinary or multi-disciplinary team (Rianthavorn, Ettenger, Malekzadeh, Marik, & Struber, 2004). Within this context, they have an opportunity to gather information from multiple sources about the severity and prognosis of the CKD, expectations for various treatment decisions, and extent of and burden associated with adherence to medical recommendations, as well as the concerns of the team related to family dynamics, mood, behavioral problems, or adherence issues. The role of the behavioral health specialist is to take these data, as well as information gathered directly from the adolescent and/or family, and work to find solutions that respect the culture and decisions of the individual while optimizing health and quality of life. Sometimes these interventions will occur directly with individual adolescents and families and sometimes with groups of patients. At other times, the target of the intervention is to change the structure in which service is provided or the interactions among team members or between team members and families (North & Eminson, 1998).

In general, it appears important that members of the pediatric nephrology team develop relationships with both the adolescent and their family (Christensen, Raichle, Ehlers, & Bertolatus, 2002; Christensen, Wiebe, Smith, & Turner, 1994; DiMatteo, 2003, 2004; Soliday et al., 2001; Watson, 1997). Adolescents should be seen individually in order to build rapport and conduct more accurate assessments (Rianthavorn et al., 2004). This may be especially true when trying to get information about issues such as adherence, sexual history, and drug and alcohol use (Hergenroeder & Brewer, 2001). Non-judgmental attitudes and assurances of confidentiality on the part of the provider make it much more likely that the patient will be honest in answering questions and raising concerns. Individual discussions also appear to promote a sense of respect and responsibility between the adolescent and the team, which may promote adherence (Rianthavorn et al., 2004; Rianthavorn & Ettenger, 2005).

Teaching and education need to occur with both the adolescent and the family. Adolescents and family members should learn about medications, dietary requirements and restrictions, and activity and behavioral limitations. In addition, parents and older adolescents need to learn about insurance and what resources may be available to them (UNC Kidney Center, 2008). Because of previously mentioned cognitive deficits, the complexity of many adherence regimens, and the stress associated with living with a chronic illness, information should be provided multiple times in multiple formats. When appropriate, evaluations of knowledge should be conducted. While education itself may not have been proven to be a sufficient condition for compliance, it is most likely a necessary condition (Blowey et al., 1997). Knowledge of the disease, in combination with coping and problem solving capabilities, promotes self-efficacy in the self-management of the illness (Creer & Holroyd, 1997).

Assisting the adolescent in developing social supports and networks may also be an important function of behavioral health specialists working with the CKD population (Melzer, Leadbeater, Reisman, Jaffe et al., 1989). Group therapy and peer support can improve social skills, social networks, and self-esteem among teenagers with chronic kidney disease (Furr, 1998; LePontois, Moel, & Cohn, 1987; Walker, 1985). The former, in particular, appear most successful when arranged in conjunction with preexisting dialysis session.

Summer camps can also provide a good opportunity to increase social networks, gain independence, and interact with the pediatric nephrology team in a more casual setting (Leumann, Mueller, & Leumann, 1989). Adolescents should be encouraged to get involved in activities with peers (Melzer, Leadbeater, Reisman, Jaffe et al., 1989); this may require specific guidance by the nephrology team about the types of activities that may be appropriate as well as reassurance to the parent that those activities will not increase the risk to their child. Having the nephrologists and other team members ask about follow-through with and frequency of such activities will provide validity and support for the recommendation.

Behavioral contingencies and reward-based systems are frequently used by pediatric nephrology teams. Rewards can be used to shape specific behaviors, such as medication adherence, improvements in knowledge about medication, or communication with the pediatric nephrology team. In particular, adolescents on hemodialysis may receive rewards for meeting goals with regard to fluid restrictions and phosphate control. Positive reinforcement of prescribed behavior should also be a priority for all members of the team.

Of course, parents and families should not be left out of interactions with team nor should the responsibility for disease management rest solely on the adolescent. It will be important to ensure that the adolescent has a facilitating environment in which to attempt to develop independence and try new skills. Specifically, parents should be encouraged to allow their child to participate in age-appropriate activities that are not restricted due to medical reasons (Furr, 1998). Parents will also need to ensure that the practical details related to medical adherence are addressed – that their child has transportation to clinic and laboratory visits and medical appointments (Tong et al., 2008). Finally, the stressors put on the family structure need to be assessed and addressed. The behavioral health provider or pediatric nephrology team will need to address psychosocial issues within the family itself which may affect the quality of life of the adolescent. Social workers and psychologists can help strengthen family systems (Furr, 1998), which can become strained due to the emotional, physical, and financial burdens associated with dealing with chronic diseases, and work to decrease conflict and improve communication and emotional expression among family members (Soliday et al., 2000).

Methodological Considerations if Conducting Research with This Population

Among the most challenging methodological considerations in conducting research with adolescents with CKD is that of limiting the sample characteristics while maximizing sample size. Existing studies usually include wide age ranges, variable functional levels, and treatment approaches, as well as varying cognitive capacity and social economic status. Any one center may be limited in the number of potential participants it has available with a particular diagnosis or in a certain age range; for this reason, studies cannot control for significant covariates. For this reason, multicenter studies are becoming the gold standard for research with adolescents with CKD (Furth et al., 2006).

The measurement of all constructs, but particularly adherence, is of significant concern. As previously noted, great discrepancies exist with regard to rates of adherence, with rates ranging from 5 to 78% for pediatric patients with renal transplants. Part of the discrepancy results from the varying ways that noncompliance is assessed. In the studies reporting low rates, adherence is typically determined by unexplained declines in renal functioning, rejection episodes, or graft losses (Didlake et al., 1988; Gagnadoux et al., 1993; Korsch et al., 1978; Morgenstern et al., 1994; Rovelli et al., 1989). Those studies that report higher rates of noncompliance are more likely to use self-report, relatives' reports, or pill counts (Didlake et al., 1988; Rovelli et al., 1989; Schweizer et al., 1990). Determining adherence by cyclosporine trough level in the blood typically results in documenting moderate rates of noncompliance (Kiley et al., 1993; Rovelli et al., 1989). Additional assessment measure may include semi-structured interviews (Zelikovsky & Schast, 2008) or compliance with laboratory appointments or clinic visits. It is recommended that both objective measures readily available in the medical record (such as adherence to appointments and medication trough levels) and self-reports be used.

Finally, the provision of psychosocial and behavioral interventions with this population can be a challenge. Specialized pediatric nephrology programs often provide oversight and services to a large geographic area. Group interventions that require travel become problematic. Sessions must be limited in number to reduce burden on adolescent and family, limited in duration to correspond with attention spans of the target population, and scheduled so as to provide minimal interference with already stressed work and school schedules (Meade et al., 2003). When available, though, they can create powerful support networks for both the adolescent and their families. Increasingly web-based intervention may be used to fulfill the same role – however, in-person interactions between clients are still recommended to facilitate actual (rather than virtual) social networks.

Research Agenda

The next 10 years should bring about significant advances in knowledge about adolescents with chronic kidney disease. Several large-scale, multicenter studies have now been funded which promise improved assessment of physiological, cognitive, and psychosocial issues among adolescents (Furth et al., 2006; Goldstein, Graham et al., 2006). In addition, several psychosocial interventions are now being funded by the National Institutes of Health, the Agency for Health Care Research and Quality, and private foundations that have the goal of improving health and quality of life in children with chronic conditions (ClinicalTrials.gov, 2008).

The Chronic Kidney Disease in Children Study, or CKiD, is a prospective cohort study funded by the National Institutes of Health to identify risk factors for the progression of CKD and the evolution of cardiovascular disease and to characterize the impact of declining kidney function on growth, neurodevelopment, cognitive abilities, and behavior (Furth et al., 2006). The CKiD consists of 57 clinical sites and 2 clinical coordinating centers as well as several central laboratories and repositories. Five hundred and forty one children aged 1 to 16 years have been enrolled for a 24-month period and participate in six follow-up assessments of general health, kidney and cardiovascular functioning, neurocognitive status, growth and nutrition, and inflammation and bone health. A subset of 30 participants who are seen as "high risk" for developing neurocognitive difficulties based on age and GFR will undergo more extensive testing. This study is likely to provide a wealth of information about CKD in adolescents, especially in milder forms of CKD.

Additionally, attempts are being made to standardize and evaluate psychosocial programs for adolescents with CKD. For example, Dr. Maria Ferris at the University of North Carolina-Chapel Hill is now leading a team to implement and evaluate a program to facilitate transition to adult care, including creating measures to evaluate transition skills, developing educational material, and conducting standardized assessments of participants at various sites (UNC Kidney Center, 2008). Many more behavioral and psychosocial interventions exist, though, that need to be evaluated in large-scale randomized clinical trials.

Finally, electronic, Internet, and web-based interventions are likely to become increasingly prevalent. The Agency for Healthcare Research and Quality (AHRQ) is currently funding investigators at Yale New Haven Hospital to evaluate the effectiveness of web-based education programs to improve knowledge about medications and prevent medication errors in adults with renal transplantations (ClinicalTrials.gov, 2008). Such interventions may be readily translated to an adolescent population who may be more comfortable with technology. In addition, health games, educational blogs, and web-based support forums may be strategies especially well suited to the adolescent population.

Acknowledgement With thanks to Dr. Thomas Geer, for all his encouragement and support.

References

Ardissino, G., Testa, S., Dacco, V., Vigano, S., Taioli, E., Claris-Appiani, A., et al. (2004). Proteinuria as a predictor of disease progression in children with hypodysplastic nephropathy. Data from the Ital Kid Project. *Pediatric Nephrology, 19*(2), 172–177.

Bawden, H. N., Acott, P., Carter, J., Lirenman, D., MacDonald, G. W., McAllister, M., et al. (2004). Neuropsychological functioning in end-stage renal disease. *Archives of Disease in Childhood, 89*(7), 644–647.

Beck, D. E., Fennell, R. S., Yost, R. L., Robinson, J. D., Geary, D., & Richards, G. A. (1980). Evaluation of an

educational program on compliance with medication regimens in pediatric patients with renal transplants. *Journal of Pediatrics, 96*(6), 1094–1097.
Binik, Y. (1983). Coping with chronic life-threatening illnesses: Psychosocial perspectives on end stage renal disease. *Canadian Journal of Behavioral Science, 15*(4), 373–391.
Binik, Y., & Devins, G. (1986). Transplant failure does not compromise quality of life in end-stage renal disease. *International Journal of Psychiatry in Medicine, 16*(3), 281–292.
Blowey, D. L., Hebert, D., Arbus, G. S., Pool, R., Korus, M., & Koren, G. (1997). Compliance with cyclosporine in adolescent renal transplant recipients. *Pediatric Nephrology, 11*(5), 547–551.
Broyer, M., Le Bihan, C., Charbit, M., Guest, G., Tete, M. J., Gagnadoux, M. F., et al. (2004). Long-term social outcome of children after kidney transplantation. *Transplantation, 77*(7), 1033–1037.
Brunner, F., Fassbinder, W., Broyer, M., Oules, R., Brynger, H., Rizzoni, G., et al. (1988). Survival on renal replacement therapy: Data from the EDTA Registry. *Nephrology Dialysis Transplantation, 3*(2), 109–122.
Chan, J., Mendez-Picon, G. J., & Landehr, D. (1981). A 3-year survey of referral pattern and ease material in pediatric nephrology. *International Journal of Pediatric Nephrology, 2*(2), 109–113.
Christensen, A., & Ehlers, S. (2002). Psychological factors in end-stage renal disease: An emerging context for behavioral medicine research. *Journal of Consulting and Clinical Psychology, 70*(3), 712–724.
Christensen, A. J., Raichle, K., Ehlers, S. L., & Bertolatus, A. J. (2002). Effect of family environment and donor source on patient quality of life following renal transplantation. *Health Psychology, 21*(5), 468–476.
Christensen, A. J., Wiebe, J. S., Smith, T. W., & Turner, C. W. (1994). Predictors of survival among hemodialysis patients: effect of perceived family support. *Health Psychology, 13*(6), 521–525.
Clearinghouse, T. N. K. U. D. I. (2008). The National Kidney and Urological Diseases Information Clearinghouse. Retrieved 6/27/2008, 2008, from http://kidney.niddk.nih.gov/Kudiseases/pubs/kdd/index.htm
ClinicalTrials.gov. (2008). ClinicalTrials.gov. Retrieved May 9, 2008, from http://clinicaltrials.gov
Collaborative Transplant Study, (2006).
Creer, T., & Holroyd, K. (1997). Self-management. In A. Baum, S. Newman, J. Weinman, & R. West (Eds.), *Cambridge handbook of psychology, health and medicine*. Cambridge: University Press.
Devins, G. M., Binik, Y. M., Gorman, P., Dattel, M., McCloskey, B., Oscar, G., et al. (1982). Perceived self-efficacy, outcome expectancies, and negative mood states in end-stage renal disease. *Journal of Abnormal Psychology, 91*(4), 241–244.
Didlake, R. H., Dreyfus, K., Kerman, R. H., Van Buren, C. T., & Kahan, B. D. (1988). Patient noncompliance: a major cause of late graft failure in cyclosporine-treated renal transplants. *Transplantation Proceedings, 20*(3 Suppl. 3), 63–69.
DiMatteo, M. R. (2003). Future directions in research on consumer-provider communication and adherence to cancer prevention and treatment. *Patient Education & Counseling, 50*(1), 23–26.
DiMatteo, M. R. (2004). Social support and patient adherence to medical treatment: a meta-analysis. *Health Psychology, 23*(2), 207–218.
Dunn, J., Golden, D., Van Buren, C. T., Lewis, R. M., Lawen, J., & Kahan, B. D. (1990). Causes of graft loss beyond two years in the cyclosporine era. *Transplantation, 49*(2), 349–353.
Ettenger, R. B., Rosenthal, J. T., Marik, J., Grimm, P. C., Nelson, P., Malekzadeh, M. H., et al. (1991). Long-term results with cyclosporine immune suppression in pediatric cadaver renal transplantation. *Transplantation Proceedings, 23*(1 Pt 2), 1011–1012.
Ettenger, R. B., Rosenthal, J. T., Marik, J. L., Malekzadeh, M., Forsythe, S. B., Kamil, E. S., et al. (1991). Improved cadaveric renal transplant outcome in children. *Pediatric Nephrology, 5*(1), 137–142.
Fadrowski, J., Cole, S. R., Hwang, W., Fiorenza, J., Weiss, R. A., Gerson, A., et al. (2006). Changes in physical and psychosocial functioning among adolescents with chronic kidney disease. *Pediatric Nephrology, 21*(3), 394–399.
Fennell, R. S., Foulkes, L. M., & Boggs, S. R. (1994). Family-based program to promote medication compliance in renal transplant children. *Transplantation Proceedings, 26*(1), 102–103.
Fennell, R. S., 3rd, Rasbury, W. C., Fennell, E. B., & Morris, M. K. (1984). Effects of kidney transplantation on cognitive performance in a pediatric population. *Pediatrics, 74*(2), 273–278.
Fielding, D., & Brownbridge, G. (1999). Factors related to psychosocial adjustment in children with end-stage renal failure. *Pediatric Nephrology, 13*(9), 766–770.
Fine, R. N. (1987). Choosing a treatment modality for the infant, child and adolescent with endstage renal disease. *Blood Purification, 5*(1), 4–13.
Fine, R., Alonso, E., Fischel, J., Bucuvalas, J., Enos, R., & Gore-Langton, R. (2004). Pediatric transplantation of the kidney, liver and heart: Summary Report. *Pediatric Transplantation, 8*, 75–86.
Fine, R., & Ho, M. (2002). North American Transplant Cooperative Study. The role of APD in the management of pediatric patients: a report of the North American Pediatric Renal Transplant Cooperative Study. *Semin Dial, 15*(6), 427–429.
Fine, R. N., Salusky, I. B., & Ettenger, R. B. (1987). The therapeutic approach to the infant, child, and adolescent with end-stage renal disease. *Pediatric Clinics of North America, 34*(3), 789–801.
Fox, E., McDowall, J., Neale, T. J., Morrison, R. B., & Hatfield, P. J. (1993). Cognitive function and quality of life in end-stage renal failure. *Renal Failure, 15*(2), 211–214.
Furr, L. A. (1998). Psycho-social aspects of serious renal disease and dialysis: A review of the literature. *Social Work in Health Care, 27*(3), 97–118.
Furth, S., Cole, S., Moxey-Mims, M., Kaskel, F., Mak, R., Schwartz, G., et al. (2006). Design and methods of the Chronic Kidney Disease in Children (CKiD) prospective cohort study. *Clinical Journal of The American Society of Nephrology: CJASN, 1*(5), 1006–1015.
Furth, S., Garg, P., Neu, A., Hwang, W., Fivush, B., & Powe, N. (2000). Racial differences in access to the kidney

transplant waiting list for children and adolescents with end-stage renal disease. *Pediatrics, 106*(4), 756–761.
Furth, S., Gerson, A., Neu, A., & Fivush, B. (2001). The impact of dialysis and transplantation on children. *Advances in Renal Replacement Therapy, 8*(3), 206–213.
Furth, S. L., Hwang, W., Neu, A. M., Fivush, B. A., & Powe, N. R. (2003). Effects of patient compliance, parental education and race on nephrologists' recommendations for kidney transplantation in children. *American Journal of Transplantation, 3*(1), 28–34.
Furth, S., Hwang, W., Yang, C., Neu, A., Fivush, B., & Powe, N. (2002). Growth failure, risk of hospitalization and death for children with end-stage renal disease. *Pediatric Nephrology, 27*(6), 450–455.
Gagnadoux, M. F., Niaudet, P., & Broyer, M. (1993). Non-immunological risk factors in paediatric renal transplantation. *Pediatric Nephrology, 7*(1), 89–95.
Gelb, S., Shapiro, R. J., Hill, A., & Thornton, W. L. (2008). Cognitive outcome following kidney transplantation. *Nephrology Dialysis Transplantation, 23*(3), 1032–1038.
Gerson, A., Butler, R., Moxey-Mims, M., Wentz, A., Shinnar, S., Lande, M., et al. (2006). Neurocognitive outcomes in children with chronic kidney disease: Current findings and contemporary endeavors. *Mental Retardation and Developmental Disabilities Research Reviews, 12*(3), 208–215.
Gerson, A., Hwang, W., Fiorenza, J., Barth, K., Kaskel, F., Weiss, L., et al. (2004). Anemia and health-related quality of life in adolescents with chronic kidney disease. *American Journal of Kidney Diseases, 44*(6), 1017–1023.
Gerson, A. C., Riley, A., Fivush, B. A., Pham, N., Fiorenza, J., Robertson, J., et al. (2005). Assessing health status and health care utilization in adolescents with chronic kidney disease. *Journal of the American Society of Nephrology, 16*(5), 1427–1432.
Gipson, D. S., Hooper, S. R., Duquette, P. J., Wetherington, C. E., Stellwagen, K. K., Jenkins, T. L., et al. (2006). Memory and executive functions in pediatric chronic kidney disease. *Child Neuropsychology, 12*(6), 391–405.
Goldstein, S., Gerson, A., Goldman, C. W., & Furth, S. (2006). Quality of life for children with chronic kidney disease. *Seminars in Nephrology, 26*(2), 114–117.
Goldstein, S., Graham, N., Burwinkle, T., Warady, B., Farrah, R., & Varni, J. (2006). Health related quality of life in pediatric patients with ESRD. *Pediatric Nephrology, 21*(6), 846–850.
Goldstein, S., Graham, N., Warady, B., Seikaly, M., McDonald, R., Burwinkle, T., et al. (2008). Measuring health-related quality of life in children with ESRD: performance of the generic and ESRD-specific instrument of the Pediatric Quality of Life Inventory (PedsQL). *American Journal of Kidney Diseases, 51*(2), 285–297.
Gonzalez Celedon, C., Bitsori, M., & Tullus, K. (2007). Progression of chronic renal failure in children with dysplastic kidneys. *Pediatric Nephrology, 22*(7), 1014–1020.
Greco, P., Brickman, A. L., & Routh, D. K. (1996). Depression and coping in candidates for kidney transplantation: Racial and ethnic differences. *Journal of Clinical Psychology in Medical Settings, 3*(4), 337–353.
Haffner, D., Schaefer, F., Nissel, R., Wuhl, E., Tonshoff, B., & Mehls, O. (2000). Effect of growth hormone treatment on the adult height of children with chronic renal failure. German Study Group for Growth Hormone Treatment in Chronic Renal Failure. *New England Journal of Medicine, 343*(13), 923–930.
Hergenroeder, A. C., & Brewer, E. (2001). A survey of pediatric nephrologists on adolescent sexual health. *Pediatric Nephrology, 16*, 57–60.
Johansen, K. L. (2005). Exercise and chronic kidney disease: Current Recommendations. Review Article. *Sports Medicine, 35*(6), 485–499.
Kaplan-DeNour, A. (1994). Psychological, social and vocational impact of renal failure: A review. In H. M. C. Bradley (Ed.), *Quality of Life Following Renal Failure* (pp. 33–42). Switzerland: Harwood Academic Publishers.
Kasiske, B., Lakatua, J., Ma, J., & Louis, T. (1998). A meta-analysis of the effects of dietary protein restriction on the rate of decline in renal function. *American Journal of Kidney Diseases, 31*(6), 954–961.
Kiley, D. J., Lam, C. S., & Pollak, R. (1993). A study of treatment compliance following kidney transplantation. *Transplantation, 55*(1), 51–56.
Kinnaert, P., Vereerstaeten, P., & Toussaint, C. (1985). Vocational rehabilitation and sexual behavior after renal transplantation. *Transplantation, 55*(1), 51–56.
Knechtle, S. J., D'Alessandro, A. M., Sollinger, H. W., Pirsch, J. D., Friedman, A. L., Chobanian, M. C., et al. (1994). Changing spectrum of pediatric renal transplantation. *Transplantation Proceedings, 26*(1), 23.
Korsch, B. M., Fine, R. N., & Negrete, V. F. (1978). Non-compliance in children with renal transplants. *Pediatrics, 61*(6), 872–876.
Lawry, K. W., Brouhard, B. H., & Cunningham, R., J. (1994). Cognitive functioning and school performance in children with renal failure. *Pediatric Nephrology, 8*(3), 326–329.
LePontois, J., Moel, D. I., & Cohn, R. A. (1987). Family Adjustment to pediatric ambulatory dialysis. *American Journal of Orthopsychiatry, 57*, 78–83.
Leumann, C., Mueller, U., & Leumann, E. (1989). Insights gained from dialysis camps. *International Journal of Adolescent Medicine and Health, 4*(1), 29–34.
Madden, S. J., Ledermann, S. E., Guerrero-Blanco, M., Bruce, M., & Trompeter, R. S. (2003). Cognitive and psychosocial outcome of infants dialysed in infancy. *Child: Care, Health and Development, 29*(1), 55–61.
Madero, M., Gul, A., & Sarnak, M. J. (2008). Cognitive function in chronic kidney disease. *Seminars in Dialysis, 21*(1), 29–37.
Mahan, J., & Smith, H. (2008). Unpublished Results.
Mahan, J., Warady, B., & The Consensus Committee. (2006). Assessment and treatment of short stature in pediatric patients with chronic kidney disease: A consensus statement. *Pediatric Nephrology, 21*(7), 917–930.
Manificat, S., Dazord, A., Cochat, P., Morin, D., Plainguet, F., & Debray, D. (2003). Quality of life of children and adolescents after kidney or liver transplantation: Child, parents and caregiver's point of view. *Pediatric Transplantation, 7*(3), 228–235.
Masur, F. T. (1981). Adherence to health care regimens. In C. P. L. Bradley (Ed.), *Medical psychology: Contributions to behavioral medicine* (pp. 441–480). New York: Academic Press.

McDonagh, J. E., & Viner, R. M. (2006). Lost in transition? Between paediatric and adult services. *BMJ, 332*(7539), 435–436.

Meade, M. A. (1999). *The development, implementation, and evaluation of a self-management program for adolescents and children with renal transplants*. ProQuest Information & Learning, US.

Meade, M. A., Creer, T. L., & Mahan, J. D. (2003). A self-management program for adolescents and children with renal transplantation. *Journal of Clinical Psychology in Medical Settings, 10*(3), 165–171.

Melzer, S. M., Leadbeater, B., Reisman, L., & Jaffe, L. R. (1989). Characteristics of social networks in adolescents with end-stage renal disease treated with renal transplantation. *Journal of Adolescent Health Care, 10*(4), 308–312.

Melzer, S. M., Leadbeater, B., Reisman, L., Jaffe, L. R., & Lieberman, K. V. (1989). Characteristics of social networks in adolescents with end-stage renal disease treated with renal transplantation. *Journal of Adolescent Health Care, 10*(4), 308–312.

Morgenstern, B. Z., Murphy, M., Dayton, J., Kokmen, T., Purvis, J., Milliner, E., et al. (1994). Noncompliance in a pediatric renal transplant population. *Transplantation Proceedings, 26*(1), 129.

NAPRTCS. (2008). *NAPRTCS Annual Report 2007*. Document Number.

National Kidney Foundation. (2002). *Clinical practice guidelines for chronic kidney disease: evaluation, classification, and stratification. Part 4. Definition and classification of stages of chronic kidney disease*. (N. K. Foundation o. Document Number)

National Kidney Foundation. (2005). K/DOQI clinical practice guidelines for bone metabolism and disease in children with chronic kidney disease. *American Journal of Kidney Diseases, 46*(4 Suppl. 1), S1–121.

Neu, S., & Kjellstrand, C. (1986). Stopping long-term dialysis. An empirical study of withdrawal of life-supporting treatment. *New England Journal of Medicine, 314*(1), 14–20.

North, C., & Eminson, M. (1998). A review of a psychiatry-nephrology liaison service. *European Child & Adolescent Psychiatry, 7*(4), 235–245.

Parekh, R., Carroll, C., Wolfe, R., & Port, F. (2002). Cardiovascular mortality in children and young adults with end-stage kidney disease. *Journal of Pediatrics, 141*(2), 191–197.

Postlethwaite, R., Eminson, D., Reynolds, J., Wood, A., & Hollis, S. (1998). Growth in renal failure: a longitudinal study of emotional and behavioral changes during trials of growth hormone treatment. *Archives of Disease in Childhood, 78*(3), 222–229.

Rasbury, W. C., Fennell, R. S., 3rd, & Morris, M. K. (1983). Cognitive functioning of children with end-stage renal disease before and after successful transplantation. *Journal of Pediatrics, 102*(4), 589–592.

Rianthavorn, P., & Ettenger, R. B. (2005). Medication non-adherence in the adolescent renal transplant recipient: a clinician's viewpoint. *Pediatric Transplantation, 9*(3), 398–407.

Rianthavorn, P., Ettenger, R., Malekzadeh, M., Marik, J., & Struber, M. (2004). Noncompliance with Immunosuppressive Medications in Pediatric and Adolescent Patients receiving Solid Organ Transplants. *Transplantation, 77*(5), 778–782.

Rosenkranz, J., Reichwald-Klugger, E., Oh, J., Turzer, M., Mehls, O., & Schaefer, F. (2005). Psychosocial rehabilitation and satisfaction with life in adults with childhood-onset of end-stage renal disease. *Pediatric Nephrology, 20*, 1288–1294.

Rovelli, M., Palmeri, D., Vossler, E., Bartus, S., Hull, D., & Schweizer, R. (1989). Noncompliance in renal transplant recipients: evaluation by socioeconomic groups. *Transplantation Proceedings, 21*(6), 3979–3981.

Schweitzer, J. B., Hobbs, S. A. (1995). Renal and Liver Disease: End-Stage and Transplantation Issues. In M. Roberts (Ed.), *Handbook of pediatric psychology* (pp. 425–445). London: Guilford Press.

Schweizer, R., Rovelli, M., APalmeri, D., Vossler, E., Hull, D., & Bartus, S. (1990). Noncompliance in organ transplant recipients. *Transplantation, 49*(2), 209–215.

Seikaly, M., Ho, P. L., Emmett, L., & Tejani, A. (2001). The 12th annual report of the North American pediatric renal transplant cooperative study: Renal transplantation from 1987 through 1998. *Pediatric Transplantation, 5*(3), 215–231.

Siegel, E., Mahan, J & Johnson, R. (1994). Solid organ transplantation in adolescents: The blessing and the curse. *Adolescent Medicine: State of the Art Reviews, 5*(2), 293–309.

Slickers, J., Duquette, P., Hooper, S., & Gipson, D. (2007). Clinical predictors of neurocognitive deficits in children with chronic kidney disease. *Pediatric Nephrology, 22*(4), 565–572.

Soliday, E., Kool, E., & Lande, M. (2000). Psychosocial adjustment in children with kidney disease. *Journal of Pediatric Psychology, 25*(2), 93–103.

Soliday, E., Kool, E., & Lande, M. B. (2001). Family environment, child behavior, and medical indicators in children with kidney disease. *Child Psychiatry & Human Development, 31*(4), 279–295.

Tan, K. K. C. (1992). Therapy with cyclosporine following solid organ transplantation in children. *Current opinion in pediatrics, 4*(3), 467–470.

The National Kidney Foundation of Ohio. (2008). The National Kidney Foundation of Ohio. Retrieved 6/15/2008, from http://www.kidney.org/site/kidneyDisease/indes.cfm?ch = 310

Tong, A., Lowe, A., Sainsbury, P., & Craig, J. C. (2008). Experiences of parents who have children with chronic kidney disease: A systematic review of qualitative studies. *Pediatrics, 121*(2), 349–360.

Tossani, E., Cassano, P., & Fava, M. (2005). Depression and renal disease. *Seminars in Dialysis, 18*(2), 73–81.

UNC Kidney Center. (2008). Smooth Transition to Adulthood with Renal Disease (STARx). Retrieved June 20, 2008, from http://unckidneycenter.org/hcprofessionals/transition.html

USRDS. (2008). *United States Renal Data Service (USRDS) Annual Report of 2007*. Document Number.

Viner, R. (1999). Transition from paediatric to adult care. Bridging the gaps or passing the buck?. *Archives of Disease in Childhood, 81*(3), 271–275.

Viner, R. (2000). Effective transition from paediatric to adult services. *Hospital Medicine (London), 61*(5), 341–343.

Viner, R. (2001). Barriers and good practice in transition from paediatric to adult care. *Journal of the Royal Society of Medicine, 94* (Suppl. 40), 2–4.

Viner, R. (2003). Bridging the gaps: Transition for young people with cancer. *European Journal of Cancer, 39*(18), 2684–2687.

Viner, R. M. (2008). Transition of care from paediatric to adult services: one part of improved health services for adolescents. *Archives of Disease in Childhood, 93*(2), 160–163.

Viswanathan, R. (1991). Helping patients cope with the loss of a renal transplant. *Loss, Grief, & Care, 5*(1–2), 103–113.

Waite, E., & Laraque, D. (2006). Pediatric organ transplant patients and long-term care: A review. *Mount Sinai Journal of Medicine, 73*(8), 1148–1155.

Walker, L. (1985). Adolescent dialysands in group therapy. *Social Casework, 66*, 21–29.

Warady, B. (2002). Neurodevelopment of infants with end-stage renal disease: It is improving. *Pediatric Transplant, 6*, 5–7.

Washington, A. W. (1999). Cross-Cultural Issues in Transplant Compliance. *Transplantation Proceedings, 31*(Suppl 4A), 27S–28S.

Watson, A. R. (1996). Chronic renal failure in childhood. *British Journal of Hospital Medicine, 55*(6), 329–331.

Watson, A. R. (1997). Stress and burden of care in families with children commencing renal replacement therapy. *Advances in Peritoneal Dialysis, 13*, 300–304.

Watson, A. R. (2005). Problems and pitfalls of transition from paediatric to adult renal care. *Pediatric Nephrology, 20*(2), 113–117.

Welch, G. (1994). Assessment of quality of life following renal failure. In H. M. C. Bradley (Ed.), *Quality of life following renal failure* (pp. 55–97). Switzerland: Harwood Academic Publishers.

Will, E., & Johnson, J. (1994). Options in the medical management of end-stage renal failure. In H. M. C. Bradley (Ed.), *Quality of Life following renal failure* (pp. 55–97). Switzerland: Harwood Academic Publishers.

Wingen, A., Fabian-Back, C., Schaefer, F., & Mehls, O. (1997). Randomized multicentre study of a low-protein diet on the progression of renal failure in children. European study group of nutritional treatment of chronic renal failure in childhood. *Lancet, 349*(9059), 1117–1123.

Zelikovsky, N., & Schast, A. (2008). Eliciting accurate reports of adherence in a clinical interview: Development of the medical adherence measure. *Pediatric Nursing, 34*(2), 141–146.

Sickle Cell Disease

Lamia P. Barakat, D. Colette Nicolaou, Emily A. O'Hara, and Sarah Levin Allen

Background

Sickle cell disease (SCD) is a collection of autosomal recessive genetic disorders involving the abnormal production of hemoglobin. In SCD, red blood cells are short-lived and brittle, assuming a "sickled" shape that hinders their ability to effectively deliver oxygen throughout the body. In addition, impaired red blood cells often aggregate to occlude smaller blood vessels and significantly reduce the amount of oxygenated blood to the lungs and other tissues (Serjeant, 1997). Several SCD variants of graded severity exist including homozygous SCD (HbSS), which is noted to be the most severe, and heterozygous SCD associated with more benign symptoms. In addition, three heterozygous thalassemia deviations occur with varying degrees of clinical manifestation (Helps, Fuggle, Udwin, & Dick, 2003). Individuals who carry the sickle cell trait generally do not experience symptoms associated with the disease (Rees et al., 2003).

Epidemiology

In the United States, SCD is diagnosed in approximately 1 in every 400–500 live births for African Americans (Kral, Brown, & Hynd, 2001) and 1 in every 1,200 live births among Hispanics and those of Caribbean descent (Driscoll, 2007). It is also noted to be found among ethnic groups originating around the Mediterranean Sea, including Italy, Greece, Turkey, Saudi Arabia, and India at similar incidence rates (Nagal, 1994). Comprehensive neonatal screening for SCD has been widely adopted in order to provide early education, intervention, and support for infants and families (Henthorn, Almeida, & Davies, 2004). While mortality rates have significantly declined as a result of treatment advances and early management, life expectance rates continue to fall below that of the general population (Platt et al., 1994). The primary cause of death prior to adulthood is bacterial infection; however, early prophylactic penicillin has greatly reduced this risk (Kral et al.; Platt et al.). Strokes are also associated with premature death. In addition to acute mortality risks, individuals with SCD can experience a number of chronic symptoms and cumulative clinical manifestations that impact health and quality of life.

Symptoms

Young prior infants rarely experience symptoms due to the protection conferred by fetal hemoglobin (HbF), which is present at birth (Helps et al., 2003). Once production of HbF declines at 6 months, individuals are at risk for a number of SCD-related complications. The primary symptom associated with SCD is pain resulting from vasoocclusive episodes. Acute pain episodes are often unpredictable in nature and generally last between 3 and 14 days, yet they can be exacerbated by changes in temperature, infection, dehydration, high altitude, stress, fatigue, or

L.P. Barakat (✉)
Children's Hospital of Philadelphia and University of Pennsylvania School of Medicine, Philadelphia, PA, USA
e-mail: barakat@email.chop.edu

W.T. O'Donohue, L.W. Tolle (eds.), *Behavioral Approaches to Chronic Disease in Adolescence*,
DOI 10.1007/978-0-387-87687-0_19,

menstruation (Yaster, Kost-Byerl, & Mazwell, 2000). While some adolescents never experience painful episodes, others require frequent hospitalizations for pain management. Pain localization varies; however, it is most commonly described as limb pain, headaches, abdomen pain, chest pain, and lower back pain (Roth-Isigkeit, Thyen, Stoven, Schwarzenberger, & Schmucker, 2005). In addition, male adolescents often experience priapism, in which red blood cells occlude vessels in the penis resulting in painful erections potentially lasting several days (Powars & Johnson, 1996). Severe vasoocclusion can lead to ischemic tissue damage in multiple body organs, including the spleen, liver, kidney, bone, and bone marrow. Additional complications can include leg ulcers, yellow jaundiced eyes, short stature, delayed puberty, fatigue, and physical limitations. Furthermore, acute chest syndrome is one of the more significant complications resulting from pulmonary infarction, and if left untreated can result in heart failure, pulmonary edema, cardiovascular collapse, and death (Vichinsky et al., 1997).

Additional complications can result when vasoocclusion occurs in the central nervous system. For example, 7–17% of youth with SCD will experience at least one stroke or cerebral vascular accident (CVA) (Brown et al., 2000; Cohen, Branch, McKie, & Adams, 1997). After an initial stroke, findings suggest a 50–70% chance of reoccurrence within 3 years (Balkaran, Char, Morris, Serjeant, & Serjeant, 1992; Powars, Wilson, Imbus, Pegelow, & Allen, 1978). More subtle CVAs, deemed "silent strokes," can occur with no obvious outward clinical manifestations but with potentially deleterious effects on brain structure. Armstrong et al. (1996) detected brain abnormalities through magnetic resonance imaging (MRI) in 12–16% of their sample with no previously reported history of CVAs. Both silent and overt strokes typically occur during the first decade of life (Kral et al., 2001).

Medical Treatment

There is currently no universal cure for SCD, so treatment is most notably palliative and focuses on reduction in frequency, severity, and duration of pain. Several early prophylactic interventions begun during infancy and early childhood help to reduce the risk of bacterial infections, including penicillin administration and immunization with pneumococcal vaccines. Screening evaluations for organ damage and stroke risk are considered part of standard care throughout adolescence and adulthood (Driscoll, 2007). In addition, parental education and support can help families sustain ongoing medical management, detect early symptoms, and address complications more effectively.

Subsequent to preventative interventions, several medical treatments are employed based on the severity of symptoms. Pain episodes are most commonly addressed through analgesic agents of varying strength, while several less invasive strategies are often used to address SCD pain, including hydration, heat, and massage. Although these approaches have little empirical research to support their use, anecdotal reports suggest that hydration increases blood flow and heat serves as a vasodilator to ease vasoocclusion in the microcirculation (Yaster et al., 2000). Psychosocial interventions have been found to address pain management, including relaxation training, hypnosis, and family interventions. Transfusion therapy is intermittently used after severe vasoocclusive events, and prior to general anesthesia and surgical procedures (Lane et al., 2001), and chronic transfusions can be used to prevent stroke. Despite the relative effectiveness of transfusion, frequent use can be associated with iron overload and other significant complications (Driscoll, 2007). Given the antisickling effects of HbF observed during infancy, research continues to investigate the use of hydroxyurea, a pharmacologic agent found to increase hemoglobin as well as HbF, for patients faced with severe SCD complications. Its use must be closely monitored by medical staff. It is important to note that while hydroxyurea is FDA approved for use among adult populations, investigations among infants, children, and adolescents are ongoing.

While the clinical presentation of adolescents with SCD can vary greatly, ongoing comprehensive care is necessary to ensure healthy development into adulthood. Most adolescents with SCD in the United States are eligible for health-care coverage by commercial insurance agents or government-sponsored programs (Lane et al., 2001). Regardless of provider, specialized medical care must be obtained through trained professionals who are sensitive to the presenting symptomatology, the long-term complications, and the sociocultural context of SCD. Routine screening for disease complications, growth and development, and psychosocial needs is central to comprehensive care, and adolescents should be aware of local facilities offering emergency care for SCD as well as have an understanding of their medical history.

Developmental and Disease-Related Considerations

Due to medical advances that have provided better care and have increased life expectancy in individuals with SCD, there has become a need to understand psychosocial factors that influence their lives. Adolescence is a particularly challenging time as youth with SCD not only deal with the medical nature of their illness but also the difficult transition into adulthood involving physiological, personal, familial, and social maturation (Gil et al., 2003). For example, patients with SCD are at risk for treatment nonadherence as they reach adolescence, which may be the result of stress due in part to the burden of poverty that disproportionately affects African Americans and increased psychosocial and academic problems related to SCD (Baskin et al., 1998). To better understand how psychosocial factors influence adaptation for youth with SCD, risk-and-resistance models have been used (Barakat, Lash, Lutz, & Nicolaou, 2006; Brown, Doepke, & Kaslow, 1993). Risk factors (such as gender, socioeconomic status, functional ability, and stigma) are circumstances that place adolescents at risk for health-related or psychosocial problems. Resistance factors (such as self-esteem, social support, and family functioning) are influences that promote adaptation.

Risk Factors

Gender

Girls with SCD are more at risk for difficult peer relationships as compared to boys. Noll et al. (1996), using sociometric measures, found that females with SCD showed more problems with sociability and leadership abilities and were less likely to be chosen as a best friend by their peers. Males were found to be less aggressive and disruptive compared to a normative sample, suggesting that their behavior may be influenced by fatigue and other SCD complications. Although for other chronic illnesses females tend to report higher pain levels than males (List, Wahlund, Wenneberg, & Dworkin, 1999; Sallfors, Hallberg, & Fasth, 2003), mixed results have been found in studies of children with SCD (Conner-Warren, 1996; Kell, Kliewer, Erikson, & Ohene-Frempong, 1998; Wagner et al., 2004). For example, Kell et al. found that adolescent boys reported more somatic symptoms than girls due to sickle cell pain, challenging the literature on gender and pain reporting among adolescents with chronic illnesses. On the other hand, Wagner and colleagues found that girls with SCD reported more severe pain supporting gender differences on pain reports.

Socioeconomic Status

Research examining the relationship between health and socioeconomic status (SES) documents that adolescents from families of lower SES have more health problems including poorer diet, lower levels of physical activity, and higher rates of cigarette smoking (Hanson & Chen, 2007). When compared to families with higher SES, youth with SCD from families of lower SES were described by parents as having less positive moods, higher levels of anxiety and depressive symptoms, and poorer academic functioning (Barbarin, Whitten, Bond, & Conner-Warren, 1999). Negative thinking and pain reports (Barakat, Schwartz, Simon, & Radcliffe, 2007) as well as functional disability (Hoff, Palermo, Schluchter, Zebracki, & Drotar, 2006) were also found to be higher among youth with SCD of lower SES. In contrast, another study, with siblings comprising the comparison group to control for SES, noted that children and adolescents with SCD reported lower self-esteem, showed less academic competence, and were less liked by peers than their healthy siblings (Brown, Kaslow et al., 1993).

Functional Abilities

Functional ability limitations, arising from SCD complications, may have a significant impact on psychosocial aspects of adolescent functioning (Palermo, Witherspoon, Valenzuela, & Drotar, 2004). Many youth with SCD are able to overcome these limitations. Yet, there are some who miss a considerable amount of school, have limitations on activities, such as household chores and social activities, and experience emotional distress (Gil et al., 2000; Palermo, 2000).

Stigma

Jenerette and colleagues suggested that stigma may contribute to depression among adults with SCD (Jenerette, Funk, & Murdaugh, 2005); however, the literature on stigma in pediatric SCD is limited. A pilot study examining perception of discrimination in health care among parents of children with cancer or hematological disorders, including SCD, found that African American caregivers did not perceive discrimination but did worry about the role of race in receiving professional support (Williams, 1993). It has also been suggested that some caregivers may be cautious of newborn screening because of anticipated prejudice that might be associated with genetic disorder affecting mostly African Americans (Radcliffe, Barakat, & Boyd, 2006). Further investigation of perceptions of stigma and discrimination within the community and health care system is warranted.

Resistance Factors

Self-Esteem

Disease-related symptoms can impact the development of self-esteem among children with chronic illness (Vitulano, 2003), and self-esteem in adolescents has been linked to positive adjustment outcomes among different populations (Meijer, Sinnema, Bijstra, Mellenbergh, & Wolters, 2002; Pidgeon, 1989; Ritchie, 2001). Studies have shown that adolescents with SCD with higher self-esteem were less likely to experience symptoms of depression (Burlew, Telfair, Colangelo, & Wright, 2000). A study examining adaptation among 55 children and adolescents with SCD using the risk-and-resistance model suggested that self-esteem, as rated by caregivers, may play a role in predicting child adjustment (Brown, Lambert et al., 2000). It has also been suggested that higher self-esteem may protect against the self-consciousness and body image dissatisfaction that can arise due to delayed puberty for adolescents with SCD (Alao & Cooley, 2001).

Social Support

Adolescents with SCD who perceive more social support reported fewer SCD complications and higher functional abilities than adolescents with lower perceived social support (Hurtig, Koepke, & Park, 1989). Also, teens with SCD who rely on social assertiveness and social support as coping mechanisms reported less trait anxiety; reduced trait anxiety was in turn associated with higher self-esteem and greater perception of a social family supportive environment (Burlew et al., 2000). For adolescents with SCD, social support may serve as a vehicle to build self-confidence, self-esteem, and communication skills (Pinckney & Stuart, 2004), yielding skills needed to cope with living with a chronic illness.

Family Environment

Behavior health specialists should be cognizant of the impact SCD can have on the entire family, including unpredictable interruptions in family routines, financial burden, the potential to overlook the needs of siblings, at-home pain management patterns, and marital stress (Burlew, Evans, & Oler, 1989; Collins, Kaslow, Doepke, Eckman, & Johnson, 1998). On the other hand, extended family among African Americans, including grandparents, aunts, uncles, cousins, neighbors, and other community members, often play an integral part in the life of an adolescent with SCD (Kaslow et al., 1997). Given that many families are faced with additional stressors, including unstable home environments and limited transportation, a child's emotional well-being, or physical symptoms, may not be a family priority at all times (Kaslow et al.).

Adolescents with SCD with strong family cohesiveness and supportiveness have a more favorable adjustment (Pinckney & Stuart, 2004). Also, higher competence in families was related to fewer behavior and emotional problems for youth with SCD, after controlling for sociodemographic and medical variables (Kell et al., 1998). Moreover, it has been shown that SCD knowledge may not be as important as a supportive and dependable family environment for the transition to adulthood in terms of disease management outcomes (Burlew et al., 2000). The family environment may have a significant impact on the adolescent's current disposition and also his or her transition to adulthood.

Behavioral Interventions

The role of the behavior health specialist in the comprehensive care of adolescents with SCD encompasses a broad range of services, including pain management, psychosocial support, assistance with cognitive impairments, health-care access and utilization, and familial issues. While we focus on disease management and school functioning in this chapter, practitioners should conduct thorough intake assessments to examine an adolescent's medical, academic, family, socioemotional, and behavioral history as a means of obtaining a broad contextual understanding of an individual's circumstances and life experiences to promote more effective interventions.

Disease Management

Adolescence is a time of social, emotional, and physical maturation. Youth with SCD must incorporate medical care (including management of potentially increased pain and other complications) and physical limitations (such as delayed puberty) with typical adolescent tasks of individuation, identity formation, and autonomy (Baskin et al., 1989). Special attention, therefore, should be placed on the transition to adulthood to address the potential impact of SCD on developmental outcomes.

Assessment

Initial steps to address the needs of youth with SCD include well-validated assessment tools employed within a culturally sensitive framework. In terms of pain measurements, the Adolescent Pediatric Pain Tool (Savedra, Tesler, Holzemer, & Ward, 1989) and the parent and child/adolescent versions of the Varni/Thompson Pediatric Pain Questionnaire (Varni & Thompson, 1985) have been used among SCD populations (Barakat, Schwartz et al., 2007; Franck, Treadwell, Jacob, & Vichinsky, 2002; Graumlich et al., 2001; Walco & Dampier, 1990). Others note the value of self-reported pain diaries among children and adolescents in order to monitor frequency and intensity of pain episodes as well as at-home pain management techniques (Barakat et al., in press; Dampier, Ely, Eggleston, Brodecki, & O'Neal, 2004). In addition, a number of psychosocial measures are available to assess adolescents' quality of life including the Child Health Questionnaire (CHQ), Parent and Child Forms (Palermo, Schwartz, Drotar, & McGowan, 2002; Panepinto, O'Mahar, DeBaun, Rennie, & Scott, 2004), and the Miami Pediatric Quality of Life Questionnaire (Armstrong et al., 1999; Nicolaou & Barakat, 2004). Additional measures, beyond those focused on pain and quality of life, can be employed as practitioners see fit. Addressing the specific needs of individuals, as well as relative strengths of adolescents with SCD and their families, will inform treatment plans, guide interventions, and allow for monitoring of progress over time and under different circumstances.

Interventions

Cognitive strategies. Pain management in adolescents with SCD is a primary goal, not only for the medical team but also for behavior health specialists. Research suggests that several cognitive strategies, including hypnosis, imagery, and self-calming, as well as behavioral tools, such as biofeedback and progressive muscle relaxation, can be effective methods for pain reduction (Chen, Cole, & Kato, 2004). Gil et al. (1997, 2000, 2001) conducted a series of investigations using a cognitive coping skills training program in which children and adolescents with SCD were trained in deep breathing, pleasant imagery, and calming self-talk. Audiotapes of exercises were provided to allow participants to practice strategies independently. Findings revealed less negative thinking and fewer reports of pain when exposed to a pain stimulus for youth in the training program as compared to a standard care control group. At 1 month follow-up, the intervention group exhibited more active coping. Furthermore, participants who consistently used coping strategies while in pain evidenced improved health outcomes. Behavior health specialists can model for, rehearse with, and encourage adolescents to consistently practice cognitive coping strategies such as those noted above. Employment of existing treatment manuals as needed to guide interventions, creation of audiotapes of relaxation or imagery components for ongoing independent use, and inclusion of parents and other support persons as added support when appropriate should also be considered.

Further research by Thomas, Dixon, and Miligan (1999) examined the effectiveness of group interventions involving relaxation training and health education for adolescents and young adults with SCD. In addition, participants were taught to identify pain cognitions, to reconceptualize their pain as manageable, and to utilize active coping skills. After 2 months of weekly group meetings, participants reported more positive coping strategies, more behavioral activities, higher pain management, self-efficacy, greater pain control, and lower affective pain reports as compared to both an attention placebo and standard medical care control groups. These findings suggest that behavior health specialists can utilize group formats to disseminate information and to teach skills among many adolescents with SCD.

Cozzi and Tryon (1987) conducted a small study among adolescents with SCD in which they found a regimen of electromyography (EMG) and thermal biofeedback to be associated with an overall decrease in muscle tension, lower frequency of headaches, less analgesic use, lower perceived pain intensity, fewer self-treated pain episodes, and lower state anxiety as recorded in pain diaries. Reports at 6-month follow-up suggested that participants continued to employ relaxation techniques and evidenced ongoing reductions in intensity of pain symptoms. Developmentally appropriate education regarding the process behind biofeedback as well as the equipment used should be provided (McGrath, 1990). If biofeedback is deemed an appropriate treatment, adolescents should be guided to employ biofeedback techniques prior to significant pain, at the first signs of discomfort, and during pain episodes in order to regulate pain responses.

Hypnosis is another method implemented to address sickle cell pain. In medical settings, hypnosis includes several cognitive behavioral relaxation components, including deep breathing, imagery, eye fixation, and progressive muscle relaxation. It also includes a phase of suggestion in which direct and indirect messages are relayed. Although younger children require a more sensitive approach, behavior health specialists can engage adolescents in standard induction procedures as a means of increasing relaxation states (Collins et al., 1998; McGrath, 1990). Dinges et al. (1997) conducted a small study among children, adolescents, and adults with SCD between the ages of 5 and 51 years. After 18 months of group hypnosis training intervention, participants evidenced fewer days of pain and less medication use. The authors asserted that hypnosis may help mitigate mild pain, but that it may not be as effective for moderate-to-severe pain episodes. These findings are consistent with several case studies examining self-hypnosis among 9–20 year olds with SCD (Agargun, Oner, & Akbayram, 2001; Zeltzer, Dash, & Holland, 1979).

Behavioral contracting. Behavioral contracting may serve to increase the active involvement of adolescents and family members in medical care by increasing healthy behaviors and symptom management (Chen et al., 2004). Patients, parents, and medical staff create a list of responsibilities and agree to follow through with the written agreement. As a result, adolescents gain a better understanding of their role and expectations, while developing confidence in their ability to manage pain. Preliminary data from youth with SCD and chronic pain have found behavioral contracting to be effective in reducing hospitalizations and increasing compliance to medical regimens (Burghardt-Fitzgerald, 1989; Walco & Dampier, 1990; Zeltzer, Bush, Chen, & Riveral, 1997). Therefore, well-outlined behavioral contracts, in which a series of simple steps are delineated (hydration, deep breathing, exercise, and medication dosing), may facilitate self-reliance among adolescents as they actively manage their disease (Collins et al., 1998).

Psychoeducation. In addition to promoting cognitive coping strategies and behavioral contracting, psychoeducational programs have been examined among adolescents and families facing chronic illness (Collins et al., 1998). These interventions often include a description of disease etiology, course, and treatment options. Much research among pediatric chronic illness groups suggests that disease-related knowledge and procedure-related information reduces anxiety, increases compliance, and improves overall adaptation (Collins et al.; Potter & Roberts, 1984). Psychoeducation by behavior health specialists should be delivered within a supportive framework, in which individual questions are addressed and intergenerational family myths about SCD are sensitively dispelled. Verbal and printed information should be communicated to match the developmental level of the child, as well as the cultural, educational, religious, and socioeconomic status of the family (Collins et al.; Day, Brunson, & Wang, 1992). Similarly, practitioners can provide SCD-related knowledge as a means of increasing coping strategies and reducing feelings of isolation among groups of adolescents and families (Anie, 2005).

Family interventions. Kaslow et al. (1997) emphasize the importance of family-based interventions due to the noted relationship between child adjustment and family functioning (Hurtig, 1994; Lemanek, Ranalli, Green, Biega, & Lupia, 2003), as well as the genetic basis for SCD. Furthermore, given the importance of the family unit in African American homes, family interventions can draw upon the strengths of the community in order to address specific sociocultural needs (Radcliffe et al., 2006). As noted above, Schwartz, Radcliffe, and Barakat (2007) designed a family-based intervention among adolescents with SCD and primary caregivers in which a culturally sensitive cognitive behavioral pain management intervention was compared to a psychoeducation control group utilizing culture-specific modifications to improve acceptability and effectiveness. Large-scale family interventions have yet to be empirically examined; however, pilot studies of manualized psychoeducation and cognitive behavioral family interventions yielded positive findings in terms of increased SCD knowledge, coping, and daily functioning (Kaslow et al., 2000; Powers, Mitchell, Graumlich, Byars, & Kalinyak, 2002).

School Functioning

Along with pain management for adolescents with SCD, the behavioral health professional must be concerned with school performance as youth with SCD are at risk for poor school functioning (Helps et al., 2003; Lemanek et al., 2003). There are many factors that influence decreased school performance including neurocognitive effects (Armstrong et al., 1996; Brown, Buchanan et al., 1993; Brown et al., 2000; Kral et al., 2001; Schatz, Finke, & Roberts, 2004; Wang et al., 2001), school absences (Shapiro et al., 1995), sociodemographic variables (Devine, Brown, Lambert, Donegan, & Eckman, 1998; Schatz et al., 2004; Tarazi, Grant, Ely, & Barakat, 2007), and inadequate education of school staff (Koontz, Short, Kalinyak, & Noll, 2004). When considering behavioral approaches to address school functioning, the associations among these variables and school performance must be taken into account.

Neurocognitive Effects

Children with SCD are at risk for cognitive impairments and learning problems (Helps et al., 2003). Studies of overall cognitive abilities of children with SCD have produced variable results (Armstrong et al., 1996; Brown et al., 2000; Noll et al., 2001; Wang et al., 2001). In general, the literature shows a 4–5-point decrement on IQ measures in youth with SCD with no central nervous system involvement, while youth with SCD and silent cerebral infarcts have about a 4–7-point decrement (Schatz, Finke,

Kellett, & Kramer, 2002). Variability in findings may be the result of the presence of deficits in specific areas of cognitive functioning (Schatz et al., 2002) so that neuropsychological assessment may be integral to delineating a clear, functional profile of cognitive strengths and weaknesses as well as deficits.

Indeed, neuropsychological performance of children with SCD has been more consistent throughout the literature. Children with overt and silent strokes have generally performed poorly than peers on attention tasks, and those with more functional impairments have shown overt infarcts in the frontal lobe (Brown et al., 2000). Youth with SCD show impaired attention when compared to their nondiseased siblings (Brown, Buchanan et al., 1993; Noll et al., 2001) and to those with SCD and no CNS impairment (Wang et al., 2001; see Schatz et al., 2002 for review). Neuropsychological performance has also been associated with imaging abnormalities that may be a reflection of frontal-executive dysfunction (Grueneich et al., 2004), further supporting the need for assessment of attention and executive functions. Problems with concentration and attention may be the first indication that SCD is interfering with school functioning (Taras & Potts-Datema, 2005).

Academic Achievement and School Attainment

In addition to identified deficits in neuropsychological functioning, youth with SCD have been found to have decreased academic achievement in the areas of reading, math, and spelling (Kral et al., 2001; Schatz, Brown, Pascual, Hsu, & DeBaun, 2001) and rates of learning disabilities twice that expected based on normative samples (Brown, Davis et al., 2000). A study of children with SCD and healthy siblings found that children with SCD performed poorer on reading decoding (Brown, Davis et al.). More specifically, youth with a history of overt stroke or silent stroke have poorer performance than children without stroke on math and reading achievement (Armstrong et al., 1996; Wang et al., 2001). However, no differences in academic performance were noted in a study of children with SCD compared to children without SCD matched on sociodemographic characteristics (Noll et al., 2001).

Examination of educational attainment (i.e., retention or presence of special academic services) confirms the neurocognitive problems associated with SCD. One study found that the rate of poor educational attainment in children with stroke was nine times the rate for typically developing siblings and twice as much as children with silent stroke, while those with silent cerebral stoke had four times the rate of retention or presence of special academic services as typically developing siblings (Schatz et al., 2001).

School Absences

School attendance promotes normalcy and social functioning among children with chronic conditions (Worchel-Prevatt et al., 1998), highlighting the imperative to address school absence rates among youth with SCD. In one pain diary study, patients reported being absent from school on 21% of days documented with only half of those absences on days when pain was reported (Shapiro et al., 1995). Daily increases in stress and negative mood have also been associated with increased same-day pain and school absences and with a reduction in same-day social activities (Gil et al., 2003). Moreover, poor sleep quality and quantity have been associated with pain (Shapiro et al., 1995; Valrie, Gil, Redding-Lallinger, & Daeshcner, 2007), which has the potential to impact school performance (Fallone, Acebo, Arnedt, Seifer, & Carskadon, 2001). School absence may be compounded by possible lack of full accommodation in the school setting. Although adolescents with SCD miss many days of school, the days are not necessarily consecutive (i.e., a requirement of school systems for receiving home-bound services). For instance, a study of sickle cell-related pain in children found that children tended to miss on average 2.7 days consecutively (Shapiro et al., 1995).

Sociodemographic and Disease-Related Factors

Although psychoeducational and neuropsychological testing are extremely important in identifying specific areas of concern, it is important to include analysis of sociodemographic and medical variables. For instance, Grueneich et al. (2004) reported that type of sickle cell disease and disease severity were not associated with performance on neuropsychological tests; however, lower hemoglobin level (i.e., anemia) was correlated with the presence of neuroimaging abnormalities that explained variability across scores on neuropsychological tests. Hemoglobin levels have also been associated with decreased general cognitive ability, crystallized ability, and processing speed in some studies (Schatz et al., 2004). In addition, socioeconomic status and psychosocial variables have been found to relate to neuropsychological functioning in preschool-aged children (Tarazi et al., 2007). Brown, Buchanan, et al. (1993) similarly reported that socioeconomic status accounted for some of the variance in cognitive functioning in a sample of children with a mean age of 9 years, 5 months. It has been suggested that cognitive functioning in children with SCD declines with increasing age (Wang et al., 2001); however, this finding is disputed (Noll et al., 2001). It should be noted that most studies include samples of children between the areas of 7 and 12 years (Schatz et al., 2004) and therefore, school functioning in adolescence as it relates to earlier periods of development is not clear.

Educator Training

School administrators and teachers require additional information regarding the impact of SCD on cognitive functioning, learning, and academic achievement in order to modify educational strategies and provide appropriate services (Schatz, 2004). Many teachers receive little information about SCD (Rae & Frankel, 1998) and therefore, may not be aware of cognitive problems and medical needs that may result from the disease (Finke, Kellett, Schatz, & Robinson, 2002).

School Interventions

Assessment. Not only is it important to address adolescents' needs within the hospital and home settings, given the high risk for neurocognitive delays and academic difficulties (Brown et al., 2000; Noll et al., 2001), the school environment should be considered. Research identifying specific impairments among adolescents with SCD, especially related to stroke, notes the importance of school involvement; however, few specific intervention protocols have been outlined. Although school systems can provide psychoeducational assessment, the behavior health specialist plays the important role of further analyzing school performance as problems may be related to neurocognitive deficits, sociodemographic risk, or to lack of education among families and schools as to appropriate educational supports. Cognitive and academic tests can be useful predictors of school outcomes (Schatz, 2004) and may provide information integral to education and curriculum planning for children with SCD. Also, the use of a screening battery to assess processing speed, visual-motor skills, memory, and attention-concentration skills may be beneficial in identifying CNS involvement (Armstrong et al. 1996; Brown et al., 2000). Furthermore, practitioners can work closely with schools to initiate more formal testing, augment current academic plans, establish a protocol for symptom management at school, and allow provisions for school absences.

Intervention programs. We identified two published intervention programs demonstrating the utility of collaboration between health-care and school personnel for school functioning. King et al. (2005) implemented a 30–45 minute educational presentation and discussion among 81 teachers of students with SCD between Kindergarten and 12th grade. Significant increases in SCD knowledge in terms of genetics, common complications, and strokes were observed. In another, more comprehensive randomized trial of a school training, Koontz et al. (2004) reported that teachers attributed fatigue and school absences among children with SCD to low motivation, family problems, or drug problems. Similarly, peers, who did not receive SCD education, endorsed responses that characterized SCD as "bad blood" (a term commonly used to describe syphilis and HIV/AIDS). The school intervention program included teacher information packets, in-service sessions for educators, classroom in-service sessions for peers, and follow-up evaluations with students, teachers, and family. Information provided to teachers and school administrators addressed disease-related facts as well as descriptions and specific action steps on how to manage observable SCD complications such as pain, fatigue, infection, academic difficulties, and absenteeism. Findings revealed a significant increase in SCD knowledge and fewer school absences in those receiving the intervention (Koontz et al.).

Anie (2005) noted the importance of neuropsychological rehabilitation services and education liaisons to optimize academic potential and establish educational assistance as early as 5 years old. Given the high risk for ongoing neurocognitive deficits, continued support for adolescents is necessary to aid in identification and achievement of vocational goals (Noll et al., 2001). The school interventions described in this section demonstrate that comprehensive care of children and adolescents with SCD may be improved through explicit attention to the neurocognitive complications of SCD and their association with school performance and attainment. Inclusion of school staff and peers/students in training as to the causes, treatments, and complications of this chronic condition is integral to care also.

Methodological Considerations and Future Research Directions

Transition programs have gained additional attention as an increasing number of adolescents are surviving into adulthood and often experience an exacerbation of physical symptoms during this developmental stage (Castro et al., 1994; Telfair, Alexander, Loosier, Alleman-Velez, & Simmons, 2004; Tucker & Cabral, 2005). The period of transition to adulthood and adult health-care services is not well understood in SCD and in pediatrics more generally. Telfair and colleagues suggested that youth with SCD are often not equipped with the information required to navigate through the adult medical system, including seeking medical providers, making decisions on medical care, and actively following through with medically related activities. They noted the importance of collaboration between multiple disciplines (physicians, nurses, social workers, and case managers) to address acute and chronic needs, provide ongoing explanations, negotiate health-care systems, and coordinate services as a means of seamlessly transitioning adolescents into adult SCD care. Although transition programming is provided by many sickle cell centers, these programs are not empirically based and outcomes are not rigorously studied. Work outlining adolescent health-care needs and foundational components of transition programs as well as transition issues specific to youth with SCD will serve future research in terms of program development and the framing of research questions.

Unfortunately, as can be ascertained in this review, there are few descriptive or intervention studies of youth with SCD that focus solely on adolescents as many target samples of children and adolescents or adolescents and young adults. Reasons for a lack of research focused on adolescent are numerous and include convenience sampling and efforts to increase sample sizes in a population with whom recruitment can be challenging due to mistrust of the research enterprise and presence of multiple stressors that interfere with research participation (Schwartz et al., 2007). The end result, however, is a relative lack of attention to developmental issues that are specific to adolescents with SCD, which may hamper efforts to maintain or improve disease management and school functioning at this critical period for preparing adolescents with SCD to transition to adult roles and adult health-care systems. Efforts to recruit adolescent samples and to carefully consider adolescent development and sociodemographic risks are central to the success of intervention research moving forward (Barakat et al., 2006). In particular, changes in sickle cell disease processes in adolescence as well as limitations in educational and vocational opportunities and health-care access for those of ethnic minority and/or lower socioeconomic status should be accounted for.

A recent Cochrane Review made several suggestions for future research endeavors to expand the methodologically sound literature on SCD interventions (Anie & Green, 2005). Noted as important were treatment manuals, consistent outcome measurement tools, control groups, and multicentered collaborations in order to empirically examine intervention strategies among youth with SCD. Currently, there are relatively more intervention studies of disease management in SCD than there are of school functioning. Both areas require attention, however, as pain and other SCD complications can bring about significant limitations on functional outcomes including quality of life and school functioning, particularly as youth move through adolescence and into adulthood. Although school interventions are just emerging, the empirical basis for launching efforts to promote school functioning is in place. There is increasing evidence that youth with SCD are at increased risk for problems in neuropsychological functioning and reduced school achievement and school attainment as described above (Kral et al., 2001). This is related in part not only to disease process and missed school days but also to lack of information and coordination with teachers, nurses, and administrators in school districts to provide the necessary educational supports to bring about higher levels of achievement (Finkle et al., 2002). Studies of interventions targeting school functioning suggest that training of school personnel along with early intervention may be useful. We also encourage targeting interventions directly to caregivers and teens themselves so that they may receive training and support to act as advocates within school systems for their educational needs, as families may not always understand or access the resources that are available to them.

Published studies of disease management interventions are focused primarily on pain management and targeted pain outcomes, including days with pain, pain intensity, pain interference and health care utilization. Although these intervention approaches are empirically well-established, the association of reductions in pain with broader quality of life outcomes of pain coping, functional abilities, school functioning, and peer relationships is rarely addressed and cannot be assumed. Our work comparing a cognitive behavioral pain management intervention to a disease education intervention suggests the importance of broader-based intervention programs that target the "whole" teen with SCD in the family context instead of maintaining a narrow focus on pain (Schwartz et al., 2007).

Although adolescence is a period of increasing autonomy including in disease management, we maintain that the family remains an integral resource in supporting adolescent development as well as adolescent competence and responsibility in self-care, particularly in the context of the central role of the family in the African American community (Radcliffe et al., 2006). Our own work suggests that health outcomes for adolescents with SCD require a strong foundation of family functioning that incorporates adolescents and their caregivers coming together to collaborate on disease management (Barakat et al., 2007). Others have also pointed out that although caregivers may perform fewer disease management activities as youth with chronic conditions move into adolescents, their family members remain concerned about and involved in these activities (Berg et al., 2007; Palmer et al., 2004). Because the family is a cornerstone of African American communities, attending to and including interested family members in interventions may serve to improve their effectiveness and generalizability, not only in the short but also in the long run.

As should be clear at this point, those working in clinical and research endeavors with adolescents with SCD must carefully consider not only disease variables but also the wide range of sociodemographic risk-and-resistance factors for this population. For example, empirical research informs us that the experience of pain is associated with lower socioeconomic status and that poverty and discrimination may limit opportunities for those with this potentially devastating disease (Barakat et al., 2006; Barakat, Schwartz et al., 2007). Therefore, clinical practice and research endeavors are bound to be hampered when work is conducted in a vacuum that focuses on the individual to the exclusion of the social ecological context of development for those with chronic conditions (Barakat & Boyer, 2007). Alternatively, careful attention to these issues will serve to increase involvement of youth with SCD and their families in our work and to improve the efficacy over time. In terms of behavioral interventions with adolescents with SCD, culturally sensitive components have been outlined and include family involvement, emphasis on empowerment, recognition of the stress of being an ethnic minority and the stress associated with lower SES as well as culturally sensitive content (Schwartz et al., 2007).

A multidisciplinary team approach to SCD has been recommended in order to provide comprehensive care to youth and families with SCD (Lemanek et al., 2003; Telfair et al., 2004; Treadwell & Gil, 1994) and has been found to reduce hospitalizations and emergency room visits (Vichinsky, Johnson, & Lubin, 1982). An early examination into SCD management by Vichinsky and colleagues noted that while pain is biologically based, coping strategies can impact the pain experience. They suggested that all outpatients receive a comprehensive medical-psychosocial evaluation with a multidisciplinary team in order to provide supplemental resources to augment coping, including vocational rehabilitation, school tutoring, individual counseling, support groups, and relaxation training. Similarly, Brown and Roberts (2000) emphasized that psychologists and other behavior health specialists should be integrated into standard medical practice. Because medical practitioners are often the first to interact with families, they frequently recognize signs of behavioral or emotional disturbances. Multidisciplinary teams allow for behavior health specialists to be readily available for consultation, immediate referrals, teaching opportunities, and collaborative research investigations (Brown & Roberts). In addition, families faced with ongoing financial stressors may be more apt to receive behavior health services in clinics they are familiar with, in conjunction with medical care, and among practitioners well-known by their medical team (Brown & Roberts). Given developmentally specific circumstances associated with adolescence, including puberty, autonomy, racial identity, transitioning to adult care, and long-term vocational and family planning (Baskin et al., 1989), a comprehensive team, familiar with SCD, is best suited to address the needs of teens and families alike.

References

Agargun, M. Y., Oner, A. F., & Akbayram, S. (2001). Hypnotic intervention for pain management in a child with sickle cell anemia. *Sleep and Hypnosis, 3*, 127–128.

Alao, A. O., & Cooley, E. (2001). Depression and sickle cell disease. *Harvard Review of Psychiatry, 9*(4), 169–177.

Anie, K. A. (2005). Psychological complications in sickle cell disease. *British Journal of Haematology, 129*, 723–729.

Anie, K. A., & Green, J. (2005). Psychological therapies for sickle cell disease and pain. *Cochrane Database Systematic Reviews, 2*, CD001916.

Armstrong, F. D., Thompson, R. J. Jr., Wang, W., Zimmerman, R., Pegelow, C. H., Miller, S. et al. (1996). Cognitive functioning and brain magnetic resonance imaging in children with sickle cell disease. Neuropsychology committee of the cooperative study of sickle cell disease. *Pediatrics, 97*(6), 864–870.

Armstrong, F. D., Toledano, S. R., Miloslavich, K., Lackman-Zehman, L., Levy, J. D., Gay, C. L., et al., (1999). The Miami pediatric quality of life questionnaire: Parent scale. *International Journal of Cancer, Supplement, 12*, 11–17.

Balkaran, B., Char, G., Morris, J. S., Serjeant, B. E., & Serjeant, B. G. (1992). Stoke in a cohort study of patients with homozygous sickle cell disease. *Journal of Pediatrics, 120*, 360–366.

Barakat, L. P. & Boyer, B. (2007). Pediatric psychology. In B. Boyer and Paharia, M. I. (Eds.), *Comprehensive Handbook of Clinical Health Psychology* (pp. 371–394). Hoboken, NJ: Wiley & Sons.

Barakat, L. P., Lash, L., Lutz, M. J., & Nicolaou, D. C. (2006). Psychosocial adaptation of children and adolescents with sickle cell disease. In R. T. Brown (Ed.), *Comprehensive handbook of childhood cancer and sickle cell disease: A biopsychosocial approach* (pp. 471–495). New York: Oxford.

Barakat, L. P., Patterson, C. A., Weinberger, B. S., Simon, K., Gonzalez, E. R., & Dampier, C. (2007). A prospective study of the role of coping and family functioning in health outcomes for adolescents with sickle cell disease. *Journal of Pediatric Hematology/Oncology, 29*(11), 752–760.

Barakat, L. P., Schwartz, L., Simon, K., & Radcliffe, J. (2007). Negative thinking as a coping strategy mediator of pain and internalizing symptoms in adolescents with sickle cell disease. *Journal of Behavioral Medicine, 30*, 199–208.

Barbarin, O. A., Whitten, C. F., Bond, S., & Conner-Warren, R. (1999). The social and cultural context of coping with sickle cell disease: II. The role of financial hardship in adjustment to sickle cell disease. *Journal of Black Psychology, 25*(3), 294–315.

Baskin, M. L., Collins, M. H., Brown, F., Griffith, J. R., Samuels, D., Moody, A. et al. (1998). Psychosocial considerations in sickle cell disease (SCD): The transition from adolescence to young adulthood. *Journal of Clinical Psychology in Medical Settings, 5*, 315–341.

Berg, C. A., Wiebe, D. J., Beveridge, R. M., Palmer, D. L., Korbel, C. D., Upchurch, R. et al. (2007). Mother-child appraised involvement in coping with diabetes stressors and emotional adjustment. *Journal of Pediatric Psychology, 32*(8), 995–1005.

Brown, R. T., Buchanan, I., Doepke, K., Eckman, J. R., Baldwin, K., Goonan, B. et al. (1993). Cognitive and academic functioning in children with sickle cell disease. *Journal of Clinical Child Psychology, 27*(2), 207–218.

Brown, R. T., Davis, P. C., Lambert, R., Hsu, L., Hopkins, K., & Eckman, J. (2000). Neurocognitive functioning and magnetic resonance imaging in children with sickle cell disease. *Journal of Pediatric Psychology, 25*(7), 503–513.

Brown, R. T., Doepke, K. J., & Kaslow, N. J. (1993). Risk-resistance-adaptation model for pediatric chronic illness: Sickle cell syndrome as an example. *Clinical Psychology Review, 13*(2), 119–132.

Brown, R. T., Kaslow, N. J., Doepke, K., Buchanan, I., Eckman, J., Baldwin, K. et al. (1993). Psychosocial and family functioning in children with sickle cell syndrome and their mothers. *Journal of the American Academy of Child & Adolescent Psychiatry, 32*(3), 545–553.

Brown, R. T., Lambert, R., Devine, D., Casey, R., Doepke, K., Ievers, C. E. et al. (2000). Risk-resistance adaptation model for caregivers and their children with sickle cell syndrome. *Annals of Behavioral Medicine, 22*(2), 158–169.

Brown, R. T., & Roberts, M. C. (2000). Future issues in pediatric psychology: Delphic survey. *Journal of Clinical Psychology in Medical Settings, 7*, 5–15.

Burghardt-Fitzgerald, D. C. (1989). Pain-behavior contracts: Effective management of the adolescent in sickle cell crisis. Journal of Pediatric Nursing, 4, 320–324.

Burlew, A. K., Evans, R., & Oler, C. (1989). The impact of a child with sickle cell syndromes on family dynamics. *Annals of the New York Academy of Sciences, 565*, 161–171.

Burlew, K., Telfair, J., Colangelo, L., & Wright, E. C. (2000). Factors that influence adolescent adaptation to sickle cell disease. *Journal of Pediatric Psychology, 25*(5), 287–299.

Castro, O., Chicoye, L., Greenberg, J., et al. (1994). Brighter horizons for sickle cell disease. *Patient Care, 28*, 26–44.

Chen, E., Cole, S. W., & Kato, P. M. (2004). A review of empirically supported psychosocial interventions for pain and adherence outcomes in sickle cell disease. *Journal of Pediatric Psychology, 29*, 197–209.

Cohen, M. J., Branch, W. B., McKie, V. C., & Adams, R. J. (1997). Neuropsychological impairment sin children with sickle cell anemia and cerbrovascular accidents. *Clinical Pediatrics, 33*, 517–524.

Collins, M., Kaslow, N., Doepke, K., Eckman, J., Johnson, M. (1998). Psychosocial interventions for children and adolescents with sickle cell disease (SCD). *Journal of Black Psychology, 24*, 432–454.

Conner-Warren, R. L. (1996). Pain intensity and home pain management of children with sickle cell disease. *Issues in Comprehensive Pediatric Nursing, 19*(3), 183–195.

Cozzi, L., & Tryon, W. W. (1987). The effectiveness of biofeedback-assisted relaxation in modifying sickle cell crises. *Biofeedback and Self-Regulation, 12*, 51–61.

Dampier, C., Ely, E., Eggleston, B., Brodecki, D., & O'Neal, P. (2004). Physical and cognitive-behavioral activities used in the home management of sickle pain: A daily diary study in children and adolescents. *Pediatric Blood Cancer, 43*, 674–678.

Day, S., Brunson, G., & Wang, W. (1992). A successful education program for parents of infants with newly diagnosed sickle cell disease. *Journal of Pediatric Nursing, 7*, 52–57.

Devine, D., Brown, R. T., Lambert, R., Donegan, J. E., & Eckman, J. (1998). Predictors of psychosocial and cognitive adaptation in children with sickle cell syndromes. *Journal of Clinical Psychology in Medical Settings, 5*(3), 295–313.

Dinges, D. F., Whitehouse, W. G., Orne, E. C., Bloom, P. B., Carlin, M. M., Bauer, N. K., et al. (1997). Self-hypnosis training as an adjunctive treatment in the management of pain associated with sickle cell disease. *The International Journal of Clinical and Experimental Hypnosis, 45*, 417–432.

Driscoll, M. C. (2007). Sickle cell disease. *Pediatrics in Review, 28*, 259–268.

Fallone, G., Acebo, C., Arnedt, J. T., Seifer, R., & Carskadon, M. A. (2001). Effects of acute sleep restriction on behavior, sustained attention, and response inhibition in children. *Perceptual and Motor Skills, 93*, 213–229.

Finkle, R. L., Kellett, J. M., Schatz, J., & Robinson, J. (2002). *Educator's beliefs about learning and adjustment problems in children with sickle cell disease.* Presented at the meeting of the national Sickle Cell Disease Program and Sickle Cell Disease Association of America, Washington, D.C.

Franck, L. S., Treadwell, M., Jacob, E., & Vichinsky, E. (2002). Assessment of sickle cell pain in children and young adults using the adolescent pediatric pain tool. *Journal of Pain and Symptom Management, 23*, 114–120.

Gil, K. M., Anthony, K. K., Carson, J. W., Redding-Lallinger, R., Daeschner, C. W., & Ware, R. E. (2001). Daily coping practice predicts treatment effects in children with sickle cell disease. *Journal of Pediatric Psychology, 26*, 163–173.

Gil, K. M., Carson, J. W., Porter, L. S., Ready, J., Valrie, C., Redding-Lallinger, R. et al. (2003). Daily stress and mood and their association with pain, health care use, and school activity in adolescents with sickle cell disease. *Journal of Pediatric Psychology, 28*(5), 363–373.

Gil, K. M., Porter, L., Ready, J., Workman, E., Sedway, J., & Anthony, K. K. (2000). Pain in children and adolescents with sickle cell disease: An analysis of daily pain diaries. *Children's Health Care, 29*(4), 225–241.

Gil, K. M., Wilson, J. J., Edens, J. L., Workman, E., Ready, Y., Sedway, J., et al. (1997). Cognitive coping skills training in children with sickle cell disease. *International Journal of Behavioral Medicine, 4*, 365–378.

Graumlich, S. E., Powers, S. W., Byars, K. C., Schwarber, L. A., Mitchell, M. J., & Kalinyak, K. A. (2001). Multidimensional assessment of pain in pediatric sickle cell disease. *Journal of Pediatric Psychology, 26*, 203–214.

Grueneich, R., Ris, M. D., Ball, W., Kalinyak, K. A., Noll, R., Vannatta, K. et al. (2004). Relationship of structural magnetic resonance imaging, magnetic resonance perfusion, and other disease factors to neuropsychological outcome in sickle cell disease. *Journal of Pediatric Psychology, 29*(2), 83–92.

Hanson M. D., & Chen E. (2007). Socioeconomic status and health behaviors in adolescence: A review of the literature. *Journal of Behavioral Medicine, 30*(3), 263–285.

Helps, S., Fuggle, P., Udwin, O., & Dick, M. (2003). Psychosocial and neurocognitive aspects of sickle cell disease. *Child and Adolescent Mental Health, 8*(1), 11–17.

Henthorn, J. S., Almeida, A. M., & Davies, S. D. (2004). Neonatal screening for sickle cell disorders. *British Journal of Haematology, 124*, 259–263.

Hoff, A. L., Palermo, T. M., Schluchter, M., Zebracki, K., & Drotar, D. (2006). Longitudinal relationships of depressive symptoms to pain intensity and functional disability among children with disease-related pain. *Journal of Pediatric Psychology, 31*(10), 1046–1056.

Hurtig, A. L. (1994). Relationships in families of children and adolescents with sickle cell disease. In K. Nash (Ed.), *Psychosocial aspects of sickle cell disease* (pp. 161–183). New York: Haworth.

Hurtig, A. L., Koepke, D., & Park, K. B. (1989). Relation between severity of chronic illness and adjustment in children and adolescents with sickle cell disease. *Journal of Pediatric Psychology, 14*(1), 117–132.

Jenerette, C., Funk, M., & Murdaugh, C. (2005). Sickle cell disease: A stigmatizing condition that may lead to depression. *Issues in Mental Health Nursing, 26*(10), 1081–1101.

Kaslow, N. J., Collins, M. H., Loundy, M. R., Brown, F., Hollins, L. D., & Eckman, J. (1997). Empirically validated family interventions for pediatric psychology: Sickle cell disease as an exemplar. *Journal of Pediatric Psychology, 22*, 213–227.

Kaslow, N. J., Collins, M. H., Rashid, F. L., Baskin, M. L., Griffith, J. R., Hollins, L., et al. (2000). The efficacy of a pilot family psychoeducational intervention for pediatric sickle cell disease (SCD). *Families, Systems, and Health, 18*, 381–404.

Kell, R. S., Kliewer, W., Erikson, M. T., & Ohene-Frempong, K. (1998). Psychological adjustment of adolescents with sickle cell disease: relations with demographic, medical, and family competence variables. *Journal of Pediatric Psychology, 23*(5), 301–312.

King, A. A., Tang, S., Ferguson, K. L., & DeBaun, M. R. (2005). An education program to increase teacher knowledge about sickle cell disease. *Journal of School Health, 75*, 11–14.

Koontz, K., Short, A. D., Kalinyak, K., & Noll, R. B. (2004). A randomized, controlled pilot trial of a school intervention for children with sickle cell anemia. *Journal of Pediatric Psychology, 29*(1), 7–17.

Kral, M. C., Brown, R. T., & Hynd, G. W. (2001). Neuropsychological aspects of pediatric sickle cell disease. *Neuropsychology Review, 11*(4), 179–196.

Lane, P. A., Buchanan, G. R., Hutter, J. J., Austin, R. F., Britton, H. A., Rogers, Z. R., et al. (2001). Sickle cell disease in children and adolescents: diagnosis, guidelines for comprehensive care, and care paths and protocols for management of acute and chronic complications. Annual Meeting of the Sickle Cell Disease Care Consortium, Sedona, AZ.

Lemanek, K. L., Ranalli, M. A., Green, K., Biega, C., & Lupia, C. (2003). Diseases of the blood: sickle cell disease and hemophilia. In M. C. Roberts (Ed.), *Handbook of pediatric psychology* (3rd ed., pp. 321–341). New York: Guilford.

List, T., Wahlund, K., Wenneberg, B., & Dworkin S. F. (1999). TMD in children and adolescents: Prevalence of pain, gender differences, and perceived treatment need. *Journal of Orofacial Pain, 13*(1), 9–20.

McGrath, P. A. (1990). *Pain in children: Nature, assessment, and treatment*. New York: Guilford.

Meijer, S. A., Sinnema, G., Bijstra, J. O., Mellenbergh, G. J., & Wolters, W. H. (2002). Coping styles and locus of control as predictors for psychological adjustment of adolescents with a chronic illness. *Social Science & Medicine, 54*(9), 1453–1461.

Nagal, R. L. (1994). Origins and dispersion of the sickle cell gene. (pp. 353–380). In S. H. Embury, R. P. Hebbel, N. Mohandas, & M. H. Steinberg (Eds.) *Sickle cell diseases: Basic principles and clinical practice*. Raven Press, New York.

Nicolaou, D. C., & Barakat, L. P. (2004). *Measurement of Quality of Life of Two Pediatric Chronic Illness Groups: Brain Tumors and Sickle Cell Disease*. Poster presented at the Society of Pediatric Psychology Conference on Child Health Psychology, Charleston, SC.

Noll, R. B., Stith, L. Gartstein, M. A., Ris, M. D., Grueneich R., Vannatta, K. et al. (2001). Neuropsychological functioning of youths with sickle cell disease: comparison with non-chronically ill peers. *Journal of Pediatric Psychology, 26*(2), 69–78.

Noll, R. B., Vannatta, K., Koontz, K., Kalinyak, K., Bukowski, W. M., & Davis, H. (1996). Peer relationships and emotional well-being of youngsters with sickle cell disease. *Child Development, 67*(2), 423–436.

Palermo, T. M. (2000). Impact of recurrent and chronic pain on child and family daily functioning: A critical review of the literature. *Journal of Developmental & Behavioral Pediatrics, 21*(1), 58–69.

Palermo, T. M., Schwartz, L., Drotar, D., & McGowan, K. (2002). Parental report of health related quality of life in children with sickle cell disease. *Journal of Behavioral Medicine*, 25, 269–283.

Palermo, T. M., Witherspoon, D., Valenzuela, D., & Drotar, D. D. (2004). Development and validation of the child activity limitations interview: A measure of pain-related functional impairment in school-age children and adolescents. *Pain 109*, 461–470.

Palmer, D. L., Berg, C. A., Wiebe, D. J., Beveridge, R. M., Korbel, C. D., Upchurch, R. et al. (2004). The role of autonomy and pubertal status in understanding age differences in maternal involvement in diabetes responsibility across adolescence. *Journal of Pediatric Psychology, 29*(1), 35–46.

Panepinto, J. A., O'Mahar, K., Debaun, M. R., Rennie, K., & Scott, J. P. (2004). Validity of the Child Health Questionnaire for use in children with sickle cell disease. *Journal of Pediatric Hematology/Oncology, 26*, 574–578.

Pidgeon, V. (1989). Compliance with chronic illness regimens: School-aged children and adolescents. *Journal of Pediatric Nursing, 4*(1), 36–47.

Pinckney, R. B., & Stuart, G. W. (2004). Adjustment difficulties of adolescents with sickle cell disease. *Journal of Child and Adolescent Psychiatric Nursing, 16*(4), 5–12.

Platt, O. S., Brambilla, D. J., Rosse, W. F., Milner, P. D., Castro, W., Steinberg, M. H. et al. (1994). Mortality in sickle cell disease: Life expectancy and risk factors for early death. *New England Journal of Medicine, 330*, 1639–1644.

Potter, P. C., & Roberts, M. C. (1984). Children's perceptions of chronic illness: The roles of disease symptoms, cognitive development, and information. *Journal of Pediatric Psychology, 9*, 13–27.

Powars, D. R. & Johnson, C. S. (1996). Priapism. *Hematology Oncology Clinics of North America, 10*, 1363–1372.

Powars, D. Wilson, B., Imbus, C., Pegelow, C., & Allen, J. (1978). The natural history of stroke in sickle cell disease. *American Journal of Medicine, 65*, 461–471.

Powers, S. W., Mitchell, M. J., Graumlich, S. E., Byars, K. C., & Kalinyak, K. A. (2002). Longitudinal assessment of pain, coping, and daily functioning in children with sickle cell disease receiving pain management skills training. *Journal of Clinical Psychology in Medical Settings, 9*, 109–119.

Radcliffe, J., Barakat, L. P., & Boyd, R. (2006). Family issues. In R. T. Brown (Ed.), *Comprehensive handbook of childhood cancer and sickle cell disease: A biopsychosocial approach* (pp. 496–513). New York: Oxford.

Rae, W. A., & Frankel, L. (1998). A school reentry program for chronically ill children. Journal of School Psychology, 36, 261–279.

Rees, D. C., Olujohungbe, A. D., Parker, N. E., Stephens, A. D., Telfer, P., & Write, J. (2003). Guidelines for the management of the acute painful crisis in sickle cell disease. *British Journal of Haematology, 120*, 744–752.

Ritchie, M. A. (2001). Self-esteem and hopefulness in adolescents with cancer. *Journal of Pediatric Nursing, 16*(1), 35–42.

Roth-Isigkeit, A., Thyen, U., Stoven, H., Schwarzenberger, J., & Schmucker, P. (2005). Pain among children and adolescents: Restrictions in daily living and triggering factors. *Pediatrics, 115*, 152–162.

Sallfors, C., Hallberg, L. R., & Fasth, A. (2003). Gender and age differences in pain, coping and health status among children with chronic arthritis. *Clinical & Experimental Rheumatology, 21*(6), 785–793.

Savedra, M. C., Tesler, M. D., Holzemer, W. L., & Ward, J. A. (1989). *Adolescent pediatric pain tool (APPT) preliminary user's manual.* San Francisco: University of California.

Schatz, J. (2004). Brief report: Academic attainment in children with sickle cell disease. *Journal of Pediatric Psychology, 29*(8), 627–633.

Schatz, J., Brown, R. T., Pascual, J. M., Hsu, L., & DeBaun, M. R. (2001). Poor school and cognitive functioning with silent cerebral infarcts and sickle cell disease. *Neurology, 56*, 1109–1111.

Schatz, J., Finke, R. L., Kellett, J. M., & Kramer, J. H. (2002). Cognitive functioning in children with sickle cell disease: a meta-analysis. *Journal of Pediatric Psychology, 27*(8), 739–748.

Schatz, J., Finke, R. L., & Roberts, C. W. (2004). Interactions of biomedical and environmental risk factors for cognitive development: A preliminary study of sickle cell disease. *Journal of Developmental & Behavioral Pediatrics, 25*(5), 303–310.

Schwartz, L. A., Radcliffe, J., & Barakat, L. P. (2007). The development of a culturally sensitive pediatric pain management intervention for African American adolescents with sickle cell disease. *Children's Health Care, 36*, 267–283.

Serjeant, G. (1997). Sickle cell disease. *Lancet, 350*, 725–730.

Shapiro, B. S., Dinges, D. F., Orne, E. C., Bauer, N., Reilly, L. B., Whitehouse, W. G. et al. (1995). Home management of sickle cell-related pain in children and adolescents: Natural history and impact on school attendance. *Pain, 61*(1), 139–144.

Taras, H., & Potts-Datema, W. (2005). Chronic health conditions and student performance at school. *Journal of School Health, 75*(7), 255–266.

Tarazi, R. A., Grant, M. L., Ely, E., & Barakat, L. P. (2007). Neuropsychological functioning in preschool age children with sickle cell disease: the role of illness-related and psychosocial factors. *Child Neuropsychology, 13*(2), 155–172.

Telfair, J., Alexander, L. R., Loosier, P. S., Alleman-Velez, P. L., & Simmons, J. (2004). Providers' perspectives and beliefs regarding transition to adult care for adolescents with sickle cell disease. *Journal of Health Care for the Poor and Underserved, 15*, 443–461.

Thomas, V. J., Dixon, A. L., & Miligan, P. (1999). Cognitive-behavioral therapy for the management of sickle cell disease pain: An evaluation of a community-based intervention. *British Journal of Health Psychology, 4*, 209–229.

Treadwell, M. J., & Gil, K. M. (1994). Psychosocial aspects. In S. H. Embury, R. P. Hebbel, N. Mohandas, & M. H. Steinberg (Eds.), *Sickle cell disease: Basic principles and clinical practice* (pp.517–529). New York: Raven Press.

Tucker, L., & Cabral, D. (2005). Transition of the adolescent patient with rheumatic disease: Issues to consider. *Pediatric Clinics of North America, 52*(2), 641–652.

Valrie, C. R., Gil, K. M., Redding-Lallinger, R., & Daeshcner, C. (2007). Brief report: Sleep in children with sickle cell disease: An analysis of daily diaries utilizing multilevel models. *Journal of Pediatric Psychology, 32*(7), 857–861.

Varni, J., & Thompson, K. (1985). *The Varni-Thompson pediatric pain questionnaire.* Unpublished manuscript.

Vichinsky, E. P., Johnson, R., & Lubin, B. (1982). Multidisciplinary approach to pain management in sickle cell disease. *American Journal of Pediatric Hematology/Oncology, 4*, 328–333.

Vichinsky, E. P., Styles, L. A., Colangelo, L. H., Wright, E. C.; Castro, O.; Nickerson, B. (1997). Acute chest syndrome in sickle cell disease: Clinical presentation and course: Cooperative study of sickle cell disease. *Blood, 89*, 1787–1792.

Vitulano, L. A. (2003). Psychosocial issues for children and adolescents with chronic illness: Self-esteem, school functioning, and sport participation. *Child and Adolescent Psychiatric Clinics of North America, 12*(3), 585–592.

Wagner, J. L., Connelly, M., Brown, R. T., Taylor, L. C., Rittle, C., & Wall-Cloues, B. (2004). Predictors of social anxiety in children and adolescents with sickle cell disease. *Journal of Clinical Psychology in Medical Settings, 11*(4), 243–252.

Walco, G. A., & Dampier, C. D. (1990). Pain in children and adolescents with sickle cell disease: A descriptive study. *Journal of Pediatric Psychology, 15*, 643–658.

Wang, W., Enos, L., Gallagher, D., Thompson, R., Guarini, L., Vichinsky, E. et al. (2001). Cooperative study of sickle cell disease. Neuropsychologic performance in school-aged children with sickle cell disease: a report from the cooperative study of sickle cell disease. *Journal of Pediatrics, 139*(3), 391–397.

Williams, H. A. (1993). A comparison of social support and social networks of black parents and white parents with chronically ill children. *Social Science and Medicine, 37*(12), 1509–1520.

Worchel-Prevatt, F. F., Heffer, R. W., Prevatt, B. C., Miner, J., Young-Saleme, T., Horgan, D. et al. (1998). *Journal of School Psychology, 36*(3), 261–279.

Yaster, M., Kost-Byerly, S., & Maxwell, L. G. (2000). The management of pain in sickle cell disease. *Pediatric Clinics of North America, 47* (3), 699–710.

Zeltzer, L. K., Bush, J. P., Chen, E., & Riveral, A. (1997). A psychobiologic approach to pediatric pain: Part II. Prevention and treatment. *Current Problems in Pediatrics, 27*, 261–292.

Zeltzer, L. K., Dash, J., & Holland, J. P. (1979). Hypnotically induced pain control in sickle cell anemia. *Pediatrics, 64*, 533–536.

Inflammatory Bowel Disease

Carin Cunningham and Rachel Neff Greenley

Inflammatory Bowel Disease

Inflammatory bowel disease (IBD) is a chronic relapsing condition of inflammation of the digestive tract, characterized by periods of active disease alternating with periods of disease remission. IBD is diagnosed in adolescence at a rate of 25–30% (Cuffari & Darbari, 2002) and uniquely impacts the typical biological, psychological, social, and cognitive changes of adolescence, as well as the process of autonomy development.

IBD includes three diagnostic categories: Crohn's disease (CD), ulcerative colitis (UC), and indeterminate colitis (IC). In CD, inflammation can occur anywhere in the digestive tract from the mouth to the skin surrounding the anus and involves mucosal inflammation. In UC, the inflammation is restricted to the large colon and to the inner lining of the large intestine, mucosal wall. A diagnosis of IC is given until the disease has evolved and a differentiation can be made (Rice & Chuang, 1999). In 2007, a consensus conference was held to standardize the diagnosis and classification of pediatric IBD. An algorithm was created to aid clinicians in reliably differentiating childhood UC from CD, thereby reducing variability among practitioners in how the terms are used (ESPGHAN, 2005).

IBD is often confused with irritable bowel syndrome (IBS), a functional gastrointestinal (GI) disorder, because they have certain common symptoms (e.g., abdominal pain, changes in bowel habits, cramping, and fatigue). However, there are distinct differences between these diagnoses: IBS does not cause bowel inflammation and to date no structural or metabolic abnormalities can explain IBS symptoms (Rasquin-Weber et al., 1999).

Epidemiology

The incidence of IBD is bimodal with the first peak occurring during the first to second decades of life and the second rise reported between the fifth to seventh decades (Mamula, Markowitz, & Baldassano, 2003). Kugathasan et al. (2003) found a twofold predominance in pediatric CD incidence in comparison to the incidence of UC, a significantly higher rate of CD diagnosis among boys compared to girls, a low frequency of patients with positive family histories, no regulatory impact of urbanization on pediatric IBD, and an equal distribution of IBD incidence across ethnicities. The number of patients who are diagnosed with IC is increasing (Cuffari & Darbari, 2002) and now accounts for approximately 15% of the cases that present as colitis (King, 2003).

The incidence of IBD is increasing worldwide (Carvalho & Hyams, 2007). Population-based studies indicate that IBD is unevenly distributed throughout the world, with the highest rates occurring in first-world, Westernized countries (Pappa, Semrin, Walker, & Grand, 2004). However, recent studies from Lebanon and China document a rising prevalence of IBD in these developing countries

C. Cunningham (✉)
Case Western Reserve School of Medicine, Cleveland, OH, USA
e-mail: carin.cunningham@case.edu

W.T. O'Donohue, L.W. Tolle (eds.), *Behavioral Approaches to Chronic Disease in Adolescence*,
DOI 10.1007/978-0-387-87687-0_20, © Springer Science+Business Media, LLC 2009

(Abdul-baki, 2007; Jiang et al., 2006). Approximately 1.1 million people in the United States have IBD (Loftus, et al., 2007), over 100,000 of whom are children and adolescents (Carvalho & Hyams, 2007). Kappelman et al. (2007) determined the prevalence of CD and UC in a large national sample via insurance claim examination. Results indicated a prevalence of 43 per 100,000 for CD and 28 per 100,000 for UC. The prevalence of both conditions was lower in the South, compared with the Midwest and West, and IBD appears to be more common in commercially insured individuals, compared with those insured by Medicaid. Americans of Jewish ancestry have an incidence rate three times higher than the national average (Heyman et al., 2005).

Disease Course

For most adolescents, the disease course of IBD is one of unpredictable exacerbation and remission. About 40–50% of youth with CD will relapse in the first year after the induction of disease remission (Ballinger, 2000). Only 1% will never relapse after diagnosis and initial therapy. Similarly, 70% of children with UC will enter remission within 3 months following initial therapy, and approximately 50% will remain in remission over the next year. Colectomy (removal of the colon) is curative for UC. It is required within 5 years in up to 26% of children presenting with severe disease compared with 10% of those with mild disease. A recent study of 99 children diagnosed with UC reported that in comparison to adults with UC, they were more likely to have worse symptoms and complications (Griffiths, 2008).

There is an increased risk of developing colorectal cancer in patients with long-standing UC; a rate of (3.7% of patients with UC). However, it is fivefold higher than the rate of colorectal cancer in the general population (www.ccfa.org) Patients with long-standing colonic CD have been reported to have a colon cancer risk similar to UC patients. Duration of the colitis (especially >10 years) and the extent of the colitis (pancolitis>left-sided colitis> proctitus) are the two most critical risk factors for adenocarcinoma (Hyams, 2000).

Etiology

The exact etiology of IBD is unknown. Current research proposes a multifactorial cause: the pathogenesis of IBD proceeds from a genetic predisposition coupled with specific triggers (bacteria and viruses) that interact with the body's immune system and trigger the disease (Kim & Ferry, 2004). Evidence for a genetic basis includes family aggregation studies and twin studies: a person with a relative with IBD has a risk 10–15% times greater than that of the general population for developing IBD (Achkar, 2007). Two genes are involved in the regulation of immunity and inflammation: *Nod2* (Cuffari & Darbari, 2002) and *IL23R* gene on chromosome 1p31 (Duerr et al., 2006).

The increasing incidence of CD has led to the speculation about changes in exposure to environmental or infectious agents. While attention has focused on the role of measles infection and/or vaccination in the pathogenesis of CD and UC, the World Health Organization has reported no direct correlation between measles virus or vaccines and IBD (Afzal et al., 1998). There is also no data to support diet or psychological factors as a cause of IBD (Bremner & Beattie, 2002).

Symptoms

IBD symptoms vary in frequency and severity and often interfere with daily functioning. In adolescents, the range of symptoms and the presenting signs of IBD are broad and often subtle. Poor growth and delayed sexual maturation may dominate the early clinical picture and are developmental issues unique to pediatric IBD (Mamula, Markowitz, & Baldassano, 2003). Growth delay, which is more common in CD than UC, is hypothesized to be secondary to inflammation, nutrient malabsorption, and undernutrition (Pappas, 2003). The combination of decreased intake and increased metabolic demands presents an especially large burden for the body of an adolescent with IBD. By the time most adolescents are diagnosed with IBD, they are already malnourished. When IBD is active during a critical period of growth such as adolescence, it is difficult to compensate for the increased demands with oral intake alone. Abnormalities in linear growth are a common presenting sign of CD. A fall in height velocity may also be the first indication of disease relapse and may be accompanied by only minor GI symptoms (Ballinger, 2000). In addition to growth delay, diarrhea, occasionally bloody, is seen in 50% of patients who have CD. Symptoms of CD may also include abdominal pain, rectal bleeding, rectal urgency, abdominal cramps, fever, weight loss, fistulas (abnormal connections between an organ, a vessel, or an intestine and another structure), abscesses (localized collection of pus in a cavity), and strictures (fibrous scar tissues which contract over time). Patients diagnosed with UC generally present with bloody diarrhea, rectal bleeding, rectal urgency, abdominal cramps, and fever. A diagnosis is typically made within 6 months of symptom onset (Cuffari & Darbari, 2002). Fever occurs in UC only in the presence of fulminant disease (severe disease which occurs suddenly), whereas in CD, fever may occur in the absence of severe GI symptoms (Hyams, 2000). Abdominal pain in patients with UC is usually limited to the predefecatory period.

Adolescents with IBD may also present with extra intestinal symptoms which can include mouth sores, back pain, joint complaints, and anemia and which vary from case to case. Up to 35% of pediatric IBD patients have at least one extra intestinal manifestation as a presenting sign (Mamula, Markowitz, & Baldassano, 2003). When the presenting symptoms consist mainly of extraintestinal manifestations such as anorexia, back pain, fatigue, anemia, and joint pain, making a diagnosis can be particularly difficult and it is often delayed. The mean time to diagnosis of CD in children is between 7 and 11 months, in UC between 5 and 8 months, and in IC 14 months (Mamula, Markowitz, & Baldassano, 2003).

Treatment

Management of adolescents with IBD can include pharmacologic, nutritional, and surgical interventions. Medical treatment goals include controlling the inflammatory process while minimizing medication side effects, providing adequate nutrition to promote growth, and facilitating patient participation in age-appropriate activities (Baldassano & Piccoli, 1999).

Pharmacological therapy varies by individual but may include one or more of the following categories of medications: aminosalicylates, corticosteroids, immunomodulators, antibiotics, and biological agents (infliximab). Medications focus on reducing inflammation, reducing GI bacteria, and immunosuppression and may be delivered by oral, rectal, topical, or intravenous delivery modalities. Corticosteroids are typically used only in the short term, given the significant side effects of long-term use including growth suppression, cataracts, glaucoma, osteoporosis, hypertension, and avascular necrosis. For adolescents, cosmetic side effects of corticosteroids [e.g., acne, cushingoid features (moon-shaped face due to bloating and swelling) define, weight gain, hirsutism, and striae] can offset the potential physical benefit that they provide (Banez & Cunningham, 2003). New biologic therapies target specific areas in the inflammatory process as opposed to the broad-based immunosuppressive approach of some older medications, and recent studies have shown encouraging results (Kugathasan & Werlin, 1999).

The goals of nutritional therapy are to correct nutritional deficiencies due to reduced appetite, poor absorption, and diarrhea and to promote catch-up growth. Nutritional therapy can include dietary modification, nutritional supplementation, and total parenteral nutrition (TPN) therapy. Nutritional therapy can be supplemental or the primary therapy.

Surgical treatment is necessary when (a) medication cannot control the symptoms; (b) there is an intestinal obstruction; or (c) there are other complications. More than one-third of pediatric IBD patients will require surgery within 20 years of diagnosis (Langholz, Munkholm, Krasilinikoff, & Binder, 1998). In CD, the inflamed part of the intestine is removed (resection), and the two ends of the healthy bowel are joined together (anastomoses). This surgery may provide symptom-free years; however, it is not curative because the disease can recur in other parts of the intestinal tract. Surgery for patients with UC is curative and it is now standard to perform sphincter-saving operations in patients with UC for whom medical therapy has been unsuccessful (Pappas, 2004). The need for and the timing of colectomy in adolescents are determined by weighing response to medical therapy, risks of growth impairment, and ultimate cancer risk against the prospects of surgical cure and potential adverse effects after surgery.

Treatment Costs and Insurance Issues

The medical costs of IBD in the United States have been reported as $1.4–1.8 billon dollars annually (www.ccfa.org/about/press/ibdfacts). Feagan, Vreeland, Larson, and Bala (2000) estimated the average annual charges for patients with CD as approximately $12,417. For pediatric and adolescent patients with IBD, the costs of missed work for parents and transportation costs also need to be taken into account. Medications can be a major expense. For example, an infliximab infusion costs approximately $2000 per patient (Kay & Wylie, 2001) and is not covered by all insurance plans. Insurance issues are often problematic for families with a patient with IBD. Many policies have a "pre-existing condition" clause which prevents pediatric patients from obtaining coverage should their parent's insurance carrier change. For young adults, obtaining their own insurance is often difficult as they transition to adult GI care. Finally, some medications may not be covered by a specific insurance policy or because they are deemed "experimental." Thus, some families may be forced to pay out of pocket and those who cannot afford to do so may receive the medication inconsistently or not at all.

Common Concerns Among Adolescents with IBD and Their Families

A number of issues unique to the diagnosis of IBD may contribute to additional stress for patients and families including the delay in diagnosis, the unpredictability of the illness course, the unknown etiology, the embarrassment of "bathroom-related" symptoms, the variability of the treatment regimens, and the idiosyncratic responses of patients to medications.

Depressive and Anxiety Symptoms

Rates of depressive and anxiety disorders in children and adolescents with IBD vary, with studies estimating prevalence rates at 25–60% among those with long-standing illness (Burke et. al., 1989; Engstrom & Lindquist, 1991) and 14–28% among those who have been recently diagnosed (Burke et al., 1994). Rates of internalizing symptoms (e.g., anxiety and depression) among youth with IBD have been found to be higher than among youth with cystic fibrosis (Burke et al., 1989) and healthy comparison groups (Engstrom, 1999; Mackner et al., 2006), but to be comparable to youth with chronic headaches or diabetes (Engstrom, 1999). Gold, Issenman, Roberts, and Watt (2000) reported lower rates of depressive symptoms among a sample of youth with IBD in comparison to a matched sample of youth with functional GI complaints. One study suggested no differences between youth with IBD and youth with CF in rates of anxiety disorders (Burke et al., 1989).

Results of certain studies are equivocal due to small sample sizes, lack of reliability checks for diagnoses, and cross-sectional designs. Studies utilizing larger samples report a lower incidence of psychiatric disorders (e.g., Mackner et al., 2006).

Correlates of Depression and Anxiety

Several factors have been associated with internalizing symptoms among youth with IBD. Regarding treatment regimen factors, although Akobeng et al. (1999) found that adolescents with IBD who were taking steroids exhibited more depressive symptoms than those who were not, Szigethy et al. (2004) failed to find an association between depressive symptoms and current steroid dose, steroid duration, or total steroid dose. Simlarly, Burke, Kocoshis, Chandra, Whiteway, and Sauer (1990) found that children who were more depressed were less likely to have been prescribed steroids. Finally, Burke et al. (1990) found that depressed children were less severely ill than were nondepressed youth. In contrast, Ondersma, Lumley, Corlis, Tojek, and Tolia (1997) found that greater subjective illness severity was associated with more negative affectivity but emotional symptoms were not associated with objective findings (e.g., lab values). Regarding individual factors, Szigethy et al. (2004) found that later age of diagnosis was associated with greater depressive symptoms; however, overall age was not significantly associated with depressive symptoms. Regarding family factors, greater parental depression, greater frequency of stressful life events, lower family cohesion, and higher family conflict have all been associated with more depressive symptoms (Burke et al., 1989; Szigethy et al., 2004).

Social and School Functioning

IBD has a significant impact on adolescent social functioning because symptoms and treatment regimen demands often interfere with daily functioning. The developmental tasks of adolescence include biological changes related to puberty, social development of a peer network, cognitive changes, and the development of independence from the family unit may all be affected by the diagnosis of IBD. Adolescence is a time when physical appearance and not looking "different" from peers assumes significant importance. Many adolescents with IBD experience a decrease or cessation in linear growth, slowed development of bones, and delayed sexual maturation, at a time when being and looking different from their peers is a particularly sensitive issue (Mamula, Markowitz, & Baldassano, 2003).

Development of social skills which typically occurs in the context of school or extracurricular activities for adolescents may be adversely affected by school avoidance due to pain, medication side effects, or fears of being teased. Moreover, an adolescent's daily routine is affected due to increased doctor's visits, painful procedures, medications and dietary restrictions, leaving less time for social interactions. Adolescents with IBD may be embarrassed regarding bathroom-related issues and hesitant to engage in social interactions because of possible rectal urgency or other GI symptoms. Using a validated measure of social competence, Mackner & Crandall (2007) found that in comparison to healthy children, youth with IBD had fewer close friends and participated in fewer organized activities. Similarly, Moody, Eaden, and Mayberry (1999) reported patients with IBD had a decrease in sports-related activities and problems interacting with peers due to their illness. Parents of children with IBD reported more clinically significant problems in youth social competence as compared to parents of healthy children Mackner et al., 2006). MacPhee, Hoffenberg, and Feranchak (1988) reported that adolescents with IBD were more likely to rely on their families as a support system than their peers, suggesting a potential developmental lag in social skills.

School-related concerns have been documented among youth with IBD. Ferguson, Sedgewick, and Drummond (1994) found that young adults with juvenile-onset IBD reported increased school absences, interference with exams, and problems pursuing higher education. Moody et al. (1999) reported that 66% of patients aged 6–17 had problems with school attendance, with the majority reporting academic underachievement due to their IBD. Akobeng et al. (1999) found that children with CD missed more school and participated in fewer peer-related activities.

Correlates of Social and School Functioning

Little research has focused on correlates of social functioning. However, findings from one study suggested that the timing of diagnosis was associated with decreased social functioning in adolescents. Participants who were diagnosed with IBD during adolescence had significantly lower social competence scores than those diagnosed in childhood (Mackner & Crandall, 2007)with scores clinically significant in 35% of patients diagnosed in adolescence as compared to 5% diagnosed in childhood.

Health-Related Quality of Life (HRQOL)

In the context of pediatric IBD, focus has been on both disease-specific and generic HRQOL measures. Initial studies of HRQOL reported that 31–50% of children reported limitations in social functioning (Rabbett et al., 1996) and concerns about weight gain, flare-ups in their condition, and school absenteeism (Akobeng, Mirajkar, et al., 1999; Griffiths et al., 1999). However, these studies were limited by small sample sizes and the use of nonvalidated instruments. More recent HRQOL studies have addressed many of these methodological issues and have provided mixed results. Loonen, Derkx, Koopman, and Heymans (2002) found no significant differences in HRQOL (via a generic measure) between younger children with IBD in comparison to a healthy control group. However, adolescents with IBD reported a significantly lower HRQOL in four domains HR including motor functioning, bodily complaints, autonomy, and negative emotion (Loonen, Grootenhuis, Last, Koopman, & Derkx, 2002). In another study, lower HRQOL was reported by adolescent patients with IBD than a comparison group of healthy children (De Boer, Grootenhuis, Derkx, & Last, B. (2005). The results indicated that adolescents with IBD, specifically boys, have a significantly lower HRQOL compared with healthy peers. Cunningham, Drotar, Palermo, McGowan, and Arendt (2007) using a standardized measure of HRQOL and a matched comparison group, found that children and adolescents reported worse HRQOL than physically healthy children in one domain: general health. Otley et al. (2002) conducted a large prospective study using the IMPACT, a disease-specific measure of HRQOL which found significant improvement in HRQOL during the first year following diagnosis.

Correlates of Youth HRQOL

Correlates of HRQOL have been identified in the literature. Cunningham et al. (2007) documented that youth with more frequent symptoms and greater steroidal side effects had greater limitations in HRQOL. Similarly, Otley et al. (2002) documented improvements in HRQOL during the first year following diagnosis and identified an association between disease activity and HRQOL: patients with increasing disease severity reported worse HRQOL. Regarding individual psychosocial functioning, higher self-esteem (DeBoer et al., 205) and use of positive coping strategies (e.g., having positive expectations about the disease) (H.J. van der Zaag-Loonen et al., 2004) has been associated with higher HRQOL. Finally, male gender and older age have been associated with lower HRQOL (DeBoer et al., 2005; Otley et al., 2002).

Adherence to Treatment Regimen

Promoting adherence to treatment is challenging among adolescents with IBD. Since medications must be taken continuously to maintain remission and because even when medications are taken as prescribed, the chance of relapse is high, the benefits of taking medication may not be immediately observable to all adolescents. In addition, the side effects of medications as well as the socially embarrassing nature of IBD pose additional barriers to adherence. Three published studies of adherence to treatment exist, which have all focused on oral medication adherence. Mackner & Crandall (2005) utilizing a structured interview to assess oral medication adherence among 50 preadolescents and adolescents with IBD found that 38% of parents and 48% of children reported perfect adherence to IBD medications. Similarly, Hommel, Davis, and Baldassano (2008) reported high rates of adherence (93–97%) based on patient self-report. Oliva-Hemker, Abadom, Cuffari, and Thompson (2007) reported adherence rates of 34–50% from pharmacy refill records depending upon the medication. Finally, Hommel et al. (2008) found lower adherence rates via pill counts: 52–63% depending upon the medication.

Correlates of Adherence

Individual factors such as less optimal coping strategies (e.g., fantasy-based strategies) and lower patient-perceived physical HRQOL have been associated with lower levels of adherence (Mackner & Crandall, 2005; Hommel et al., 2008). Unexpectedly, Hommel et al. (2008) also found a relationship between poorer social functioning and greater 5-ASA adherence. The authors speculated that the increased burden of the 5-ASA regimen (multiple daily doses and multiple pills at each time) may interfere with youth social activities. Finally, Oliva-Hemker et al. (2007) found that patients with greater disease activity were more likely to be adherent.

Family Functioning

IBD requires attention to daily treatment regimen and ongoing symptom monitoring and creates added demands for the family. The significant effects on the family have been reported in a number of studies (Akobeng et al., 1999; Engström, 1992; Miller, 1997).

Parental Distress

A number of studies have examined maternal functioning in the context of having a child diagnosed with IBD. Engstrom (1999) found that mothers of children with IBD reported more family dysfunction than mothers of healthy children or those with diabetes; they also endorsed more psychiatric symptoms on the Symptom Checklist-90 than mothers of healthy children. Burke et al. (1994) reported that 51% of mothers of children with IBD had a history of depression and 10% had a current diagnosis of depression, similar to the rates of mothers of children with CF. Data which focus on the functioning of fathers of youth with IBD are limited and anecdotal.

Parent QOL

Parent QOL is an important area of consideration given the role stain and added stress that parents of youth with chronic medical conditions may experience (Quittner, Davis, & Modi, 2003). Parents of adolescents with IBD reported worries regarding their child's medication, including the side effects, school absenteeism, and future plans (Akobeng et al., 1999; Miller et al., 1999; Rabett et al., 1996). Caregivers of children and adolescents with IBD reported that they experienced more emotional worry, greater impact on their personal time compared to caregivers reporting on healthy same-age children, a decrease in social activities, and changes in financial resources in the context of pediatric IBD (Engstrom, 1992; Cunningham, 2002; Cunningham et al., 2007). Using a validated QOL measure, Greenley and Cunningham (2008) reported that parents of children and adolescents with IBD evidenced higher QOL in five of eight domains when compared to a US normative population. However, greater youth disease activity and poorer youth QoL predicted lower parent QoL, suggesting a subset of parents may be at risk for impaired QoL.

Sibling Adjustment

Studies have documented that the healthy siblings of patients with IBD may be impacted by a diagnosis of IBD; however, much of this work has been descriptive in nature and has not utilized validated measures or comparison groups. Siblings of patients with IBD have reported concerns about their parents keeping them uninformed about the illness, their sibling being teased at school, and their sibling needing to be hospitalized (Akobeng et al., 1999; Miller, 1997). Wood et al. (1987) found that siblings of children with CD had higher scores on an unspecified scale of the CBCL than did the siblings of children with UC.

Correlates of Family Functioning

Difficulties with family and parent functioning have been shown to be associated with more severe disease, more bowel movements, increased pain, youth fatigue, and a greater number of behavioral and emotional symptoms (Tojek, 2002; Burke et al., 1990; Greenely & Cunningham, 2008).

Best Practices for Assessment

Recent focus has been given to evidence-based assessment in pediatric psychology (Cohen et al., 2008), given that the use of measures with sound psychometric characteristics is the critical "first step" in effective treatment. Yet assessment measures specific to IBD in youth are lacking with the exception of one measure for HRQOL, the IMPACT SCALE (Otley et al., 2002). Given the lack of disease specific measures and limited research in the area, much of what is known about assessment strategies is based on clinical anecdote.

Adolescents with IBD tend to underreport their problems and they do not want to be reminded of having IBD when feeling well (DeBoer et al., 2005; Cunningham, 2002). Clinical assessment of the following issues may facilitate adjustment to the illness (Banez & Cunningham, 2003).

1. **Knowledge of IBD**. Assessment of youth and parent knowledge of IBD is important to identify areas in which education is warranted. We recommend that knowledge assessment be an "ongoing process" beginning at the time of diagnosis. Helpful assessment questions include the following: What is the teen's/parent's understanding of IBD? What is the teen's/ parent's understanding of the cause of IBD? Does the family understand the proposed treatment regimen, including possible side effects of the medications? What are their biggest fears about having IBD? Do they think that IBD is life threatening?
2. **Adolescent Psychological functioning.** Given that adolescents with IBD may be at risk for impairments in psychosocial functioning, assessment in this domain is warranted at diagnosis and throughout the course of their illness. Since no IBD disease-specific measures exist, we recommend that clinicians select evidence-based measures as outlined by Holmbeck et al. (2008) such as Children's Depression Inventory (Kovacs, 1985) and Children's Global Assessment Scale (Shaffer et al., 1983)which have been used in pediatric IBD research and are well-established assessment methods. A clinical interview with the patient and family can also yield important information.
3. **Adolescent Social and school functioning.** Key domains for the assessment of social functioning should include consideration of the following: Are their friends aware of their having IBD? Does having IBD interfere with socializing with their peers? Are there activity limitations because of IBD symptoms or concerns? Regarding school functioning, it is important to assess whether or not the adolescent has a 504 plan to help with special needs (e.g., bathroom privileges, need to take medicine during the day, or to rest between classes), if the adolescent has missed school days or had to repeat a grade because of IBD-related symptoms, and whether or not the adolescent is able to participate in the full academic schedule given their current symptoms.
4. **Body Image and Concerns.** Little research has examined body image concerns among adolescents with IBD, but given the importance of physical appearance during adolescence, clinical assessment in this area is of value. The clinician should assess if particular body image concerns exist, the extent to which the adolescent is satisfied with his/her appearance, and whether or not body image concerns have interfered with social functioning.
5. **Youth HRQoL.** Attention to HRQoL is important given literature to suggest that youth with IBD may be at risk for impairments in this domain. Assessment of HRQoL includes attention to general domains as well as disease-specific HRQoL. The Child Health Questionnaire (Landgraf Abetz & Ware, 1996) and TACQOL (Verrips et al., 2000) are well-established assessment methods and have been used in IBD samples (Palermo et al., 2008). In addition to the assessment of generic QoL, disease-specific measures are useful in identifying which disease symptoms or treatments influence adolescent well-being. The IMPACT is a disease-specific HRQOL instrument. Research documents that it is a valid and reliable measure (Otley et al., 2002) with four-factor analytically supported domains: general well-being and symptoms, emotional functioning, social interactions, and body image (Perrin et al., 2008).
6. **Assessment of family functioning.** Assessment of family functioning should be routinely conducted and should focus on a number of domains. It is important to determine the role of different family members in various aspects of the treatment regimen. In addition, identification of the family's support system, the presence of financial pressures or insurance concerns, and whether other family members have a diagnosis of IBD are important data that will help in determining a more robust assessment. Assessment of parent functioning is important with attention to clinical and subclinical levels of psychological

distress, parent QoL, and parent coping skills. Adelfer et al. (2007) offer guidelines for selection of evidence-based measures of parent and family functioning. Finally, attention to sibling adjustment is warranted. We have found anecdotally that obtaining the following information is useful: Do they understand what IBD is? Are they afraid that they will "get" IBD? Are they functioning well in their daily activities? Are they jealous of the extra attention that their sibling receives?

7. **Assessment of Adherence.** Multiple methods of adherence assessment exist including self-report measures (e.g., questionnaires, structured interviews, daily diary methods), electronic monitors, prescription refill documents, and biochemical assays (Drotar, 2000). To maximize the assessment of adherence, Quittner, Modi, Lemanek, Ievers-Landis, & Rapoff (2007) recommend (1) multiple methods of adherence assessment be utilized; (2) electronic data (when available) be used to "correct" self-report measures of adherence data; (3) barriers to adherence be assessed; and (4) patient and family knowledge and skill related to the treatment regimen be assessed.

Self-reported measures are well suited for clinical practice since they are relatively inexpensive, easy to administer, can be conducted quickly, and do not require the advanced training of the patient or the assessor. However, they are subject to social desirability biases and correlate only minimally with objective indices of adherence (i.e., bioassay, pill counts). One parent and adolescent report interview of adherence to IBD medication, developed by Mackner & Crandall (2005), holds promise, as initial data support the measure's validity based on moderate correlations between parent and youth reports of adherence. Additionally, the Medication Adherence Measure (MAM; Zelikovsky, 2001) scores predicted teen reported QOL in sample of teens with IBD (Hommel et al., 2008).

Daily diary methods allow for data collection in either real time (e.g., PDA) or within the recent past. Anecdotally, we have found that having patients and/or parents keep a daily log of medication taking can be useful clinically both in documenting rates of adherence and in identifying antecedents of nonadherence.

Pill counts and pharmacy refill data are generally more accurate than self-reports (Epstein & Cluss, 1982) and can be incorporated into clinical care. However, neither method confirms ingestion nor do they provide information in real time. Pharmacy refill records can be difficult to obtain and assume that when prescriptions are filled corresponds to when the pills are actually needed.

Electronic monitoring devices (e.g., MEMS caps, Aardex, LTD) record the date and time a pill bottle is opened and offer the potential to obtain objective assessments of when medication was dispensed, rather than relying on patient recall. However, these devices do not provide conclusive information on medication ingestion, only whether or not the bottle was opened (Quittner et al., 2007), and the cost of the devices ($120–$150 per cap plus software costs) may be prohibitive for clinical use.

Bioassays are becoming a popular method of adherence assessment, since they confirm medication ingestion. Only certain IBD medications have blood metabolites that can be detected and used as a proxy for adherence. However, given the invasiveness and the expense of performing blood draws, bioassays are often impractical for clinical use.

Identification of barriers to adherence in multiple domains including intraindividual factors, family factors, and health professional relational factors is important (Lemanek, Kamps, & Chung, 2001; Litt & Cuskey, 1984; Hazzard, Hutchinson, & Krawiecki, 1990) Components of the medical regimen including longer duration of the regimen, greater regimen complexity, and more side effects of the medication have also been linked with lower levels of adherence (Lemanek et al., 2001). Several scales have been developed to assess barriers to medication taking (e.g., the Medication Adherence Measure, Zelikovsky & Schast, 2008 Parent and Adolescent Medication Barriers Scales; Simons & Blount, 2007) and have relevance for use with youth with IBD.

Evidence-Based Treatment

The treatment literature for psychosocial interventions involving adolescents with IBD is largely anecdotal with the exception of treatment of depression.

Interventions for Depression

Szigethy et al. (2007) used a manual-based CBT approach with adolescents with IBD and depression. Results indicated that the use of the Primary and Secondary Control Enhancement Training (PASCET) manualized treatment may be an efficacious intervention for subdromal depression in adolescents with IBD.

Interventions to Address Other Psychosocial Concerns

There are no evidence-based treatments specific for IBD for anxiety, social functioning, or school functioning. Anecdotal reports suggest that psychosocial treatment is helpful at strategic points: at diagnosis, at recurrence, and around treatment-related issues (Cunningham & Banez, 2006).

One study examined the effects of a camp experience for youth with IBD. Results indicated a positive effect on HRQOL and improvement in social functioning, better acceptance of symptoms, and less distress regarding their treatment regimen (Shepanski, 2005). There is no research data to support the benefit of psychotherapy, behavioral techniques, complimentary medicines, or psychotropic medications to affect the long-term medical course of IBD in youth.

Interventions to Promote Adherence

No published studies on enhancing adherence in pediatric IBD exist. Among other pediatric chronic medical conditions, organizational strategies (i.e., altering clinic and or regimen characteristics), cognitive behavioral and behavioral strategies, and multicomponent strategies have demonstrated evidence for their effectiveness (Lemanek et al., 2001). Anecdotally, we have found that many of the above strategies have been successful, including having written treatment plans, visual reminders, storing pills in a visible location, setting cell phone reminders, and formulating plans in advance for how to have medication available when away from home.

Interventions to Improve Parent and Family Functioning

There are no evidence-based treatments to improve parent, family, or sibling functioning in pediatric IBD. Clinically we have found that parent support groups are helpful as is meeting with parents and the whole family to provide support and answer questions during an inpatient admission.

General Suggestions for Clinical Care of Adolescents with IBD

1. Familiarize yourself with the medical aspects of IBD, including presenting symptoms, diagnostic procedures, treatment modalities, and medication side effects.
2. Introduce psychosocial services at the time of diagnosis since an approach that includes education, anticipatory guidance, and a multidisciplinary team can set a model for treatment which recognizes the psychosocial impact of IBD on youth.
3. Clarify misconceptions about the patient or family's knowledge regarding the etiology, treatment, and prognosis of IBD. Provide families with local and national information such as pamphlets and web sites. Ongoing education for patients and families is needed because of the chronic and unpredictable nature of IBD. Information distribution with youth and parents was documented as an important component of the management of pediatric and adolescent patients with IBD (Day, Whitten & Bohane, 2005), and education was described as an "ongoing process." Web sites were also cited as helpful.
4. Normalize patient and family reactions to dealing with IBD and the treatment regimen. Knowing that their fears about bathroom issues or medication side effects are common for patients with IBD may help to decrease their anxiety.
5. Facilitate the transition of adolescent patients to adult care. Adolescents need preparation to assume responsibility for their own medical care, including familiarity with medications, warning signs of a disease flare, recognition of

emergencies, and how to access care and support systems. Hait Arnold and Fishman (2006) offer a timeline to facilitate this transition process. Effective transitioning could result in improved compliance with therapy and effective planning of long-range needs. Implementations of such programs could also address the needs for a benefits package to be designed covering issues of continuing health insurance, life insurance, and disability (Mamula & Markowitz, 2003).

Methodological Considerations When Conducting Research in Pediatric IBD Populations

Obtaining an Adequate Sample Size and Narrowing Population of Focus

Identifying large populations of adolescents with IBD within a small geographic region can be challenging given prevalence rates. An even greater challenge can be obtaining adequate samples of youth who are relatively homogenous with respect to disease characteristics (disease severity, time since diagnosis, age, etc.). Studies with small sample sizes may lack power to detect significant findings.

IBD is a broad category in which heterogeneity is the rule rather than the exception. Distinct differences do exist which can have implications for research design. It is important to consider whether to (1) focus on patients with only one type of IBD or if the research questions of interest have relevance across different types of IBD and (2) focus on recently diagnosed patients, patients with long-standing diagnoses, or both. Additionally, variability exists in terms of disease location and disease behavior, both across individuals and within the same individual over time. The extent to which heterogeneity may confound study findings is important to consider in the planning phases of research development.

Decisions about demographic differences are of interest and/or may be relevant to understanding study findings. Past research did not target subgroups (e.g., by age, SES, ethnicity) because of difficulties in identifying large samples at single sites; however, understanding differences in adjustment or adherence as a function of cultural or economic factors is of value in identifying subgroups that may need targeted intervention.

Choice of Comparison Group

An additional consideration is whether or not a comparison group is warranted, and if so, what is the most appropriate comparison group? A healthy matched comparison group may be appropriate for research questions examining if IBD poses unique challenges for adjustment above those challenges encountered by all adolescents. A matched sample of adolescents with another chronic medical condition may be useful, for example, in examining the impact of being diagnosed with a chronic illness during adolescence. In this case, a comparison group of youth diagnosed with a chronic medical condition at birth (e.g., cystic fibrosis) or in early childhood (e.g., diabetes) may be appropriate. In contrast, if the research question relates to examining whether youth with IBD have a better functioning than youth with other chronic illnesses, then a comparison group may need to match youth based on age, sex, and age of diagnosis.

Measure Selection

Few measures have been developed or validated for pediatric IBD populations. As such, utilizing multiple measures of similar domains is useful. For example, The Family Assessment Device (Kabacoff, Miller, Bishop, Epstein, & Keitner, 1990), a well-established measure of general family climate, has been utilized in research with adolescents with IBD (Alderfer et al., 2007). In contrast, the Negative Impact on Family Scale (Stein & Jessop, 2003) provides specific information about the impact of the child's chronic illness on the family and may be more sensitive to the unique impact of the child's condition. Obtaining assessments from multiple reporters both within (e.g., youth, parents) and outside (observational strategies) of the family is advantageous (Holmbeck, Li, Schurman, Friedman, & Coakley, 2002). Guidelines on the selection of evidence-based measures of youth QoL, psychosocial functioning, coping and stress, adherence, pain, and family functioning have been published (Cohen et. al., 2008) and we recommend that practitioners seek to use evidence-based assessments when possible.

Follow-Up Interval

Researchers need to address if participants will be followed longitudinally and if so, for how long. Existing research on pediatric IBD is largely cross-sectional in nature, and little is known about how psychosocial functioning changes over time. Moreover, little is known about interrelationships of medical or disease-related factors and psychosocial functioning over time. Given the increasing prevalence of CD among children, it is important to undertake longitudinal studies to understand the developmental implications of being diagnosed with a chronic medical condition at different developmental periods (childhood versus adolescence). Longitudinal studies allow for examination of the extent to which normal developmental trajectories (e.g., social development) may be altered by the presence of IBD.

Research Agenda

The expansion of psychosocial research on pediatric IBD in six major priority domains including (1) psychopathology; (2) QOL; (3) psychosocial issues; (4) adherence; (5) neuropsychiatric aspects of IBD; and (6) behavioral health prevention and intervention is a priority of the Crohn's and Colitis Foundation of America (CCFA; Bousvaros et al., 2006).

In the area of psychopathology research, the committee recommends comprehensive assessment of the prevalence of psychiatric diagnoses, as well as research on factors that predict the development of anxiety and depressive symptoms. Epidemiological data on the prevalence of depressive and anxiety disorders among children and adolescents with IBD and comprehensive data on developmental or gender differences in rates of psychopathology or psychosocial adjustment problems are needed.

The need for examination of QOL in pediatric IBD compared to other chronic illnesses in order to better understand the extent to which pediatric IBD may pose additional risk for impairments in QOL relative to other pediatric chronic conditions is highlighted. Also important is the assessment of QOL via the use of developmentally appropriate and psychometrically sound measures. For example, no disease-specific QOL measures have been validated for use with youth younger than age 11. The routine assessment of QOL as an outcome in psychosocial intervention trials is seen as an important domain for future research development, to document relationships between changes in disease activity and youth QOL, and to determine the impact of treatment on youth QOL. Greater attention to parent QOL in the context of pediatric IBD is needed since only one published study has examined this using a validated measure (Greenley & Cunningham, 2008).

Deficiencies in our knowledge of key domains of psychosocial functioning exist including adolescent academic performance, social functioning, and family functioning (including mother, father, and sibling adjustment) in the context of pediatric IBD. Additionally, our knowledge base with respect to risk factors for adjustment difficulties is limited. Little is known about individual and systemic (e.g., family, social) factors that protect against the development of psychosocial adjustment problems in youth with IBD. To this end, prospective longitudinal studies, which incorporate the perspective of multiple family members are also needed. Longitudinal studies would also be valuable in elucidating salient developmental issues in adapting to IBD (i.e., are there differences in adjustment of prepubertal versus post pubertal youth?) and would allow for temporally meaningful investigations of moderators and mediators of psychosocial adjustment in this population. Finally, studies that utilize matched comparison samples of youth with and without chronic illnesses would help advance our understanding of the unique impact of IBD on adolescent adjustment.

Research on adherence in pediatric IBD is in its infancy. Little is known about the psychosocial and developmental factors that influence adherence behaviors. Moreover, few tools designed to assess adherence in this population exist. Although the impact of medication nonadherence has been well documented in the adult IBD literature (Kane, Huo, Aikens, & Hanauer, 2003; Moody, Jayanthi, Probert, MacKay, & Mayberry, 1996), the impact of nonadherence on adolescent psychosocial functioning, medical functioning, health-care utilization, and future health risk is not well understood. Finally, expansion of adherence research to examine adherence rates and barriers to adherence in domains outside of oral medication adherence [e.g., adherence to dietary recommendations, adherence to medications delivered via other modalities (topically, rectally, via infusion)] is also warranted.

Our current knowledge is limited in several domains regarding neuropsychiatric aspects of IBD, including the prevalence and significance of pain among youth with IBD, links between genetics and psychiatric symptoms or disorders, the understanding of long-term side effects of steroid treatment, the impact of growth failure or pubertal delay on adolescent psychosocial adjustment, and neural substrates for depression and anxiety. Research on each of these areas is recommended.

Finally, the committee notes the importance of future research on interventions to prevent or treat psychosocial and psychiatric problems among youth with IBD. Our current knowledge is limited by a lack of treatment algorithms for different psychiatric symptoms or conditions, an absence of longitudinal studies of treatment effectiveness over time, and little data on mediators and moderators of treatment outcome. We know little about the effectiveness of different modalities of intervention (with the exception of individual CBT for depression; Szgeithy et al., 2007) including family- or group-based preventive or intervention efforts. Although RCTs are considered the gold standard in intervention research, other intervention modalities are also of value including developing and testing behavioral health interventions in clinical practice settings such as case studies and case series (Drotar, 2006). Such interventions would establish the feasibility and utility of interventions in real-world settings, as well as provide valuable data on the cost-effectiveness of behavioral health interventions implemented in clinical settings.

The management of IBD in children and adolescents presents many challenges from a biopsychosocial perspective. As the rates of children and adolescents with IBD increase, maximizing the functioning in all areas of their lives of adolescent patients with IBD will become an increasing health-care priority. Research that determines the most efficacious assessment and treatment procedures is critically needed in order to meet this challenge, and pediatric psychologists adhering to evidence-based practice suggestions can play an important role in maximizing the adjustment of these youth.

References

Abdul-Baki, H., ElHajj. I., El-Zahabi, L. M., Azar. C., Aoun, E., Zantout, H., et. al. (2007, April). Clinical epidemiology of inflammatory bowel disease in Lebanon. *Inflammatory Bowel Disease, 13*(4), 475–480.

Achkar, T. (2007). New Vistas in Inflammatory Bowel disease. Crohn's and Colitis Foundation of Northeast Ohio Education seminar, Independence, Ohio.

Afzal, M. A., Minor, P. D., Begley, J., Bentley, M. L., Armitage, E., Ghosh, S., & Ferguson, A. (1998). Absence of measles-virus genome in inflammatory bowel disease. *Lancet, 351*(9103), 646.

Akobeng, A., Miller, V., Firth, D., Suresh-Babu, M. V., Mir, P., & Thomas, A. G. (1999). *Quality of Pediatric Gastroenterology and Nutrition, 28*, S40–S42.

Akobeng A. K., Mirajkar, B., Suresh-Babu M. V., Firth D., Miller, D., Mir, P., et al. (1999). Quality of life in children with Crohn's disease: A pilot study. *Journal of Pediatric Gastroenterology and Nutrition, 28*, S37–S39.

Alderfer, M. A., Fiese, B. H., Gold, J., Cutuli, J., Grayson, J. A., Holmbeck, N. et al. (2007). Evidence-based assessment in pediatric psychology: Family measures. *Journal of Pediatric Psychology. 33*(9), 1046–1061.

Baldassano, R. N., & Piccoli, D. A. (1999). Inflammatory bowel disease in pediatric and adolescent patients. *Gastroenterology Clinics of North America, 28*, 445–458.

Ballinger, A. B. (2000). Epidemiology, natural history and prognosis of inflammatory bowel disease. In D. Ramptain (Ed.), *Inflammatory bowel disease* (pp. 59–70). Martin Dunitz.

Banez, G. A., & Cunningham, C. (2003). Pediatric gastrointestinal disorders: Recurrent abdominal pain, inflammatory bowel disease, and rumination disorder/cyclic vomiting. In Roberts, M. C. (Ed.). *Handbook of Pediatric Psychology* (3rd ed., pp. 462–480). New York, NY: Guilford.

Bousvaros, A., Sylvester, F., Kugathasan, S., Szigethy, E., Fiocchi, C., Colletti, R., et al. (2006). Challenges in pediatric inflammatory bowel disease. *Inflammatory Bowel Disease, 12*, 885–913.

Bremner, A. R., & Beattie, R. M. (2002). Theory of Crohn's disease in childhood. *Expert opinions in Pharmacology, 3*(7), 809–825.

Burke, P., Kocoshis, S. A., Chandra, R., Whiteway, M., & Sauer, J. (1990). Determinants of depression in recent onset pediatric inflammatory bowel disease. *Journal of the American Academy of Child and Adolescent Psychiatry, 29*(4), 608–610.

Burke, P., Meyer, V., Kochoshis, S., Orenstein, D., & Sauer, J. (1989). Obsessive–compulsive symptoms in childhood inflammatory bowel disease and cystic fibrosis. *Journal of the American Academy of Child and Adolescent Psychiatry, 4*, 525–527.

Burke, P., Meyer, V., Kocoshis, S., Orenstein, D. M., Chandra, R., Nord, D. J. et.al. (1989). Depression and anxiety in pediatric inflammatory bowel disease and cystic fibrosis. *Journal of the American Academy of Child and Adolescent Psychiatry, 28*, 948–951.

Burke, P. M., Neigut, D., Kocoshis, S., Chandra, R., & Sauer, J. (1994). Correalates of depression in new onset pediatric inflammatory bowel disease. *Child Psychiatry and Human Development, 24*(4) 275–283.

Carvalho, R., & Hyams, J. S.(2007). Diagnosis and management of inflammatory bowel disease in children. *Seminar in Pediatric Surgery, 3*, 164–171.

Cohen, L. A., Blount, R., Lemanek, K., Dahlquist, L., Lim, C., Palermo, T., Mckenna, K., & Weiss, K. (2008). Introduction to special issue: Evidenced-based assessment in pediatric psychology. *Journal of Pediatric Psychology, 33*, 939–957.

Crohn's and Colitis Foundation of America. (1999). How Many Americans have IBD?

Cuffari, C., & Darbari, A. (2002). Inflammatory bowel disease in the pediatric and adolescent patient. *Gastrenterology Clinics of North America, 31*, 275–291.

Cunningham, C. (2002). *Talking with teens: A pediatric Crohn's disease and ulcerative colitis seminar*. Independence, Ohio.

Cunningham, C., & Banez, G. A. (2006). *Pediatric gastrointestinal disorders: Biopsychosocial assessment and treatment* (pp. 31–54). New York, NY: Springer.

Cunningham, C., Drotar, D., Palermo, T., McGowan, K., & Arendt, R. (2007). Health related quality of life in children and adolescents with inflammatory bowel disease. *Children's Health Care, 36*, 29–43.

Day, A. S., Whitten, K. E., & Bohane, T. D. (2005). Childhood inflammatory bowel disease: Parental concerns and expectations. *World Journal of Gastroenterology, 11*(7), 1028–1031.

De Boer, M. A., Grootenhuis, M., Derkx, B., & Last, B. (2005). Health-related quality of life and psychosocial functioning of adolescents with inflammatory bowel disease. *Inflammatory Bowel Disease, 11*, 400–406.

Desir, B., & Seidman, E. G. (2003). Transitioning the pediatric IBD patient to adult care. *Best Practices res Clinical Gastroenterology, 17*(2), 197–212.

Drotar, D. (2000). *Promoting adherence to medical treatment in chronic childhood illness.* Mahwah, NJ: Lawrence Erlbaum Associates, Publishers.

Drotar, D. (2006). *Psychological interventions in childhood chronic illness.* Washington, DC: American Psychological Association.

Duerr, R. H., Taylor, K. D., Brant, S. R., Rioux, J. D., Silverberg, M. S., Daly, M. J. et al. (2006). A genome-wide association study identifies IL23R as an inflammatory bowel disease gene. *Science, 1; 314*(5804), 1403–1405.

Eiser, M.C., & Morse, R. (2001). Can parents rate their child's health-related quality Of life? The results of a systematic review. *Quality of Life Research, 10*, 347–357.

Engstrom, I. (1992). Mental health and psychological functioning in children and adolescents with inflammatory bowel disease: A comparison with children having other chronic illnesses with health children. *Journal of Child Psychology and Psychiatry, 33*, 563–582.

Engstrom, I. (1999). Inflammatory bowel disease in children and adolescents: Mental health and family functioning. *Journal of Pediatric Gastroenterology and Nutrition, 28*, S28–S33.

Engstrom, I., & Lindquist, B. L. (1991). Inflammatory bowel disease in children and adolescents: A somatic and psychiatric investigation. *Acta Paediatric Scandinavia, 80*(67), 640–647.

Epstein, L. H., & Cluss, P. A. (1982). A behavioral medicine perspective on adherence to long-term medical regimens. *Journal of Consulting and Clinical Psychology, 50*, 950–971.

Feagan, B. G, Vreeland, M. G., Larson, L. R., & Bala, M. V. (2000). Annual cost of care for Crohn's disease: A Payor perspective. *American Journal of Gastroenterology, 8*, 1955–1960.

Ferguson, A., Sedgwick, D. M., & Drummond, J. (1994). Morbidity of juvenile-onset inflammatory bowel disease: Effects on education and employment in early adult life. *Gut, 35*, 665–668.

Gold, N., Issenman, R., Roberts, J., & Watt, S. (2000). An alternate view of children with inflammatory bowel disease and functional gastrointestinal complaints. *Inflammatory Bowel Disease, 6*, 1–7.

Greenley, R., & Cunningham, C., (2008). Parent quality of life in the context of pediatric inflammatory bowel disease. *Journal of Pediatric Psychology, 34*(3), 129–136.

Griffiths, A. M. (2008). Recent research in ulcerative colitis. Northeast Ohio Crohn's and colitis foundation of America, 6, 1.

Griffiths, A. M., Nicholas, D., Smith, C., Munk, M., Stephens, D., Durno, C., et al. (1999). Development of a quality of life index for pediatric inflammatory bowel disease: Dealing with differences related to age and IBD type. *Journal of Pediatric Gastroenterology and Nutrition, 28*, S46–S52.

Gryboski, J. D. (1994). Crohn's disease in children 10 years old and younger: Comparison with ulcerative colitis. *Journal of Pediatric Gastroenterology and Nutrition, 18*, 174–182.

Hait, E., Arnold, J. H., Fishman, L. N. (2006). Educate, communicate, anticipate-practical recommendations for transitioning adolescents with IBD to adult health care. *Inflammatory Bowel Disease, 12*, 70–73.

Hazzard, A., Hutchinson, S. J., & Krawiecki, N. (1990). Factors related to adherence to medication regimens in pediatric seizure patients. *Journal of Pediatric Psychology, 15*, 543–555.

Heyman, M. B., Kirschner, B. S., Gold, B. D., Ferry, G., Baldassano, R., Cohen, S. A., et al. (2005). Children with early-onset inflammatory bowel disease (IBD): Analysis of a pediatric IBD consortium registry. *Journal of Pediatrics, 146*(1), 35–40.

Holmbeck, G. N., Li, S. T., Schurman, J. V., Friedman, D., & Coakley, R. M. (2002). Collecting and managing multisource and multimethod data in studies of pediatric populations. *Journal of Pediatric Psychology, 27*, 5–18.

Hommel, K., Davis, C. M., & Baldassano, R. N. (2008). Medication adherence and quality of life in pediatric inflammatory bowel disease. *Journal of Pediatric Psychology Advance Access*, Mary 11, 1–8.

Hyams, J. (2000). Inflammatory bowel disease. *Pediatrics in Review, 21*, 291–295.

Hyams, J. S., Ferry, G. D., Mandel, F. S., Gryboski, J. D., Kibort, P. M., Kirschner, B. S., et al., (1991). Development and validation of a pediatric Crohn's disease activity index. *Journal of Pediatric Gastroenterology and Nutrition, 12*, 439–447.

IBD Working Group of the European Society of Pediatric Gastroenterology, Hepatology, and Nutrition (ESPGHAN) (2005). Inflammatory bowel disease in children and adolescents: recommendations for diagnosis-the Porto criteria. *Journal of Pediatric Gastroenterology and Nutrition, 1*(1), 1–7.

Jiang, L., Xia, B., Li, J., Ye, M., Yan, W., Deng, C., et al. (2006, March). Retrospective survey of 452 patients with inflammatory bowel disease in Wuhan city, central China. *Inflammatory Bowel Diseases, 12*(3):212–217.

Kabacoff, R. I., Miller, I. W., Bishop, D. S., Epstein, N. B., & Keitner, G. I. (1990). A psychometric study of the McMaster Family Assessment Device in psychiatric, medical, and nonclinical samples. *Journal of Family Psychology, 3*, 431–439.

Kane, S., Huo, D., Aikens, J., & Hanauer, S. (2003). Medication nonadherence and the outcomes of patients with quiescent ulcerative colitis. *The American Journal of Medicine, 114*, 39–43.

Kappelman, M. D., Rifas-Shiman, S. L., Kleinman, K., Ollendorf, D., Bousvaros, A., et al. (2007). The prevalence and geographic distribution of Crohn's disease and ulcerative colitis in the United States. *Clinical Gastroenterology and Hepatology, 12*,1424–1429.

Kim, S. C., & Ferry, G. D. (2004). Inflammatory bowel disease in pediatric and adolescent patients: Clinical, therapeutic and psychosocial considerations. *Gastroenterology, 126*, 1550–1560.

King, R. A. (2003). Pediatric inflammatory bowel disease. *Child and Adolescent Psychiatric Clinics of North America, 12*, 967–995.

Kugathasan, S., Judd, R. H., Hoffmann, R. G., Helkenen, J., Telega, G., Khan, F. et al. (2003). Epidemiologic and clinical characteristics of children with newly diagnosed inflammatory bowel disease in Wisconsin: A statewide population-based study. *Journal of Pediatrics, 143*, 525–531.

Kugathasan, S., & Werlin, S. L. (1999). Measurement of pANCA (antineutrophil cytoplasmic antibodies) and ASCA (anti-*Saccharomyces cerevisiae*) in screening for IBD in young children. *Inflammatory Bowel Disease, 4*, 283–284.

Langholz, E., Munkholm, P., Krasilinikoff, P. A., & Binder, V. (1998). Inflammatory bowel diseases in children. *Ugeskrift for Laeger, 160*, 5648–5464.

Lemanek, K. L., Kamps, J., & Chung, N. B. (2001). Empirically supported treatments in pediatric psychology: Regimen adherence. *Journal of Pediatric Psychology, 26*(5), 253–275.

Lindberg, E., Lindquist, B., Homquist, L., & Hildebrand, H. (2000). Inflammatory bowel disease in children and adolescents in Sweden, 1984–1995. *Journal of Pediatric Gastroenterology and Nutrition, 30*, 259–264.

Litt, I. F., & Cuskey, W. R. (1984). Satisfaction with health care: A predictor of adolescents' appointment keeping. *Journal of Adolescent Health Care, 5*, 196–200.

Loftus, C. G., Loftus, E. V. Jr., Harmsen, W. S., Zinsmeister, A. R., Tremaine, W. J., et al., (2007). Update on the incidence and prevalence of Crohn's disease and ulcerative colitis in Olmsted County, Minnesota, 1940–2000. *Inflammatory Bowel Disease, 3*, 254–261.

Loonen, H. J., Derkx, B. H. F., Koopman, H. M., & Heymans, H. S. A. (2002). Are parents able to rate the symptoms and quality of life of their offspring with IBD? *Inflammatory Bowel Diseases, 8*, 270–276.

Loonen, H. J., Grootenhuis, M. A., Last B. P., Koopman, H. M., & Derkx, H. H. F. (2002). Quality of life in paediatric inflammatory bowel disease measured by a generic and a disease specific questionnaire. *Acta Paediatrica, 91*, 347–354.

Mackner, L. M., & Crandall, W. V. (2005). Long-term psychosocial outcomes reported by children and adolescents with inflammatory bowel disease. *American Journal of Gastroenterology, 100*, 1386–1392.

Mackner, L. M., & Crandall, W. V. (2005). Oral medication adherence in pediatric inflammatory bowel disease. *Inflammatory Bowel Disease, 11*, 1006–1012.

Mackner, L. M., & Crandall, W. V. (2007). Psychological factors affecting pediatric inflammatory bowel disease. *Current Opinion in Pediatrics, 19*, 548–552.

Mackner, L. M., Crandall, W. V., & Szigethy, E. M. (2006). Brief report: Psychosocial functioning in pediatric inflammatory bowel Disease. *Inflammatory Bowel Disease, 12*, 239–244.

Mackner, L. M., Sisson, D. P., & Crandall, W. V. (2004). Review: Psychosocial issues in pediatric inflammatory bowel disease. *Journal of Pediatric Psychology, 29*, 243–257.

MacPhee, M., Hoffenberg, E. J., & Feranchak, A. (1988). Quality-of-life factors in adolescents inflammatory bowel disease. *Inflammatory Bowel Disease, 4*, 6–11.

Mamula, P., Markowitz, J. E., & Baldassano, R. N. (2003). Inflammatory bowel disease in early childhood and adolescence: Special considerations. *Gastroenterology Clinics of North America, 32*, 967–995.

Moody, G., Eaden, J., & Mayberry, J. (1999). Social implications of childhood Crohn's disease. *Journal of Pediatric Gastroenterology and Nutrition, 28*, S43–S45.

MEMS 6 electronic monitor [Software]. Zug, Switzerland: Aardex LTD.

Moody, G. A., Jayanthi, V., Probert, C. S., MacKay, H., & Mayberry, J. F. (1996). Long-term therapy with sulphasalazine protects against colorectal cancer in ulcerative colitis: a retrospective study of colorectal cancer risk and compliance with treatment in Leicestershire. *European Journal of Gastroenterology and Hepatology, 8*, 1179–1183.

Oliva-Hemker, M. M., Abadom, V., Cuffari, C., & Thompson, R. E. (2007). Nonadherence with thiopurine immunomodulator and mesalamine medications in children with Crohn Disease. *Journal of Pediatric Gastroenterology and Nutrition, 44*, 180–184.

Ondersma, S. J., Lumley, M. A., Corlis, M. E., Tojek, T. M., & Tolia, V. (1997). Adolescents with inflammatory bowel disease: The roles of negative affectivity and hostility in subjective versus objective health. *Journal of Pediatric Psychology, 22*, 723–738.

Otley, A., Smith, C., Nicholas, D., Munk, M., Avolio, J., Sherman, P. M. et al. (2002). The IMPACT questionnaire: A valid measure of health-related quality of life in pediatric inflammatory bowel disease. *Journal of Pediatric Gastroenterology and Nutrition, 35*, 557–563.

Pappa, H. M., Semrin, G., Walker, T. R., & Grand, R. J. (2004). Pediatric inflammatory bowel disease. *Current Opinion in Gastroenterology*, 20, 333–340.

Perrin, J. M., Kuhlthau, K., Chughtai, A., Romm, D., Kirschner, B. S., Ferry, G. D., et al. (2008). Measuring quality of life in pediatric patients with inflammatory bowel disease: Psychometric and clinical characteristics. *Journal of Pediatric Gastroenterology and Nutrition, 46*, 164–171.

Quittner, A. L., Davis, M. A., & Modi, A. C. (2003). Health-related quality of life in pediatric populations. In M. C. Roberts (Ed.), *Handbook of pediatric psychology* (pp. 696–709). New York, NY: The Guilford Press.

Quittner, A. L., Modi, A. C., Lemanek, K. L., Ievers-Landis, C. E., & Rapoff, M. (2007). Evidence-based assessment of adherence to medical treatments in pediatric psychology. *Journal of Pediatric Psychology, 33*, 916–936.

Rapoff, M. A. (1999). *Adherence to pediatric medical regimens*. New York: Kluwer Academic.

Rabbett, H., Elbadri, A., Thwaites, R., Northover, H., Dady, I., & Firth, D. (1996). Quality-of-life in children with Crohn's disease. *Journal of Pediatric Gastroenterology and Nutrition, 5*, 528–533.

Rasquin-Weber, A., Hyman, P. E., Cucchiara, S., Fleisher, D. R., Hyams, J. S., Milla, P. J., et al. (1999). Childhood functional gastrointestinal disorders. *Gut, 45*(Suppl. 2), 1160–1168.

Rice, H. E., & Chuang, E. (1999). Current management of pediatric inflammatory bowel disease. *Seminars in Pediatric Surgery, 8*, 221–228.

Shepanski, M. A., Hurd, L. B., Culton, K., et al., (2005). Health-related quality of life improves in children and adolescents with Inflammatory Bowel Disease after attending a camp sponsored by the Crohn's and Colitis Foundation of America. *Inflammatory Bowel Disease, 11*, 164–170.

Simons, L. E., & Blount, R. L. (2007). Identifying barriers to medication adherence in adolescent transplant recipients. *Journal of Pediatric Psychology, 32*, 831–844.

Stein, R. E. K., & Jessop, D. J. (2003). The impact on family scale revisited: Further psychometric data. *Journal of Developmental and Behavioral Pediatrics, 24*, 9–16.

Szajnberg, N., Krall, V., Davis, P., et Al. (1993). Psychopathology and relationship measures in children with inflammatory bowel disease and their parents. *Child Psychiatry and Human Development, 23*, 215–232.

Szigethy, E., Kenney, E., Carpenter, J., & Hardy, D. M. (2007). Cognitive-behavioral therapy for adolescents with inflammatory bowel disease and subsyndromal depression. *Journal of the American Academy of Child and Adolescent Psychiatry, 46*(10), 1290–1298.

Szigethy, E., Levy-Warren, A., Whitoon, S., Bousvaros, A., Gauvreau, K., Leichtner, A. M., Beardslee, W. R. (2004). Depressive symptoms and inflammatory bowel disease in children and adolescents: a cross sectional study. *Journal of Pediatric Gastroenterology and Nutrition, 39*, 395–403.

Tojek, T. M., Lumley, M. A., Corlis, M., et al., (2002). Maternal correlates of health status in adolescents with inflammatory bowel disease. *Journal of Psychosomatic Research, 52*, 173–179.

van der Zaag- Loonen, H. J., Grootenhuis, M. A., Last, B. P., & Derkx, H. H. F. (2004). Coping strategies and quality of life of adolescents with inflammatory bowel disease. *Quality Life Research, 13*, 1011-–1019.

Verrips, G. H., Vogels, A. G., den Ouden, A. L., Paneth, N., & Verloove-Vanhorick, S. P. (2000). Measuring health-related quality of life in adolescents: Agreement between raters and between methods of administration. *Child Care Health and Development, 26*(6), 457–469.

Wood, B., Watkins, J. B., Boyle, J. T., Nogueira, J., Zimand, E., & Carroll, L. (1987). Psychological functioning in children with Crohn's disease and ulcerative colitis: Implications for models of psychobiological interaction. *Journal of the American Academy of Child and Adolescent Psychiatry, 26*, 774–781.

Zelikovsky, N., & Schast, A. P. (2008). Eliciting accurate reports of adherence in a clinical interview: Development of the medical adherence measure. *Pediatric Nursing, 34*, 141–146.

Websites and Resources for Families and Patients

Crohn & Colitis Foundation of America, 386 Park Avenue South, New York, NY 10016-8804, (800) 826-0826. www.ccfa.org

North American Society for Pediatric Gastroenterology, Hepatology and Nutrition, PO Box 6, Flourtown, PA 19031, (215) 233–0808. www.naspgn.org

The Crohn's and Colitis Foundation's Information Resource Center, 1-888.MY.GUT.PAIN phone line with professionals who can answer questions Monday to Friday 9am–5 pm EST.

This is a free online community where patients and family members can participate in discussion boards and receive support. www.ccfacommunity.org

This is a website for children and adolescents where they can share, stories, tips and chat. www.UCandCrohns.org

United Ostomy Association, Inc., 19772 MacArthur Boulevard, Suite 200, Irvine, CA 92612-2405. www.uoa.org

Chronic Fatigue Syndrome

M. Elena Garralda

Description of Chronic Fatigue Syndrome

Chronic fatigue syndrome (CFS) in young people may be regarded as a modern disease. The syndrome became an established part of clinical paediatric practice in western countries over the turn of the 20th century. Interest has grown speedily however, and now a number of countries have developed guidelines for assessment and treatment. Chronic fatigue syndrome is a disorder characterised by severe, persistent, impairing fatigue together with a number of other symptoms, all of which are unexplained by a medical or psychiatric disorder. Over the past two decades, a concerted effort was made to rigorously define the basic features of the disorder to aid both clinical work and research. This has resulted in the development of a well-defined chronic fatigue syndrome meeting all diagnostic criteria and a subsyndromal chronic fatigue-*like* state meeting most but not all diagnostic criteria. In clinical practice, the differentiation between the two is not always clear-cut, and this chapter will consider both chronic CFS and chronic fatigue-*like* states.

The status of chronic fatigue syndrome as a medical disorder has been debated because there is no recognised pathophysiology and there is a strong psychological component. The main symptom is fatigue, which is commonly seen in a variety of medical, surgical and psychological disorders. Fatigue is also a normal everyday experience following physical exercise, psychological stress, mental exertion or a sleepless night, though too much sleep can also lead to fatigue. In chronic fatigue syndrome, the primary patient experience is one of poor physical health and of physical symptoms leading to substantial impairment in everyday life. In spite of the uncertain nature of the syndrome within medicine, patients generally regard it as having a biological cause and to be within the remit of physical rather than psychological medicine (Garralda & Rangel, 2002; Garralda & Chalder, 2005).

The Controversy

Few medical conditions generate such controversy that even the name is debated. Chronic fatigue syndrome (CFS) and myalgic encephalopathy (ME) both refer to the same disorder and set of symptoms. Whereas most doctors – in the absence of an organic cause – prefer the term CFS and fatigue is undoubtedly the central component, many patients and their families would rather use the term ME because they believe the disorder must be due to some illness affecting the muscles and neurological system.

Biological abnormalities may well occur in CFS (for example, glandular fever sometimes precedes it, and some immune and hormonal abnormalities can be seen in association), but no single physical cause or pathology has yet been identified. Evidence so far suggests that CFS involves a complex interaction between physical, psychological and environmental factors, all of which need to be considered and worked on as part of treatment.

M. Elena Garralda (✉)
Imperial College London, London, UK
e-mail: e.garralda@imperial.ac.uk

W.T. O'Donohue, L.W. Tolle (eds.), *Behavioral Approaches to Chronic Disease in Adolescence*,
DOI 10.1007/978-0-387-87687-0_21, © Springer Science+Business Media, LLC 2009

The controversy about CFS stems partly from the fact that it is poorly understood and the symptoms can be diverse, but also because whereas the presentation is primarily through physical symptoms, the lack of an organic substrate can carry the implication that the symptoms are "all in the mind" and the unwarranted assumption that it is a sign of a deranged mind, or criticism of the child's moral fibre and parenting. Instead the term ME is seen as carrying the power and strong aura of organic illness and makes the disorder more "respectable".

In practice, rather than debating whether the problem is physical *or* psychological – a perceived division of mind and body, which is unhelpful in understanding *any* illness – it is far more useful for the clinician to direct the discussion towards how the problem can best be managed.

Description of the Condition in Adolescents

Epidemiology

Typical age of onset: When it strikes before adulthood, chronic fatigue syndrome is typically a disorder of adolescents. It is rarely seen in early childhood and two onset peaks have been noted: at around 11 years of age, which coincides in some countries with the move to secondary or high school, and at a more established adolescent stage at around 13–14 years of age. The disorder is more prevalent in females than males.

Progression: By definition, the disorder is chronic: adult CFS diagnostic criteria state that impairing symptoms must have been present for at least 6 months for a CFS diagnosis to be considered. However, this criteria has been questioned for paediatric CFS on the grounds that waiting 6 months to put a management plan into practice is thought to be an unnecessary and unacceptable delay, as children may become increasingly more impaired, miss out on important life experiences, and become established in a sedentary lifestyle that might be more difficult to break the longer it lasts. Once established, childhood CFS can last for months or years, and some severely affected children do not recover.

Population affected: Community and primary care-based studies in adults have reported CFS prevalence rates of 0.2–2.6%. The rates vary according to the rigour with which diagnostic criteria have been applied and are, therefore, lower for CFS and higher for CFS-*like* states. They are also generally higher in females but comparable in people from different socioeconomic and ethnic groups. There are some exceptions with some general population studies finding higher levels among ethnic minorities and lower occupational status. Conversely, among patients attending specialist services there is a predominance of patients from higher socioeconomic groups, although this could be because affluent patients are more likely to seek specialist medical opinions (Gallagher et al., 2004).

What about the prevalence in young people? Questionnaire community surveys in the United States have reported CFS-*like* syndromes in 2% of children and adolescents: in a typical large secondary school with 1000 pupils, therefore, about 20 pupils may be expected to be absent from school with fatigue symptoms otherwise unexplained by a medical or psychiatric disorder. In a British population study, one-third of 11–15 years olds stated that they were currently tired at the time of the study; however, only 0.6% said that they were *chronically* fatigued, and even fewer (0.19%) met criteria for chronic fatigue syndrome (in a typical large secondary school only two children would be so affected). A parental belief that the child had a medically explained chronic fatigue syndrome (called ME, or meningoencephalitis, implying inflammation of the nervous system as a cause) was noted in only 0.04% of the parents in this study.

We know very little about how the, presumably milder, forms of CFS identified in these large community studies compare with the severe problems seen in specialist clinics, because empirical research has tended to be based on young people from high socioeconomic groupings seen by specialists. Therefore, most of what follows is based on our knowledge of more severe clinical cases.

Diagnostic Criteria

The mostly commonly used diagnostic criteria in the United States or CDC criteria were outlined by Fukuda et al. (1994). Although other diagnostic criteria have been also developed, they are all on broadly comparable lines (REEVES et al., 2003). The Fukuda criteria are applicable to children and young people, except for the criterion of 6-month duration which is thought to be too stringent. They include the presence of new-onset fatigue lasting at least 6 months and the presence of at least four of eight other physical symptoms. CFS is defined as (1) clinically evaluated, unexplained persistent or relapsing chronic fatigue that is of new or definite onset (has not been lifelong), is not the result of ongoing exertion, is not substantially alleviated by rest; and results in substantial reduction in previous levels of occupation, education, social or personal activities; and (2) the concurrent occurrence of four or more of the following symptoms, all of which must have persisted or recurred during six or more consecutive months of illness and must not have predated the fatigue: self-reported impairment in short-term memory or concentration severe enough to cause substantial reduction in previous levels of occupational, educational, social or personal activities; sore throat; tender cervical or axillary lymph nodes; muscle pain, multijoint pain without joint swelling or redness; headaches of a new type, pattern or severity; unrefreshing sleep, and post extertional malaise lasting more than 24 hours.

Diagnostic assessment involves a full and comprehensive medical history and examination, as well as investigations to screen for blood disorders, glandular fever indicators, thyroid, liver and urinary function tests. In markedly impaired cases additional specialist neurological investigation may be helpful. Recurrent infection episodes may call for full investigation of immunology and infectious status.

A full psychiatric history and mental state of the child are equally relevant to diagnosis. Differential diagnosis will consider primary depressive or anxiety disorders including school phobia and eating disorders. This assessment will also reveal the presence of co-morbid treatable psychiatric disorders such as mood disorders, which may arise in the course of CFS and impede its treatment.

Symptoms

Onset and frequency: The condition typically starts with an acute illness episode such as a "flu"-type illness or glandular fever, but it can also start gradually. The biological start of illness in many cases is a potent reason why parents ascribe a medical cause to the disorder. Sometimes fatigue is both the initial and the main continuing symptom, but this is not always the case. There are occasions when young people present with symptoms such as headaches, abdominal pains or limb pains: only gradually does fatigue become a main symptom. Typically children complain of severe fatigue or overwhelming exhaustion, physical and mental, in association with headaches or disrupted sleep, though occasionally hypersomnia is present instead. A number of other physical symptoms may be present including sore throats, lymph node tenderness, joint paints, fever, diarrhoea, anorexia, nausea and dizziness. Less commonly reported symptoms include feeling too cold or hot, hypersensitivity to light or sound, weight gain or loss and muscle weakness. Some of these will be secondary to inactivity. Symptoms are subjective and not all are visible, and some young people will appear healthy and alert, though if inactivity is prolonged they may come to look pale and lacking in vitality.

The symptoms tend to occur daily and fatigue is not improved by rest, but there can also be fluctuations in severity over the course or the day or over longer time periods. On occasions young people feel able to engage fully in educational, sporting or other activities for a day or two, or more rarely for weeks, only to feel exhausted and even more impaired and despondent about their symptoms afterwards.

Life interference: A central feature of the syndrome is marked inactivity and impairment, which is higher than observed for many other severe chronic paediatric disorders. Some children do not feel able to get up from bed before midday and will then have several rest periods throughout the day, remaining generally physically and mentally inactive. This often leads to missing school, and some of the more severely affected young people are reduced to using a wheelchair and/or being bedbound for prolonged periods. Of special developmental importance in these cases is the prolonged continuing absence from school and the loss of contact with peer groups.

Disruption of family activities can be very marked with family life and relationships revolving round the need to accommodate the child's symptoms and impairment. Children can become anxiously dependent on their parents, and mothers can become highly attentive to, and emotionally involved with, their ill children. Family disruption, parental mental distress and high levels of emotional involvement with the child have been found to be more pronounced in this than in other chronic paediatric disorders.

Duration: Chronic fatigue syndrome is not regarded as life threatening, and we know that even in severely affected cases, half to three quarters of young people may be expected to become free of the disorder eventually. However, the duration of the illness can be very protracted. Some studies report the length of "worst illness episodes" and school non-attendance stretching to more than 1 year, with time to full recovery being as long as 3 years. Moreover, even after recovery from the syndrome some young people continue to experience uncomfortably high levels of fatigue symptoms, and there is a likely increase in the risk of developing psychiatric disorders following recovery from CFS. The increased likelihood of recovery has been linked to well-defined physical triggers of the illness such as a definite infectious disease, as well as to better socioeconomic circumstances, good mental and physical family health, and possibly also to personality features that protect from excessive reactivity to everyday stresses.

Complications: Inactivity, both physical and mental, is a significant complication of CFS. Whilst extreme exercise may lead athletes to experience fatigue as part of the over-training syndrome (10% of college swimmers in the United States have been described as "burning out" every year), the converse, namely inactivity, results in alterations to bodily systems and is in itself a potent cause of fatigue.

It is generally recognized that *reduced physical activity* and prolonged rest affect physiological mechanisms. A period of rest for as little as 1 week may result in a measurable loss of muscle volume, and 4–6 weeks' rest results in substantial loss of muscle strength. Prolonged bed rest also results in reduced bone mineral density and in immunological consequences such as an effect on T lymphocyte function. In severe cases, inactivity and prolonged bed rest can lead to muscle weakness and/or contractures, poor appetite and weight loss. Exercise after a period of prolonged rest may also lead to exhaustion as the body tries to compensate for these deficits.

Inactivity also results in impaired neuro-psychological performance, altered autonomic regulation leading to deficits in postural blood pressure control, impaired balance and consequent dizziness on standing, as well as impaired thermoregulation. In CFS, a vicious circle develops whereby fatigue leads to rest, which in itself leads to more fatigue.

In addition, many young people who develop fatigue states have been highly active and successful, academically and socially, prior to the onset of CFS. Some are involved in competitive sports. They may have had prior difficulty in efficiently modulating the usual daily activity/rest cycles that are a necessary requirement for smooth daily life and have a tendency to get involved in activities excessively intensely. Their efforts to combat the increasing fatigue might also be excessive and lead to more fatigue at crucial initial stages of the disorder. Eventually, the experience of failing to control activity/fatigue cycles efficiently can in itself become deeply demoralizing. Conversely, other young people will settle comfortably into a life pattern involving few demands with few requirements to face the usual life stresses, and they will resist efforts to help them go back to a more demanding lifestyle.

Treatment Regimen for Adolescents and Families

CFS in young people affects the whole family and clinical management is therefore normally family based. Management is inextricably linked to the process of diagnosis. Because the diagnosis of CFS is partly one of exclusion, the first step is a full paediatric assessment to exclude explanatory medical disorders. This should also incorporate a full psychiatric assessment to exclude any possible explanatory psychiatric disorders such as eating, anxiety or depressive disorders.

A number of management guidelines have been developed in different countries, incorporating comparable principles as described here (Garralda, 1999; Royal College of Peadiatrics and Child Health, 2004, Chalder & Hussain, 2002).

Medically, a thorough examination is called for, including a general physical examination, height and weight measurements, a neurological examination including gait and signs of muscle wasting, checking for lymph node/liver/spleen/tonsillar enlargement, lying and standing blood pressure and heart rate, because some young people will have postural hypotension. Blood and urine tests are carried out to exclude anaemia, iron deficiency and leukaemia, autoimmune disease and chronic infection, diabetes mellitus, renal impairment, muscle disease, thyroid or liver dysfunction and urinary tract infection, as well as current or recent EBV (glandular fever) infection.

When a diagnosis is made it is important that the reasons for a diagnosis of CFS are carefully explained to the patient and family, and that parents' illness beliefs and reactions to the diagnosis are taken note of and addressed. This does not however mean endorsing possibly unfounded theories of aetiology.

The main aim of the rehabilitation approach to CFS in young people is to enable them, with the help of their family, to carry out their own rehabilitation with support and guidance from a health professional. In practice, this can be a family doctor or a paediatrician. In more established, severe or protracted cases, more intensive treatment will be required possibly from a physiotherapist, occupational therapist, nurse therapist, or psychologist working with the young person and his or her family. A team effort of different professionals including teachers and other mental health workers may be required.

Developing a rapport with the family and establishing an empathetic relationship is essential to the success of the management plan. During the early stages of treatment, it is helpful for the therapist to be explicit in conveying belief in the real and physical nature of the symptoms that are not "all in the mind". Some families find the use of terms such as "psychological" objectionable. It is useful to direct the discussion not towards how the problem arose, but rather to how it can best be managed, taking into account physiological, behavioural and cognitive factors.

General management strategy: Problems requiring more than paediatric supervision and guidance can be amenable to therapeutic input through family work or behavioural family therapy, and some young people can benefit from being seen individually for guidance on cognitive behavioural principles whilst their parents are seen separately for behavioural advice and guidance. At the same time, liaison with teachers may be appropriate to attend to educational requirements. When seen for therapy, a good pattern to aim for is one of fortnightly visits totalling 15 hourly sessions of face-to-face treatment. Follow-up may be carried out at 3–6 months and then at 1 year, in order to monitor progress and tackle any residual problems. Questionnaires are useful to assess fatigue and disability before and after treatment and at follow-up.

It is helpful to negotiate both long- and short-term targets. It is also helpful to anticipate problems and rehearse appropriate strategies for dealing with them. Parents should be encouraged to praise their child – and young people to praise themselves – for small achievements, because some have high expectations and a tendency to disregard and not acknowledge small but important personal achievements.

The cornerstone of treatment is *activity management*. This entails establishing a baseline activity level and introducing gradual increases as appropriate. In addition, parallel advice should be offered where necessary about symptomatic treatment for other symptoms, such as sleep programme, pain management and dietary advice, as well as management of any anxieties about the treatment. The important principle is that any increases in activity should be gradual, starting from current activity levels: brusque increases in activity or wide fluctuations are to be avoided.

A number of young people will be reluctant to engage in increased activity, fearing that this will result in symptom deterioration, or to engage in a change of routine and a more demanding lifestyle, fearing an increase in symptoms of anxiety or stress. Early stages of treatment will therefore often deal with these concerns. The best motivator for continuing engagement is a recognition of change for the better, so it is important that fatigue levels are monitored regularly and that even small changes are acknowledged at early stages in treatment.

Activity scheduling goals usually include a mixture of social, school and leisure-related activities. Short walks or tasks carried out throughout the day are ideally interspersed with rests. The emphasis is on consistency and breaking the association between experiencing symptoms and stopping activity. The goal for someone who is not very disabled may be walking for 10 minutes three times a day, which is gradually built up as tolerance increases. Fatigue levels do not necessarily decrease very much initially, but will do so gradually. Tasks such as reading or school work, which require concentration, should also be included.

Details of a Graded Exercise Training and Activity Scheduling Programme

Details of a graded exercise training programme have been described in the NICE (2007) guidelines and can be adapted for use with children by involving parents and sometimes school in supporting the treatment. It involves planned increases in the duration of physical activity, based on the person's current level of activities (such as physical activity, daily routines and sleep patterns), educational factors and individual goals as outlined in an activity diary. It also involves sleep and relaxation strategies. It is important that the young persons do not get involved in a "boom-and-bust" cycle before they increase the time spent in exercise and discuss ultimate goals that are important and relevant to them, such as involvement in sport or other activities. It is equally important to recognize that it can take weeks, months or even years to achieve goals and explain symptoms and benefits of exercise in a physiological context. Increases in activity have to be sustainable, independent of daily fluctuations in symptoms, aware of the fact that this may mildly increase symptoms for a few days. When low-intensity exercise can be sustained for 5 out of 7 days, the duration should be reviewed and increased if appropriate by 20%.

Activity management should include understanding that activities have physical, emotional and cognitive components. As with graded exercise it involves keeping a diary that records cognitive and physical activity, daytime rest and sleep, establishing a baseline and gradually increasing activity above the baseline in agreement with the young person, planning daily routines to allow for a balance and variety of different types of activity, rest and sleep, spreading out the difficult or demanding tasks such as school work over the day or week, splitting activities into small achievable tasks, regularly reviewing activity levels and goals and preparing for the likelihood of setbacks and relapses, as progress often takes the form of "two step forwards and one step backwards".

Management of sleep difficulties: Sleep difficulties – either sleeping excessively or difficulties in sustaining a good sleep routine – are very common. It is helpful to establish the nature of the problems by keeping a diary of bedtime, sleep time, wake-up time, and get up time. The total number of hours spent asleep is calculated and a variety of strategies can then be used to improve both quality and quantity of sleep. Establishing a routine of going to bed and getting up at pre-planned times, whilst simultaneously cutting out daytime sleeping, gradually helps to improve both hypersomnia and insomnia.

Negative and unhelpful thinking. As already noted, many young people and their families will have misgivings about a programme of increasing activity levels. Whereas the main improvement in this area will come from behavioural change and realisation that improvement is possible in spite of more activity, as the patient becomes more active and confident it can be helpful to discuss explicitly with families their concerns and correct misleading information they might have about the condition. Explanations regarding the physiological effects of inactivity can help patients understand the rationale for activity scheduling.

Young people can be encouraged to record negative thoughts about their muscles being damaged by exercise, together with alternative more positive views. Perfectionist traits might make it difficult for them to accept small changes as worthwhile, and this can also be tackled during sessions to help increase motivation for treatment.

Pain and other physical symptoms: Simple analgesics may be used for joint and muscle pains or headaches, but these are often unhelpful and when that is the case, symptoms are best dealt with in the general rehabilitation programme, as they often decrease alongside improvements in fatigue symptoms.

Education: School non-attendance or concerns about education and peer relationships in school are very common in young people with chronic fatigue syndrome. Although negotiating a return to formal education is an aspect of treatment, several factors need to be considered, including the patient's age and degree of fear about school return, degree of disability, plans for the future, the school's view and their degree of support. As part of rehabilitation some adolescents will attend school part-time, some will have home tuition, some will be working at home independently and liaising with the school, while others will not be in a position to receive any education at all at initial stages of treatment. It can be helpful to meet to discuss progress and set realistic expectations and supports with the school or home tutor to ensure that all involved are being supportive and working towards similar goals. The child may need considerable encouragement, especially at early stages of change.

In practice, the longer a child is away from school, the more confidence will be lost and the further behind with their work they will become, making a return even more difficult. Exploring the possibility of reducing the number of exams undertaken can bring relief. As with previous problems, challenging perfectionism and "all-or-nothing" thinking can be useful in relation to academic issues.

Other Treatment Considerations

Illness beliefs and coping mechanisms are an important component of treatment. Young people with CFS tend to underestimate normal adolescent fatigue levels and by implication overestimate their own tiredness. This might be part of a perfectionist tendency whereby nothing short of high activity performance is felt to be acceptable. In some children, however, it will be part of a mindset in the child characterised by viewing themselves as "sickly", with a tendency to overemphasise physical symptoms and to withdraw from social responsibilities in response to them. A number of young people who develop CFS have a prior history of unexplained somatic symptoms, including abdominal pains, muscle pains or fatigue. Conversely, others are described as especially active and high achieving prior to illness onset, with difficulties in their ability *to regulate* activity/rest periods. It is useful to explore fully and aim to modify these views and expectations if they get in the way of engaging in treatment.

Young people with CFS and their families have been found to display an enhanced tendency to believe in the presence of disease in spite of medical evidence and reassurance to the contrary. This can lead to requests for secondary specialist opinions and to seeking help from alternative health practitioners. Excessive medical investigations might ensue. These can maintain anxious parental expectations, undermine parents' confidence and delay the introduction of potentially efficacious interventions. In one sample of young people seen in a specialist paediatric clinic, the mean number of professionals seen was nearly 7 with a range of 2–22.

Unhelpful coping mechanisms may also need to be addressed. There is some evidence that young people with CFS use more emotional regulation and resignation to cope with illness and/or disability compared to those with other paediatric problems. This can result in relinquishing some of the problem-solving techniques they use successfully to cope with other difficulties in their life.

Other Treatment Options and Frequency of Necessary Medical Attention

In contrast to the activity management programme described above, an "organic" school of thought exists that regards CFS as a purely medical disorder with a to-date unidentified biological substrate. It therefore favours a "pacing"-based treatment, which is an energy management strategy in which patients are encouraged to achieve an appropriate balance between rest and activity and to accept and adapt to life within the limitations imposed by the illness, rather than aiming to achieve change and improved levels of activity. In some cases, when other more efficacious approaches have been tried and found ineffective, this might be the only alternative left.

Drug-based treatments such as gamma globulin infusions have been tried and found to result in small gains, but these are not substantial enough to recommend this treatment in routine clinical practice.

Young people with CFS who are severely incapacitated by their symptoms will require specialist treatment and sometimes hospital admission to correct biological anomalies that may derive from insufficient food intake or profound inactivity.

The necessity for medical attention is variable. Mild cases may respond to medical support and guidance and benefit from sporadic or monthly appointments, but when active treatment is instituted, initial weekly sessions can be followed by biweekly or monthly sessions.

Common Problems Seen in Adolescents with CFS

Stigma

Concerns about stigma often feature highly among young people with CFS and their families. The physical presentation leads many parents, and some clinicians, to believe that there must be a physical cause, for example, an encephalopathy, and a preference for the term ME (myalgic encephalomyelitis) rather than CFS to designate the problem. Nevertheless, CFS is preferred by many clinicians as more in line with current empirical evidence. For proponents of the term, ME is seen as carrying the power and strong aura of an organic illness and as "protective" against a psychiatric misdiagnosis such as a depressive or anxiety disorder. It is also thought by some that because chronic fatigue disorder does not have a clear-cut organic aetiology it is not medically respectable, and is not treated with respect by doctors. The associated underlying belief is that the reality of illness has to be substantiated by insisting that it is a medical illness. In young people, the advice to engage in more activity or go to school may be seen as proof that the problem is not taken seriously and that the doctor believes the child is "putting the symptoms on" and that they are modifiable by the child at will.

Some young people may experience a deep sense of shame about their symptoms. Children are often deeply sensitive to how they may be perceived by teachers and fellow pupils, and some fear that they will be thought of as exaggerating their illness in order to gain the privilege of staying at home and avoiding school activities they find irksome. They may react to these perceptions with anger and frustration and may fear exposure to such attitudes upon return to school.

Managing the fear of stigma entails acknowledging real and perceived negative evaluations on the part of others and discussing ways in which perceived negative evaluations may be tackled.

Co-Morbidity

Emotional distress and mood changes are commonly reported in children with CFS, and psychiatric co-morbidity – in particular mood disorders – have higher prevalence rates than in other chronic paediatric disorders. The same applies to certain personality features: adolescents with CFS have been shown to be specially sensitive and vulnerable. Some are also anxiety prone, with a tendency to conscientiousness. As desirable as some of these qualities are, they may compromise adaptation to everyday stresses including common infections and social and educational pressure.

Mood changes can be marked enough to constitute emotional or psychiatric disorders worthy of treatment in their own right. Emotional disorders can be differentiated from the mood symptoms common in the course of CFS, because the emotional disorder symptoms are severe, persisting and impairing. Emotional disorders can stop a young person from becoming involved in the rehabilitation process. For example, anxiety symptoms can make it difficult for children to face difficult situations such as attending school or certain lessons, and depression is often linked to despondency and despair that they will recover from CFS.

One reason that depressive and anxiety disorders are so common in young people with CFS may be shared vulnerability features such as predisposing personality styles. Some of the enduring personality traits seen prior to illness onset in young people with CFS are comparable to those among individuals predisposed to having emotional disorders. These features may also act as maintenance factors for CFS, since a trend for poorer CFS outcome has been noted in children with personality features that are strong enough to be impairing.

Young people with severe depression co-morbid with CFS may benefit from specific cognitive behavioural therapy or the use of antidepressants. Some, however, will find that their mood improves with activity scheduling and cognitive restructuring management strategies. When anxiety disorders predominate, discussion about common physiological aspects can be helpful. Many adolescents and their parents are unaware of how physically exhausting stress and anxiety can be: providing information about the nature of autonomic arousal can help explain the patient's experience of intrusive, frightening somatic sensations.

Social Support

Because concerns about educational and social performance are often encountered in CFS, it is important to explore ways in which they may be assuaged. As they become ill, children often lose confidence in their ability to perform educationally and socially to their aspired level of achievement and this, in addition to any existing stressors – individual, familial or social – may militate against successful rehabilitation and recovery.

Treatment will therefore often involve liaison with school, provision of wheelchair access if necessary, gradual return to school via lessons the child finds easier to cope with, extended into full attendance at a rate the child can accommodate. In severely affected children, attendance at a special school for children with disability or a school with good disability provision may be appropriate. Some children will require a period of home tuition, or time in a small tutorial unit with individual support, before they are ready to consider returning to mainstream school.

Family Conflict

Many families find themselves becoming highly involved in the child's illness. At early stages in the disorder, they may have disregarded the child's symptoms and encouraged the young person to return to school as usual. This can create tensions between resisting children and encouraging parents. Alternatively, parents may have conflicting attitudes towards management. As the disorder progresses, they may have confidence in an assertive, encouraging approach, as they come to believe that this may have an adverse effect on the child's condition. This can lead to lack of confidence and a yielding to the young person's request to be left to rest and sleep.

High levels of parental mental distress and emotional over-involvement with the child's problem might have the unintended result of over-emphasising the physical symptoms and rewarding their continuation, as drawing attention to physical symptoms can enhance their impact. As already noted, disruption of family activities is often very pronounced, and in severe cases family life can be seen to revolve around the need to accommodate the child's symptoms and impairment.

Another complication derives from the fact that fatigue symptoms and syndromes have a family aggregation. If other family members have had similar problems or are experiencing unpleasant excessive tiredness and fatigue, they might find it more difficult to provide the child with an optimistic view of the problem and to support active attempts at rehabilitation. This is made even more difficult if – as is often the case – children have become anxiously dependent on their parents and their parents are highly emotionally involved with the child and the condition.

Treatment Adherence Issues

As a result of the misgivings families often have about engaging in a treatment based on active rehabilitation, adherence can be a significant problem. Some families reject this approach completely, and young people can deteriorate into states of withdrawal and total inactivity. In such extreme cases, professionals need to discuss a comprehensive treatment plan, which might even involve consideration of child protection procedures. More commonly, the young person's motivation will waiver and motivation techniques will need to be put into place to encourage continuation of the rehabilitation work. The expectation of "two steps forward, one step backward" is a good metaphor for how progress is likely to take place.

Cultural Considerations

Chronic fatigue syndrome, as seen in specialist clinics, has until comparatively recently been described primarily in young people in northern European and American countries. Medical clinicians in other countries have wondered about the lack of CFS within their patient group. However, more recently the disorder is being described more globally. It is possible that secular trends influence its manifestation. It has been argued that the stress and exhaustion that doctors are seeing in their patients reflects problems in adaptation from an industrial culture to one dominated by globalisation and quick technological change, especially in the area of information accessing and sharing, and that similar changes were seen in middle-class England in the late 18th and 19th centuries as a response to industrialisation. Different countries would have engaged with these secular changes to various degrees or have different means of adapting to them, thus influencing national CFS rates. However, this is highly speculative. The increase in CFS/ME diagnoses in the last decade has also been ascribed to changes in diagnostic fashion and practice, in response to the increased legitimisation and awareness of the syndrome.

Chronic fatigue in children attending specialist clinics in western countries tends to identify White populations predominantly, but this may reflect socioeconomic status bias in clinic attendees.

How a Behavioural Health Specialist, Working Within an Integrated Team, Can Most Effectively Target Adolescents with CFS

A behavioural health specialist is likely to have a role when young people fail to respond to general advice and guidance by their doctor, or when psychological symptoms are prominent. Because of the prevailing health beliefs and the significant school concerns in the majority of affected young people, the behavioural health specialist's work will need to be closely integrated with that of medical doctors and teachers, as well as of other therapists involved, for example, physiotherapists, dieticians and occupational therapists.

Work by the behavioural specialist may involve setting up an activity programme, working on motivational issues, instituting cognitive behavioural family therapy or cognitive behavioural therapy with the young person. It may also involve joint work with psychiatrists or other mental health specialists with experience in this area of work.

What are the Best Practices for Assessment and Treatment?

Few rigorous research efficacy trials have been conducted with young people with CFS, though a number have been carried out in adults with the disorder. These have shown that in the context of a supportive relationship, cognitive behaviour therapy and/or graded exercise improve disability and symptoms. In young people a number of case studies, case reports and open treatment studies indicate that an effective approach involves a combination of behavioural interventions linked to family therapy or work. A randomised controlled study of 10 sessions of cognitive behaviour therapy for adolescents with CFS has demonstrated significantly greater decrease in fatigue severity and in functional impairment, including school attendance, in patients receiving therapy compared to a waiting-list control group (Stulemeijer et al., 2005).

Methodological Considerations when Conducting Research with This Population

Research into CFS requires adhering to rigorous diagnostic criteria with the exclusion of possible medical or environmental explanations for the fatigue through standardised medical and psychiatric examination. Epidemiological studies tend not to provide good evidence for exclusion of underlying disorders, and therefore normally report on CFS-*like* conditions. Most studies of CFS proper meet this requirement and are conducted with markedly affected participants attending specialist centres.

Treatment studies would ideally need to report on outcomes of patients unwilling to enter the treatment study, in addition to conducting a full "intent to treat" analyses of those who do. Excluding a high percentage of cases because of unwillingness to consider a rehabilitation approach greatly weakens the conclusions of studies demonstrating good outcomes, if patients agreeing to take part represent only a small proportion of those eligible.

Research Agenda

Future research could usefully address the study of genetic mechanisms, biological and personality vulnerabilities and their interactions in young people with CFS. It would be helpful to understand better the reasons why so many young people with CFS and their families reject the possibility of a psychosocial contribution to the disorder, by exploring attitudes related to concepts of stigma and their origins. In terms of treatment, research on motivational approaches to facilitate therapeutic engagement would be highly appropriate, as would trials comparing active and passive therapeutic approaches to the management of CFS in young people. There is still work to be done to clarify to what extent clinical features, psychiatric co-morbidity and risk factors overlap in cases presenting at different severity levels, in CFS-*like* as opposed to full CFS.

References

Chalder, T., & Hussain, K. (2002). *Self help for chronic fatigue syndrome: A self help for young people*. Blue Stallion Publications.

Fukuda, K., Straus, S. E., Hickie, I., Sharpe, M. C., Dobbins, J. G., Komaroff, A., et al. (1994). The chronic fatigue syndrome: A comprehensive approach to is definition and study. *Annals of Internal Medicine, 121*, 953–959.

Gallagher, A. M., Thomas, J. M., Hamilton, W. T., & White P.D. (2004). Incidence of fatigue symptoms and diagnoses presenting in UK primary care from 1990 to 2001. *Journal of the Royal Society of Medicine, 97*, 571–575.

Garralda, M. E. (1999). *Chronic fatigue syndrome: Helping children and adolescents* (Rep. No. Occasional paper 16). London: ACPP.

Garralda, M. E., & Chalder, T. (2005). Practitioner review: Chronic fatigue syndrome in childhood. *Journal of Child Psychology and Psychiatry, 46*, 1143–1151.

Garralda, M. E., & Rangel, L. A. (2002). Annotation: Chronic fatigue syndrome in children and adolescents. *Journal of Child Psychology and Psychiatry, 43*, 169–176.

NICE. (2007). Chronic fatigue syndrome / Myalgic encephalopathy diagnosis and management. National Institute for Clinical Excellence.

Reeves, W. C., Lloyd, A., Vernon, S. D., Klimas, N., Jason, L. A., Bleijenberg, G. et al. (2003). Identification of ambiguities in the 1994 chronic fatigue syndrome research case definition and recommendations for resolution. *BMC Health Services Research, 3*, 1–9.

Royal College of Paediatrics, & Child Health. (2004). *Evidence based guidelines for the management of CFS/ME (Chronic fatigue syndrome/Myalgic encephalopathy) in children and young people* London: RCPCH.

Stulemeijer, M., de Jong, L. M., Fiselier, T. J., Hoogveld, S. W., & Bleijenberg, G. (2005). Cognitive behaviour therapy for adolescents with chronic fatigue syndrome: randomised controlled trial. *British Medical Journal, 330*, 14–17.

Adolescents Living with HIV/AIDS

Maureen E. Lyon and Lawrence J. D'Angelo

Epidemiology

Worldwide, approximately half of all new HIV infections occur among youth aged 10–24 years (WHO, 2005). With improvements in treatment and accessibility, these youth can expect to live well into adulthood. Of equal importance is the fact that the majority of perinatally infected children now have an excellent chance of surviving into adolescence and young adulthood. Thus, behavioral treatments to prevent HIV transmission and chronic illness self-management for HIV-infected adolescents are critical for the well-being of youth living with HIV/AIDS (YLWHA).

To date, risk behavior intervention research on YLWHA is just beginning in middle-income countries (Rongkavilit et al., 2007; Thato, Jenkins, & Dusitsin, 2008). Unfortunately, other biologically based prevention interventions such as a vaccine or a highly effective microbicide have had disappointing results in their early phases of development. In the absence of such measures, Lagakos and Gable (2008) recommend that "With so many lives at stake, it is imperative to prioritize the identification and implementation of effective behavioral ... interventions."

Since the first cases of AIDS were reported in 1981, the epidemiology of HIV infection in adolescents and young adults has been characterized by a series of overlapping "miniepidemics." In the 1980s, the majority of infected youth were hemophiliacs and patients who had received blood transfusions. By the late 1980s and into the early part of the 1990s, the majority of cases were seen in those adolescents who looked the most like their older counterparts with the infection: men who had sex with men and teens who injected drugs. Shortly thereafter, however, there was a rapid shift and we began seeing large numbers of cases (and in some locales even the majority of cases) in young women who had had sex with older males. This group became predominant until the late 1990s when substantial number of young gay men began to reemerge in the HIV and AIDS case counts. Finally, the new millennia introduced us to steadily growing numbers of youth who had acquired their infection at birth and lived until adolescence and well beyond. Today, in many HIV clinics in the United States, more than half of the adolescent and young adult patients who are living with HIV/AIDS were perinatally infected (Rogers, 2006).

Progression of HIV infection depends on many factors. The virus attacks the body's immune system in such a way as to leave the infected host susceptible to a variety of other illnesses. Therefore, for most patients, it stands to reason that the longer they have been infected, the more likely they are to have experienced significant suppression of their immune system. This is more or less true, but there are exceptions. Certain long term survivors appear to have a genetic makeup that allows their immune system to resist the inevitable progression from infection to immunosuppression to AIDS. Other adolescents may be infected with strains of virus that are inherently more or less aggressive. Finally, the availability of highly active antiretroviral therapy (HAART) since the mid-1990s has put a

M.E. Lyon (✉)
Children's National Medical Center, Washington, DC, USA
e-mail: mlyon@cnmc.org

W.T. O'Donohue, L.W. Tolle (eds.), *Behavioral Approaches to Chronic Disease in Adolescence*,
DOI 10.1007/978-0-387-87687-0_22,

premium on being able to take medications on a regular schedule. Adolescents and young adults who were able to adhere to complicated regimens involving three to five different medications were more likely to survive and live on into adulthood. While recent changes in how some of these medications are formulated have lessened the demands on the patient, the rate of disease progression still is influenced by age of acquisition, type of virus, medication regimen, and adherence to these regimens.

Since the beginning of the epidemic, 42,929 youth aged 13–24 years have been diagnosed with AIDS. This represents only 4.2% of all diagnosed cases of AIDS in the United States. Of the entire population in the United States who died from AIDS, 10,096 or 1.8% of these were aged 13–24 years. In 2006, the last year for which figures are available, 2143 youth received a diagnosis of AIDS (CDC, 2008). This represents 5.6% of persons diagnosed that year. Overall, a total of 19,979 young people are now living with AIDS, a 19% increase from 2003 when 16,817 young people were living with AIDS. Of course, counting cases of AIDS significantly underestimates the real impact HIV infection has on this population group because it measures only those most severely compromised by their HIV infection. To date, however, surveillance of all of those individuals who are HIV infected has been incomplete, reflecting counts from only 33 states. With universal reporting of all HIV cases now mandated in this country, this discrepancy will be corrected soon.

Some cities in the country are disproportionately affected by the epidemic. For example, the age-adjusted death rates for HIV disease in 2003 in the District of Columbia (DC) were 43.3 per 100,000, the highest in all states (DC Department of Health, 2007). The total US rate is 4.7 per 100,000 (CDC, 2008).

Significant racial disparities exist in diagnosis and prognosis. Although black Americans represent 13% of the population, in 2006, they represented 49% of new cases of AIDS reported in the United States. Of persons aged 13 to 25 years diagnosed with HIV/AIDS in 2006, 61% are black. This is 10 times the rate for whites. In many urban centers, HIV-infected teens are primarily black or non-white Hispanic (Kaiser HIV/AIDS Policy Fact Sheet, July, 2007).

Prognosis for HIV/AIDS has improved dramatically since the mid-1990s, coincident with the advent of highly active antiretroviral therapy (HAART). HAART has changed HIV/AIDS from a death sentence to a chronic disease, enabling many young people to live into adulthood. Unfortunately, compounding the discrepancy of the occurrence of the infection itself, the prognosis for black Americans is poorer than for white Americans. From 1997 to 2004 a smaller proportion of blacks, 66% were alive after 9 years, compared to 77% of whites (CDC, 2008).

Symptoms

The symptoms experienced by HIV-infected individuals are directly related to the stage of their disease. These stages are defined by either the degree of immune suppression the virus has inflicted on the infected host or the presence of infections defined as "opportunistic infections", infections or health conditions which more commonly occur in individuals with severely compromised immune systems. While individuals acutely infected with HIV may experience a flu-like illness with associated rash, fatigue, and lymphadenopathy (swollen lymph nodes), after this initial "seroconversion illness," prolonged periods can go by with no symptoms. While patients are experiencing essentially no symptoms, the virus has been replicating in the host and helping establish the underlying failure of the immune system later on in the infection.

When symptoms do appear, they are often the result of the above-mentioned "opportunistic infections". They can affect the central nervous system (meningitis, encephalitis, dementia, peripheral neuropathy, etc.,), lungs (pneumonia), or result in "disseminated infection" with no particular single organ system targeted.

In their classification of HIV infection, the Centers for Disease Control has long used the presence of such *opportunistic infections* to define when an HIV-infected individual has proceeded to the point in their illness that they are classified as having AIDS. These include, but are not limited to, *Candida* (a fungus) infection of esophagus, trachea, bronchi, or lungs; cytomegalovirus infection;

cryptococcal meningitis (another fungus); herpes simplex >1 month duration; *Mycobacterium tuberculosis*; *Pneumocystis jirovecii* pneumonia; and toxoplasmosis. Other health conditions more commonly seen in immunosuppressed individuals are also included in the list of illnesses which mark the transition from HIV infection to AIDS. These include cervical cancer, dementia, wasting (weight loss >10% of baseline), and lymphoma of the central nervous system (CDC, 1993).

At this time, HIV infection must be considered an otherwise "incurable" infection. However, even before highly effective treatment was available, the median time from infection to meeting the immunologic or infectious complication definition of AIDS was 8–12 years. The treatment regimens that have now been established have transformed HIV infection into a chronic, albeit serious and still often fatal, disease. Nonetheless, since 1981, of the almost one million US residents who have been diagnosed as having AIDS, almost 60% have died (CDC, 2008).

As noted above, the complications of HIV infection usually involve the acquisition and expression of another infection or other health condition. Any one of these conditions can become life-threatening. At a minimum, these conditions often also interfere with adaptive functioning because of missed school or work for medical visits or long hospitalizations.

Because of the more direct affect it can have on behavior, the neurologic consequences of HIV can be significant. Infections such as fungal meningitis are easier to diagnose with appropriate testing than are other neurologic conditions. CNS-mediated depression and dementia, while less common than some HIV-related illnesses, are often difficult to diagnose. In two hospital-based clinics for HIV-infected adolescents during the post-HAART period, 8% of 76 YLWHA and 18.2% of 33 YLWHA were diagnosed with encephalopathy (Lyon, Marsh, Trexler, Crane, & D'Angelo, 2007; Shanbhag et al., 2005).

While other complications of HIV are usually fairly equally distributed by gender and race/ethnicity, one in particular, renal failure, appears to be overly represented in African-Americans (Lucas et al., 2008). While this is now considered a treatable complication with diet and dialysis, it is sometimes painful and exhausting.

Treatment Regimen for Adolescents

The treatment of HIV infection has evolved dramatically in the past 20 years. When HAART became the standard for treating HIV infection in the mid-1990s, patients were often faced with medication regimens that consisted of upward of 8–14 pills that needed to be taken up to four times daily. Fortunately, as new medications were developed and we gained a better understanding of those that already existed, we have been able to reduce this "pill burden" to the point where the most common starting regimen consists of one pill (which combines three separate drugs) taken once daily.

This beneficial change in our approach to treating HIV has enabled more HIV-positive individuals to attain "undetectable" levels of the virus in the blood. However, attaining an "undetectable" level of the virus in the blood does not mean that an HIV-infected individual is cured, only that the virus is suppressed and cannot be measured in the blood. Virus is still maintained in many organs throughout the body.

A new and controversial study (Bernard, 2008; Vernazza, Hirschel, Bernasconi, Flepp, 2008) led the Swiss National AIDS Commission after reviewing the scientific data to state that "An HIV-infected individual without an additional STD and on an anti-retroviral therapy (ART) with completely suppressed viremia ... is sexually non-infectious, i.e. he/her cannot pass on the HIV-virus through sexual contact as long as the following conditions are fulfilled:

- The HIV-infected individual complies with the anti-retroviral therapy (ART), the effects of which must be evaluated regularly by the treating physician;
- The viral load has been non-detectable for at least six months (viral load in the blood is suppressed < 40 copies/ml);
- There are no additional sexually transmitted diseases (STD) present."

The Commission compared the current data to that for kissing in 1986 when the statement that HIV could not be transmitted by kissing was published and communicated, even though it could never be proven. The reader is referred to the Australian Web site in which links with English translations and discussion of the controversy are available (http://www.ashm.org.au/news/280/11/).

The Centers for Disease Control responded to this study with the recommendation that all HIV-positive individuals continue to use condoms, regardless of viral suppression.

When to start treatment is debated among practitioners. Early on in the epidemic it was thought best to "hit hard and hit early." However, the adverse side effects and long-term toxicities associated with HAART regimens have led the Department of Health and Human Services to recommend modifying this approach to treatment and postponing initiation until there is clear evidence that the immune system has been affected by the virus and that there is significant amount of virus circulating in the patient's blood. Multidrug treatments (usually at least three drugs) and treatments including drugs from multiple classes of medications, especially non-nucleoside reverse transcription inhibitors (NNRTIs) or protease inhibitors (PIs), appear to be the best in that they are most effective in dramatically lowering the amount of virus and least likely to cause resistant virus to emerge (Bangsberg, 2008). For YLWHA who are experiencing neurocognitive changes, starting earlier is recommended (Antinori et al.,2007).

Once treatment is initiated, patients need close follow-up (every 4–6 weeks) to determine any side effects of the medication and to allow an assessment of level of adherence to therapy. Once stabilized, this visit frequency can become every 8–12 weeks.

The rapid and continual replication of the virus in the infected host makes development of mutant strains of the virus that are resistant to the medications a patient is taking likely. The best way to avoid this is to completely suppress (to the degree possible) replication of the virus. This is the major reason to insist on high levels of patient adherence, so that medication levels remain high enough to stop replication. The emergence of resistance can signal a major change in the illness and make therapy quite challenging. It usually means that some or all of medications in use with this patient need to be switched and can ultimately lead to the inability to stop the progression of HIV replication and further suppression of the immune system.

A surprising number of adolescents have ongoing difficulty in swallowing pills. Specialized training on pill swallowing and the use of liquid formulations is often necessary to ensure adherence. Side effects from HAART include but are not limited to depression, nausea, diarrhea, and malaise or a general run-down feeling. There are also more serious toxicities associated with HAART medications, which require monitoring with routine lab testing. During advanced disease, outpatients are seen weekly. An excellent summary of medical care for HIV-infected teens is provided by Dr. D'Angelo in the book *Adolescents HIV and AIDs: The Voices of Teens Living with the Virus* (2006).

HAART medications are expensive, thousands of dollars a month. But in resource-rich countries like the United States, medications may be covered by private health insurance, Medicaid, and Ryan White funding to cover those without insurance.

Stigma and Disclosure

All epidemics raise fears of transmission. Learning to live with the HIV epidemic and how to interact in a safe and sensitive way with persons infected with HIV (Krauss, Godfrey, O'Day, Freidin, & Kaplan, 2006) is a challenge. Stigma causes psychological distress and may interfere with HIV-positive adolescents' efforts to cope with their illness, including medication adherence. Adolescents may not want to be observed taking their medications for fear friends will ask what is wrong. Often they do not want school nurses to administer their medications for fear the health history will not be kept confidential. Fear of discrimination or outright rejection results in many newly infected teens not disclosing their HIV diagnosis to family, friends, or sexual partners. It is not unusual for those infected since birth to be told by their caregivers to not disclose their HIV status to their friends or classmates. Disclosure of HIV status may inadvertently disclose the status of one or more family members, while failure to disclose HIV status can have the unintended consequence of further isolating the adolescent or putting sexual partners at risk. In a study in which teens were asked, "What are the "complications" of living with HIV?" a question intended to elicit medical complications, HIV-infected teens often mentioned the need to keep their diagnosis a secret and the feeling that they are living a lie (Lyon, McCarter, Briggs, D'Angelo, 2008, May).

Despite these negative consequences, several existing studies suggest that disclosure of their HIV status to significant others increases immune functioning and social support. This is a process that varies by gender, ethnicity, sexual orientation, and age (see review for adolescents in Wiener & Lyon, 2006). Children who told their HIV diagnosis to friends had significantly higher immune functioning (higher CD4 cell %) than children who had not yet told their HIV status to friends (Wiener, 2004). Among the adolescents in the Reaching for Excellence in Adolescent Care and Health (REACH), those who disclosed their HIV status to family and friends reported better psychosocial adjustment and a strong sense of social support (D'Angelo, Abdalian, Sarr, Hoffman, & Belzer, 2001). In contrast, HIV-positive children and adolescents who responded to invitations from the media to talk about living with HIV often experienced greater social dysfunction and lower perceived self-competence than those who said no to these requests (Wiener, Battles, & Heilman, 2000).

More worrisome in terms of secondary prevention of transmission of HIV is the fact that 32–40% of YLWHA do not tell their sexual partners their serostatus (Koenig et al., Adolescent Living with HIV or AIDS (ALPHA) study, 2007; Lyon, Brasseux, & D'Angelo, 1999). Adolescents must judge whether the benefits of disclosure will outweigh the potential costs. Adolescents can benefit from training in ethical decision-making to help them cope with the complexities, challenges, and pitfalls of disclosure.

Whether a licensed professional has the legal right to disclose the patient's HIV status to others is a matter of law which varies from state to state. Behavioral health specialists working in medical settings need to be familiar with their state laws, their agencies' regulations regarding disclosure of protected information, their professional guidelines, as well as the medical ethics principles of autonomy, beneficence, do no harm, fidelity, and justice. Clinical situations will arise in which the law, agency policies, professional guidelines, and medical ethics principles are in conflict. The American Psychological Association's Office on AIDS (janderson@apa.org) provides training in ethical decision-making. Consultation with colleagues and malpractice insurance attorneys is often critical to a well-reasoned and professional outcome.

Comorbidity

Similar to other viral infections, HIV can cause persistent and progressive changes in emotional and cognitive functions (Kopnisky, Bao, & Lin, 2007). Primary HIV-1 virus is found in both the subcortical region and the basal ganglia of the brain. Research efforts are indicating that the mediators of psychiatric illness, substance abuse, and HIV neuropathogenesis use similar brain structures, neurocircuitry, and receptor symptoms.

With highly active antiretroviral therapy (HAART), the incidence of HIV-dementia (HIV-D) has decreased, while the prevalence of HIV-associated neurocognitive disorders (HAND) has persisted (Antinori et al., 2007), despite viral suppression (Shanbhag et al., 2005). Revised definitional criteria for HAND gives greater priority to cognitive aspects of impairment, compared to deficits in psychomotor speed, mood, or behavioral regulation (Antinori et al., 2007).

To our knowledge, few data are available on screening for or assessment of the prevalence of adolescent HAND (Drs. Lucy Civitello, Donna Futterman, Marvin Belzer, personal communication). In the first decade of the epidemic, an estimated 50–90% of HIV-infected children developed encephalopathy. Our experience with adolescents has been somewhat different in that we identified encephalopathy in 8% of 76 adolescent patients. All of these teens were males who were perinatally infected (Lyon et al., 2007), suggesting that they may be a particularly vulnerable population requiring close monitoring. Two of the six adolescents with encephalopathy did not have advanced disease, but had CD4 cells between 200 and 500. A study (Shanbhag et al., 2005) of children, with a median age of 8.1 years, found that despite the decreased prevalence of HIV encephalopathy in perinatally infected children born before 1996 (29.6%, N=113), those born since 1996 had an 18.2% (N=33) prevalence of all encephalopathy. Clearly, encephalopathy can interfere with adaptive functioning, especially the ability to perform at school or work or to remember to adhere to complex medication regimens. Adolescents with HIV being treated with HAART who maintain viral suppression may be at risk for developing CNS disease. Screening or comprehensive neuropsychological assessment to assess for changes from baseline over time, using the revised criteria (Antinori et al., 2007), is critical to optimum outcomes.

It is estimated that more than 60% of HIV-infected individuals will suffer from at least one major psychiatric disorder during the course of infection (Kopnisky et al., 2007). This finding is consistent with findings in a small study of YLWHA in which 65% met criteria for a psychiatric diagnosis using a structured diagnostic interview (Pao et al., 2000). There is an effort to understand these viral-induced imbalances in neuronal network functioning thought to be associated with precipitating or accentuating psychiatric conditions in individuals with HIV and genetic vulnerabilities (Kopnisky et al., 2007).

Psychiatric symptoms are complicated by the fact that HAART medications can cause side effects that mimic depressive symptomatology (e.g., fatigue, sleep disturbance, and weight loss). Medication for psychiatric symptoms/syndromes is appropriate, generally safe, and helpful. Dosing recommendations are to "go low, go slow and monitor" (Maryland Pao, MD, personal communication). Psychotropic treatment of psychiatric symptoms improves the overall care and functioning of YLWHA. Behavioral manifestations of the disease process may also remit with effective adherence to HAART.

One of the tragedies of HIV/AIDS is that often more than one family member is infected. Bereaved adolescents who have lost a parent to AIDS experience significant difficulties with adjustment. Rotherham-Borus, Weiss, Alber, and Lester (2005) found that these adolescents suffered significantly more emotional distress, negative life events, and contact with the criminal justice system when compared to nonbereaved adolescents. Immediately following the death of the parent, bereaved adolescents had more depressive symptoms and sexual risk behaviors than nonbereaved adolescents.

Adherence

The World Health Organization (WHO, 2003) has estimated that if all individuals living with a chronic illness were adherent to their medication regimens, the results would be equal to curing cancer. WHO warns against blaming the patient for failures in adherence to medication regimen. There are many systems issues that pose barriers to adherence, such as lack of access to care or distrust of the doctor or medical establishment. Furthermore, HIV regimens are often complex and always lifelong. Adhering to HAART regimens is even more challenging than that found with other illnesses.

New research suggests that the old belief that effective treatment requires 90–95% adherence is incorrect. Rather the effectiveness of viral suppression interacts with adherence and the nature of the HAART regimen and whether or not it is a boosted regimen (Bangsberg, 2008). Ironically, on some earlier less-potent regimens, 100% adherence was more likely to cause resistance (Bangsberg, 2008). With the introduction of once a day dosing, adherence rates are expected to improve. Medication side effects and toxicities can also interfere with adherence. Patients need to be educated about when to speak with their practitioner about side effects. Stigma, lack of disclosure, and secrecy are additional barriers to adherence to medication (for a review of barriers to adherence, see Koenig & Bachanas, 2006). There are also cultural barriers to ability and willingness to take medication. In Thailand, for example, adherence rates for adolescents are close to the ideal of 95% (Rongkavilit et al., 2007) in contrast to adherence rates for adolescents in the United States.

In the most recent published study describing HAART adherence among 120 adolescents in the United States, the PACTG 381 study team (Flynn et al., 2007) found that the majority of adolescents started on HAART stopped treatment (63%) within the 3-year period of observation. Only 24% of behaviorally infected adolescents (29/120) who were started on a HAART regimen achieved and maintained undetectable viral loads over 3 years. Those who maintained adherence had immune functioning that appeared to be as good as non-infected adolescents on measures of CD4 counts and viral load. Poorer adherence, higher baseline viral load, and CD8 naïve counts predicted virologic failure for the remaining 13% (15/120) who stayed on medication for the 3 years of observation. Adherence during the first 16 weeks on medication appeared to be critical for achieving undetectable viral loads.

These results confirm those from the REACH (Reaching for Excellence in Adolescent Care and Health) in which only 28.3% of HIV-positive adolescents (N=161) in 13 US cities reported having missed no doses in the previous month (Murphy et al., 2005). These results are also consistent with those from substance-abusing adolescents (Rotheram-Borus et al., 2004).

How can we improve adherence? Going beyond the context of institutional and community variables, there are very few published interventions aimed at increasing adherence to medication in YLWHA. One of the first (Lyon et al., 2003) found that self-reported adherence and satisfaction with treatment increased in a 12-session pilot study of a multifamily "HAART" group (N=46; 23 families). The intervention alternated six "family group" psychoeducational sessions with six "adolescent only" support sessions for a total of 12 sessions for YLWHA and 6 sessions for the family which included the adolescent. Participants discussed the dynamics of HIV, why they should take therapy, how to manage side effects, and how to communicate with doctors. Most (78%) of the 46 participants (adolescents and treatment buddies/family members) completed the intervention; 91% of the adolescents reported increased adherence. Four adolescents experienced a one-log reduction in viral load to undetectable levels at the end of the 12-week intervention. At 6-month evaluation, two of four participants who had not been taking any medication started HAART. Two adolescents continued to decline antiretroviral medications. One adolescent died during the intervention. One lesson learned was that in the future study, family members as well as adolescents should receive reimbursement and incentives. Participants said that what they gained most from the group were connectedness and decreased isolation. Family/treatment buddies rated the overall program as highly helpful, citing social support as most valuable. An unanticipated benefit was an increase in other health behaviors, including medical and dental appointments, hepatitis B and influenza immunizations, and referrals to mental health and substance abuse treatment. Games and prizes were used to review the content of the six educational/skill sessions. Participants tested five devices to help them take their medication, rating a multiple alarm watch as the best aid.

The TREAT (Therapeutic Regimens Enhancing Adherence in Teens) program (Rogers, Miller, Murphy, Tanney, & Fortune, 2001) was an 8-week intervention. It was designed to prepare teens who had never taken HAART by providing them with education through written materials and a video. Contrary to the hypothesis, 40% of the 79 participants were found to be at stages of readiness that did not match with their treatment stage or their actual adherence behavior. The lesson learned from this trial was not to use stage of readiness as a reason to deny access to medication.

Teens Linked to Care (TLC) is the only adherence intervention to be evaluated in a clinical trial (Rotheram-Borus et al., 2001). Because of poor attendance, it was modified to be delivered as one-to-one counseling, offered either in person or by phone. Unfortunately, despite decreases in risk behavior, the intervention did not significantly improve medication use or adherence (Rotheram-Borus et al., 2004).

A randomized clinical trial funded by the CDC to improve adherence to treatment and to reduce risk behaviors for YLWHA at three sites, Adolescent IMPACT, is currently in the data analytic phase with dissemination of results expected soon (Lyon, Marhefka, Abramowitz, Koenig, LaGrange & ADIMPAT Team, 2008).

The first community-level intervention aiming to reduce HIV incidence and prevalence among urban youth is Connect to Protect. This intervention includes components of structural change and community mobilization. It is a 6-year project under the Adolescent Trials Network funded through the National Institutes of Health. It is in the initial planning phases with intentions to lay groundwork for the intervention in multiple cities throughout the United States. A qualitative review of adherence recommendations for research and clinical management in pediatrics is provided by Simoni et al. (2007).

Cultural Considerations

Psychotherapy and interventions with HIV-positive adolescents and youth need to be culturally sensitive so that when we offer services our patients will come. There are strategies for health specialists working in medical settings to engage, for example, HIV-positive African-American teens in mental health and support services in nonstigmatizing ways (Lyon & Woodward, 2003). Ethnicity and related racial disparities, sexual orientation or identity, gender as well as the needs of the community usually require adaptation of evidence-based treatments (Bell et al., 2007).

Role of Behavioral Specialist Working with an Integrated Team

Psychologists working in a medical setting with an HIV treatment team (1) provide comprehensive psychological and neuropsychological assessment; (2) provide individual psychotherapy, family, and group therapy; (3) develop, obtain funding, and implement interventions based on sound scientific theory and evidence; (4) train staff about psychosocial issues of YLWHA and around ethical decision-making; (5) act as a consultant with staff in coping with difficult cases; (6) provide individual support to the staff and devise programs to help prevent burnout and to enhance morale; and (7) conduct research in priority areas.

A behavioral specialist in a medical setting needs to maintain their professional identity. Participating in professional organizations or peer consultation is one of the few ways to do this. The role of the behavioral specialist can be broadened to include advocacy, for example, by participating in the multidisciplinary Society for Adolescent Medicine (SAM) or the American Psychological Association's Committee on Psychology and AIDS (COPA), which advocates for policy changes or maintenance of current policies that benefit YLWHA within the political system. For example, SAM and COPA were very active in supporting funding for Abstinence Plus education as opposed to increasing funding for Abstinence Only education, which had not been demonstrated to be effective in protecting teens from risky sexual behavior (Santelli et al., 2006).

Psychological and Neuropsychological Assessment

A baseline comprehensive psychological assessment is critical to identifying the cognitive, psychological, social, and educational needs of YLWHA. Several batteries have been proposed for assessing people at varying stages of HIV infection for cognitive impairment, some comprehensive and others abbreviated. For a list of appropriately normed tests and confounding factors in assessing neurocognitive impairment, see the *Neurology*® Web site, www.neurology.org

Because HIV/AIDS can involve neurological complications discussed earlier, the battery of tests should include an assessment of HIV-associated neurocognitive disorders (HAND) (Antinori et al., 2007). Antinori et al. revised the American Academy of Neurology definitional criteria to recognize the following three conditions: (1) asymptomatic neurocognitive impairment (ANI); (2) HIV-associated mild neurocognitive disorder (MND); and (3) HIV-associated dementia (HAD). Patients can develop ANT even on HAART and with normal or near-normal CD4 cell counts (Lyon et al., 2009; Shanbhag et al., 2005).

Full-scale intelligence testing provides a baseline against which to assess changes in cognitive functioning over time, which can lead to identification of neurological complications. Also important is identifying adolescents who may be developmentally delayed, but not receiving appropriate services. Achievement testing in reading and mathematics provides an opportunity to identify teens with learning disabilities who have been overlooked and underserved in the public school system. Advocacy of appropriate services is important. Furthermore, assessment of literacy in reading and math is important to the health-care provider who will need to spend more time with a teen who is illiterate or functionally illiterate (reading at 4th–6th grade level) in reviewing treatment recommendations, for example, use of a pill box or other tools to help with medication adherence or having the teen drop by once a week to check in until the regimen is mastered. Paper and pencil screening measures for attention problems can later be followed up when indicated for a full assessment for attention-deficit hyperactivity disorder. Screening measures for anxiety, depression, and externalizing behaviors should also be included with appropriate referrals made for a fuller assessment.

What Do We Know About Programs that Work?

The Centers for Disease Control (CDC) has several Web sites where evidence-based programs in adolescent HIV prevention are featured: (1) Prevention Research Programs (PRS: see http://www.cdc.gov/hiv/topics/research/prs/index.htm); (2) Replicating Effective Programs (REP: see http://www.cdc.gov/hiv/projects/rep/default.htm); (3) Diffusion of Effective Behavioral Interventions to provide training for diffusing programs (DEBI: see http://effectiveinterventions.org/); (4) Technical Assistance Resources, Guidance, Education and Training Center (TARGET: see http://careacttarget.org/).

Recent reviews of the core characteristics of evidence-based programs for adolescents in general (Evans et al., 2005), as well as those at risk for (DiClemente & Crosby, 2006) or living with HIV (Galbraith et al., 2008; Ingram, Flannery, Elkavich, & Rotheram-Borus, 2008; Malow, Kershaw, Sipsma, Rosenberg, & Devieux, 2007; Tevendale & Lightfoot, 2006), have identified essential elements of programs that work:

Theoretically grounded – with regard to causes of outcomes and mechanisms of change.

More hours – more effective – concerns about attrition of effects over time suggest that spreading the sessions out over time or offering booster sessions may help.

Earlier is better – put the program in place before the target behavior is set, e.g., prior to the onset of sexual activity for decreasing high-risk sexual behaviors.

Structured – clear goals, ongoing monitoring are essential, as are agenda setting and trained facilitator(s).

Accurate – accurate education not pushed by political/religious agenda.

Delivery vehicle – dyadic, family, and community programs have explained more variance in risk outcomes than traditional, individual-level interventions (DiClemente & Crosby, 2006). Very few controlled studies demonstrate the efficacy of individual psychotherapy for people living with HIV/AIDS and there are none to our knowledge with adolescents. Family-based interventions that support parental monitoring and supervision, parental warmth and support, and improve parent–child communication are effective in reducing and delaying sexual risk behaviors. To our knowledge, there are few evidence-based studies of group or family psychotherapy with HIV-positive adolescents. Rather research has focused on group and family interventions described earlier under programs that work. Group interventions, when they are cohesive and supportive of self-disclosure while encouraging fun through humor, games, or refreshments, are potent.

Target several systems simultaneously – change was most effective when multiple levels, e.g., home, school, community, were targeted particularly with respect to norms.

Active engagement/skills focused – skills targeted-to the outcome through experiential activities and role plays increased effectiveness. Activities were interactive and competency building (and fun). Cognitive behavioral principles, problem-solving techniques, and decision-making skills were most useful. Competency building through increasing self-control, delaying gratification, developing an internal moral code, and increasing a sense of responsibility in relationship with others were also critical.

Culturally and socially relevant – tailored to participants through community consultation (Community Advisory Boards or Focus Groups with adolescents, their families, and/or community leaders). Facilitators from the same ethnic group.

Developmentally appropriate – Effective programs promoted moral values and set social rules, fostered the development of responsible intimate relationships, and focused on the future applying learning in real-life settings (work, home, and school) within the context of a developing social identity and a sense of empowerment and self-care.

Sexual Abuse History

YLWHA with a history of sexual abuse, estimated to be about 50% of the behaviorally infected population (Pao et al., 2000; preliminary data from ADIMPACT unpublished), are at particular risk because of difficulties with affect regulation and dysfunctional thinking that are thought to be sequelae of the abuse. These difficulties can lead to impulsivity and failure to assertively set limits in sexual situations. Cognitive behavior therapy (CBT: Beck, 1983) has frequently been employed in the treatment of abused children and adolescents, and a variant of this, dialectical behavior therapy (DBT) (Linehan, 1999), has been applied to abused adults. DBT may be useful as a framework for addressing affect dysregulation and dysfunctional thinking specific to sexuality within an HIV prevention intervention for abused adolescents (Lescano, Brown, Puster & Miller, 2005; Koenig, Doll, O'Leary, Pequegnat, 2004). Other forms of therapy may also be effective, but they have not been studied.

What Has Worked to Decrease Risk Behaviors?

Research on interventions for HIV-infected youth worldwide is in its infancy. Rotheram-Borus and colleagues implemented a 2-intervention module/23-session small-group intervention to target risk behaviors in HIV-infected youth in the United States. The intervention was successful in reducing unprotected sex and substance use (Rotheram-Borus et al., 2001). However, there were no effects on adherence as defined by keeping appointments. One-third of youth did not attend any session. Retention in group interventions may be difficult because of fears of stigmatization. A brief intervention or individual sessions may be more feasible and suitable for HIV-infected youth. Naar-King et al. (2006), Ellis, Naar-King, Cunningham, and Secord (2006) were able to retain HIV-infected youth in a study of MET, and youth receiving MET had significantly greater condom use and greater improvements in viral load than youth in standard care.

Family-Centered Advance Care Planning

Although HIV is now managed as a chronic illness, death rates continue to be relatively high in Washington, DC, New York City, California, Florida, and Puerto Rico, particularly for African-Americans (Kaiser, 2007). Many African-American HIV-positive teens who live in these areas have friends who have died from AIDS and have thought about their own death. When asked what they want, YLWHA have said that they want to have conversations early in the course of their illness and their families have asked for help "breaking the ice" (Lyon, McCabe, Patel, D'Angelo, 2004). Yet, despite the wishes of adolescents and their families and the recommendations from the Institute of Medicine (Field & Behrman, 2002) and the American Academy of Pediatrics (2000) that adolescents with life-threatening illnesses have these conversations integrated into their care and that they be included in these discussions, these recommendations have not been put into practice. Standard of care continues to wait until there is a life-threatening medical crisis. In large part, this is because these conversations are anxiety-provoking and sad, and no structured program exists for adolescents and families to help families speak directly and honestly about end-of-life care.

Children who die of AIDS rarely have DNR/hospice enrollment (Lyon, Williams et al., 2008). Quality of life was found to be significantly lower for those with DNR/hospice than those without across most domains, not surprising as this measure includes physical symptoms. Of note, psychological status was in healthy ranges for both groups of children, those who did have a DNR order or hospice enrollment and those who did not, suggesting that having a DNR or hospice enrollment does no harm.

One theoretically based and evidenced-based structured program, Family-Centered Advance Care Planning, has been developed (Lyon et al., 2007, July) and implemented (Lyon, McCarter, Briggs et al., 2008; Lyon, McCarter, Briggs, He, D'Angelo, 2008) to create a facilitating environment for these conversations with HIV-positive teens and their families. This randomized controlled clinical trial was feasible and acceptable to families recruited from two hospital-based clinics (Lyon, Garvie,

Birggs, et al., 2009). Surrogates in the intervention were significantly more likely to know what their adolescent's wishes were for end-of-life care than controls (Lyon, Garvie, Briggs, et al., (April, 2009).

Methodological Considerations

HIV-positive transgender, gay, drug users, juvenile offenders, school dropouts, runaways, homeless, and migrant youth are especially vulnerable. They may be excluded from research protocols, because they are often hard to reach and may be reluctant to access to health-care systems in which research is conducted. Youth in the neglect system or those with developmental delays are also unlikely to be represented in research because of concerns about exploitation or decision-making capacity. As a consequence, the results of many of the evidence-based programs presented here may not be generalizable to these adolescents. Community-based participatory research and community consultation with these groups is one key to engaging these youth in care and in research protocols. Other barriers to participation are transportation, missed school/work, and distrust of research.

Research Agenda

We agree with Malow et al. (2007), the Institute of Medicine (Field & Behrman, 2002), and the NIH Workshop (Kopnisky et al., 2007) that when conducting comorbidity research, biological data need to be included in order to keep pace with the progress on psychosocial determinants of high-risk behaviors. Biologic outcomes could include, for example, laboratory testing of STDs. New methodologies should be used to allow investigation of the molecular mechanisms or pathways through which genes act so that there is a greater understanding of the mechanism of action in an intervention and study populations' biologic antecedents.

We also agree with Evans et al. (2005) on the need to develop a research base on the effectiveness of treatments for youth with more than one problem, delivering services within complex service systems. We need to continue outreach efforts to marginalized youth in order to ensure that all youth have access to medical as well as mental health care. We need to ensure that all studies of treatment development and delivery include the perspectives of families and providers.

Facilitating the transition of chronically ill adolescents to adulthood and to adult health care remains a problem. Development of a transition model program is supported by major policy documents in the United States. Despite the policy recommendations, to our knowledge, structured, evidence-based programs to transition YLWHA to adult health care or adulthood do not exist in the United States. While disease knowledge and skills have been emphasized as important components for successful transition, there is little empirical data to support this and a lack of attention to the psychosocial complexities of the transition process. Insurance barriers and privacy laws in the United States make the necessary longitudinal follow-up a daunting challenge. Future research should strive to overcome the institutional barriers to ensure optimum health and psychological care to chronically ill youth as they reach adulthood.

Conclusion

YLWHA and their providers are learning to live well with HIV. As new cohorts of youth reach adolescence and the risks associated with transmission, researchers and medical health specialists need to remain vigilant in providing effective behavioral preventive interventions specific to their needs, until such time as a vaccine or a cure is found. Loving with care is the foundation of this effort.

References

American Academy of Pediatrics, Committee on Bioethics and Committee on Hospital Care. (2000). Palliative care for children. *Pediatrics* 106, 351–357.

Antinori A., Arendt G., Becker, J. T., Brew, B. J., Byrd, D. A., Cherner, M., et al. (2007). Updated research nosology for HIV-associated neurocognitive disorders. *Neurology, 69*, 1789–1799.

Bangsberg, D. (2008, May). The importance of adherence: resistance, viral fitness, and adherence patterns in determining outcomes. Grand rounds George Washington University HIV/AIDS Institute.

Beck, A. T. (1983). Cognitive therapy of depression: new perspectives. In P. Clayton & J. E. Barrett (Eds.), *Treatment of depression: Old controversies and new approaches* (pp. 265–290). New York: Raven Press.

Bell, S. G., Newcomer, S. F., Bachrach, C., Borawski, E., Jemmott, J. L., Morrison, D. et al. (2007). Challenges in replicating interventions. *Journal of Adolescent Health*, 40(6), 514–520.

Bernard, E., (2008) Swiss experts say individuals with undetectable viral load and no STI cannot transmit HIV during sex Link to report: Aidsmap Wednesday, January 30, 2008 http://www.aidsmap.org/en/news/4E9D555B-18FB-4D56-B912-2C28AFCCD36B.asp

Centers for Disease Control. (1993). 1992 revised classification system for HIV infection and expanded surveillance case definition for AIDS among adolescents and adults. Mortality and Morbidity Weekly Reports Recomm Rep 41 (RR-17), 1–19.

Centers for Disease Control and Prevention. (2008). HIV/AIDS surveillance report, 2006. Vol. 18. Atlanta: U.S. Department of Health and Human Services, Centers for Disease Control and Prevention.

D'Angelo, L. J., Abdalian, S. E., Sarr, M., Hoffman, N., & Belzer, M. (2001). Disclosure of serostatus by HIV infected youth: the experience of the REACH study. Reaching for Excellence in Adolescent Care and Health. *Journal of Adolescent Health, 29*(suppl. 3), 72–79.

DiClemente, R. J. & Crosby, R. A. (2006). Preventing HIV infections in adolescents: What works for uninfected teens. In. M. E. Lyon & L. J. D'Angelo (Eds.), *Teenagers HIV and AIDS: Insights from youths living with the virus* (pp. 143–161). Westport, CT: Praeger Publishers.

District of Columbia Department of Health HIV/AIDS Fact Sheets. Revised November 2007. www.doh.dc.gov

Ellis, D. A., Naar-King, S., Cunningham, P. B., & Secord, E. (2006). Use of multisystemic therapy to improve antiretroviral adherence and health outcomes in HIV-infected pediatric patients: evaluation of a pilot program. *AIDS Patient Care & STDS, 20*, 112–121.

Evans, D. L., Foa, E. B., Gur, R. E., Hendin, H., O'Biren, C. P., Seligman, M. E. P. et al. (Eds.). (2005). *Treating and preventing adolescent mental health disorders: What we know and what we don't know: A research agenda for improving the mental health of our youth.* New York: Oxford University Press.

Field, M. J., Behrman, R. E. (Eds.). (2002). *When children die: Improving palliative and end-of-life care for children and their families.* Washington, DC: Institute of Medicine, National Academy Press.

Flynn, P. M., Rudy B. J., Lindsey, J. C., Douglas, S. D., Lathey, J., Spector, S. A. et al., & PACTG 381 Study Team. (2007). Long-term observation of adolescents initiating HAART therapy: Three-year follow-up. *AIDS Research and Human Retroviruses, 23*(10), 1208–1214.

Galbraith, J. S., Stanton, B., Boekeloo, B., King, W., Desmond, S., Howard, D., et al. (2008). Exploring implementation and fidelity of evidence-based behavioral interventions for HIV prevention: Lessons learned from the focus on kids diffusion case study. *Health Education & Behavior*, 0: 1090198108315366v1

Ingram, B. L., Flannery, D., Elkavich, A., & Rotheram-Borus, M. J. (2008). Common processes in evidence-based adolescent HIV prevention. *Aids Behavior, 12*(3), 374–383.

Kaiser HIV/AIDS Policy Fact Sheet, Black Americans and HIV/AIDS. July, 2007.

Koenig, L. J. (2007, July). Addressing drug use in a sexual transmission risk reduction intervention for adolescents with HIV: The Adolescent Impact Study. Presented at the Joint Meetings on Adolescent Treatment Effectiveness. Washington, D. C.

Koenig, L. J., & Bachanas, P. J. (2006). Adherence to medications for HIV: Teens say, "Too many, too big, too often." In. M. E. Lyon & L. J. D'Angelo (Eds.), *Teenagers HIV and AIDS: Insights from youths living with the virus* (pp.45–65). Westport, CT: Praeger Publishers.

Koenig, L. J., Doll, L. S., O'Leary, A, & Pequegnat, W. (Eds.). (2004). *From child sexual abuse to adult sexual risk: Trauma, revictimization, and intervention.* Washington, D. C.: American Psychological Association.

Kopnisky, K. L., Bao, J., & Lin Y. W. (2007). Neurobiology of HIV, psychiatric and substance abuse comorbidity research: Workshop report. *Brain, Behavior and Immunity, 21*, 428–441.

Krauss, B. J., Godfrey, C., O'Day, J., Freidin, E., & Kaplan, R. (2006). Learning to live with an epidemic: Reducing stigma and increasing safe and sensitive socializing with persons with HIV. In. M. E. Lyon & L. J. D'Angelo (Eds.), *Teenagers HIV and AIDS: Insights from youths living with the virus* (pp. 83–103). Westport, CT: Praeger Publishers.

Lagakos, S. W. & Gable A. R. (2008). Challenges to HIV prevention –; seeking effective measures in the absence of a vaccine. *New England Journal of Medicine, 358*(15), 1543–1545.

Lescano, C. M., Brown, L. K., Puster, K. L., & Miller, P. M. (2005). Sexual abuse and adolescent HIV risk a group intervention *Framework HIV/AIDS Prevention in Children and Youth, 6*(1), 43–57.

Linehan, M. M. (1999). Development, evaluation, and dissemination of effective psychosocial treatments: Stages of disorder, levels of care, and stages of treatment research. In M. G. Glantz & C. R. Hartel (Eds.), *Drug abuse: Origins and interventions.* (pp. 367–394). Washington, DC: American Psychological Association.

Link to English translation of the report *HIV-positive individuals without additional sexually transmissible diseases (STD) and on effective anti-retroviral therapy are sexually non-infectious*: http://www.ternyata.org/books/wisdom/swiss_english.pdf

Lucas, G. M., Lau, B., Atta, M. G., Fine, D. M., Keruly, J., & Moore, R. D. (2008). Chronic kidney disease incidence, and progression to end-stage renal disease in HIV-infected individuals: A tale of two races. *Journal of Infectious Diseases, 197*(1 June), 1548–1557.

Lyon, M., Brasseux, C., & D'Angelo, L. J. (1999). Who should I tell? Disclosure of HIV status by infected adolescents. *Journal of Adolescent Health, 24*, 20.

Lyon, M. E., Garvie, P. A., Briggs, L., McCarter, R., D'Angelo, L., et al. (2009). Development of a Family-Centered (FACE) Advance Care Planning Intervention for adolescents with HIV. *J Palliative Medicine, 12*(4). In press.

Lyon, M. E., Garvie, P. A., Briggs, L., McCarter, R., He, J., & D'Angelo, L. (2009). Who will speak for me? Improving end-of-life decision-making for adolescents with HIV and their families. *Pediatrics, 123*(2), e1–e8.

Lyon, M. E., Marhefka, S. L., Abramowitz, S., Koenig, L. J., LaGrange & ADIMPACT Team. (2008, August). Psychosocial issues of adolescents with HIV infection acquired at birth and later in life. Symposium. Annual Meeting of the American Psychological Association. Boston.

Lyon, M. E., McCarter, R., & D'Angelo, L. (2009). Detecting HIV associated neurocognitive disorders in adolescents: What is the best tool? *Journal of Adolescent Health.* DOI: 10.1016/j.jadohealth.2008.06.023 and *44*(2), 133–135.

Lyon, M. E, McCabe, M. A., Patel, K., & D'Angelo, L. J. (2004). What do adolescents want? An exploratory study regarding end-of-life decision-making. *Journal of the Adolescent Health. 35*(6), 529. http://journals.elsevierhealth.com/periodicals/jah

Lyon, M. E., McCarter, R., Briggs, L., & D'Angelo, L. (2008, May). Creating a facilitating environment for family-centered advance care planning. In (Chair, Mary Ann Cohen) *A Biopsychosocial Approach to AIDS: Update for Dynamic Psychiatrists.* Symposium conducted at the meeting of the *American Academy of Psychoanalytic and Psychodynamic Psychotherapy Symposium on HIV AIDS,* Washington, D.C.

Lyon, M. E, McCarter, R., Briggs, L., He, J., & D'Angelo, L. J. (2008, August). *A Pilot Study of Family-Centered Advance Care Planning in Adolescents.* Poster session to be presented at the annual meeting of the American Psychological Association, Boston, MA.

Lyon, M. E., Trexler, C., Akpan-Townsend, C., et al. (2003). A family group approach to increasing adherence to therapy in HIV-infected youths: results of a pilot project. *AIDS Patient Care & STDS, 17,* 299–308.

Lyon, M. E., Williams, P. L., Woods, E. R., Hutton, N., Butler, A. M., Sibinga, E., et al. (2008). Do not resuscitate orders and/or hospice care, psychological health and quality of life among children/adolescents with AIDS. *Journal of Palliative Medicine, 11*(3), 459–469. PMID:18363489

Lyon, M., & Woodward, K. (2003). Nonstigmatizing ways to engage HIV-positive African-American teens in mental health and support services: A commentary. *Journal of the National Medical Association, 95*(3), 196–200.

Malow, R. M., Kershaw, T., Sipsma, H., Rosenberg, R., & Devieux J. G. (2007). HIV preventive interventions for adolescents: A look back and ahead. *Current HIV/AIDS Reports, 4*(4), 173–180.

Murphy, D. A., Belzer, M., Durako, S. J., Sarr, M., Wilson, C. M., & Muenz, L. R. (2005). Longitudinal antiretroviral adherence among adolescents infected with human immunodeficiency virus. *Archives of Pediatric and Adolescent Medicine, 159*(8), 764–770.

Naar-King, S., Wright, K., Parsons, J., Frey, M., Templin, T., Lam, P., et al. (2006). Healthy choices: Motivational enhancement therapy for health risk behaviors in HIV-positive youth. *AIDS Education & Prevention, 18*(1), 1–11.

Pao, M., Lyon, M., D'Angelo, L. J., Schuman, W. B., Tipnis, T., & Mrazek, D. A. (2000). Psychiatric diagnosis in adolescents seropositive for the human immunodeficiency virus. *Archives of Pediatrics and Adolescent Medicine, 154*(3), 240–244.

Rogers, A. S. (2006). HIV in youth: How are they different? In. M. E. Lyon & L. J. D'Angelo (Eds.), *Teenagers HIV and AIDS: Insights from youths living with the virus* (pp. 3–20). Westport, CT: Praeger Publishers.

Rogers, A. S., Miller, S., Murphy, D. A., Tanney, M., & Fortune, T. (2001). The TREAT (Therapeutic Regimens Enhancing Adherence in Teens) program: theory and preliminary results. *Journal of Adolescent Health, 29*(Suppl. 3), 30–38.

Rongkavilit, C., Naar-King, S., TChuenyam, T., Wang, B., Wright, K., & Phanuphak, P. (2007). Health risk behaviors among HIV-infected youth in Bangkok, Thailand. *Journal of Adolescent Health, 40*(4), 358 e1–;e8.

Rotheram-Borus, M. J., Lee, M. B., Murphy, D. A., Futterman, D., Duan, N., Birnbaum, J. M. et al. (2001). Efficacy of a preventive intervention for youths living with HIV. *American Journal of Public Health, 91*(3), 400–405.

Rotheram-Borus, M. J., Swendeman, D., Comulada, S., Weiss, R. E., Lee, M., & Lightfoot, M. (2004). Prevention for substance-using HIV-positive young people: Telephone and in-person delivery. *Journal of Acquired Immune Deficiency Syndrome, 37S,* 68–77.

Rotherham-Borus, M. J., Weiss, R., Alber, S., & Lester, P. (2005). Adolescent adjustment before and after HIV-related parental death. *Journal of Consulting and Clinical Psychology, 73*(2), 221–228

Santelli, J., Ott, M., Lyon, M., Rogers, J., Summers, D., & Schleifer, R. (2006). Abstinence and abstinence-only policies and programs: A position paper of the Society for Adolescent Medicine. *Journal of Adolescent Health, 38*(1), 83–87.

Shanbhag, M. C., Rutstein, R. M., Zaoutis, T., Zhao, H., Chao, D., & Radcliffe, J. (2005). Neurocognitive functioning in pediatric human immunodeficiency virus infection: Effects of combined therapy. *Archives of Pediatrics and Adolescent Medicine, 159,* 651–656.

Simoni, J. M., Montgomery, A., Martin, E., New, M., Demas, P. A., & Rana, S. (2007). Adherence to antiretroviral therapy for pediatric HIV infection: A qualitative systematic review with recommendations for research and clinical management. *Pediatrics, 119*(6), e1371–;e1383

Tevendale, H. D., & Lightfoot, M. (2006). Programs that work: Prevention for positives. In M. E. Lyon & L. J. D'Angelo (Eds.), *Teenagers HIV and AIDS: Insights from youths living with the virus.* Westport, CT: Praeger Publishers.

Thato, R., Jenkins, R. A., & Dusitsin, N. (2008). Effects of the culturally-sensitive comprehensive sex education programme among Thai secondary school students. *Journal of Advanced Nursing: Original Research, 62*(4), 457–469.

UNAIDS/World Health Organization (2005). *AIDS epidemic update: December 2005.*

Vernazza, P., Hirschel, B., Bernasconi, E., & Flepp, M. (2008) Les personnes séropositives ne souffrant d'aucune autre MST et suivant un traitment antirétroviral efficace ne transmettent pas le VIH par voie sexuelle. *Bulletin des médecins suisses*, *89*(5).

Wiener, L. S. (2004). Disclosure. In S. L. Zeichner & J. S. Read (Eds.), *Textbook of Pediatric HIV Care* (pp. 667–671). Cambridge: Cambridge University Press.

Wiener, L. S., Battles, H. B., & Heilman, N. (2000). Public disclosure of a child's HIV infection: Impact on children and families. *AIDS Patient Care STDS 14*(9):485–497.

Wiener, L. S., & Lyon, M. E. (2006). HIV disclosure: Who knows? Who needs to know? In M. E. Lyon & L. J. D'Angelo (Eds.), *Teenagers HIV and AIDS: Insights from youths living with the virus* (pp. 105–126). Westport, CT: Praeger Publishers.

World Health Organization. (2003). Adherence to Long-Term Therapies: www.who.int/chronic_conditions/adherencereport/en/

Health-Related Quality of Life Instruments for Adolescents with Chronic Diseases

Alexandra L. Quittner, Ivette Cruz, Avani C. Modi, and Kristen K. Marciel

Introduction

Over the past two decades, tremendous progress has been made in defining and measuring health-related quality of life (HRQOL) and in recognizing its importance as a health outcome (Palermo et al., 2008; Quittner, Davis, & Modi, 2003). More than 50 years ago, the World Health Organization proposed the first definition of HRQOL as "a state of complete physical, mental, and social well-being, and not merely the absence of disease or infirmity" (World Health Organization [WHO], 1947, p. 29). A consensus definition of HRQOL has now emerged, with agreement that it is multidimensional and includes four core domains: (1) disease state and physical symptoms, (2) functional status (e.g., performing daily activities), (3) psychological and emotional functioning, and (4) social functioning (Hays, 2005; Rothman et al., 2007).

More recently, the Food and Drug Administration (FDA) has formally recognized the importance of patient-reported outcomes (PROs) and their relevance to the approval of new medications and treatments (FDA, 2006). HRQOL measures are one type of PRO; however, there are others, including single-item ratings of pain and observable behaviors (e.g., ability to walk). A PRO instrument is defined as any measure of a patient's health status that comes directly from the patient and assesses how a patient "feels or functions with respect to his or her health condition" (p. 2 FDA Guidance). This may include observable behaviors or perceptions (e.g., ability to climb stairs, lack of appetite) or nonobservable outcomes known only to the patient (e.g., feelings of depression). Seeking input from patients represents a significant shift in health outcomes research and is particularly relevant for adolescents with chronic diseases, in which a more collaborative model of care is required (Von Korff, Gruman, Schaefer, Curry, & Wagner, 1997).

Efforts to develop reliable and valid PROs have been very successful, leading to their use for several different purposes: (1) as primary or secondary outcomes in clinical trials, (2) to evaluate new pharmaceutical and surgical interventions, (3) to describe the impact of illness on patient functioning, (4) to analyze the costs and benefits of medical interventions, and (5) to aid in clinical decision-making (Fayers & Hays, 2005; Quittner et al., 2003; Revicki et al., 2000). Regardless of the measure's structure or complexity, in order to utilize a PRO in a clinical trial as a primary or a secondary endpoint, the instrument must meet rigorous psychometric criteria, including evaluation of the conceptual framework on which the instrument is based and evidence of its reliability and validity.

There are several types of reliability and validity that must be established, including internal consistency (Cronbach's alpha), test–retest reliability, and cross-informant reliability. Validity includes concurrent or predictive (associations between the measure and other outcomes the measure was expected to predict), convergent validity (correlations between the target measure and associated variables), and discriminant validity (a lack of

A.L. Quittner (✉)
Department of Psychology & Pediatrics, University of Miami, Miami, FL, USA
e-mail: aquittner@miami.edu

W.T. O'Donohue, L.W. Tolle (eds.), *Behavioral Approaches to Chronic Disease in Adolescence*,
DOI 10.1007/978-0-387-87687-0_23, © Springer Science+Business Media, LLC 2009

association between the target measure and variables that should not be related). These tests of validity combine to produce evidence that the "construct" being targeted is being measured by the instrument. In addition, the minimal clinically important difference (MCID) score, which establishes the smallest change that can be detected by respondents, must be determined (Guyatt et al., 2002; Wyrwich et al., 2005). The MCID provides an empirical method for interpreting the clinical significance of the observed effects (Quittner, Modi, Wainwright, Otto, Kirihara, & Montgomery, in press).

In this chapter, we review the HRQOL measures available for the chronic conditions discussed in this book. Using the American Psychological Association, Division 54 (Pediatric Psychology) guidelines on empirically supported assessment (Cohen et al., 2008), we have highlighted those measures that are "well-established." To be classified as "well-established," the measure must have demonstrated good reliability and validity and have been used in published studies by more than one investigator (see Palermo et al., 2008 for a comprehensive review). Reliability of the scale (internal consistency) should range from 0.60 for a developing scale to 0.70 and higher for an established scale; test–retest reliability coefficients should indicate stability and be statistically significant with a relatively small sample (e.g., 30 participants); the measure should converge with generic measures of HRQOL or with relevant clinical parameters (e.g., respiratory symptoms with pulmonary function); and the measure should discriminate between patients on the basis of disease severity or other hypothesized relationships (e.g., age, gender). The names, age ranges, and summaries of the psychometric properties of the instruments reviewed in this chapter appear in Table 1.

Developmental Considerations

Few studies have provided guidelines about the development and use of HRQOL measures for adolescents. In this brief section, three major issues are highlighted for consideration when developing and administering HRQOL measures to adolescents: (1) What are the cognitive and emotional abilities of the adolescent? (2) Is the item content relevant for adolescents? and (3) How should adolescent self-report and parent-proxy reports be integrated? In contrast to the development of HRQOL instruments for young children (e.g., simple and developmentally appropriate language, fewer response options, use of pictorial representations), fewer guidelines have been established for the development and use of these instruments for adolescents. Developmental theories suggest that, in general, adolescents have more well-developed cognitive skills (Inhelder & Piaget, 1958), can better evaluate their own thoughts and feelings (Harris, 1983; Quittner et al., 2003), and understand more complex concepts related to health than their younger counterparts (Bibace & Walsh, 1980). One important implication is that adolescents are generally capable of completing measures of HRQOL independent of their caregivers.

The content of items in the HRQOL instrument should also be developed specifically for adolescents. Inclusion of items that are developmentally appropriate provides a clearer understanding of how a chronic disease affects typical adolescent development. For example, items for younger children in the domain of social functioning often elicit information about the ability to play with same-aged peers, whereas items for adolescents should focus on the ability to form and sustain long-term friendships. The developmental emerging adulthood literature suggests that engaging in activities, such as work and romantic relations, is predictive of adult success in similar domains (Roisman, Masten, Coatsworth, & Tellegen, 2004). Thus, it is important to assess these aspects of HRQOL in adolescents. Recently, Modi and Zeller (2008) developed a parent-proxy, obesity-specific HRQOL measure (i.e., Sizing Them Up), in which they incorporated an Adolescent Developmental Adaptation Module. This module assesses participation in extracurricular activities, work, romantic relations, and concerns about the future for adolescents who are obese.

In the pediatric literature, both self-report and parent-proxy reports are frequently used (Eiser & Morse, 2001; Quittner et al., 2003; Turner, Quittner, Parasuraman, & Cleeland, 2007). The use of proxy raters of HRQOL is particularly important in situations in which it is the only means of measuring the child's HRQOL. For adolescents, this might include those who are developmentally delayed or in the

Table 1 HRQOL instruments for adolescents with chronic diseases

Instrument	Age Range	Respondent	Reliability	Validity
Diabetes				
Audit of Diabetes-Dependent QoL – Teen	13–18 years	Adolescent	α	α
Diabetes Self-Management Profile	6–15 years	Child/Adolescent	α	α
Diabetes Quality of Life Measure	13–17 years	Adolescent	α	α
Obesity				
Impact of Weight on Quality of Life-Kids	11–19 years	Adolescent	α	α
Sizing Them Up	5–18 years	Parent proxy	α	α
Cystic fibrosis				
Cystic Fibrosis Quality of Life Questionnaire	14 years–adult	Adolescent/adult	α	α
Cystic Fibrosis Questionnaire – Revised (CFQ-R)	6 years–adult	Child/adolescent/adult	α	α
Questions on Life Satisfaction – Cystic Fibrosis	16years–adult	Adolescent/adult	α	α
Asthma				
About My Asthma (AMA)	6–12 years	Child	α	α
Adolescent Asthma Quality of Life Questionnaire (AAQOL)	12–17 years	Child	α	α
Childhood Asthma Questionnaires	4–7 years	Child	α	α
	8–11 years	Youth		
	12–16 years	Adolescent		
Children's Health Survey for Asthma (CHSA)	7–16 years	Child	α	α
	5–12 years	Parent		
Pediatric Asthma Quality of Life Questionnaire	7–17 years	Child/adolescent	α	α
Pediatric Asthma Caregiver's Quality of Life Questionnaire	7–17 years	Parent	α	α
Asthma-Related Quality of Life Scale (ARQOLS)	6–13 years	Child	α	α
TACQOL-Asthma	8–16 years	Child & Parent	α	α
PedsQL-Asthma Module	5–18 years	Child	α	α
	2–18 years	Parent		
Life Activities Questionnaire for Childhood Asthma	5–17 years	Child	α	α
How Are You?	8–12 years	Child	α	α
Integrated Therapeutics Group Child Asthma Short Form	2–17 years	Parent	α	α
Headaches				
24-hour Adolescent Migraine Questionnaire	12–18 years	Adolescent & parent	α	α
PedMIDAS	6–18 years	Child	α	α
Quality of Life Headache in Youth	12–18 years	Adolescent & parent	α	α
Epilepsy				
Quality of Life in Epilepsy Inventory for Adolescent	11–17 years	Adolescent	α	α
The Child Self-Report Scale & Parent-proxy Response Scale	8–15+ years	Child/adolescent	α	α
	6–15 years	Parent		
US Version – Quality of Life in Childhood Epilepsy Questionnaire	4–18 years	Parent-proxy	α	α

Table 1 (continued)

Instrument	Age Range	Respondent	Reliability	Validity
Cancer				
Behavioral, Affective and Somatic Experiences Scale (BASES)	2–20 years	Child, parent, and nurse	α	α
The Miami Pediatric Quality of Life Questionnaire	1–18 years	Child and parent	α	α
The Minneapolis-Manchester Quality of Life	8–12 years	Youth	α	α
	13–18 years	Adolescent		
The Pediatric Cancer Quality of Life Inventory	8–18 years	Child and parent	α	α
The Pediatric Oncology Quality of Life Scale	5–17 years	Parent	α	α
PEDSQL Cancer Module	8–12 years	Child	α	α
	13–18 years	Adolescent		
Play Performance Scale for Children	6 months–16 years	Parent	N/A	α
Quality of Life-Cancer Survivors Questionnaire	16–29 years	Adolescent/adult	α	α
The Royal Marsden Hospital Pediatric Oncology Quality of Life Questionnaire	3–19 years	Youth and parents	α	α
Sick lecell disease				
– No available measures for children and adolescents				
Juvenile rheumatoid arthritis				
Juvenile Arthritis Quality of Life Questionnaire	2–18 years	Youth	α	α
HIV/*AIDS*				
Aids Clinical Trials Group	12–20 years	Child/adolescent	N/A	α
	0–4 years	Parent		
	5–11 years	Parent		
ChronicPain				
McGill Pain Questionnaire	10–Adult	Youth/adult	N/A	α
Quality of Life Questionnaire for Adolescents with Chronic Pain	12–18 years	Adolescent	N/A	N/A

terminal stages of an illness. In these cases, proxy respondents provide a critical window into the adolescents' level of functioning. In contrast, for adolescents who can complete self-report measures, it is not clear whether parent-proxy measures are needed. Furthermore, valid self-report and parent-report measures are not available for all chronic conditions. For example, in cystic fibrosis (CF), a parent-proxy measure was not developed for adolescents (e.g., Cystic Fibrosis Questionnaire-Revised Teen-Adult Form; Quittner, Buu, Messer, Modi, & Watrous, 2005), and self-report was considered the best and most accurate assessment of an adolescent's HRQOL. When both are available, they can and should be used as complementary tools. Although studies have found discrepancies between caregivers and youth on emotional and social domains (Modi & Quittner, 2003; Theunissen et al., 1998; Verrips, Vogels, den Ouden, Paneth, & Verloove-Vanhorick, 2000), parent reports can "contribute to the overall understanding of the child's quality of life" (Sherifali & Pinell, 2007, p.95).

Generic Quality of Life Measures

Generic HRQOL measures utilize general items that are applicable to a variety of chronic illnesses and typically assess functioning across several domains. A number of "well-established" HRQOL measures are available for children and adolescents: the Child Health and Illness Profile (CHIP; Starfield, Riley, & Green, 1999), the Child Health Questionnaire (CHQ; Landgraf, Abetz, & Ware, 1996); the Pediatric Quality of Life Inventory (PedsQL; Varni, Seid, & Rode, 1999), and the Youth Quality of Life (YQOL; Edwards, Huebner, Connell, & Patrick 2002; Patrick, Edwards, & Topolsaki, 2002). These measures have all demonstrated good reliability and validity (Palermo et al., 2008). Internal consistency has ranged from 0.63 to 0.97, indicating good reliability. Test–retest has only been demonstrated for the YQOL, with coefficients of 0.74–0.85 over a 1-week period. All of the generic measures listed above have shown that they can discriminate between healthy and chronically ill populations and are correlated with disease severity. Normative data have also been gathered for the CHQ and PedsQL. The MCID for the PedsQL has been determined. Note that some generic HRQOL measures include disease-specific modules (e.g., PedsQL). The major advantage of generic measures is that scores can be compared across adolescents with different chronic illnesses. However, the major disadvantage of these measures is that they lack the precision and sensitivity to detect change over time, and often their results do not translate easily into treatment recommendations (Quittner et al., 2003).

In contrast, disease-specific HRQOL measures focus on the domains most relevant for a particular disorder and its treatments and thus have greater clinical relevance to patients and families. A growing body of research also indicates that disease-specific measures are able to detect small, but clinically meaningful changes. In addition, they have recently been recognized by the FDA as important primary or secondary endpoints in clinical trials (FDA, 2006). A disease-specific HRQOL measure for CF was recently used as the primary endpoint in an efficacy trial of a new. Inhaled antibiotic, with approval expected in the fall of 2008 (McCoy et al., 2008; Retsch-Bogart et al., in press). This is an area of instrument development that is likely to grow considerably over the next decade.

Disease-Specific HRQOL Measures

Endocrinology

Diabetes

Diabetes Quality of Life for Youth (DQOLY; Ingersoll & Marrero, 1991) has adequate psychometric properties, takes between 15 and 20 minutes to complete, and has been used in a number of studies. This 52-item measure was developed in the Diabetes Control and Complication Trial (DCCT), with satisfactory reliabilities, ranging from 0.82 to 0.85, for all of the scales: Diabetes Life Satisfaction, Diabetes Impact, and Disease-Related Worries. No test–retest reliability has been reported and the MCID has not been determined. Validity data indicate that better HRQOL by adolescent report has been associated with better health outcomes (HbA1c) in families with more structure (Grey, Sullivan-Bolyai, Boland, Tamborlane, & Yu, 1998). Ingersoll and Marrero (1991) recommended that the DQOLY be used as an outcome measure for diabetes education programs; however, no changes on this measure were observed after a 6-month-long weekly diabetes nurse educator telephone intervention (Lawson, Cohen, Richardson, Orrbine, & Pham, 2005). The DQOL is available in 15 languages. Test–retest reliability has not yet been established, thus, this tool is considered "approaching well-established."

The Audit of Diabetes-Dependent QoL – Teen (ADDQoL; McMillan, Honeyford, Datta, Madge, & Bradley, 2004) is a 25-item measure with excellent internal consistency (e.g., $r = 0.91$). The ADDQoL can be completed in 10–15 minutes. No test–retest reliability has been evaluated. Evidence of construct validity was supported by ratings of the impact of diabetes on quality of life. The ADDQoL measures only the impact of diabetes on the adolescent and the adolescent's interaction with other people. The majority of teens (61.8%) reported that diabetes negatively affected their lives; however, cross-sectional data indicated that older adolescents reported less impact than younger adolescents. Sundaram et al. (2007) found that increased depressive symptoms were related to lower HRQOL scores, which provides some supportive evidence for convergent validity. The MCID has not been established.

The PedsQL-Diabetes Module (PedsQL-DM; Varni et al., 2003) is a 28-item scale that can be used with the generic PedsQL core scale and requires 5–10 minutes to complete. It has demonstrated good internal consistency, ranging from 0.63 to 0.81, and good construct and content validity. The MCID has not been determined. The PedsQL-DM evaluates HRQOL across several domains including symptoms, treatment barriers, treatment adherence, worry, and communication. In a recent review of four generic and five disease-specific HRQOL measures, the PedsQL-DM was rated as the most practical tool for clinical use because of its brevity and inclusion of both generic and disease-specific domains (de Wit, Delemarre-van de Waal, Pouwer, Gemke, & Snoek, 2007). This module has been translated into 12 languages.

None of the disease-specific measures for diabetes meet all of the criteria for well-established instruments. However, we would recommend the use of the DQOLY because it is currently the measure that comes closest to meeting the APA criteria.

Obesity

To date, two weight-specific HRQOL measures have been developed. The first is a self-report measure specifically designed for adolescents, the Impact of Weight on Quality of Life-Kids (IWQOL-Kids©; Kolotkin et al., 2006). This measure has strong internal consistency, with coefficients ranging from 0.88 to 0.95. However, test–retest reliability and the MCID have not been determined. Convergent validity between this instrument and the PedsQL has been reported and it has discriminated between adolescents in different body mass index groups. This measure has shown responsivity to change in adolescents who lost weight through a weight-loss camp (Kolotkin et al., 2006). However, the measure is not specific to obesity and was validated on adolescents across the weight spectrum, from underweight to extremely obese. As a result, items selected during the validation study may not apply exclusively to those who are obese.

The second HRQOL measure, Sizing Them Up (Modi & Zeller, 2008), is an obesity-specific measure that uses parents as proxy respondents. Sizing Them Up has demonstrated adequate psychometric properties. Internal consistency coefficients ranged from 0.52 to 0.90, test–retest reliability ranged from 0.57 to 0.80, and this measure showed good convergence with body mass index and other quality of life measures. It has shown responsiveness to change in adolescents who have undergone bariatric surgery. MCID values ranging from 5.10 to 13.29 have been established. One unique strength of this measure is the Adolescent Developmental Adaptation Module, which examines parents' perceptions of the impact of weight on their adolescents' engagement in developmentally appropriate activities (e.g., dating, participation in activities) and concerns related to these activities. To date, this measure has not been evaluated in overweight (non-obese) or community samples.

Based on our review, we recommend the IQWOL-Kids because it assesses HRQOL from the adolescent's own perspective. However, Sizing Them Up, the parent-proxy measure had stronger reliability and validity data. Sizing Them Up was also the only measure to establish MCIDs for children who are obese.

Pulmonology

Cystic Fibrosis

Three disease-specific HRQOL measures for adolescents with CF are available: the Cystic Fibrosis Questionnaire-Revised (CFQ-R; Modi & Quittner, 2003; Quittner et al., 2005), the Cystic Fibrosis Quality of Life Questionnaire (CFQoL; Gee, Abbot, Conway, Etherington, Webb, 2000), and Questions on Life Satisfaction – Cystic Fibrosis (FLZM-CF; Goldbeck, Schmitz, Henrich, & Herschbach, 2003). All three measures assess functioning and symptoms in a variety of domains, including respiratory symptoms, treatment burden, and social functioning.

The CFQ-R is currently the most widely used HRQOL instrument for CF (Goss & Quittner, 2007) and was classified as "well-established" in a recent review of HRQOL measures (Palermo et al., 2008). There are three versions: a child version for ages 6–13, a parent version for this same age group, and a teen/adult version for ages 14 through adulthood. A preschool version using a pictorial format is currently being validated. Reliability and validity have been extensively documented (Quittner et al., 2005; Quittner, Modi, & Cruz, 2008). Internal consistency ranged from 0.60 to 0.76 for the child version and from 0.67 to 0.94 for the teen/adult version, with the exception of the Treatment Burden scale which reported lower internal consistency. Test–retest reliability has also been reported ranging from 0.45 to 0.90 for the teen/adult version. Good cross-informant agreement between the parent and the child subscales has also been reported (0.27 to 0.57). Furthermore, an MCID of 4 points out of 100 was established for the CFQ-R Respiratory Symptom Scale (Quittner et al., in press, 2005). Significant associations have been found between CFQ-R domain scores and pulmonary functioning, height, weight, and body mass index (Modi et al., 2007), suggesting good discriminant validity. In addition, convergent validity between this measure and the SF-36 and the PedsQL have been reported. The CFQ-R has also demonstrated responsivity in several clinical trials (Donaldson et al., 2006; Elkins et al., 2006) and was the primary endpoint in a successful study of an inhaled antibiotic awaiting FDA approval (Retsch-Bogart et al., in press; McCoy et al., 2008). The CFQ-R has been translated into 25 languages (Quittner et al., 2008).

The CFQoL is a 52-item HRQOL measure for adolescents and adults, which assesses nine domains of functioning, including physical, interpersonal relationships, body image, and career. Good internal consistency (α ranging from 0.72 to 0.92) and test–retest reliability ($r > 0.74$) have been reported. In addition, this measure has demonstrated strong validity; it has been shown to discriminate between patients with mild and moderate disease severity. Convergent validity between this instrument and the SF-36 has been reported and this measure has also demonstrated sensitivity to change following IV antibiotics (Gee et al., 2000). The MCID has not been established.

The FLZM-CF is the briefest HRQOL measure for adolescents with CF, consisting of nine items that are rated for importance and satisfaction. This measure has reported good internal consistency ($\alpha = 0.80$) and test–retest reliability ($r = 0.69$). However, reliability was calculated on the aggregated CF-specific and generic life satisfaction items, indicating that these items are not independent. The FLZM-CF has also demonstrated adequate validity and sensitivity to change. This instrument discriminates between patients who have different levels of disease severity and correlates with pulmonary functioning and time spent doing treatments (Goldbeck et al., 2003). It has also demonstrated sensitivity to change following an inpatient rehabilitation program. However, this measure has two limitations. First, it relies on a single set of questions to represent each domain. This may be useful for screening purposes but is not adequate to assess more complex constructs (e.g., problems in eating, maintaining normal routines). The second limitation is the 4-week recall interval. Ideally, recall periods should be no longer than 2 weeks because of increased error and recall bias (Schwarz & Sudman, 1996).

Based on this review, we recommend both the CFQ-R and the CFQoL as "well-established" measures. They are comprehensive, reliable, and valid instruments for adolescents and adults with CF; however, only the CFQ-R has established an MCID. For studies of younger children with CF, the CFQ-R is the only measure that has been validated for children and parent-proxy respondents. The FLZM-CF is a good screening tool and is very brief but would not meet the criteria established by the FDA for PROs.

Asthma

Twelve disease-specific HRQOL measures have been developed for asthma. At present, the Pediatric Asthma Quality of Life Questionnaire (PAQLQ; Juniper et al., 1996a) is the most widely used HRQOL measure for children and adolescents with asthma and has been classified as "well-established." Internal consistency ranged from 0.54 to 0.89 and intraclass coefficients ranged from 0.84 to 0.95; however, test–retest reliability has not been reported. Validity has also been established. Specifically, the PAQLQ is associated with physician ratings of asthma severity and patient-reported "feeling" thermometers. Furthermore, it has demonstrated responsiveness to change following an intervention to treat and control asthma symptoms has an established MCID of 0.5 on a 7-point scale, and has been used in several clinical trials. The Pediatric Asthma Caregiver's Quality of Life (PACQL; Juniper et al., 1996b), the parent-proxy version, has also demonstrated adequate reliability, with intraclass correlation coefficients ranging from 0.80 to 0.85. This measure also discriminates among disease severity groups and is responsive to change. No data have been reported on parent–child agreement. The PAQLQ and the PACQL are available in over 30 languages.

The Adolescent Asthma Quality of Life Questionnaire (AAQOL; Rutishauser, Sawyer, Bond, & Bowes, 2001) was specifically developed for adolescents with asthma. It is a brief measure that takes approximately 5–7 minutes to complete. This measure assesses symptoms, medication, physical activities, emotions, and social interactions. Adequate reliability and validity have been reported. Internal consistency ranged from 0.70 to 0.93 and test–retest reliability ranged from 0.76 to 0.93. Convergent validity has also been reported with the PAQLQ. Additionally, weak-to-moderate correlations with patient reports of symptom severity and number of hospitalizations have been reported, suggesting adequate discriminant validity (Rutishauser et al., 2001).

The Childhood Asthma Questionnaire (CAQ; Christie, French, Sowden, & West, 1993; French, Christie, & Sowden, 1994) is a brief self-report HRQOL measure for children and adolescents with asthma. Three versions are available: (1) for children 4–7 years of age, (2) for children 8–11 years of age, and (3) for adolescents 12–16 years of age. Adequate reliability, test–retest, and validity have been reported for all versions. Internal consistency ranged from 0.50 to 0.84 across all versions and intraclass correlation coefficients ranged from 0.59 to 0.84. Test–retest has also been reported, ranging from 0.59 to 0.84. The CAQ discriminates between children with and without asthma and correlates with parental ratings of asthma severity.

The Children's Health Survey for Asthma (CHSA; Asmussen, Olson, Grant, Fagan, & Weiss, 1999; Olson et al., 2007) is a 25-item instrument that assesses physical health, emotional health, and child activities in children and adolescents with asthma. There is also a parent version for children ages 5–12 years. Adequate internal consistency ($\alpha = 0.61$–0.93) and test–retest ($r = 0.57$–0.96) reliabilities have been reported for both versions. In addition, the parent version is correlated with disease severity as measured by symptom activity (i.e., wheezing, coughing, tightness of chest) and medication use. It is also correlated with treatment burden as measured by the Asthma Symptoms Day-14, indicating convergent validity (Mitchell et al., 1997). The MCID has not been established.

The TACQOL-Asthma (Flapper, Koopman, ten Napel, & van der Schans, 2006) and the PedsQL-Asthma Module (Varni, Burwinkle, Rapoff, Kamps, & Olson, 2004) were developed for children and adolescents and have parent versions as well. Both measures have reported adequate internal consistency and good parent–child agreement. Internal consistency for the TACQOL-Asthma ranged from 0.60 to 0.85 and 0.74 to 0.91 for the PedsQL-Asthma Module across both the parent and child versions. Convergent validity between both measures and the PAQLQ has also been reported. In addition, both measures have reported discriminant validity; the TACQOL-Asthma discriminates between levels of disease severity and the PedsQL-Asthma Module has been shown to discriminate between children with and without asthma. Furthermore, the PedsQL-Asthma Module was shown to be sensitive to change in a small study aimed at improving adherence to medications (Varni et al., 2004). The MCIDs for these measures have not been reported.

The Life Activities Questionnaire for Childhood Asthma (Creer et al., 1993) assesses seven domains, including physical, work, emotional, and eating. It has demonstrated good internal consistency ($\alpha = 0.97$) and test–retest reliability ($r = 0.76$); however, no validity data have been reported. One disadvantage of this measure is its length – 71 questions, which may be difficult for adolescents to complete.

The About My Asthma (AMA; Mishoe, Baker, Poole, Harrell, Arant, & Rupp, 1998), the How Are You? (HAY; le Coq, Colland, Boeke, Bezemer, & Eijk, 2000), and the Asthma-Related Quality of Life Scale (ARQOLS; Chiang, Tzeng, Fu, & Huang, 2006) are several less well-established HRQOL measures for children and younger adolescents with asthma. The AMA and the HAY can be completed by teens up to age 12 and the ARQOLS can be used with teens up to age 13. All three measures have reported adequate internal consistency, ranging from 0.93 for the AMA, 0.61 to 0.83 for the HAY, and 0.81 to 0.96 for the ARQOLS. Test–retest reliability has also been reported for the AMA ($r = 0.57$). Intraclass correlation coefficients for the HAY ranged from 0.11 to 0.83, indicating poor stability on some domains. The AMA and the HAY have also reported good validity. Convergent validity between the AMA and the PAQLQ has been reported. Moreover, the AMA has demonstrated responsiveness to change following a week-long asthma day camp. Furthermore, the HAY discriminates between children with and without asthma in terms of their physical and social activities and has been responsive to change following treatment. No validity data are available for the ARQOLS. One limitation of the AMA is that it provides only a total score, which precludes analyses of functioning in specific domains. MCIDs have not been established for these measures.

Finally, a parent-proxy measure for adolescents, the Integrated Therapeutics Group Child Asthma Short Form (ITG-CASF; Bukstein, McGrath, Buchner, Landgraf, & Goss, 2000; Gorelick, Brousseau, & Stevens, 2004), was specifically developed to measure outcomes for children with acute asthma treated in the emergency room. Internal consistency ranged from 0.84 to 0.92; however, no test–retest reliability has been reported. The ITG-CASF is responsive to change and correlates with asthma severity and number of days missed at school, indicating good discriminant validity.

There are several reliable and well-validated HRQOL measures for adolescents with asthma; however, we recommend the PAQLQ because it is the most widely used and best-established measure.

Neurology

Headaches

Currently, there are three disease-specific HRQOL measures for adolescents with chronic headaches: (1) the Quality of Life Headache in Youth (QLH-Y; Langeveld, Koot, & Passchler, 1997; Langeveld, Koot, Loonen, Hazebroek-Kampschreur, & Passchi, 1996), (2) the 24-hour Adolescent Migraine Questionnaire (24-hour AMQ; Hartmaier, DeMuro-Mercon, Linder, Winner, & Santanello, 2001), and (3) the PedMIDAS (Hershey et al., 2001).

The QLH-Y is a 71-item HRQOL measure for adolescents with headaches. There is also a parent-proxy version which has demonstrated good parent–child agreement. This questionnaire measures functional status, physical, psychological, and social functioning. Good reliability and validity have been reported and it was recently classified as "well-established" (Palermo et al., 2008). Internal consistency ranged from 0.66 to 0.87. Test–retest ranged from 0.44 to 0.66 over a 2-week period and 0.31 to 0.60 over a 4-week period. This measure has shown good discriminant validity between adolescents who have headaches versus those who do not.

Furthermore, changes in headache frequency and intensity were related to changes in self-reported HRQOL within all subdomains (Langeveld et al., 1997, 1996). However, one limitation of this instrument is its length, which creates a larger response burden for adolescents. However, the trade off is that this measure provides a broader picture of how migraine headaches affect adolescents' psychosocial and physical functioning.

The 24-hour AMQ was specifically developed to assess adolescent functioning during and immediately following an acute migraine attack. The authors developed this questionnaire specifically for use in clinical trials to assess the potential benefits of acute migraine therapy. Adequate to good internal consistency coefficients ranging from 50 to 0.84 have been reported (Hartmaier et al., 2001). No test–retest or validity data are available on this instrument.

The PedMIDAS is a brief 6-item HRQOL measure that was modified from an adult version of the tool (Hershey et al., 2001; Stewart, Lipton, Dowson, & Sawyer, 2001). Adequate internal consistency ($\alpha = 0.78$) and test–retest ($r = 0.80$) reliability have been reported. The PedMIDAS also correlates with headache frequency, severity, and duration, indicating good discriminant validity. Moreover, it has been responsive to change following treatment. However, the MCID has not been established.

Based on the review, we would recommend the QLH-Y. This measure is the only one that has been classified as "well-established;" however, it may be burdensome because of its length. The PedMIDAS is a shorter questionnaire with strong reliability and validity and may be a useful alternative.

Epilepsy

Four measures have been developed to assess epilepsy-specific HRQOL. The first instrument, the Quality of Life in Epilepsy Inventory for Adolescents (QOLIE-AD-48; Cramer et al., 1999), was developed in 1999 and was modeled on an adult epilepsy-specific measure (Devinsky et al., 1995). The authors recognized the need to address the developmental needs of adolescents and not only modified the items but also added more developmentally sensitive items (e.g., school functioning). The QOLIE-AD-48 has strong internal consistency, with the exception of the Health Perception scale (α ranged from 0.52 to 0.94). Adequate test–retest has also been reported ($r = 0.83$). In addition, HRQOL scores have been associated with seizure severity, indicating discriminant validity, and specific scales have been shown to correlate with measures of self-efficacy and self-esteem. This measure also includes both generic and disease-specific questions, which allows for cross-disease comparisons. The MCID has not been established.

The next two measures were developed by Ronen and colleagues (Ronen, Streiner, & Rosenbaum, 2003) and include both a self-report for children and adolescents, The Child Self-Report Scale, and a parent-proxy version, the Parent-proxy Response Scale. Items for these measures were developed using qualitative and quantitative methods, yielding measures that are brief in nature and can be used as complementary tools. Internal consistency coefficients ranged from 0.63 to 0.84 for the child version and 0.59 to 0.69 for the parent version. Test–retest for the child version ranges from 0.59 to 0.69 and 0.60 to 0.81 for the parent version. Good convergence with health outcomes, such as seizure frequency, days in hospital, and use of antiepileptic medications, has also been reported. The MCID has not been established.

The last measure is the Quality of Life in Childhood Epilepsy Questionnaire, which is a parent-proxy instrument. Although this instrument has demonstrated good internal consistency ($\alpha = 0.76$–0.97), it lacks test–retest reliability data and the MCID has not been determined. This measure covers several domains of functioning relevant to children and adolescents with epilepsy, such as physical activity, general feelings, cognitive processes, and social activity. However, this has resulted in a 79-item measure which takes about 25–30 minutes to complete. Convergent validity between this measure and the CHQ has been reported. In addition, this measure discriminates between inpatient and outpatient populations.

Based on our review, we recommend the QOLIE-AD-48 for adolescents with epilepsy because of its developmentally appropriate items and strong psychometric data. The QOLIE-AD-48 is also the most widely used HRQOL measure for adolescents with epilepsy and has been used in both research and clinical practice.

Hematology/Oncology

Cancer

The Pediatric Oncology Quality of Life Scale (POQOLS; Goodwin, Boggs, & Graham-Pole, 1994) is considered a "well-established" measure (Palermo et al., 2008). This 21-item parent-report measure assesses physical functioning and role restrictions, emotional distress, and reactions to current medications in children and adolescents being treated for cancer. This measure demonstrated good internal consistency (e.g., $\alpha = 0.68$–0.87), as well as concurrent and discriminant validity. This measure discriminates between patients in active treatment compared to those in remission (Goodwin et al., 1994). High interrater reliability was found ($r = 0.89$) between mother and father report. Test–retest reliability was not reported and the MCID has not been established.

The Miami Pediatric Quality of Life Questionnaire (MPQLQ; Armstrong et al., 1999) was derived from interviews with children and adolescents with cancer. The final measure includes 56 items on domains, such as self-competence, emotional stability, and social competence. The MPQLQ has demonstrated adequate internal consistency ($\alpha = 0.76$–0.88) and good test–retest reliability over 1 month for the parent-report version ($r = 0.38$–0.94). In terms of validity, this measure discriminates between patients with brain tumors compared to those with other types of cancers. One limitation of this measure is the absence of scales that assess physical functioning and the impact of treatment. The MCID has not been established. Although this measure is not yet "well-established," its psychometric properties suggest that it is a "promising" tool.

The PedsQL Cancer Module (Varni, Burwinkle, Katz, Meeske, & Dickinson, 2002) is a 27-item module which includes items about pain, nausea, procedural anxiety, treatment anxiety, worry, cognitive problems, perceived physical appearance, and communication. A large validation study indicated that the Cancer Module has good internal consistency ($\alpha = 0.72$). Test–retest reliability was not reported. Adequate agreement was found between patient and parent reports ($r = 0.30$–0.57). Differences were found between those on versus off cancer treatment on the Nausea, Treatment Anxiety, and Worry Scales (Varni et al., 2002). The MCID has not been established.

The Pediatric Cancer Quality of Life Inventory (PCQL; Varni et al., 1998) is a 32-item measure evaluating five domains of HRQOL in children and adolescents with cancer. This measure has demonstrated adequate internal consistency ($\alpha = 0.69$–0.83) and marginal agreement between patient and parent reports ($r = 0.21$–0.34). Test–retest reliability was not reported. In terms of validity, this measure discriminated between patients who were on treatment compared to those who were not. The MCID has not been established. In addition to the original measure, a 15-item subscale with items assessing pain and nausea is also available (Seid, Varni, Rode, & Katz, 1999).

The Behavioral, Affective and Somatic Experiences Scale (BASES; Phipps, Dunavant, Jayawardene, & Srivastiva, 1999) is an HRQOL measure for children and adolescents, aged 2–20 years, with cancer and has a patient, parent, and nurse version. The BASES has demonstrated adequate internal ($\alpha = 0.77$) and cross-informant consistency between nurses ($r = 0.87$). Test–retest reliability was not reported. Discriminative validity has also been shown between patients receiving allogeneic and autologous bone marrow transplantation (Phipps et al., 1999). The MCID has not been established.

The Minneapolis-Manchester Quality of Life instrument (MMQL; Bhatia et al., 2002) consists of 32 items and evaluates domains of outlook/family dynamics, physical symptoms, physical functioning, and psychological functioning. The MMQL has adequate internal consistency ($\alpha = 0.85$), good test–retest reliability over a 2-week period ($r = 0.56$–0.79), and discriminates among patients undergoing treatment, survivors, and controls. In contrast to most measures of HRQOL for cancer, this measure can be used to assess HRQOL both during and after treatment. This provides opportunities to evaluate HRQOL longitudinally. The MCID has not been established.

Royal Marsden Hospital Pediatric Oncology Quality of Life Questionnaire (Watson et al., 1999) is a 78-item parent-proxy form. This measure has demonstrated adequate internal consistency ($\alpha = 0.65$–0.85) and sensitivity to changes in physical symptoms from baseline to 2 months post-treatment. Test–retest reliability was not reported. The authors noted this parent-proxy measure was influenced by the parent's mental health status. Child and adolescent report forms are needed. The MCID has not been established.

The Quality of Life-Cancer Survivors (QOL-CS; Ferrell, Dow, & Grant, 1995) is a 41-item visual analog scale for adolescents and young adults who have been successfully treated for cancer. Despite evidence of internal consistency ($\alpha = 0.71$–0.89), test–retest reliability ($r = 0.89$), and concurrent validity ($r = 0.44$–0.74, with another measure of HRQOL), the authors suggested that this measure needs additional revisions due to the lack of association among some of the scales (Zebrack & Chesler, 2001). For example, the spiritual well-being scale was not associated with physical well-being or psychological distress. The MCID has not been established.

There are several good measures of HRQOL for adolescents with cancer. However, based on this review, two measures are recommended. The POQOLS is a "well-established" measure, but is available only for parent report. For adolescents with cancer, the MPQLQ is a "promising" tool, which includes both parent and self-report. Thus, both of these measures are recommended, depending on the availability of the adolescent to complete the self-report measure.

Sickle Cell Disease

There are currently no disease-specific HRQOL measures for adolescents with sickle cell disease. Despite the prevalence of this disease (1 in 600 African-Americans and 1 in 1000–1400 Hispanic Americans; National Heart, Lung, and Blood Institute, 2003) and its significant impact on adolescents, there is only one recently published measure for adults, the Sickle Cell Impact Measurement Scale (SIMS; Adams-Graves, Lamar, Johnson, & Corley, 2008). Future research should focus on the development of an HRQOL measure for pediatric patients with sickle cell disease.

Immunology

Juvenile Rheumatoid Arthritis

There is one disease-specific HRQOL measure for adolescents with JRA, the Juvenile Arthritis Quality of Life Questionnaire (JAQQ; Degotardi, 2003). The JAQQ is a 74-item instrument with four domains: gross motor function, fine motor function, psychosocial function, and general/systematic symptoms. There are two versions: a self-report form for children older than 9 years and a parent-proxy version for children 2–18 years of age. These measures take approximately 20 minutes to complete and use a 2-week recall period. Good internal consistency has been reported across the four domains with α ranging from 0.88 to 0.97 (Shaw, Southwood, Duffy, & McDonagh, 2006). Test–retest reliability was not reported because this measure was designed to be responsive to changes in functional status. The MCID has not been established. This measure has also demonstrated convergence with ratings of disease severity, such as number of active joints, number of limited joints, pain, and erythrocyte sedimentation count. Responsiveness to change following drug treatment and good parent–child agreement has also been reported. The JAQQ is available in French and Dutch.

HIV/AIDS

There is one HRQOL measure for adolescents with HIV, the General Health Self-assessment from the Aids Clinical Trials Group (ACTG; Testa & Lenderking, 1995). This 49-item measure covers the following domains: physical functioning, psychological functioning, social and role, disease-related symptomology, general health perceptions, and physical resilience. This measure can be completed by adolescents aged 12 years and older and there is a parent-proxy version for children birth to 11 years (General Health Assessment for Children, GHAC; Gortmaker et al., 1998). Good internal consistency ($\alpha = 0.80$–0.91) was found on the adolescent self-report version; internal consistency ranged from adequate to good for the parent-report version ($\alpha = 0.59$–0.97; Lee et al., 2006). The adolescent measure takes about 10 minutes to complete, however, the recall period is 4 weeks, which is not ideal (Lenderking, Testa, Katzenstein, & Hammer, 1997). Test–retest reliability was not reported. Discriminative validity was demonstrated by comparing adolescents who received antiretroviral medications to those who were not on medication. As expected, the group not receiving treatment reported worse symptoms and health perceptions than the treated group (Lee et al., 2006). The MCID has not been established. Translations are available in Spanish, French, and Creole (Lenderking et al., 1997).

Pain

A recent review of HRQOL measures did not identify any condition-specific pain measures for children and adolescents (Vetter, 2007). However, two general pain measures are available for adolescents, the Quality of Life Pain-Youth (QLP-Y) and the McGill Pain Questionnaire (MPQ).

The QLP-Y (Hunfeld et al., 2001) is a 71-item measure based on the Quality of Life Headache-Youth (QLH-Y) questionnaire. In terms of validity, both higher pain frequency and intensity were related to lower HRQOL (Hunfeld et al., 2001). Further, the QLP-Y demonstrated stability across yearly assessments during a 3-year follow-up study (r = 0.40–0.90; Hunfeld et al., 2002). The QLP-Y was then shortened and renamed the Quality of Life Questionnaire for Adolescents with Chronic Pain (QLA-CP; Merlijn, Hunfeld, van der Wouden, Hazebroek-Kampschreur, & Passcier, 2002). This revised instrument consists of 44 items and has demonstrated adequate internal consistency (α = 0.64–0.88) and significant associations with other measures of functional health (Merlijn et al., 2006). The MCID has not been established.

The MPQ (Melzack, 1975) is a 20-item pain measure for individuals 10 years of age and older who have acute and/or chronic pain. The MPQ assesses dimensions of pain, including sensory (e.g., location and temperature of pain), affective (i.e., autonomic, emotional experience of pain), and evaluative (i.e., intensity of pain) and discriminates among different types of pain (Reading, 1984). Intercorrelations across categories were high ($r >$ 0.90). The MPQ can be completed in 15–20 minutes and has been translated into more than 20 languages. The MPQ Short Form has 15 items, takes 2–5 minutes to complete, and is sensitive to treatments for pain, such as analgesic drugs, epidural blocks, and transcutaneous electrical nerve stimulators (Melzack, 1987). Internal consistency, test–retest reliability, and MCID were not reported. Concurrent validity between long and short forms of the MPQ was reported (r = 0.65–0.94).

The QLP-Y is recommended currently because it has better established psychometric properties than the other measure available.

Conclusions

In sum, over the past decade there has been tremendous growth in the development and validation of HRQOL measures for adolescents with chronic conditions. This interest reflects a shift in health care more generally toward inclusion of patients in shared decision-making and more collaborative relationships between health-care providers and patients with chronic conditions. It also dovetails with the movement toward evidence-based practice and assessment. HRQOL measures offer a standardized method for assessing both the impact of a chronic illness on the patient's daily functioning and the effects of new treatments or behavioral interventions on their quality of life. The importance of these measures has recently been emphasized by the FDA, which now recommends the inclusion of these instruments in clinical trials for patients with chronic diseases. Psychologists, who have a strong background in psychometrics and assessment, are in an ideal position to contribute to these developments.

References

Adams-Graves, P., Lamar, K., Johnson, C., & Corley, P. (2008). Development and validation of SIMS: An instrument for measuring quality of life of adults with sickle cell disease. *American Journal of Hematology, 83*(7), 558–562.

Armstrong, F. D., Toledano, S. R., Miloslavich, K., Lackman-Zeman, L., Levy, J. D., Gay, C. L., et al. (1999). The Miami pediatric quality of life questionnaire: Parent scale. *International Journal of Cancer, Supp 12*, 11–17.

Asmussen, L., Olson, L. M., Grant, E. V., Fagan, J., & Weiss, K. B. (1999). Reliability and validity of the children's health survey for asthma. *Pediatrics, 104*, 1–10.

Bhatia, S., Jenney, M. E., Bogue, M. K., Rockwood, T. H., Feusner, J. H., Friedman, D. L., et al. (2002). The Minneapolis–Manchester quality of life instrument: Reliability and validity of the Adolescent Form. *Journal of Clinical Oncology, 20*(24), 4692–4698.

Bibace, R., & Walsh, M. E. (1980). Development of children's concepts of illness. *Pediatrics, 66*(6), 912–917.

Bukstein, D. A., McGrath, M. M., Buchner, D. A., Landgraf, J., & Goss, T. F. (2000). Evaluation of a short form for measuring health-related quality of life among pediatric asthma patients. *Journal of Allergy & Clinical Immunology, 105*, 245–251.

Chiang, L., Tzeng, L., Fu, L., & Huang, J. (2006). Testing a questionnaire to measure asthma-related quality of life among children. *Journal of Nursing Scholarship, 38*, 383–386.

Christie, M. J., French, D., Sowden, A., & West, A. (1993). Development of child-centered disease-specific questionnaires for living with asthma. *Psychosomatic Medicine, 55*, 541–548.

Cohen, L. L., La Greca, A. M., Blount, R. L., Kazak, A. E., Holmbeck, G. N., & Lemanek, K. L. (in press). Introduction to special issue: Evidence-based assessment in pediatric psychology. *Journal of Pediatric Psychology, 33*(9), 911–915.

Cramer, J. A., Westbrook, L. E., Devinsky, O., Perrine, K., Glassman, M. B., & Camfield, C. (1999). Development of the quality of life in epilepsy inventory for adolescents: The QOLIE-AD-48. *Epilepsia, 40*(8), 1114–1121.

Creer, T. L., Wigal, J. K., Kotses, H., Hatala, J. C., McConnaughy, K., & Winder, J. A. (1993). A life activities questionnaire for childhood asthma. *Journal of Asthma, 30*, 467–473.

Degotardi, P. (2003). Pediatric measures of quality of life. *Arthritis & Rheumatism, 49*, S105–S112.

Devinsky, O., Vickrey, B. G., Cramer, J., Perrine, K., Hermann, B., Meador, K., et al. (1995). Development of the quality of life in epilepsy inventory. *Epilepsia, 36*(11), 1089–1104.

de Wit, M., Delemarre-van de Waal, H. A., Pouwer, F., Gemke, R. J. B. J., & Snoek, F. J. (2007). Monitoring health related quality of life in adolescents with diabetes: A review of measures. *Archives of Disease in Childhood, 92*, 434–439.

Donaldson, S. H., Bennett, W. D., Zeman, K. L., Knowles, M. R., Tarran, R., & Boucher, R. C. (2006). Mucus clearance and lung function in cystic fibrosis with hypertonic saline. *New England Journal of Medicine*, 354, 241–250.

Edwards, T. C., Huebner, C. E., Connell, F. A., & Patrick, D. L. (2002). Adolescent quality of life, part i: Conceptual and measurement model. *Journal of Adolescence, 25*, 275–286.

Eiser, C., & Morse, R. (2001). Quality-of-life measures in chronic diseases of childhood. *Health Technol Assess, 5*(4), 1–157.

Elkins, M. R., Robinson, M., Rose, B. R., Harbour, C., Moriarty, C. P., Marks, G. B., et al. (2006). A controlled trial of long-term inhaled hypertonic saline in patients with cystic fibrosis. *New England Journal of Medicine*, 354, 229–240.

Fayers, P., & Hays, R. (2005). *Assessing quality of life in clinical trials* (2nd ed.) Oxford, England: Oxford University Press.

Ferrell, B. R., Dow, K. H., & Grant, M. (1995). Measurement of the quality of life in cancer survivors. *Quality of Life Research, 4*(6), 523–531.

Flapper, B. C.T., Koopman, H. M., ten Napel, C., & van der Schans, C. P. (2006). Psychometric properties of the TACQOL-asthma, a disease-specific measure of health related quality of life for children with asthma and their parents. *Chronic Respiratory Disease, 3*, 65–72.

U. S. Food and Drug Administration. (2006). Guidance for Industry: Patient-Reported Outcome Measures: Use in Medical Product Development to Support Labeling Claims. Retrieved May 31, 2008, from http://www.fda.gov/cder/guidance/5460dft.pdf.

French, D. J., Christie, M. J., & Sowden, A. J. (1994). Reproducibility of the childhood asthma questionnaires: Measures of quality of life for children with asthma aged 4–16 years. *Quality of Life Research, 3*, 215–224.

Gee, L., Abbot, J., Conway, S. P., Etherington, C., & Webb, A. K. (2000). Development of a disease specific health related quality of life measure for adults and adolescents with cystic fibrosis. *Thorax*, 55, 946–954.

Goldbeck, L., Schmitz, T. G., Henrich, G., & Herschbach, P. (2003). Questions on life satisfaction for adolescents and adults with cystic fibrosis. *Chest*, 123, 42–48.

Goodwin, D. A. J., Boggs, S. R., & Graham-Pole, J. (1994). Development and validation of the Pediatric Oncology Quality of Life Scale. *Psychological Assessment, 6*(4), 321–328.

Gorelick, M. H., Brousseau, D. C., & Stevens, M. W. (2004). *Annals of Allergy, Asthma, & Immunology, 92*, 47–51.

Gortmaker, S. L., Lenderking, W. R., Clark, C., Lee, S., Fowler, M. G., Oleske, J. M., & the ACTG 219 Team. (1998). Development and use of a pediatric quality of life questionnaire in AIDS clinical trials: Reliability and validity of the General Health Assessment for Children. In D. Drotar (Ed.), *Measuring Health-Related Quality of Life in Children and Adolescents: Implications for Research and Practice* (pp. 219–235). Mahwah, New Jersey: Lawrence Erlbaum Associates.

Goss, C. H., & Quittner, A. L. (2007). Patient-reported outcomes in cystic fibrosis. *Proceeding of the American Thoracic Society, 4*, 378–386.

Grey, M., Sullivan-Bolyai, S., Boland, E. A., Tamborlane, W. V., & Yu, C. (1998). Personal and family factors associated with quality of life in adolescents with diabetes. *Diabetes Care, 21*(6), 909–914.

Guyatt, G. H., Osoba, D., Wu, A. W., Wyrwich, K. W., Norman, G. R., & The Clinical Significance Consensus Meeting Group. (2002). Methods to explain the clinical significance of health status measures. *Mayo Clinic Proceedings*, 77, 371–383.

Harris, P. (1983). Children's understanding of the link between situation and emotion. *Journal of Experimental Child Psychology, 36*, 490–509.

Hartmaier, S. L., DeMuro-Mercon, C., Linder, S., Winner, P., & Santanello, N. C. (2001). Development of a brief 24-hour adolescent migraine functioning questionnaire. *Headache*, 41, 150–156.

Hays, R. (2005). Developing and evaluating questionnaires. In: P. Fayers & R. Hays (Eds.), *Assessing Quality of Life in Clinical Trials* (pp. 3–8). Oxford, England: Oxford University Press.

Hershey, A. D., Powers, S. W., Vockell, A. L. B., LeCates, S., Kabbouche, M. A., & Maynard, M. K. (2001).

Development of a questionnaire to assess disability of migraines in children. *Neurology, 57*, 2034–2039.

Hunfeld, J. A. M., Perquin, C. W., Bertina, W., Hazebroek-Kampschreur, A. A. J. M., van Suijlekom-Smit, L. W. A., Koes, B. W., van der Wouden, J. C., & Passchier, J. (2002). Stability of pain parameters and pain-related quality of life in adolescents with persistent pain: A three-year follow-up. *The Clinical Journal of Pain, 18*, 99–106.

Hunfeld, J. A. M., Perquin, C. W., Duivenvoorden, H. J., Hazebroek-Kampschreur, A. A. J. M., Passchier, J., van Suijlekom-Smit, L. W. A., & van der Wouden, J. C. (2001). Chronic pain and its impact on quality of life in adolescents and their families. *Journal of Pediatric Psychology, 26*(3), 145–153.

Ingersoll, G. M., & Marrero, D. G. (1991). A modified quality-of-life measure for youths: Psychometric properties. *Diabetes Education, 17*(2), 144–148.

Inhelder, B., & Piaget, J. (1958). *The growth of logical thinking from childhood to adolescence: An essay on the construction of formal operational structures*. New York: Basic Books.

Juniper, E. F., Guyatt, G. H., Feeny, D. H., Ferrie, P. J., Griffith, L. E., & Townsend, M. (1996a). Measuring quality of life in children with asthma. *Quality of Life Research*, 5, 35–46.

Juniper, E. F., Guyatt, G. H., Feeny, D. H., Ferrie, P. J., Griffith, L. E., & Townsend, M. (1996b). Measuring quality of life in the parents of children with asthma. *Quality of Life Research*, 5, 27–34.

Kolotkin, R. L., Zeller, M., Modi, A. C., Samsa, G. P., Quinlan, N. P., Yanovski, J. A., et al. (2006). Assessing weight-related quality of life in adolescents. *Obesity (Silver Spring), 14*(3), 448–457.

Landgraf, J. M., Abetz, L., & Ware, J. E. (1996). *Child Health Questionnaire (CHQ): A user's Manual* (1st ed.). Boston, MA: The Health Institute, New England Medical Center.

Langeveld, J. H., Koot, H. M., Loonen, M. C., Hazebroek-Kampschreur, A. A., & Passchier, J. (1996). A quality of life instrument for adolescents with chronic headache. *Cephalalgia, 16(3)*, 183–196.

Langeveld, J. H., Koot, H. M., & Passchler, J. (1997). Headache intensity and quality of life in adolescents. How are changes in headache intensity in adolescents related to changes in experienced quality of life? *Headache*, 37, 37–42.

Lawson, M. L., Cohen, N., Richardson, C., Orrbine, E., & Pham, B. (2005). A randomized trial of regular standardized telephone contact by a diabetes nurse educator in adolescents with poor diabetes control. *Pediatric Diabetes, 6*(1), 32–40.

le Coq, E. M., Colland, V. T., Boeke, A. J.P., Bezemer, D. P., & van Eijk, J. T.M. (2000). Reproducibility, construct validity, and responsiveness of the "how are you?" (HAY), a self-report quality of life questionnaire for children with asthma. *Journal of Asthma, 37*, 43–58.

Lee, G. M., Gortmaker, S. L., McIntosh, K., Hughes, M. D., Oleske, J. M., & Pediatric AIDS Clinical Trials Group Protocol 219C Team. (2006). Quality of life for children and adolescents: Impact of HIV infection and antiretroviral treatment. *Pediatrics, 117*(2), 273–283.

Lenderking, W. R., Testa, M. A., Katzenstein, D., & Hammer, S. (1997). Measuring quality of life in early HIV disease: The modular approach. *Quality of Life Research, 6*, 515–530.

McCoy, K. S., Quittner, A. L., Oermann, C. M., Gibson, R. L., Retsch-Bogart, G. Z., & Montgomery, A. B. (2008). Inhaled aztreonam lysine for chronic airway *Pseudomonas aeruginosa* in cystic fibrosis. *American Journal of Respiratory and Critical Care Medicine, 178*(9), 921–928.

McMillan, C. V., Honeyford, R. J., Datta, J., Madge, N. J. H., & Bradley, C. (2004). The development of a new measure of quality of life for young people with diabetes mellitus: The ADDQoL-Teen. *Health and Quality of Life Outcomes, 2*, 61–74.

Melzack, R. (1975). The McGill pain questionnaire: Major properties and scoring methods. *Pain, 1*, 277–299.

Melzack, R. (1987). The short-form McGill pain questionnaire. *Pain, 30*, 191–197.

Merlijn, V. P., Hunfeld, J. A., van der Wouden, J. C., Hazebroek-Kampschreur, A. A., & Passcier, J. (2002). Shortening of a quality of life questionnaire for adolescents with chronic pain and its psychometric qualities. *Psychological Reports, 90*, 753–759.

Merlijin, V. P., Hunfeld, J. A., van der Wouden, J. C., Hazebroek-Kampschreur, A. A., Passcier, J., & Koes, B. W. (2006). Factors related to the quality of life in adolescents with chronic pain. *The Clinical Journal of Pain, 22*(3), 306–315.

Mishoe, S. C., Baker, R. R., Poole, S., Harrell, L. M., Arant, C. B., & Rupp, N. T. (1998). Development of an instrument to assess stress levels and quality of life in children with asthma. *Journal of Asthma, 35*, 553–563.

Mitchell, H., Senturia, Y., Gergen, P., Baker, D., Joseph, C., McNiff-Mortimer, K., et al. (1997). Design and methods of the national cooperative inner-city asthma study. *Pediatric Pulmonology, 24*, 237–252.

Modi A. C., Lim, C. M., Driscoll, K. A., Koumoutsos, J., Piazza-Waggoner, C., Messer, M. A., et al. (2007) Intravenous antibiotic treatment of a pulmonary exacerbation: Effects on child and adolescent health-related quality of life. [Abstract] *Pediatric Pulmonology, S30*, 344.

Modi, A. C., & Quittner, A. L. (2003). Validation of a disease-specific measure of health-related quality of life for children with cystic fibrosis. *Journal of Pediatric Psychology, 28*(8), 535–545.

Modi, A. C., & Zeller, M. H. (2008). Validation of an obesity-specific parent-proxy measure of health-related quality of life: Sizing Them Up. *Obesity,16* (12), 2624–2633.

National Heart, Lung and Blood Institute of the National Institutes of Health and US Dept of Health and Human Services. (2003). NHLBI: Sickle Cell Anemia. Retrieved May 31, 2008, from http://www.nhlbi.nih.gov/health/dci/Diseases/Sca/SCA_WhatIs.html.

Olson, L. M., Radecki, L., Frintner, M. P., Weiss, K. B., Korfmacher, J., & Siegel, R. M. (2007). At what age can children report dependably on their asthma health status. *Pediatrics, 119*, e93–102.

Palermo, T. M., Long, A. C., Lewandowski, A. S., Drotar,D., Quittner, A. L., & Walker, L. S. (2008). Evidence-based assessment of health-related quality of life and functional impairment in pediatric psychology. *Journal of Pediatric Psychology, 33* (9), 983–996.

Patrick, D. L., Edwards, T. C., & Topolski, T. D. (2002). Adolescent quality of life, part ii: Initial validation of a new instrument. *Journal of Adolescence, 25*, 287–300.

Phipps, S., Dunavant, M., Jayawardene, D., & Srivastiva, D. K. (1999). Assessment of health-related quality of life in acute in-patient settings: Use of the BASES instrument in children undergoing bone marrow transplant. *International Journal of Cancer Supplement, 12*, 18–24.

Quittner, A. L., Buu, A., Messer, M. A., Modi, A. C., & Watrous, M. (2005). Development and Validation of the Cystic Fibrosis Questionnaire (CFQ) in the United States: A Health-Related Quality of Life Measure for Cystic Fibrosis. *Chest, 128*, 2347–2354.

Quittner, A. L., Davis, M. A., & Modi, A. C. (2003). Health-related quality of life in pediatric populations. In M. C. Roberts (Ed.), *Handbook of pediatric psychology* (3rd ed., pp. 696–709). New York: Guilford Publications.

Quittner, A. L., Modi, A. C., & Cruz, I. (2008). Systematic review of health-related quality of life measures for children with respiratory conditions. *Paediatric Respiratory Reviews, 9*, 220–232.

Quittner, A. L., Modi, A., Wainwright, C., Otto, K., Kirihara, J., & Montgomery, A. B. (in press). Determination of the minimal clinically important difference (MCID) scores for the Cystic Fibrosis Questionnaire-Revised (CFQ-R) Respiratory Symptom scale in two populations of patients with CF and chronic *Pseudomonas aeruginosa airway infection. Chest.*

Reading, A. E. (1984). Testing pain mechanisms in persons in pain. In P. D. Wall & R. Melzack (Eds.), *Textbook of pain* (pp. 195–204). Edinburgh: Churchill Livingstone.

Retsch-Bogart, G. Z., Quittner, A. L., Gibson, R. L., Oermann, C. M., McCoy, K. S., Montgomery, A. B., Cooper, P. J. (in press). Efficacy and safety of inhaled aztreonam lysine for airway *Pseudomonas* in cystic fibrosis. *Chest.*

Revicki, D. A., Osoba, D., Fairclough, D., Barofsky, I., Berson, R., Ledidy, N. K., et al. (2000). Recommendations on health-related quality of life research to support labeling and promotional claims in the United States. *Quality of Life Research, 9*, 887–900.

Roisman, G. I., Masten, A. S., Coatsworth, J. D., & Tellegen, A. (2004). Salient and emerging developmental tasks in the transition to adulthood. *Child Development, 75*(1), 123–133.

Ronen, G. M., Streiner, D. L., & Rosenbaum, P. (2003). Health-related quality of life in children with epilepsy: Development and validation of self-report and parent proxy measures. *Epilepsia, 44*(4), 598–612.

Rothman, M. L., Beltran, P., Cappelleri, J. C., Lipscomb, J., Teschendorf, B., the Mayo/FDA Patient-Reported Outcomes Consensus Meeting Group. (2007). Patient-reported outcomes: Conceptual issues. *Value in Health, 10*, S66–S75.

Rutishauser, C., Sawyer, S. M., Bond, L., Coffrey, C., & Bowes, G. (2001). Development and validation of the adolescent asthma quality of life questionnaire (AAQOL). *European Respiratory Journal, 17*, 52–58.

Schwarz, N., & Sudman, S. (1996). *Answering questions: Methodology for determining cognitive and communicative processes in survey research.* San Francisco, CA: Jossey-Bass Inc.

Seid, M., Varni, J. W., Rode, C. A., & Katz, E. R. (1999). The Pediatric Cancer Quality of Life Inventory: A modular approach to measuring health-related quality of life in children with cancer. *International Journal of Cancer Supplement, 12*, 71–76.

Shaw, K. L., Southwood, T. R., Duffy, C. M., & McDonagh, J. E. (2006). Health-related quality of life in adolescents with juvenile idiopathic arthritis. *Arthritis & Rheumatism, 55*, 199–207.

Sherifali, D., & Pinelli, J. (2007). Parent as proxy reporting: Implications and recommendations for quality of life research. *Journal of Family Nursing, 13*(1), 83–98.

Starfield, B., Riley, A. W., & Green, B. F. (1999). *Manual for the child health and illness profile: Adolescent edition (chip-ae)*. Baltimore: The Johns Hopkins University.

Stewart, W. F., Lipton, R. B., Dowson, A. J., & Sawyer, J. (2001). Development and testing of the Migraine Disability Assessment (MIDAS) Questionnaire to assess headache-related disability. *Neurology, 56*, S20–S28.

Sundaram, M., Kavookjian, J., Patrick, J. H., Miller, L. A., Madhavan, S. S., & Scott, V. G. (2007). Quality of life, health status and clinical outcomes in Type 2 diabetes patients. *Quality of Life Research, 16*(2), 165–177.

Testa, M. A., & Lenderking, W. R. (1995). Quality-of-life considerations in AIDS Clinical Trials. In D. Finkelstein, & D. Schoenfeld (Eds.). *AIDS clinical trials* (pp. 213–241). New York, NY: Wiley-Liss.

Theunissen, N. C., Vogels, T. G., Koopman, H. M., Verrips, G. H., Zwinderman, K. A., Verloove-Vanhorick, S. P., et al. (1998). The proxy problem: Child report versus parent report in health-related quality of life research. *Quality of Life Research, 7*(5), 387–397.

Turner, R., Quittner, A. L., Parasuraman, B. M., & Cleeland, C. S. (2007). Patient-reported outcomes: Instrument selection issues. *Value in Health, 2* (Suppl. 2), S86–S93.

Varni, J. W., Burwinkle, T. M., Jacobs, J. R., Gottschalk, M., Kaufman, F., & Jones, K. I. (2003). The PedsQL in type 1 and type 2 diabetes. *Diabetes Care, 26*, 631–637.

Varni, J. W., Burwinkle, T. M., Katz, E. R., Meeske, K., & Dickinson P. (2002). The PedsQL in pediatric cancer: Reliability and validity of the pediatric quality of life inventory generic core scales, multidimensional fatigue scale, and cancer module. *Cancer, 94*(7), 2090–2106.

Varni, J. W., Burwinkle, T. M., Rapoff, M. A., Kamps, J. L., & Olson, N. (2004). The PedsQL in pediatric asthma: Reliability and validity of the pediatric quality of life inventory generic core scales and asthma module. *Journal of Behavioral Medicine, 27*, 297–318.

Varni, J. W., Katz, E. R., Seid, M., Quiggins, D. J. L., Friedman-Bender, A., & Castro, C. M. (1998). The Pediatric Cancer Quality of Life Inventory (PCQL). I. Instrument development, descriptive statistics, and cross-informant variance. *Journal of Behavioral Medicine, 21*(2), 179–204.

Varni, J. W., Seid, M., & Rode, C. A. (1999). The PedsQL: Measurement model for the pediatric quality of life inventory. *Medical Care*, 37, 126–139.

Verrips, G. H., Vogels, A. G., den Ouden, A. L., Paneth, N., & Verloove-Vanhorick, S. P. (2000). Measuring health-related quality of life in adolescents: Agreement between raters and between methods of administration. *Child Care Health Development, 26*(6), 457–469.

Vetter, T. R. (2007). A primer on health-related quality of life in chronic pain medicine. *Anesthesia & Analgesia, 104*(3), 703–718.

Von Korff, M., Gruman, J., Schaefer, J., Curry, S. J., & Wagner, E. H. (1997). Collaborative management of chronic illness. *Annals of Internal Medicine, 127*, 1097–1102.

Watson, M., Edwards, L., Von Essen, L., Davidson, J., Day, R., & Pinkerton, R. (1999). Development of the royal marsden hospital paediatric oncology quality of life questionnaire. *International Journal of Cancer*, (Suppl. 12), 65–70.

World Health Organization. (1947). The constitution of the World Health Organization. *WHO Chronicles, 1*, 29.

Wyrwich, K. W., Bullinger, M., Aaronson, N., Hays, R. D., Patrick, D. L., Symonds, T, et al. (2005). Estimating clinically significant difference in quality of life outcomes. *Quality of Life Research*, 14, 285–295.

Zebrack, B. J., & Chesler, M. A. (2001). A psychometric analysis of the Quality of Life-Cancer Survivors (QOL-CS) in survivors of childhood cancer. *Quality of Life Research, 10*, 319–329.

Index

B

MIX
Papier aus verantwortungsvollen Quellen
Paper from responsible sources
FSC® C105338

If you have any concerns about our products,
you can contact us on
ProductSafety@springernature.com

In case Publisher is established outside the EU,
the EU authorized representative is:
Springer Nature Customer Service Center GmbH
Europaplatz 3, 69115 Heidelberg, Germany

Printed by Libri Plureos GmbH
in Hamburg, Germany